A primer of fundamental food facts and nutrition concepts for everyone.

FOOD HEALING
FOR
MAN

Volume I, "Man" Series

Bernard Jensen, PhD
Clinical Nutrition

Bernard Jensen, Publisher

First Edition

Copyright 1983 Bernard Jensen
ALL RIGHTS RESERVED

BERNARD JENSEN, Publisher
Route 1, Box 52
Escondido, CA 92025

Library of Congress Card Catalog Number 83-083144
ISBN 0-9608360-0-4

Dedication

I dedicate this book to the great pioneers of food healing:

Christiaan Eykman	Max Warmbrandt
Casimir Funk	Otto Carque
Robert McCarrison	Herbert Shelton
Weston Price	John Christopher
Clive McCay	Eugene Christian
J. H. Tilden	Alfred McCann
George Weger	Adelle Davis
Joseph Goldberger	Tom Spies
R. Swinburne Clymer	Roger Williams
V. G. Rocine	Emanuel Cheraskin
Dr. Bircher-Benner	Norman Walker
Dr. Thrall	William Howard Hay
Sir Arbuthnot Lane	Benjamin G. Hauser
Stanford Claunch	Arne Waerland
John Harvey Kellogg	Henry Lindlahr

and to all others who have labored to awaken mankind to the knowledge that man's foods must be whole, natural and pure to sustain life at the wonderful level of health that Nature and Nature's creator intended.

Bernard Jensen, Ph.D.

Acknowledgment

I wish to give Sudi Oliver my special thanks for organizing and arranging much of the material in this book in such a lively, interesting, wholesome way and also wish to express my great appreciation to the many others who have assisted in its preparation.

Biography

Dr. Bernard Jensen has had one of the most remarkable careers of any professional in the health arts, traveling, teaching and lecturing in 52 countries all over the world and maintaining one of the most successful sanitarium practices in the United States.

Born on March 25, 1908, to parents of Danish descent, Bernard Jensen experienced the healing power of foods firsthand when his health failed soon after graduation from West Coast Chiropractic College. Given up to die after doctors diagnosed advanced bronchiectasis, he turned to a Seventh Day Adventist physician, who took him off all junk foods and gave him a special diet of natural foods, high in fresh raw fruits and vegetables. Slowly, but surely, his health returned, and his lungs eventually healed completely.

Confident of the value of nature-cure methods, Dr. Jensen studied with many of the great nature cure physicians of his time, such as Dr. John Harvey Kellogg of Battle Creek, Michigan; Dr. Benedict Lust of Butler, New Jersey; Dr. Ralph Benner of the Bircher-Benner Sanitarium in Zurich, Switzerland; Dr. John Tilden of Denver, Colorado; Dr. George Weger of Redlands, California; Dr. Randolph Stone, Dr. Major DeJarnette, Dr. Max Gerson, Dr. S. Claunch and Dr. Robert Jackson of Canada.

One of the major influences on his life and work was a Norwegian homeopath named V. G. Rocine, who became his teacher and life-long friend. Rocine, fluent in several languages, had studied the works of Europe's foremost food chemists, and had already come to the conclusion that a well-balanced body chemistry, dependent upon a variety of natural, pure and whole foods, was the key to good health and mental vigor, while the science of Nutrition was still in its infancy. Rocine also believed that most chronic disease was caused by chemical deficiencies.

Recognizing that Rocine's work was far ahead of its time, Dr. Jensen studied the chemical elements with him until he knew the role of each of the 16 major biochemicals in human nutrition, the symptoms of deficiency and excess and which foods were richest in each element. Then it was time for the student to take on the mantle of teacher.

Dr. Jensen, following in the footsteps of some of the nature-cure men with whom he had studied, opened his first health sanitarium in Ben Lomond, California. Later, he operated sanitariums in Altadena, California and Escondido, California. Throughout his sanitarium work, Dr. Jensen put Rocine's ideas into practice, adding what he had learned from his other studies and from foreign travels, until people from all over the United States and from many other countries came to his sanitariums in search of health and rejuvenation.

Almost side by side with his nutrition studies, iridology has played a major role in Dr. Jensen's career. Dr. J. Haskel Kritzer, MD, encouraged him in the 1930s to study iridology, a method of analyzing tissue states in the body as reflexly represented in the eyes. *The Science and Practice of Iridology*, a textbook published in the 1950s, established Dr. Jensen as the world's foremost authority on the subject. In 1982, he published *Iridology: The Science and Practice in the Healing Arts, Volume II,* which has been acclaimed as the finest textbook on iridology ever published.

Iridology and nutrition, Dr. Jensen found, work as a complementary team—each supporting and proving the validity of the other. Using iridology, the doctor could tell if his nutrition program was working for individual patients. Using nutrition, he could see changes being made in the irides of his patients, which showed the accuracy and reliability of iridology as a means of monitoring chemical change and rejuvenation of the tissues in the body. If the regimen he designed for a patient wasn't bringing the right improvements as shown in the iris, he changed it until it did. "My patients have been my textbooks." Dr. Jensen has said. "The real proof of any health regimen is in the healing of patients."

In the 1960s and 1970s, Dr. Jensen traveled all over the world in search of the secrets of longevity, in hopes that interviewing men and women well over 100 years of age would disclose keys to good health in addition to those he already knew. One of the highlights of his travels was staying as a guest of the Mir of Hunza's palace for ten days. A professional film titled *World Keys to Health and Long Life*, narrated by Dennis Weaver, was made of these travels.

Changing from his sanitarium practice in 1980, Dr. Jensen turned his energy and priorities to writing, speaking and teaching. This book is the first in his five-volume "Man" series, covering the natural processes by which disease can be prevented or overcome and high-level well-being maintained. The second volume in the series is *The Chemistry of Man*. The rest are *The Healing Essence of Man* (in two volumes) and *Arise and Shine: The Spiritual and Mental Healing of Man*. At his Ranch, classes are held on Tissue Cleansing,

Rejuvenation and Iridology. He teaches at the University of Humanistic Studies, where he received his Ph.D. at the age of 75.

Awards and Recognition

In 1954, Dr. Jensen was named Doctor of the Year in Portland, Oregon. He was presented the Ignatz Von Peczely International Iridology Gold Medal award at a ceremony in San Remo, Italy in 1973, and the following year, he was honored at a congress of health professionals at Aix-en-Province, France, for his "valuable contribution in the field of iridology." In 1975, the International Naturopathic Association recognized him for his contributions to the fields of health, iridology and nutrition.

At a special ceremony in New York City, Dr. Jensen was knighted into the Order of St. John of Malta in 1978 for his humanitarian work in the field of health.

This Order is the oldest chivalric organization in the world, tracing its origin back to the time preceding the first Crusade.

The Agnes Arbor Distinguished Service Award was presented to him in 1981 at the 5th Annual Herb Symposium in Santa Cruz, California, for his contributions to the current "herb renaissance."

In 1982, Dr. Jensen was recognized by the National Health Federation with its Pioneer Doctor of the Year award at the Organization's annual convention in Long Beach, California.

Later in the same year, Dr. and Mrs. Jensen were honored by the Pax Mundi Academy in Brussels, Belgium with the 1982 Dag Hammarskjold award. The award, for "exceptional services rendered to collective humanity," was the first given in the category of scientific merit to any practitioner of the natural healing art. The doctor was personally congratulated by U.S. Ambassador, Charles Price.

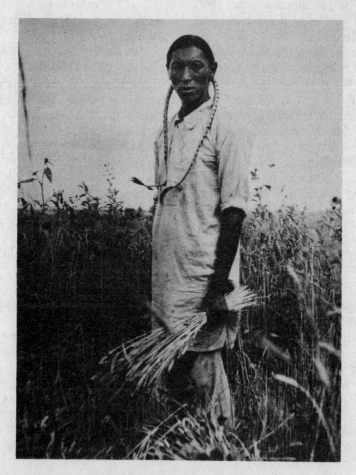

Nature knows best.

Foreword

There is a renaissance in this day and age, bringing back the health methods that were once part of our natural heritage. People today are looking for an easier and more natural way of getting well. Somehow or another, we have gotten off the track, and there have been so many failures, we have come to the place where people are looking for an alternative. We have been told so much about what Nature can do and what our potentials are in the body, yet no one seems to be teaching us how this new day program can be put into effect.

A new wind is blowing, a new consciousness is arising, and man is beginning to accept the idea that there is much he can do for himself in his own home, his own lifestyle, in his own mind, to take care of his own health. Research into the many facets that bring us a full, healthy, long life has contributed importantly to our knowledge of how to stay well. We do not have to constantly face doctor bills. We can prevent hospital expenses using the doctor only in dire emergency. We advocate living in such a way as to prevent disease, having the doctor take proper care of us before any chronic condition has shown up in the body, before malignancy develops. It takes 20 years to develop cancer or other chronic diseases, but if we live right from the start, they will not develop.

The idea from years past that the working man and the housewife could take care of themselves has been gradually replaced by the notion that we have to depend on advanced medical technology for diagnosis and treatment. In other words, our health has been taken out of our hands through the assumption that medical technology will have a complete cure, a breakthrough any day now for whatever disease we may have. So, it is all right to get diseases, if that is true. But, we all know it is not true. The cure we are chasing is not "just" around the next corner.

Nutritionists today talk about RNA factors, SOD, DNA, CHT, amino acids, prostaglandins, enzymes and a whole host of other health factors. You have to be a specialist these days to really know how to build health. Yet, when I talked to Hunzans in their 120s and more, they did not know any of these things and they were perfectly healthy. I never heard one of them mention tryptophan or lysine. They did not talk to me about vitamin and mineral supplements, yet they had every tooth still in place and would remember events that took place over 100 years before.

I wonder if we have not taken the natural healing art and tried to follow the same technical complexity Western medicine is following. A man who has a cold can go to the doctor and he has no cure for it. But if that man developed pneumonia overnight, the doctor has treatments and cures galore to care for that condition. We have specialists now in taking the foods apart, making it almost impossible to understand for the farmer, worker, housewife and the person on the street. The idea is implied that we cannot take care of ourselves unless we go to a specialist in the health food work to get the right advice about what foods and supplements to buy and how much of each to take. Nutrition, like medicine, is being placed more and more in the hands of experts when it should be taught to everyone.

We have to get back to natural principles, simple principles. Most of my work has been slanted toward one direction and that is to help the average person, the nonexpert, the sincere person who wants to know how to live. The average person cannot afford $36,000 for a transplant or a heart operation that has been proclaimed absolutely necessary.,

In dealing with the prevention of disease, we must consider the expense of buying specialty foods and supplements that have been extracted, refined and repackaged into the simplest form through our technology. The average natural health seeker possibly takes more pills than those who are really sick. We must get back to the simplest way of right living. We have to get back to the place where we are dealing first of all with the soil. Then plant life, then the supermarket, then the kitchen and finally our digestive system. We have to consider the physical and spiritual, psychological processes. We have to put a lifestyle together. And, unless we succeed in putting a healthy lifestyle together, we will forever be waiting for science to discover the one cure that is going to help us.

The day is coming when Alzheimer's disease will be taken care of by a nutritional supplement extracted from natural substances. Other diseases will be overcome similarly. Science has shown us how to break foods down to their nutritional components, but until we understand the larger perspective, a vitamin here and an amino acid there is not going to help us. We need to stop thinking about meeting all the body's needs one nutrient at a time, one supplement capsule at a time.

We find there are small things that get people well and there are big things that get people well. I visited

Charlie Smith, the oldest man in the United States, when he was 135 years of age. He had been living for 30 years on sardines and crackers. Most people would shun such a diet. And yet, he had a memory clear enough to sing many songs he learned in his childhood. He could relate experiences of his youth that were just unbelievable at his age. What was in the sardines that could have been any good? There is a possibility that they had something very few people think of. I would never have thought of sardines as natural, pure, free of pollution, complete enough to take care of all the chemicals needed by the body. But they were. I found out something else—the RNA, the ribonucleic acid—which is the long life factor—is very high in sardines. At one time, yeast was considered the highest food in RNA. Then 10 years later, it was found that the sardine has 10 times as much RNA as yeast. Here, the old man was living on something that was naturally just keeping him well, giving him a clear, active mind and an active body well past the century mark. It may not work for everyone, but it is something to think about.

Do we have to wait for new discoveries? I believe vitamin B-6 will be found to be one of the most important individual nutrients among all foods.

Vitamin B-6 is necessary in protein metabolism, hemoglobin formation and the production of neurotransmitters in the brain and peripheral nervous system. kIt is found in organ meats such as liver, and in wheat germ, whole grains, soybeans, peanuts and brewer's yeast.

I think it is well to turn back to basic principles and to those food ideas that have been passed along to us by the older, food-wise persons who have lived in certain parts of the world, demonstrating that living a certain lifestyle has produced good health. I think we ought to follow their wisdom until the sciences come up with some better answers.

A suggestion for the future: We need to come up with better ways of purification of the body. We need to learn what it is to "come clean" in more directions than one. We have to have a mental philosophy that is not breaking us down. We have to know how to keep our nerve system at the highest functional ability possible, but not overstrained and over stressed. We are going to have to take this knowledge into our homes, into our pantries and develop a program that the body can live with in wellness.

Introduction

Man Is A Seeker

All human progress is based on discovery, lessons that come forth from the work and insight of the few whose vision and understanding have prepared them to discover important facts, facts that can benefit all mankind. But, memory is a fickle creature. We have lost sight of many tremendous discoveries of the past that would be of great help to us today. Perhaps it is time to rediscover these discoveries.

Here we have brought forth landmark nutritional discoveries from the past and a great deal of current work that will be of special interest and practical use to the seeker, the person who would like to discover a new continent, a new land, a new body of water, a new lifestyle. If we are to get out of our present-day problems and troubles, it is necessary to realize that the way we are living is not good enough to meet the needs of the normal human body.

Many times, I have stood before audiences and held up a "poison" pickle in one hand and a ripe apricot in the other. "Which would you rather have?" I ask them. Instinctively, I believe, most people know that the natural thing is the right thing.

Why, then, has modern man departed so far from what is natural in foods and living habits? We could name many things such as convenience, pleasure, money, advertising, peer-group pressure and we would be partly right. But, the Bible speaks of those who have eyes and see not, those who have ears and hear not. Is it possible that living in the most affluent nation in the world has made most of us blind and deaf to basic principles of good health? Yet, without good health affluence means nothing.

A few historical events, now mostly forgotten or ignored, are actually dramatic eye-opening discoveries that show us why the natural way in foods is best and why packaged, processed, refined foods are dangerous. Nature seems willing to share her secrets with seekers, and there is much in nature to find out and to hold dear, for our bodies were designed to go the natural way. Keep searching. Keep discovering these things.

We need to realize that what we are deepest, we really are. And, it is in our deeper self that wholeness is born or disease is born. Those who believe a lie live a lie, and the fruit of living a lie is dis-harmony, dis-ease. The problem can be simply that of discernment. Do you read the labels on the products you buy? Are you searching for the cheapest bargains instead of quality foods? Is taste more important to you than nutritional value? Are you always in such a rush that junk foods have become a big part of your lifestyle?

The problem is, the longer we have abused these wonderful bodies of ours, the more our understanding and perception seem to deteriorate. We become satisfied with low-level health, as long as we can still have our coffee, donuts and cigarettes. But, what is our vision for if not to pick out foods that are beautiful, glorious, natural, whole and pure, as found in our fruit and vegetable kingdoms? What is our understanding for if not to discriminate between what is good for us and what is not? Don't you feel you deserve the very best in life?

We've all heard the expression, "I smell a rat," meaning someone senses a bad situation. Is there any reason we can't smell out a good situation? Natural, pure, whole foods are best for us. Junk foods, refined carbohydrates, caffeine drinks, fried foods—unnatural, impure and altered—are harmful to our bodies.

McCarrison and Sansom produced diseases at will in test animals by giving them the kinds of foods the modern housewife buys in the supermarkets. Can't we wake up to these things?

There is a responsibility that rests squarely on the shoulders of doctors: treating a patient after he or she has acquired a disease is too late. We should have been able to intervene earlier by getting at the cause. We are not getting in at the beginning. Our major responsibility should be prevention, and treatment should be a secondary thing.

In what follows, we present stories of several classic landmark discoveries in nutrition. There are important lessons in them for all of us. What we are trying to do here is to point out that there is a right way of doing things, a natural way, a healthy way.

Where Healing Begins

I cannot help a person who does not want to help himself. I will not take a patient who does not desire to get well. Picking up the natural work, we start first with the mental process. When we follow the natural way, it is not a matter of just getting rid of a pain, an ache, a problem that has developed into a discharge, boils, pimples or skin troubles.

There is law we follow called Hering's law of cure. This states that all disease is cured from within out, from the head down and in reverse order as it has built up in the body. If you have degerminated starch in one knee, pickles in your shoulder and 63 artificial ice cream flavors in another part of your body, this has to be washed out. You have to become clean.

New tissue has to take the place of old tissue, and there is one thing I can say that with all the assurance obtained from 54 years in sanitarium work. True healing only comes when we replace old tissue that is not functioning satisfactorily with healthy new tissue. This comes through taking the proper foods and through higher-evolved living. The body repairs itself and gets rid of disease by replacing old tissue with new and by throwing off old toxic material.

One lady told me that I had done so much for her neighbor that she was going to "try" me. "I'm alright," I said. "You're not going to try me." She was the one on trial. I am wondering if we realize that everybody is looking for a good doctor. My view is entirely opposite. I've always looked for good patients, people so motivated to get well that they will cooperate with me. Before I retired, I used to carefully observe a patient's attitude on the first visit. I wanted to know whether they were willing and able to wait and let the body make the changes, a slow, often trying—but reliable—approach.

Repair of any organ in the body depends on the time it takes to put new tissue in place of the old. This is the path of true healing. This is for the person who wants to change his life, who is willing to change his lifestyle in order to rejuvenate his body. We must know that the body molds to coffee and doughnuts or it molds to a salad. It can only use what we put in it.

We know that the body is self rejuvenating, self repairing and self building and is ready to move into a new situation the moment our attitude changes, the moment our mind sees a new path, the moment we take on a knowledge of how to live correctly.

The diet is the foremost consideration in any therapy. We may take any other type of treatment or combination of treatments, but without the proper nutrition, it will come to nothing. Only food builds new tissue. Most therapies today take care of pains, aches and other symptoms. But, how much of the doctor's advice, counseling and treatment works toward making a new body? This is why I tell people it is going to be a year before they overcome their troubles, before they wash out the old that is in the tissue and exchange it for new. It cannot be done overnight. You have to work for it. You learn and you ear good health.

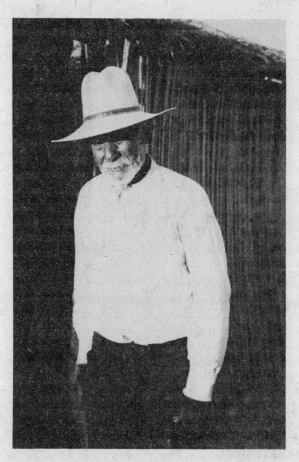

Food healing for man.

Notice of Error: All Index References to pages following page 287 are two pages back. Example: Ginseng 317, 318 should be 315, 316. There may be others, but God only knows how we tried to do it right.

Dr. B. Jensen and Staff

Contents

III. *The art of food preparation*   *230*

IV. A well being   328

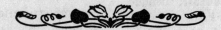

I

Food as a healer

"When we open up our consciousness and dwell in the beauties of Nature, we allow healing to enter our lives."

We find there are some things man does not understand or appreciate until they are gone, and health is one of those things. When life is going well, when we wake up in the morning glad to be alive and feeling wonderful, we hardly give a thought to what is making that possible. But when there is an ache in the shoulder, a pain in the stomach, a stiffness in the back—then we appreciate health. Then we start thinking about what we can do to bring it back.

Pain makes us into philosophers; pain makes us think.

When we stop and think about it, we realize there was no pain, no disease, no suffering in the Garden of Eden. Nor were there any hospitals, drugstores or doctor's offices. Why not? Because all the food in that Garden was fresh, whole, natural and pure—delicious and ready to eat in its natural state. The berries, nuts, fruits and vegetables in the Garden of Eden were more than sufficient to sustain life and chemical balance in the body.

Eve didn't need a can opener, a toaster, a range or refrigerator. She didn't need a microwave oven. Everything in the Garden tasted wonderful. If there had been a French restaurant there, it would have gone out of business.

Now, in the 20th century, we have millions of people in the industrialized nations dying of heart disease, cancer, kidney disease, cirrhosis of the liver and other diseases. Millions of others have arthritis, asthma, bronchitis, hypoglycemia, venereal disease, dental problems and mental illness of various kinds.

Could all of these be avoided with a Garden of Eden diet and lifestyle?

It may seem strange to ask such a question, but the question isn't hypothetical at all.

Some years ago, I visited the Hunza Valley in Pakistan, and my wife and I were invited by the Mir of Hunza to be his palace guests. In our walks around the Valley, we met people over 120 years old who had every tooth in their heads, clear minds and remarkable memories and who still worked in the fields every day. Like the Garden of Eden, there were no drugstores, hospitals, police stations, prisons, doctors, lawyers or police—because there was no substantial problem with disease or crime.

The Hunza people farmed a valley with rich black soil, through which a clear, cold river made its way, fed by the melting snows of surrounding mountains. They raised a large quantity of fruit, including grapes, mulberries and apricots; they raised vegetables, millet and other grains. The average diet included milk and a very little meat. Many of the steep hillsides had been terraced for raising grapes and other crops.

Only one road led into the Hunza Valley at the time of my visit, and it was closed nine months of the year due to snow and ice. Because of the expense and difficulty of transportation, little trade took place. So, the Hunza people had no access to white sugar, white flour, cola drinks, coffee, donuts or other civilized amenities. Instead, they ate the kinds of foods we might expect to have found in the Garden of Eden.

In a 1922 lecture in Pittsburg, Sir Robert McCarrison, the British surgeon who brought the magnificent health of the Hunza people to world attention, said, "During the period of my association with these people, I never saw a case of asthenic dyspepsia, of gastric or duodenal ulcer, of appendicitis, of mucous colitis, of cancer." Yet, in the late 1970s, the road to the Hunza Valley was widened, and "civilized foods" such as white sugar and white flour were brought in. Recent reports tell of cases of tuberculosis and a dramatic increase in dental caries, signs of weakening of the Hunza's constitutions.

Can we learn a lesson from this?

Isn't it time for us to understand that the food we eat either sustains health or tears it down? The best medical technology in the world cannot save the health of nations and people who choose to eat wrong foods.

My travels in over 52 countries of the world have brought me in contact with some of the world's oldest living citizens. They knew little or nothing of vitamins, minerals, amino acids, fiber, calories and so forth. But, they lived long, healthy lives because they ate whole, pure, natural foods, had plenty of physical exercise and a clean lifestyle.

There is *Food Healing for Man* in the right foods—and that is what this book is all about. We need to know a right way to live, to reach high-level well-being, to feel wonderful. The choice is ours.

Chapter 1

Nutrition and body defenses

Spiritual and mental aspects of life are always to be considered together with our delving into the physical realm. Food is not everything — for the body, that is. The spirit, soul, and body require special nourishment, and they are all interrelated as we will find in exploring the principles of nutrition and the functioning of body defenses.

How do you feel? We'll start with this because in taking care of the body we will find that it is necessary for us to start feeling good before we start taking proper care of the body.

There's a lot of resistance in life to taking care of the body. Why should we take care of the body? If you're religiously inclined, to be absent from the body and to be present with the Lord or the Law is what I call truth and good. And after all, the Lord is only interested in truth anyway; so what we're after is truth and when we get that developed well and going in the right direction, then we are identifying ourselves with the Lord, or any religious idea. I don't care if it's Buddha, I don't care if it's Christ . . . Oh yes I do! We find that these masters of the past are the ones we want to identify ourselves with, to identify ourselves with as much truth as we possibly can.

Body Defenses Win the War

We must realize, that the defenses in the body are necessary to win a war. The defenses of a country win. We must be strong in our defenses spiritually, mentally and physically.

In fact, other factors come into this. We've got to be strong in our resources . . . we've got to be strong in still another thing and that's our reserves, because there are pressures to use up these reserves, and if we don't have adequate reserves, we die. We actually become burned out. I have seen people who have no more reserves. They have burned the silicon out of their body. They say, "I've gone as far as I can go . . . I just can't go anymore." They need more reserves.

The Christ tells you to turn the other cheek, and sometimes when you get it slapped on both sides, you're finished, you're ready to fight. You don't know that you're supposed to go 70 times 7, and maybe 70 times 700.

There is no end, and so we only put an end to things because we don't have any more reserves. We don't have a reserve mentally, or even from a spiritual standpoint. Some of us need a larger spiritual reserve. Some of you have to realize that there are "many mansions in my Father's house," and we must go through many different rooms. Many people don't know that they are being tested. You're being tried. This is a life of schooling and you're going through one examination after another. You learn a little bit and the first thing you know you're going to have to use what you have learned. If you don't know how to do things better, Nature comes along and tells you that you need a lesson.

Disease Is A Lesson

Do you know that disease is a terrible lesson people earn and bring on themselves? Disease is not natural. Some people do not realize this, but good health is natural. I think we earn both of them, and some of you have had a very good time getting dis-ease. Some of you have enjoyed everything you've done—the beer, the pretzels, the Christmas candies, barber shop stick candy. When you come to me, I see a body in front of me with creamed cereal in one knee and pancakes in one shoulder, and I begin to think . . . "Well, what am I going to do with this kind of body?" But I realize, too, that the body is in a state of flux; it's in a state of change. You grow new skin in the palm of your hand every day. But if it has been built of "coffee and doughnuts," you're complaining about it, because it's got eczema. I know it's dry. I know it isn't clean. I know there's trouble perspiring, I know that a lot of complaints you have can be transposed into deficiencies in your life, hungers in your life. You haven't learned the lifestyle you should live within.

Health Is Extremely Demanding

I don't like to tell you these things, but I have to tell you the truth. Everybody goes to church on Sunday morning between eleven and twelve to get the truth, so it would be terrible if I told you something that wasn't right. But you can depend on me, because what I'm telling you now is not so personal that we can't both accept it for what it is. I don't like this health business. It's demanding: It takes a lot of discipline; it takes a lot of discrimination and I have to get "wised up," and sometimes I don't like that! I sometimes like to do the same old things that I've been doing a long time, right or wrong, because it doesn't take any effort, any energy, so why should I move?

Get Out of That Rut

You're going to have to move; you're going to have to get out of this rut. You know what a rut is, don't you? It is a grave with the ends kicked out. That's all it is. You're going to have to move; yes, you'll have to move. Move into something better than you've had before. The only way you can get out of this rut is to see that there's a better life to live. You can't be like the worm in the horseradish. He thinks it's the sweetest place in the world because he's never been anyplace else. I've seen people who don't know what it is to feel wonderful. Many people don't know what it is to really experience high-level well-being.

Don't Ask People How They Feel

I'm going to go back and forth telling you how to build these defenses. First of all, people can wear you out. So you're not going to listen to people's troubles and problems anymore. In fact, you're not even going to ask anybody how they feel. Because if you do, they're going to tell you and you're going to have an organ recital for 15 or 20 minutes. The first thing you know, they'll tell you about their headache and that opens the door to you telling them about your headache. Then you'll have two headaches going back and forth. You don't get well discussing headaches. You don't get well living on negative applications in life. Do you know what's behind all of this? Do you know what's listening all the time? Do you know what is feeling all the time? You! Your nervous system! Your digestion. . .and even your elimination. Some people can be constipating, too. Some people can tie you up in knots. I can end up in the bowel. It's just as well that you do not have some people's company. Or, haven't you ever eaten with people who made you feel so sad that you didn't enjoy your meal? Why, certainly you have or you haven't lived.

A Wise Man Chooses Good Friends

Your next thought is this — you've got to pick out the people you're going to associate with. The wise man picks the friends he's going to have. Why should you run around with anybody? Get away from these people who live on Main Street. They're not going to do you any good! There's company for them but not you because

you have decided to get out of this rut or you wouldn't be reading this. They say that many are called but few are chosen. You choose yourself.

A Master can come along and teach you the finest lessons in the world, but if you're not ready for it, it's going to pass over you like a floating cloud. You've got to make yourself ready, too. I hope you really get sick of being sick. That's the time you move — or do you understand that? I don't know how far down you want to go. The point is. . .there is a better way to live, and it's available in the lifestyle you create for yourself. You want to do something nice. You learn to reach for the better things in life. The nicer people, the nicer thoughts, good foods, natural foods, Godly pursuits. How can I put it any better? Or, do you think you're all finished? Do you think you know it all? Don't you think this is a school? Why, certainly! Then let's get in and learn.

Refuse to Honor Negatives

So, the first thing you refuse in life is to associate with negative influences that are around you all the time. That reminds me of Pasadena, California, where they have what they call "Suicide Bridge." Eighty-seven people have jumped off that bridge. They have had to put up a big fence so people can't climb over and kill themselves. I have the records of these people. Do you know why they jumped off? They had a disappointment with their boy friend, a disappointment with their girl friend, or their love went to pot, or their marriage didn't work out. They were sick and they thought there was no hope. They wanted to end it all. They wanted to get out of this world. There is a lot to end in this world, which reminds me of a story about a boy who was on "suicide bridge" and wanted to end it all. He was climbing up the fence, and a patrol car came along. A couple of policemen got there just in time and were pulling the boy down and one policeman said, "Say, son, what are you trying to do here, and why are you trying to end it all? Come on down here and let's talk it over." I understand they talked it over about half an hour and both jumped off.

Step Up to the Positive

We can associate with things that get us to start fighting. You're going to fight with people who are constantly giving you negative vibrations. Why do I say this? At the very beginning of this "class," I think you have to start creating a path. Good health depends upon the path you go. This is the whole story.

I had a little boy here, Peter, from Albuquerque, New Mexico. You should have seen this boy, four or five years ago. They had to carry him in with asthma. He couldn't breathe without fighting for his breath. He was here all by himself, getting hold of life. He couldn't see well because he was even allergic to light. His eyes were running badly. He had been from one doctor to another, but they were always symptom-minded, treating his eyes, treating the wheezing, treating the condition of his lungs. They said his digestion didn't have anything to do with it, elimination didn't have anything to do with it. Change this idea. This body is built as a whole. The first thing you take care of is the body, totally and wholistically.

What Does Feeling Good Feel Like?

A little boy came here with asthma at one time. He was 11 years old, and he said, "Doctor, I just want to tell you something." I said, "What is it, John?" And he said, "I just wanted to tell you I never knew it felt so good to feel good." I have always remembered that. There is something very wonderful in that statement.

A woman came in and said, "I just can't tell you what you've done for me. For the first time in years I've gone three weeks without being on a respirator constantly for my asthma."

Rebuild Your Life Today for Tomorrow

What has happened? These people are living differently. They came here hungry and they were so satisfied with their first taste of a new life that they took it up permanently. I don't like to see people who have waited so long for this but I tell you that the body is ready to change as soon as you are. As soon as you begin living another life, your body is going to be re-made. Your body is made according to the life you live. I can't put it any stronger or any better. Much of this life is not good, but you can start creating a new life.

You want to live this life better than you found it, perhaps despite what your parents have taught you. Many parents don't understand their children. Children can many times teach their parents a lesson. Little Peter's family is living differently due to what I taught Peter. They have to live differently and even the family is finding that they are feeling better now. It is just a matter of an elevation.

I went to Tacoma, Washington, some time ago and lectured. They had the headlines in the newspaper, DOCTOR DROPS A BOMB IN TACOMA. I wouldn't drop a bomb or hurt anybody. But, on the other hand, you might be surprised to read what they said . . . "The doctor says 75% of all healing in the future will come out of an educational department and not out of a doctor's office."

Doctors Prosper on Man's Ignorance

Now, that's a bomb to some people. That would shake some people up. But you know, doctors make a living on your living . . . and they make a living on what you know and what you don't know. If you go the next step on that, they make a living on sick, ignorant people — crippled mentally. Wouldn't you say this was dreadful? I'm interested in getting you well because I feel bad to see you not feeling good. But you can alter this. The funny part of it is, I can't heal. I can't do a thing. I know that Nature heals, but she needs an opportunity, and the only one who can give her an opportunity is you. Nature cures; doctors get the fees. Healing has become a business these days and this has become a big dollar business too. I don't mind it being a business, but sometimes we find it's become a horrendous thing. For instance, I can give you one example.

Preventive Medicine Is Long Overdue

To sell an X-ray machine to a doctor or clinic, the salesman says, "You can add another $10,000, $15,000, $20,000 or even $25,000 to your income by having X-rays. The plate only costs a dollar, and you can charge $15.00 for the X-ray." This certainly adds up, and then sometimes I wonder if we need 20 or 30 X-rays. I wonder about the side effects and cumulative effects. How many people have X-ray effects in their bodies? How many X-rays are really necessary.

Today people are sued so much, doctors are sued so much, because people are suit happy. To protect themselves, doctors tend to go to the extreme. "I have proof that you had this; I have proof that I did the right thing; I have proof that they did the right thing, you're going to pay for it." I wonder if you realize what you've been paying for? There are many factors that we must remove ourselves from. The only way you're going to get out of drugstores, doctors' offices and hospitals is with what we call preventive medicine.

Doctors Have to Find an Ailment

A couple of patients recently made life difficult for me. I couldn't find anything wrong. I'm wondering what it is that I should find. I've been trained to find something wrong and I've worked very hard to find something wrong. There is something wrong with everyone, but it shouldn't be made into a mountain. And you know when you come in feeling good, it is a challenge these days for doctors to change their approach and concentrate on how they are going to keep people well, how they are going to tell people to continue to maintain health, to learn more about a better lifestyle.

This is an entirely new way of doing things. The average doctor's waiting room is waiting for sickness. Fewer than three percent of the doctors practice preventive medicine in this country. It's hard to believe. Get into this "preventive" idea. You wait and prolong your problem, eat the wrong things for twenty years and then you want it over, done, taken care of in one night, one shot. You try to pick out a doctor who's going to give you relief immediately; I'm wondering if you realize that you can't make a new body with drugs. You can't make a new liver and new tissues and well-working tissues on drug-oriented treatments. It all has to come through your living habits, and I say that's where we started the ailments.

Where Are Your Reserve Defenses?

Build up your good health! Our goal is to build good health and we're not going to treat disease. You can look for a cure for disease from here on. They're still looking for a cure for multiple sclerosis, arteriosclerosis (hardening of the arteries). They're still looking for cures for all those things and countless more. You pay the March of Dimes, and you pay to cure tuberculosis and you don't know anything about it. Do you know how to prevent those things? Have you gotten the information yet? We have health departments. Have you heard any information come out of the Health Department lately? No, they are waiting for you to get a disease, then they will tell you all about it. They're going to cure you after you get into problems and trouble. They tell the people that they are susceptible to flu, get your shot now. Shame on you if you've got a susceptibility to flu! You haven't been living on the preventive side of life. You haven't kept yourself well enough, and flu is going to walk right in.

Do you want to take this religiously? If there isn't enough God in your life, the devil has a place there. Yes, you can put it that way. I can't put it in any other way for you. How much good do you feel you can build out of junk foods? What kind of blood do you think you can build on junk food? The young people have been taught about junk foods lately. Doctors should have been taught about junk food a long time ago. These young people are seeking wonderful changes. They're making *us* think these days.

Diseases Are Winning the War

We're not leaving too good a life for those coming later. We should leave this earth better than we found it — if possible. It's "going to pot," it's deteriorating, there's more disease than ever before. They tell us in 25 years there will be such an increase in diabetes that everybody in the United States will have it. Is it possible? At one time they gave figures that in 85 years there will not be enough sane

people to take care of the insane at the rate we are increasing. Stop and think about it! You go into institutions where people are eating canned foods, and they're having fried foods, they are eating spaghetti and meat balls. From the foods they're eating, would you expect them to get well? No, I'm afraid not. I feel, too, that if you could look at some of the experiences and experiments these people have gone through, you can see that there will be no changes until we take the upper way...the higher path.

Better Health Is Your Option

This is the secret of making a new body. Seek the better things in life, the more godly things, those things approved by God, those things that are natural, those things that are as Nature would have you take it. (You can't compare a nice apricot picked ripe from the tree, with one picked six days early to allow for shipping time to market.) There are many things we should learn and put together.

I make a living on people who only live on half a loaf of bread. That's white flour, from which 40% of the original calcium is gone. You need calcium, you need silicon but every time they polish the outer husk off the grain, they're taking away the silicon; and when you have a lack of silicon your hands will perspire and you'll find that your skin will get rough and dry, your hair will get brittle and dry and many other symptoms will arise. Silicon is necessary to the whole body.

Potassium Promotes Endurance

At the University of Florida two doctors were working with three experimental groups: One group is just taking water when they run seven miles; one group is taking water and salt and running seven miles; and one group is taking potato with the potato peeling. They ran the experiments to see which group was the best in endurance tests. Those who had the peelings on the potatoes had the least fevers, the least perspiration, didn't drain their bodies, didn't come out tired, and had more endurance running the seven miles. I talk about potato peelings, and you call me a "nut." How long do you have to go before you know that it's the peeling that has 60% of the potato's potassium? Yes, in the peeling! Potassium is needed in the muscle structure of your body to keep you from having excessive perspiration and to prevent fevers. Yet, you have these things and don't know what to do about them.

Are You Soul Hungry?

Now, it's time we find the knowledge that's going to help us to be able to go through these things. I know you would like to have remedies and you'd like to have something for your body. I especially see that with people who want to learn how to live correctly. Every doctor should spend half of his life teaching his patients how to live right. That's the reason I believe in lecturing; that's the reason I believe in writing. I know you're hungry. I know you want to do the right thing, but you don't know what to do. I've spent 50 years in this work "practicing." I don't like that word because I should know what I'm doing pretty soon. We have to go the way of knowledge, of wisdom.

There are a few things I know. Some people are soul hungry. They're hungry for quiet. They just want silence. They need to go into meditation. They need to know what prayer will do for them. They should learn what love will do for the soul. That's why I say they're "soul hungry." I see things. It's an inner need that I see. It comes at any age. It doesn't have to come after you've had many experiences.

A little boy at the age of 8 had cancer and had only six months to live. People in his home town were very concerned about this boy. "What is it you would like to do?" they asked him. "Is there something we can do for you? What would you like to do more than anything else in this world?" This little boy said, "I just want to see an astronaut land." He was given that privilege. That was many years ago, and he doesn't have cancer today. I am wondering what brought about this change. Have you ever asked yourself what you would really like to do more than anything else in the world?

We Are All Seekers

I think many people's lives would change if they did some of the things they really would love to do. The heart is sick today. Some people are heartsick. Some people are lonesome. People need to be fed. We all have hearts. There are many things to take care of a yearning for love, to be touched by someone. The heart has to be cared for, too. People are often heartsick when they come into my office. They're hungry. When a person's wife passes away and somebody says, "I can see you don't feel well." I have a cup of tea here that's good for the heart." In that case a cup of tea doesn't satisfy the need of the heart. Tea is for physical things. In order to mend the heart, we have to mend other things.

Of course, the mind needs knowledge. We are all seekers. We're all after the finer things in life and we seek these things. You can't be satisfied living at the age of 20 all your life. That's why very shortly, I'm not going to be doing the things that I've been doing the last 50 years. I'm going to act my age. I'm going to be doing some of the things that I'm now wise enough to do and that I should be doing. Why shouldn't I get in and do something now at my age? I'm going to leave some of the old things and

I'm going on to better and higher channels, and there's a possibility that you would like to have some of the higher and better knowledge, too. I can't keep on talking about the wonders of the slant board like I did when I was 25. I can't keep on talking about skin brushing like I did when I was 25. I have to leave this.

Healing Power of Vibrations and Color

There are new things you have to know. There are things you should know about color. There are things you should know about vibrations. There are things you should know in the photography field, because I believe that photography is going to bring in the new day of showing your actual feelings in the body. Wouldn't it be nice to photograph your aura? Wouldn't it be nice to photograph your vibrations and see how far the aura goes out when you're angry...when you hate? Wouldn't it be nice to see your vibrations come out when you love? Wouldn't you like to see your vibrations photographed when you're spiritually attuned, and when you are in a state of prayer? What a difference to see the colors that come out of your body when you love as compared to when you hate. It might awaken you. You may be led to another way of touching, and maybe I'll find another way of touching you. That's what I would like to do in my photography.

Healing the Physical Symptoms

When I look at a person physically, I can see a calcium lack. I can see a potassium lack. You don't draw the water out of your body fast enough. You perspire so much you need sodium to replace the salt you're throwing out of the body. I can see in many cases when you have varicose veins, you need an extra amount of Vitamin E. You need silicon in your body.

We Don't Need Sympathy

I can see that when a kid comes in scratching and picking his nose, he needs silicon. I can see the man that scratches his ear. He's got flaky dust coming from his ear and I know he needs phosphorous. I transpose what I see, not your hunger. All I do is transpose back to see what you need. You're really needy people and I'm in need, too. There are a lot of things I would like to do in my life, and I've made up my mind to do some of them because we all love to be pleased, don't we? Certainly we do. Stationery stores have sympathy cards because they make you feel better, but some people don't know that sympathy won't help them. It doesn't give you the knowledge, it doesn't give you the things you need to be well. When we come to foods and chemical elements, we've got to recognize that we've got to restore the body.

A lot of people go to restaurants. Do you know what restaurant means? It means "to restore." I make a living on people who live in restaurants. We have to teach you a better way; I have to bring you back to Nature. I have to bring you back to natural things. Possibly we don't restore as well as we should. One of the finest foods that I know for restoring our body, the body forces, is possibly greens. Yes, greens. This is the thing to think about. If you want to get well, think of greens. Some of you don't like this. I'm one of them. But, I do it anyway. I have to change my mind about some things. I can't live on what I learned as a child from a Danish family. I can't live on my Danish pastry anymore and be well. I've found that out.

Reroute To A Better Road

I had to take another path. I found out I didn't have a good liver when I was averaging 20 cups of coffee a day. I found out and I hope you find out pretty soon so you'll change also. You'll find that your food will be your medicine one of these days, and your medicine will be your food because it satisfies the physical hungers of the body. *All* disease is a sign of a chemical lack in the body. You can describe any disease in the body and I can tell you the chemical elements you're not putting into your body. There's a possibility you burned them out. You can burn out chemical elements by being mean, obstreperous; you can burn them out by resenting and resisting people. You cannot live this way. You've got to love people even if you don't like what they do. You have to love your enemies, even when they spit on you. That's very difficult, but when you do that, you can heal yourself.

How Sprouts Rejuvenated the Zoo Families

I wish I could take you on some of the experimental trips I've gone on, such as my trip to the Zoo in San Diego. After feeding on leftover lettuce from local restaurants for several years, the young animals couldn't carry on. Many were dying before they matured; others were dying when they were young. Somehow or another, mother's milk wasn't strong enough to give them good teeth, good digestion, good bowel elimination, etc. The Zoo had to make a change. They were losing their young monkeys, their young birds, and so forth. Do you know what they did? They changed the animal diets to sprouts. And, after giving sprouts to these birds down in the San Diego Zoo they no longer had any trouble raising their young. Many animals had lost interest in reproduction and had no sex ability. But they found by just changing them to sprouts they regained both interest and ability.

Set Your Vibratory Forces to Work

To keep your glands young, you're going after vitamin E. So, why don't you do it by eating right? It's in nice green vegetable juice. The fresh Vitamin E in food has a terrific vibratory force also, and you're going to live on that vibratory force. I can tell you what you can do.

Take television for instance; you can measure it with an instrument and tell that the television throws off an emanation. Dr. Ott in Florida has written some lovely books and one of them is, *My Ivory Cellar*. In it, an experiment is described in which animals were put in front of a television — mice and guinea pigs. Their pituitary glands degenerated and grew smaller. The animals became stunted, lost their fur and did not have good digestion. This man brought these experiments to the U.S. Government, and twelve thousand television sets of a particular brand name were recalled by the government because they found the filters were not strong enough to take out the harmful rays.

Counteracting A Polluted Environment

I'm going to tell you something very nice. You can put grass right below a television and you'll find out when you test it with a gauge, you can't get any reading. The grass absorbs the radiation. This is something else for you to think about. You don't get the effects from that television. You reduce radiation effects on the body by using grass juice and other green juices. The chlorophyll helps you get rid of these toxic effects. Green juice is one of the greatest healers you can put in the body. If you'll study color, you'll begin to see the various values of these colors in the body. What are we doing? We're building up the defenses in our body. We're building up good health in this body.

When my son Art was young, we had a birthday party for him and had twelve boys over. I remember Art passing out 12 cookies. He got down to the 12th boy and there was only one cookie left. He looked at this cookie for awhile and said, "You know, I think I'll eat this cookie because I have been living on health foods. I can take it."

Nature's Powers Are Infinite

I'm wondering if this means anything to you. You're never going to do the perfect thing even if I teach it to you. But, get as much of it as you can. The healthier you become, that'll keep you in good stead, for problems yet to come. We've got a lot of problems in this life. The foods you buy are not too good. I'm going to tell you the nice things to have but I doubt if you can have all of them. You may not be able to get ripe raspberries, ripe blackberries. It is difficult to get ripe fruit because they don't pick it ripe for sale in the supermarkets. It's so wonderful to taste a ripe apricot off the tree, and to taste a nice ripe blackberry right off of the bush. It's something you never tasted in the city when you bought them from the store.

Seek Higher Spiritual and Mental Paths

Our possiblities with nature are just boundless. We find there is a spiritual way, and we find there's a mental way. I can't help but think about my visit once to the Virgin Islands. People walk in the street and you can hear a little rattle sound in their pocket. On the inside of this little box they carry is what they call a "worry stone." They take out the worry stone with a shallow depression on it and they just rub this to get rid of their worries. You know, I thought it was wonderful for them to think of a useful stone like this. The stones only cost $5 or so. "It was worth it...it only cost me $5 and imagine, to get rid of my worries for $5. Sure beats paying a psychiatrist $50 an hour." If I could give you an untroubled mind for $5, I'd have a rush here. You can get these Virgin Island "worry stones" in different colors and different materials — green, jade and other compositions.

Cultivate A Better Philosophy

We had the Health Minister here from India and he told me that in India they are not allowed to buy or sell tiger claws anymore. These tiger claws are something that you have to think about. Tigers are not legally hunted anymore. In India, he told me, they use tiger claws to solve an interesting problem. When kids are afraid of the dark, they hang a tiger claw around their neck, and it cures them. It works because people believe it will work. We live by our beliefs, and I'm only telling you that if it only costs you $5.00 to get rid of your worries, buy a "worry stone."

You don't really have to do it that way. There are other ways of directing your intelligence so you can get over worries. If to overcome is a battle for you, then you'll never get well. You'd just as soon waste your energy in overcoming and not have to battle it. If you have to labor over your worries, then you'll kill yourself. The labor will kill you. You've got to learn to run and not become weary. You've got to love some of the things that you have to do and not always do the things that you love to do. There is a philosophy you take up. As Mother used to say, "It isn't what you give up in life, it's what you take up in life that counts." There's no such thing as a vacuum in your mind or in what you are doing. So, if you wish to get rid of the old, start taking up something new that is beautiful, that is wonderful. I don't feel sorry for the man who dies. I feel sorry for the man who never has lived.

A Time to Listen; a Time to Act...

There's a time when we have to turn to advice. There's a time when we have to change our life and this may be the moment when we do this. I'd like to start out with maybe the thought of my old friend, Yogananda. I remember one day standing with him — the most unusual day I've ever sepent with any man in my life. To train himself, he put adhesive tape over his mouth so he wouldn't say anything that day. Nobody would talk to him because he wasn't going to answer. To spend a day with him not saying anything, was very difficult to do, but you see I have learned something that I can't forget and it's just one little thing in the world: we recuperate in silence. "Be still and know." Silence is the greatest thing in the world. That's one of the things I learned from Yogananda which means so much to me.

Resistance Is Deadly

So, when we come back into the Christian religion again, we find that it says to "Resist not evil." I am convinced that evil never hurt us as much as resistance to it. Oh, how people resent things and how people resist things and wear themselves out resisting. You can't live in resistance. You die in resistance.

Are You Dying to Get Well?

A lady came in recently and said, "I'm just dying to get well." And, she had been doing all the dying things to get well. I doubt she is going to get well because she is busy dying too fast. In putting these things together, I want you to recognize that we are embarking on a new path, one to build the positive forces in our life. We are going to take in foods that are going to add something of a positive nature to our body. I think you would all exchange anything for good health, wouldn't you? Well, let's build good health. What does good health mean? "Cleanse and purify thyself and I will exalt thee to the throne of power." This is what you get in good health.

Onward to a Victorious Day

When you're working with me, when you are working in the path I encourage people to follow, you're going to cleanse yourself. Not only that, but you are going to have better health working in your body. When you build this health principle, disease begins to leave. You'll find if you nourish the roses they will grow; however, if you nourish weeds they will grow. You've got to put your attention on the roses, get them to grow, and let the weeds go. This life is created as we exchange one moment for another. You're going into a new moment every moment. But now, don't crowd this moment with the problems and troubles of the past and don't take on things that are unborn as yet. Stop and take a few moments out to see how you can change your life.

Black Can Turn to White

Through my iridology work we change the black that we find in the iris of the eyes to light. It is said in Germany that black is compared to the devil of Hell while white is compared to the angels of Heaven. What we're going to do is to go the upper way. We're going to go the approved way.

A Body Is the Mind's Servant

There's no one who can say we shouldn't eat a ripe apricot in preference to a green one; to have a nice salad in place of spaghetti and meat balls. No one has any objections to natural foods compared to junk foods. If any doctor tells you that food makes no difference, he simply doesn't know any better. We find that your body is a mold, your body molds to the food you eat. The body is a servant to your mind, a servant to your spirit. This body is in your hands, to be molded as you will.

You find that you can will it into any disease you wish. Dr. Sanson of the Sanson Clinic in Santa Barbara produced hemorrhoids in rabbits by giving them coffee. He was able to produce certain diseases, diabetes, for instance, by giving laboratory test animals white sugar and white flour. You make these diseases, you eat them. You drink them. You think them. And, you bring them into existence within yourself.

Purge those Negative Tendencies

What you should do now is to seek knowledge, wisdom and guidance. You should be trying to get rid of the black, the negative things. Those things are meant for people who don't know any better. And, you find that you're on your way up. You're an advised person. Whether you are wiser or not depends on what you put into action. I'll know you by your deeds and not by the faith you say you have. What did you do after you got off your knees? You find it's the work you do that counts.

Every Gift Returns Full Cycle

Put this all together. We've done our thinking. But don't stop there. Get going again. When we put up our defenses and begin to develop a good body, we are going to take everything we possibly can to build better health. We're going to be clean; we're going to come clean now. We're going to have a clean mind. We're going to unfold into a lovely life so the body can mold to it. We're going to realize that what pours out of our body nourishes us. We live on what we pour out. If we pour out hate, the vibrations from that will kill us.

The Martyr Suffers Least

A man shot one of my employees. Of course it upset us all for awhile, but we found out he was going to be all right. We've got to realize that it isn't the man who is shot or the man who is killed who's going to do the suffering, it's the man who does the killing or the shooting. He is the one who is going to suffer. This goes into the higher laws of life. So, let us reach for some of these higher gifts of life. You really deserve them. You deserve the finer aspects in life.

Inward Calm — Long Life's Key

All I can tell you is the greatest lesson I have learned from a man who lived to 256 years of age, Li Chung Yun, who died in 1930. This man was asked before he died what he attributed his long life to. He said he had lived on herbs, such as ginseng and fo-ti-tieng. He'd lived on all the better herbs. He played tennis when he was 196 which he thought was one of the things that shortened his life. But when I look at all of these things, I wonder what is most important. Just before he died, he said, "You know, you asked me what I attributed my long life to and I would like to tell you in a very short sentence. . .it's inward calm."

I think you can go through life as a calm person and not get mixed up with everything that is disheartening, that has a breakdown nature. Get out of remorse, get out of sorrow, take care of your mind, take care of your body as it should be taken care of. Then, I know you people will be working toward the light and all I can tell you is that you need more light. Pray for enlightenment. My mother used to say, and I believe it, "Give a man light and he'll find his own way."

Dr. Herman Bundeson, Chief of Chicago Health Department said, "57 artificially-fed babies are lost for every death among breast-fed infants."

Chapter 2

Recipe for a healthy life

Awaken a New You

I think there's a destiny that is set up for us but I feel that we add to this destiny. I also feel we can hurry the good things that can possibly come to us. We are going to have experiences whether we want them or not, aren't we? Realization of what you can get out of these experiences really belongs to you. This is your job. It is your problem. All I can do for you is to awaken you. In your awakening stage you'll have progress, elevation and ecstasy; you'll have harmony, peace, the good things of life. You will find out how to reach for it, touch it, and to know that it's always there and it is always available. It is not a fleeting thing. It is not like the human being... moody. The truth never gets moody. It is always there, always in that perfection stage.

Christ put it so wisely, "Even before Abraham, I WAS." In other words, the truth existed long before many things you see today.

Step Up to Health Consciousness

We've got to get connected with these truths. Now, what has this got to do with diet? With food? There is no use having a spiritual philosophy and being miserable as far as this body is concerned. The better you are physically, the better your memory is, the better your awareness is, the less you have to lean on other people, the less you have to beg someone to hold your hand. You must learn to be more independent. You can be self-sufficient. Sick people do not have these qualities. They are in need of help, begging. Help me! God save me! I want you to get out of this stage. Get into the stage of body health, stage of higher consciousness, something you really want! I want it myself. You must ask for growth and enlightenment. Because you'll find that in every stage of consciousness you have problems and troubles.

Spiritual, Mental, Physical Food Laws

The same principle exists within the physical realm. I am going to tell you about good foods and how you can get them. People can interfere with Nature's original foods. We have man-made foods, mishandled foods, super-market foods, dollar foods, eternal life foods, and they are all bad. When foods are made incapable of spoil-ing, their value is gone. You must learn this. In going through the physical things, there are laws to follow, as we go mentally there are laws to follow, and spiritually there are laws to follow. If you are just going to go through life seeking the physical things, that is all you have in your consciousness. If all you are looking for to marry is a man or woman with 72 heartbeats per minute, then you're not living. You really haven't got much if you marry a man or woman for physical reasons, and that takes in sex and all other physical characteristics.

Life's Endless Growth Process

There are greater and finer things such as putting your mind and heart on a higher level. Everything in life is a matter of growth. If you've gone through the seventh grade then you are ready for the eighth grade. My hope is that I can help you one step above where you are now. Nature cures but she needs an opportunity. Man could be a Master if he used all his opportunities. There are those who go through life feeling that life owes them a living. You must work for everything you get! In other words, earn it!

Every Wise Man Was Once a Fool

Some come into the world with an old soul. Some people don't have to learn the same lessons I have had to learn. I feel too, that Christ came as an old soul. He must have, to be all things to all men. We're all on our way to a Mastership, whether we like it or not. We go through grade school, high school, college receiving a Bachelor of Arts Degree, or a Master of Arts Degree. Then perhaps there will come a time when you are able to be of help to people. The fool doesn't know what is in the wise man's head, but the wise man knows what's in the fool's head because he was once a fool himself. This is growth. Wise men are not born, they're made, and wise men do in the beginning what the fool does in the end. The diet work I teach is only for the sincere people. For those who do not care, I have nothing. This may sound dreadful, but I can't care for everyone because some won't let me. But, I'll go out of my way to help you if you want me to.

Begin with Mental Optimism

So, we start with desire, motivation. One must have a good mental philosophy. The diet that I am going to prescribe to you is the finest you can get. It should be taught in colleges. It should be taught with the idea that all food has a spiritual background, that food should build a perfect body to enable you to go through life and do perfect things with your body. Food should not build a body to harm other people, to kill or to destroy. Food has a divine purpose in life. I started in the health work years ago with the purpose of serving. Many people feel that if they just drink carrot juice that will answer all their problems. But, I have seen people suffering from financial problems, and diets did them no good whatsoever.

One man I knew with high blood pressure had lost his money in the 1929 stock market crash. He was afraid to work for fear of getting a stroke. A mental stress can become a physical ailment. So we must view this from the mental aspect and also the spiritual aspect, since I will be giving you materials relating to a hungry stomach, hungry cell life, hungry bones that are porous, arthritic bones and arteries that are hardening. They all need help. Some people could be starving for music; other people could be starving for friendship. There are many types of hungers in life. We must learn to feed them right.

Love Your Enemies For Your Benefit

First, we must realize that we are responsible for our own life. We can bathe our body with any kind of thoughts possible hoping we can get ourselves in order. It is well to stop at the beginning of the day and tell yourself that this is going to be a fine day. I am going to be good to myself and also to other people. Love your enemy and the greatest good will come to you. Your enemy may not need your love, but you need to love him for your own good.

Enemies: Hate, Jealousy and Resentment

We are all seeking advice, all seeking remedies. One lady came in the other day and said, "You've done so much for my neighbor, I'm going to try you." I said, "Darling, you're not going to try me, I'm all right." I said, "You're on trial." So this trying business must be changed to knowing business. We get mixed up with human feelings. We resent, we resist, hate, live in jealousy. These mental conditions must be corrected. Everything is not nutrition, food.

It's like the man who went to the psychiatrist and told him how depressed he was. The psychiatrist said, "Why don't you go to the circus? "There's a clown over there who's got people rolling in the aisles with laughter." The man looked at him and said, "Doctor, I'm that clown."

We must hold onto these good things. Some people go to church on Sunday and wake up like devils on Monday. The nice things don't carry one. Monday morning a little boy wakes up and he makes faces at the bulldog and his mother says, "Don't make faces at the bulldog." The boy replied, "Well, he started it."

Depend on Yourself — Nobody Else

Don't live other people's lives; get out of this mental attitude. Don't live other people's opinions, asking people how to cure a cancer, how to cure this and that. Get good knowledge, true knowledge and leave other people alone. Don't ever expect to get happy with people because we find that people are as a rule not happy and are also seeking something for themselves. Don't give people advice. People always like to tell others what to do.

I recall sitting down at a counter where a man was eating fried bacon, fried eggs, fried potatoes. I reached over and said, "One of these days you are going to have an ulcer, bowel problems and constipation." I was repaid for my sage advice by the statement, "Mind your own business." Since then, I have found that salt and advice are two things that are never wanted until you are asked for them.

Nutrition is Disease Prevention

Dr. Tom Spies, honored by the medical profession for his work in diet, stated that all diseases are caused by chemicals, all diseases can be cured by chemicals, all chemicals used by the body (except for the oxygen we breathe and water we drink) are taken in through foods. With the proper nutrition all diseases could be prevented. This is a powerful statement. However, he is a doctor who actually works with food. He has contributed much to healing in the food regimen.

He continues to say that tissues become damaged when they lack the chemicals required in good nutrition. They do not have what he called "tissue integrity," and become prematurely old. There are people of forty whose brains and arteries are senile. If we can help tissues repair themselves by correcting the dietary deficiencies, we can make old age wait. The problem is to keep ourselves well enough so that when we do come to old age we will be young enough to enjoy life minus sickness or disease.

Return to Garden of Eden Nutrition

I'd like to share a few incidents from my own life. First of all, I was given up to die as a young man. I know how it feels when a doctor tells you that you have only about three weeks to live and says all you can do is to rest.

I said "Doctor, it sounds as if I'm going to rest a long time. Isn't there something else I can do?" He told me of a doctor who was a dietitian, a nutritionist, a Seventh Day Adventist. He was a man who had studied foods. I recall this man coming in and sitting down on my bed and giving me a one hour lecture on the values of certain foods, natural foods. He told me about how natural foods were necessary in the scheme of life, even telling me about the Garden of Eden. I wasn't particularly interested in any religious ideas but when I saw from his talk how we had strayed away from the wonderfulness we had in the beginning and what a mess the people are in today and how I was brought into it, why, I was ready for the change. I was open and I felt this and I know this is true: when the student is ready, the teacher appears. This man was a master, and I don't even remember his name; but he was my master at that moment. Do you understand? It was a fleeting knowledge that I grasped and held on to and it saved my life. This doctor told me about eating only fish that had white meat, fins and scales. It is different from shellfish, and I never realized until later that shellfish causes much of the food poisoning that we have in California.

I found out, too, that people starve themselves without realizing it when they eat the wrong foods. Some people don't know any better until ten years after they've depleted their bodies to a diseased state. Then they awaken to the better life.

After this, he went into the background of the lung disease I had developed. I told him I had lived for four years on four milk shakes a day. He pointed out it came from a mental problem because I was called "shrimp" in school. I was the smallest, skinniest kid in school. I could run between the shower drops and never get wet. I was only interested in one thing and that was putting on weight. If I could get some weight on, even fat, I thought I would be all right. So, I found a place where they made milkshakes eighteen inches high with whipped cream, nuts and a nice red cherry on top. Do you know what they called these milkshakes? "The Idiot's Delight!" I was the idiot if there ever was one. I tell you, it takes experience to awaken, but I did wake up. I changed my diet...I began to see a change in my body.

Vital foods are the answer. One of my first patients was a woman with thirteen open ulcers on her legs from calcium deficiency. She had seen many doctors. To stimulate healing of those ulcers, they gave her calcium; to control the calcium they gave her thyroid. Three months here, three months there, she ran around to different places in the United States...looking for someone who could help her. I was just beginning in my work but I knew she needed calcium. I remembered the people in the Hunza Valley who had perfect bones and teeth as described in the book, *The Wheel of Health* by G.T. Wrench, a London medical doctor. It told about the Hunza Valley, where they had no doctors, no diseases, no hospitals, no dentists.

What a wonderful place to find out how to live right.

And then this girl came in here with leg ulcers, and what could I do? Doctors had tried to give her calcium. Where was I going to get calcium she could assimilate? I thought about the Hunza people who lived to 120 and over, with every tooth in their heads. That was calcium! No rickets, no pronated ankles, no calcium diseases. They had calcium. Their children weren't in need of calcium. I began to see something, how they lived on sunshine vegetables. I found out that sixty-seven percent of their diet was made up of greens, tops of vegetables, outside vegetables, foods grown in the sunshine. By comparison, only sixteen percent of the American diet is made up of sunshine vegetables. What a difference!

I put her on raw greens for three weeks. This was before we had electric juicers, before we ever had the idea of making vegetable juice. I chopped up vegetable tops, tops of nine green vegetables, put them in distilled water, squeezed the mixture and gave the juice to her.

In three week's time those leg ulcers were completely gone. I was a chiropractor but I never touched that girl. I never gave her an adjustment. Remember the power Nature puts in the green vegetables! This is what I'm trying to show you.

Arthritis Can Be Conquered

Another lady from Long Beach, California came to me with a spine like a corkscrew. At the age of 35, doctors told her she'd have to have a brace and spend the rest of her life in a wheelchair. She had arthritic spurs on her spine as big as your thumb nail. They told her it was incurable. They said, "We can't cure arthritis. Do you understand that? We can only relieve it. We just try to reduce the pain."

She was averaging forty-eight aspirin tablets a day. I found out that when you have arthritis, you're lacking sodium, a bio-chemical element that helps dissolve calcium deposits in the body. I found that she had calcium out of solution, so I gave this girl a lot of sodium. In one year's time her spine was as straight as a die. X-rays from the hospital showed that she had no arthritic spurs remaining on her spine. This is something to think about. Do I believe in foods? Do I believe food can be your medicine? I have "seen the light," and I'm a believer.

Improve Your Body with Proper Diet

I deal with this physical body as the temple of the living God. Our body is in a state of change constantly. You're making new skin on the palm of your hand every twenty-four hours, and if you don't like the skin in the palm of your hand, you can get rid of it. If you want a better skin than you have now, you have to elevate your way of life. You have to go into a new life style entirely. So your job here is to find a right way of life, a way of living, a healthy way as far as eating is concerned and this is important to see.

Now in working with diet, we must realize something. I say "Get off of these diets!" Everybody is on a diet! People have come to me on a grapefruit and peanuts diet, on a grape diet, on a carrot juice diet. Or, they're on a fast and that's not a diet but you find fasts have their purpose and do a lot of good, but only for a certain length of time. The one thing you'll really have to seek is a healthy way of living. This is the most important thing I can tell you. Don't look for a healthy diet; find a healthy way to live. I bring this up because there's such a thing as a pretzel and ice cream diet. You understand?...people live on these things. That's the diet you're on, but it's a diet, and when I find cream of wheat in the right shoulder and white flour in the left knee, I've got to get rid of it. I can get rid of it. It can flow out. It will change. How? I'm going to put something in its place that builds a perfect body. To get this perfect body we have to go back to what the meaning of health is.

The Origin of Health

Health came from the old Teutonic language meaning "our salvation" and it tells you to have that salvation is found in wholeness, and in what is natural, pure and whole. Isn't that something to think about? That's the basis for my diet work. Food must be natural, pure and whole.

At the Ranch, we served Chinese peas so patients could get the pea pods along with the peas. One of these days you may realize that watermelon seeds are one of the finest things for the kidneys, a wonderful help for hypertension in the body. And what do people do? They spit the seeds out. We don't use them. Yet again when you're sick, you may go down to an herb store and buy watermelon seed powder for the kidneys.

We've got to have pure foods. We cannot live well on food grown on artifical soil. I mean, I go down to the valley where I live, and they've got the most luscious looking strawberries you'd ever want to see, but in the spring of the year they fertilize heavily with inorganic chemical fertilizer, the artifical stuff. Those strawberries may look wonderful, but they are neither natural nor pure. Mine don't look as nice, but they are grown Nature's way, and I end up with a pure food.

Don't you have a little laboratory on the inside of you that tells you what is right and wrong? My neighbors were picking strawberries before mine even had much growth. But you see, when their strawberries were developing, the plants were weakened from the stress of rapid growth on artificial fertilizer, and the bugs really went after them. So they had to use a toxic spray to kill all the bugs. And as we begin to look at this way of growing crops, we find out that every stage is artificial in some way. It's not salvation to have artificial foods. When we eat these synthetic wonders, accepting substitutes for what Nature meant us to eat, we have to pay for it. Substitutes will let you down faster than a strapless gown. When you're looking for substitutes, it's like bargain hunting, trying to get something for nothing. If you try to get something *good* for nothing, you'll get something good for *nothing*. You have to pay for good foods, and that's what I tell my wife. I don't care how much it costs. If you don't spend money for good foods, you'll spend more on a doctor. I make a living on your living. All doctors do. And I don't feel entirely comfortable about it. On the other hand, too, I'm trying to help you change. I'm dedicated to teaching change as much as I possibly can because I feel things aren't right and when things aren't right, it's time for a change. That's the way I feel.

Now in working out our food routine, we have to find out what a whole body needs. We have to get off diets where we expect a lettuce leaf to build a good brain structure. It won't do it. It hasn't any brain food in it. Well, it may have enough brain substance in it to build a good brain for an ox.

You are human...you're godly...built in the image of God. So, you must eat godly foods. There's food for sheep; there's food for horses and there's food for human beings. If we could just follow the "uncivilized" Indian of many years ago who never went to college, probably we'd be better off. He often lived over a hundred years of age, and the average doctor only lives to the age of 49. Did you know that? A farmer lives to the average age of 79. I've been practicing 50 years now. I should have been dead a long time ago. But I feel this...that's it's time for doctors to learn to live as well as anyone else.

Make It Natural, Pure and Whole

When we come to foods, we start off natural, pure and whole, and I'd like to start out with the other laws that we have to think about. I call this food regimen "law" because it has worked so well for thousands of my patients over many years.

You have to have six vegetables a day and two fruits a day — that's the proportion you should have. I feel that you need the vegetables more than the fruits because you often can't get tree-ripened fruits, good fruits. If you want to live on a fruitarian diet, you have to grow your own fruits. Or, you have to live where the fruits grow. Of course, you can go down in the tropics and live around the equator with all the fruits you can possibly eat. There you probably can live a fruitarian life. I visited these people who live that fruitarian life, and I've even been with people who wanted to live a breatharian life. They don't even want to live on food. But, if you want to live that kind of life, then you shrink away to a body that does not invent, create, develop, progress anymore. You understand that? You have to have a brain where there's any challenge in this life, and the brain needs more than fruit.

Civilization is a challenge. People are a challenge. A family is a challenge. Work is a challenge. When you have a child, when a child is born to you, he or she knows nothing. That's a real challenge because you have to prepare them for that time when they grow up and are ready to leave. So you have all of this to do in life. We know little about getting along with one another; we know little about the foods we should eat because we don't have the Garden of Eden anymore. You've got a supermarket and you'd better know what you're going to do in these because you're going to come out with a basketful of disease if you don't. That grocery basket could be full of biochemical deficiencies. You understand? You cannot tell what you're going to come out with unless you know right from wrong.

Know Your Fruits and Vegetables

So, I feel the six vegetables today are most important. Six vegetables. Let me tell you the difference between vegetables and fruits. Fruits have a maturity date and when you study the sunshine, and the stars, and the natural earth and moon rhythms and find out how fruits grow from the earth, you will realize that fruit has to have sun until it's finished. The sun is a sodium star. Venus is a calcium star. If you want calcium, to make sure the calcium is there, when Venus comes over it will fix calcium in the ground for the vegetables in a biochemical form fit for human consumption. We find out that without sufficient sunshine we get green fruits. Green apricots that are not ripe. An overripe apricot isn't "ripe" either. To have it just right, that maturity time for that fruit must be right on target. There's a perfection point there that you have to live by to get nourishing fruit.

But we don't need that perfection point in vegetables. You can have young string beans or old string beans. You can have young beets or old beets. The maturity is not critical in the vegetables, and this way I don't have to be seeing patients because they have green citric acid in their system, in their joints. I don't have to deal with green apples or cramps in the stomach or ulceration. Can you understand that you've gotten into troubles because you didn't know any better? You didn't live according to the sun and the stars. You didn't live according to the earth. You didn't plant properly. You just didn't know. You grew up like Topsy.

Raise Your Consciousness to Better Health

And then you go to a doctor who treats all the diseases and never sets you right. You come in one door with a certain state of consciousness, certain knowledge to live by; you get your treatment and you go out another door with the same state of consciousness and the same level of living. That's why every operation the doctor does leads to another. People seldom do anything to stop this recycling of ignorance.

Diets Have A Season: Winter and Summer

When we have the two fruits and the six vegetables in our program, we can follow this for the whole year. You don't have to gorge on fruit in the summertime (with resulting elimination problems) and go without it in the wintertime. Why not have a body that works well all the time? That's why some people are entirely different in the wintertime than in the summertime.

Now there are winter foods. There are summer foods. . .and we'll discuss those. A person who wants to make changes in his diet should do it at the beginning of every winter and the beginning of every summer. That's when you should change your diet. Spring comes along, and you get Spring fruits and vegetables for elimination purposes. Now we want to eliminate that. We want a thinner body. We want a little thinner blood to take care of the heat that's coming through. People are not as well able to work; the heat gets them. Well, that's because they're filled with 41 flavors of ice cream, and I tell you this keeps us from being able to mold to the seasons. Now your body can cope if you can mold to the seasons. You find the seasons are there for a purpose. The nice red strawberries come in first, the highest sodium food you can have and sodium helps you to thin the blood. Sodium helps you to cool the blood. Something to think about, isn't it? And red is the first color of the rainbow.

And then we come in with the nice yellows. Yellows are always laxative foods. We need to clean this bowel in the spring and in the summer. We find out we've gone through sedentary occupations during the winter. We've been inside the house for a long time. We haven't been eliminating through the skin and kidneys as well as we should. Then we get into these cleansings.

At the end of summer, the following comes. Grapes. . .grapes at the end of the season. It's the last opportunity for cleansing. You're elevating yourself and getting yourself ready for wintertime. It's the summertime when you should take care of the cleansing of your body.

The Less Cooking the Better

I want you to be able to know when to cook on all burners and when not to cook at all. I want you to know you don't have to cook in the summer as much as you do in the winter. There is a time for cooking and there is a time for not cooking. There are some foods that should be cooked. I feel if you want to be totally a raw-fooder, you could be. But you have to know what you're doing. This is why we're working out this knowledge, so we can work it out well.

Get Off Those Diets

All right now we find we need one starch a day. We need one protein a day. I do not want to be responsible for you if you want to go on grapefruit and peanuts. We had a man come to the Ranch who was on the grapefruit diet and it did much for his sinuses. Then he had the idea, "Why not go on carrot juice? It's high in Vitamin A." Certainly it's all right to go on three weeks of carrot juice, but when he got finished he wanted to go three weeks on watermelon, because it's high in silicon. When he got finished with that he wanted to go three weeks on grapes because it's a good bowel elimination food. This man was always on a diet.

What I say is "Get off these diets!" Cream of wheat, pickles and ice cream are a diet. A bad diet. There are reducing diets that are good. There are building diets that are good. There are many forms of diets that we can have and we may have to mold them to your type and your temperament, the size, the shape, how you've been born, your weaknesses, the problems that you have now, whether it's going to be solved, whether you're healthy in type and can take lettuce and chew it and really break it down.

Some people are born with stomachs of iron. They can digest nails, but those people don't come to me. We have mentally oriented people who come here with a poor digestive system and a lack of force in the body, a lack of nerve force to stimulate good digestion. They have a very poor digestion.

I'm bringing this thing out because types and temperaments are important things to study. To "Know Thyself," to know who you're feeding, is vital. It's very important. I've seen many a man cooked onto the operating table by the wife's culinary art. She says, "I eat it. Why shouldn't he?" There are no two people who act alike, work alike or digest alike. I've seen people who are so intense they wear out all of their nerve energy just talking to one another. Some people are so slow, they remind me of a master I sat with once in India. Six hours. He winked his eyebrow twice. He didn't need any food because he didn't need any animal heat. I mean he had a different body, and he didn't waste energy moving.

I have a son who is very fast, so he needs a lot of protein. I have another son who is very slow. Takes a lot of time to think it over and sometimes I think he doesn't need much food for the mind. I remember I was shaving one morning and David came in. He was about eight or nine years old and he stood up next to me and said, "Dad...I think you'd better go up to the sanitarium." I look around and said, "What makes you think I ought to go up to the sanitarium?" He said, "It's...on...fire."

Well, we have people who are slow and we have people who want to do things in a hurry, and if you want anything done, come around and see me. I'll get it done. I'll do it fast. I have a lot of joy in accomplishment and getting it off my mind, and that's the kind of person I am.

And you find if you've got a heavy body loaded with water, you can't drink a lot of water. These are people who can gain water right out of the air. In fact, ask them. A hydro type can drink half a glass of water and gain five pounds.

Some people are silicon types. Some people are calcium types. All the old people that I visited around the world were calcium types. They were earthy people, plodders. They just repair and rebuild the tissue they break down every day. They go to bed every night at 10. And they watch for 10:00 to come around. They know just exactly the time to get up in the morning because they know when the vegetables need water, they've got to have it. They're people of the earth, close to the soil. They work with earth. They use the same kind of a plow they did hundreds of years ago. They're not inventors. They're not thinkers or artists.

There are mind foods, brain foods. And, there are muscle foods found in proteins and starches. That's why you cannot live on fruits and vegetables alone.

If you want to become a vegetarian you can, but it will change your whole life entirely. To want to be a vegetarian is an admirable thing, and I respect vegetarianism. I went 25 years as a strict vegetarian and I mean strict. I've gone through Ehretism. I was in the Ehret Club in 1923 before most of you were born. I know what it is to go through the extreme ways of eliminating catarrh because that's one of the things I was given up to die with. You drink four milk shakes every day for four years and you'll find out you're a catarrh factory. But, I eliminated it.

Ehretism was a wonderful stepping stone. And I don't mean that it's the whole business. Ehret was a man who never worked. Ehret was a man who lived off whatever he could pick off trees as he went through life; he was a Naturist. He didn't need anything. He was self-sufficient...He never hated anybody. It turned out that mentally he was all right, and we have people like that. But you can't say, "Look at me; I did it and I eat this way, so you can too." We're all different. Many can starve to death without the proper amount of protein. Don't ask me to guess how much protein you can have because we're all different. Don't ask me how much starch you should have because we're all different. In fact, don't ask me how much you should eat.

The Threefold Healing Art

All right, so now if we put this diet together and have these vegetables and fruits, remember that we have to take care of our hair; we have to take care of sex; we have to take care of the glands; we have to take care of our eyes; we have to take care of our memory; we have to take care of the muscle structure. We also have to take care of the heat in our body. We have to have heat in the body to break down, digest and assimilate foods in this natural energy factory we have inside us.

If you're a vegetarian and have been cheating yourself out of some of the heat giving foods, you'll find out you've got cold feet, cold hands and a cold head. You don't get enough blood to the head because it takes starches and proteins to take care of that. We have to have a body with enough heat.

Practically all sick people have cold feet, cold hands. Their circulation is poor. That's why we teach circulation here. Their circulation is sluggish. You should partake in games, foot baths, nice walks, and so forth, grass walks; get that circulation in your legs. You'll never get enough blood in the head if you don't have circulation in the legs. So we have to take care of the legs, keep the blood flowing; but you have to have circulation with it and that's through exercise.

No one gets well on nutrition alone. It's a one sided healing art, but I think it's the first of all the things we should learn in the healing arts. Always start with food and nutrition, FIRST. I've used chiropractic, adjusted people given them the perfect nerve supply through the stomach and they've gone home and lived on coffee and donuts and never gotten any good results. Can you understand good nerve supply and a poor diet will never do you any good? But if you fell out of a two-story window and you had the best diet in the world, you may need chiropractic adjustments. You may need spinal replacement or your may need joint replacement. There are times when we must take care of the mechanical things.

"We've got to have a balanced mind to see what directions we must go. Some people are mentally unbalanced. Some people need stabilization; some people need security. Did you know that? Some people are flitting around because they've only got a dime to their name. You'll find out that when you only have a dime to your name, that's when you really need a spiritual philosophy. And when you really have a spiritual philosophy, you can go down to only a dime to your name and you'll be all right. But you see, some people live on the fear that one of these days they will get there. So, they live in greed. They live in hoarding. They live in other various abnormal things. So let us be careful now in all of our getting that we understand that we need to get a good balance.

A balanced diet now is more important. People come in to see me. They are know about diets, but they don't know anything about a healthy way of living. I seldom have ever set a person on a diet until I know they live correctly. I've seen people go 30 or 40 days on a diet, or on a fast, and when they get off they don't know how to live. They tried this tangent and that wild goose chase after all the sacrifice they'd gone through. They spoil everything they've done in their fasting. So learn how to live right and that's what I'm teaching you now, And by the way, half of my diet is eliminating. Half of my diet is building. And if you never went on a diet, you'd get well on my food program. It may take a little longer.

Fasting is the fastest way to getting your health. But maybe you have to go the longer way until you know better.

We can add juices between meals. We can have our vegetable juice at 10 and we can call it a mineralizing time. And you must have a nice juice in the middle of the afternoon for mineralizing. In the afternoons at 3 or so you have herb tea or a punch made from herb tea. Make sure the herb tea fits what you need in life.

Variety Is Health's Only Path

If you need a lot of silicon think about oat straw tea. If your nails aren't right, if you hair isn't right, then the nerves aren't right, so use a nice oat straw tea and then you can put in your concentrate. You can put in apple juice, prune juice, any kind of juice that you want. If you have only five vegetables instead of six, it's all right, but patients had as many as twelve a day at my Ranch. You'll just have to measure your sprouts, two of these vegetables in your salad, one or more cooked vegetables at noon and another cooked vegetable or two at night. It isn't hard to get twelve vegetables a day.

The next thing we have to remember is that we are building a body. And, it's made out of the dust of the earth, the whole earth. That doesn't mean a clump of earth that probably has too much calcium and not enough iron in it. It's got to be all the elements, so we need variety. That's the second law. We must have variety. And you can't be like my aunt; she has carrots and peas. That's the only variety she ever has. She has vegetables but that's all she ever has. You can't live on just carrots and peas.

Diets for All Ages

As you grow older, two proteins a day may be good and one starch. Young kids, people who are working on tractors, outside life, putting a lot of effort into life and using their body a lot probably could use two starches a day and one protein. It won't hurt you a bit to have two starches a day and two proteins a day. If you are a mental worker and use your mind strenuously, you need proteins. You could have more protein.

Food Combining Is Essential

We have both starches and proteins for breakfast at the Ranch. You can have them both, but at lunch time we have starches and in the evening we have a protein so that you're having two starches a day and two proteins. If you want to leave out the starch for breakfast and have your two proteins a day and starch for lunch, it's all right. If your growing child wants the starches for breakfast, starches at noon, proteins at night, it's perfectly all right. But when you have a protein habit, when you have a starches habit, don't fool around with half starches, half protein. Know your starches, know your proteins. I'm going to tell you now what the proteins and starches are. They are necessary to know. I'm dealing a bit with combinations there. If the combinations are not right for breakfast, you'll get it. That's only one-third of the day. You do two-thirds right and Nature will do the rest. Don't be too finicky with these separations because Nature never made a pure starch, Nature never made a pure protein. They're all mixed with starches and proteins together. There are a few that are close to a complete protein.

Know Your Proteins

Here they are. The most complete protein that you can get is found in meat and that means lean meat, no fat, (no pork), poultry and fish — white meat fish that has fins and scales. The next protein is milk, and that's whole milk, raw milk — goat milk if you can get it. Goat milk is an excellent food, balanced chemically almost like mother's milk. The next one I recommend is eggs. In fact, I could put eggs first because all proteins are evaluated by professional nutrition scientists in comparison to the egg yolk. The egg yolk is considered the perfect protein.

There are many cults, many studies, many Indian philosophies that tell you the egg yolk isn't good. They can tell you all kinds of stories about it. But, I'm interested in the chemical elements right now.

Diseases Signify Bio-Chemical Shortages

It is the biochemicals that I get people well with because every disease is a sign of a chemical shortage in your body. You can mention any symptoms, and I can tell you what chemicals are lacking. That's what doctors should know.

There's a reason for sticky perspiration. There's a lack of certain biochemical elements. Find out what they are. You may not correct it in a day by adding the missing element because it will most likely take you a whole year to get the elements you need in the body. It'll take you a year to get the reserve built up in your body so that you can get well. You've got to have reserves to draw on. What I give you today you may use up so fast that you still are not getting well. You're not getting rid of your symptoms yet but you've got to build up a reserve and as soon as that reserve is built up you can get going. Keep after it and keep working. This knowledge is indispensable.

The Case for the Egg Yolk

Now when we speak about the egg, I speak about the egg yolk as the perfect protein. A lot of people say you can't take the egg yolk because there's too much cholesterol in it. Well, I'll tell you, most doctors have never studied eggs. Half of them only know what a fried egg is. That's all they've ever had. Most have never gone into diet; most have never gone into nutrition. They don't know anything about nutrition, natural nutrition. We find out that the egg yolk is one of the highest foods in cholesterol. BUT we also find that Nature has added a certain amount of cholesterol to some foods because it is necessary in the human body. Don't think that all cholesterol is bad in the body. Let me ask you this one question. If you wanted to dissolve cholesterol what would you do it with? Lecithin, of course. Do you know what is one of the highest lecithin foods in Nature? An egg yolk. God put that lecithin right next to the cholesterol so you get the balance. God didn't make mistakes, but we do. So I tell you now that if you don't destroy that lecithin by frying it or by putting it in bread and baking it, the lecithin will balance the cholesterol. High heat destroys lecithin. And that's why you can get cholesterol. Eggs must be taken soft boiled, poached or raw.

Cholesterol deposits (arteriosclerosis) are made in people who live too much on fried foods — fried eggs, doughnuts, Danish pastries (which I know so much about) and baked goods. I'm giving you a very vital thought here, and the same thing goes for oils. I never recommend cooking with oils. They're cholesterol producing. You have to be careful. They've got to be raw [cold pressed], otherwise you're into trouble.

The egg yolk has lecithin, vitalin, cholesterol, phosphates, iron and iodine. The chemical balance is lovely. The phosphates go to the brain and nervous system. Use the egg white sparingly and aerate it when you use it. It is high in albumin that is difficult to digest. Soft boil the egg or use the yolk raw; the temperatures above boiling destroy Vitamin E and lecithin. The white of the egg contains heavy albumin that the kidneys have to take care of. It builds feathers on chickens and you don't need feathers. But in the egg yolk we feed the nervous system, the eye structure, the bony structure, the structure of the *whole* body. Do you understand that? This is one of the finest foods I know. It builds a *whole* body.

Now you don't have to eat eggs. They're not necessary. But if you go into Chinese lore, you'll find out that the egg is the most important thing in their life. They even use 200-year-old eggs for a gourmet delicacy. I wish I could tell you some of the stories from China about how these birds give eggs to human beings. Do you think animals are here just for themselves? They're here to serve you. And when I get milk from my goat, why that's a blessed goat. Do you understand that? We're in business of living together. She's saving my life and I'm saving hers. Can you understand that...? We have to look at this animal business maybe a little differently, too.

Raw Milk and Raw Milk Products

Animal products supply the amino acid proteins and brain and nerve matter of a higher order than you find in fruits and vegetables. Egg yolk and raw goat milk are foods that provide animal heat for the body. Raw milk and raw milk products are a *whole* food — pasteurized milk isn't.

Cow's milk produces catarrh; it isn't made like mother's milk or goat milk. Goat milk has almost the same chemical balance of mother's milk while cow's milk is different. It has too much calcium — the material that builds horns, hooves and hide.

There is a great controversy about the difference between raw and pasteurized milk, and there is a difference. Randleigh Farms, New York, ran experiments with thousands of rats and mice that showed every one that was fed pasteurized milk died of disease. Those fed raw, natural milk didn't die from disease — not a single death. The scrawny animals with the poorest digestive systems, the poorest teeth were on pasteurized milk. I see it happening with human beings as well, so I have raw goat milk in my diet. Goat milk costs more in the store, but it's worth it. I can give it to my asthmatic cases and bronchial cases and they don't have catarrhal troubles.

Are we going to need a certain amount of the acidophilus bacterial culture? Certain foods break down the "friendly bacteria" in the colon — chocolate is probably one of the worst offenders. Pasteurized products and cultures don't have the "friendly bacteria"; they have been destroyed by heat. Aged cheeses that crumble help build the acidophilus bacteria in the intestinal tract. I don't believe in cheese spreads or cheese foods manufactured overnight. Get a raw cheese or raw goat cheese if you can. These are a good protein, and cheese is not a *whole* food unless it is uncooked and unprocessed. This is why I don't believe in too much yogurt; it has been heated. The old

men of the world had clabbered milk culture every day and it was their special drink.

Gland Proteins: Seeds and Nuts

All right, now we get down to the next one. That's seeds and nuts as a protein and we find that they are fattening foods. They're high in oil and it's hard to use these seeds and nuts and reduce on them. We find that these can be hard on the liver especially if you've got a small liver, or if your liver has been diseased. You have to be careful of nuts. It takes a healthy person to handle nuts and seeds whole.

On the other hand, seeds and nuts can be broken down into nut milk drinks. That's what we're going to learn. Nuts go through the body in about 10 hours, so they should be soaked for several hours in honey water or fruit juice to soften them so they can be assimilated. Sick persons have cold stomachs, heads and so on, so they don't handle cold proteins like seeds and nuts well. That's why we use the seed and nut drinks, butters and meals. These are non-catarrh forming milk substitutes, and so is soy milk powder.

The champion seed is the sesame, and the sunflower seed is next. Turkey is known for the strength of its people. They make tahini (sesame butter) and halvah. Why, the man who once headed the Turkish wrestling team was 75! I believe that in seeds we get strength, tissue power and good muscular development. Seeds are also a gland food, and we find out that the long life people have wonderful glandular systems. They come from the seed. They say you are as young as your glands, and one man I met at age 153 had his last child at 123. This is something for you to think about. The average man going into the doctor's office today is worried at 60. He hasn't got the glandular force; he hasn't got the sexual energy. Seeds have all the chemical elements for all the glands, and that's not just for procreation — we're reproducing our bodies all the time. The person who doesn't have the glands, the hormones to do this properly dries out. That's why this country has become a hormone prescribing nation. We find that everybody is taking hormones these days, and we've gone hormone crazy.

The next best protein is the nut and the almond is the king. It is the alkaline nut. It is close to the apricot kernal, which is what the Hunzas live on so much. It's one of their proteins. When you choose nuts have the hard-shelled variety, and don't buy nuts with paper-thin shells, like paper-shelled pecans or almonds. The oil is gone from these and so is the lecithin — the brain and nerve food. The Missouri Black Walnut is the best because its shell is so hard and it's rich in manganese for the memory. These oils are an excellent gland food and if we don't have good glands the rest of the body will deteriorate, degenerate and break down. Vitamin E is another important oil in them that is good for the heart and helps tissues that get flabby. It helps bring oxygen to the brain and who doesn't need that? If you have varicose veins you need Vitamin E — it isn't just a sex vitamin.

Legumes Are Valuable Proteins, Too

Then after the seeds and nuts come the legumes — peas, beans, lentils, garbanzos. We find the lentil is the king of all the legumes, the easiest to digest. The hull is the easiest to take care of in the intestinal tract and causes the least gas. It is the hull of the bean that causes intestinal gas. Loma Linda University has taken the hulls from soybeans, for instance, and given them to people and they don't get gas. It's the shell that causes the trouble. Split pea soup doesn't cause gas.

Recapping the List of Proteins

Many people who come here want to go on an all natural, raw food program, with nuts and seeds. But the body can't handle it because it doesn't have enough heat; a sick body can't handle and assimilate cold proteins. It's too low in temperature, digestion, etc. If you make nuts and seeds into butters and drinks — nut and seed milk drinks — the weak body can handle it. I'm working with sick people, not healthy people. Proteins are for the brain and nervous system and don't forget that. You have to feed these systems with heating proteins, magnetic proteins from the animal kingdom. I might add that I don't approve of shell fish because they are scavengers; they live on the droppings of other fish. They have found that most of the food poisoning in California comes from shell fish. Meat is the highest protein food we have, but I don't say you have to eat it.

So we've gone down the list of proteins. They say you can't have meat because it's putrefactive; you can't have fish because it ferments in the bowel; you can't have eggs because they're hard on the liver; you can't have milk because it produces catarrh; you can't have cheese because it's binding to the bowel. (That's why we serve whey with cheese; it's laxative and it was removed in making the cheese.) What have you got left? Nuts and seeds, cold proteins. You have to be careful how far down the list to go. But if you have good bowels and can move things along well and can have foods that take care of putrefaction and fermentation such as papaya, whey, it helps to build the friendly bacteria and you can handle some of these foods all right. Fried foods are out. If you have meat and fish have it broiled, baked or roasted.

Muscle-Building Rye (Starch)

Starches...the best of all the starches are found in these four starches — rye, yellow cornmeal, rice and millet — and which is the best one really doesn't matter. But these four starches produce no catarrh and will produce no weight gain in fat. Wheat puts on fat; rye puts on muscle. Nobody needs fat. You do need muscle if you're going to run through life with me. Do you understand? You've got to have the power and energy to work with in the muscle structure. Finland uses a lot of rye and the greatest Olympic runners we've ever known have come from Finland.

Yellow Cornmeal: The Laxative Starch

We go down now to the second starch that's so good for us and that's yellow cornmeal. If you go down to Central and South America, you'll find they live on a good deal of yellow cornmeal. It's the most laxative food you can put in the bowel, the highest food in magnesium which is a bowel element, and I have very few people coming to me who have good bowels. I think you should have yellow cornmeal at least twice a week. And, you can have it if you have colitis. You can get it down to a gruel if you want to. You can liquefy it after it's steam cooked if you want to or before it's cooked.

If you study the ancient Aztecs of Mexico, they knew how to live close to Nature and they reaped her rewards. Their strength in warfare was attributed to yellow cornmeal. They were known to feed the Spaniards the foods that pleased them and to save the strengthening corn for themselves. The corn and the cactus foods were reserved for them only. The Aztecs were well aware of the fact that their physical power came from their fields of yellow corn.

Asia Survives on Brown Rice

And then rice...You never saw a fat Chinese man and we find out that all of Asia lives on rice. The body moves more slowly on rice and it is good for high blood pressure.

Our greatest experiment to show us the wonderful value of Vitamin B is in the rice polishings. They took off the rice polishings and fed rice to pigeons in the polished form. In four days' time the pigeons flapped backwards and died on rice without the polishings, but just before they died they could be given rice polishings and be brought back to life. That's how vital it is.

When you go to Japan they take rice polishings and make a nutritional syrup for sick children. You can go to Turkey and you find it's a law that they can't take all the bran off the wheat. You can't get white flour there. They have to have a certain amount of the silicon and the

Vitamin B on the outside of the grain. But look at all the sick children, and I have to put them on rice bran syrup that's made from rice polishings. We are chasing a cure because we didn't do the right thing in the first place.

Millet: Longevity Secret of the Hunza

All right, the other one is millet. You look in these countries where people are using millet and they've got beautiful bodies, not fat ones. I went over to the Hunzas and took photographs, the most beautiful pictures, and they are in my book *World Keys To Health and Long Life*. You'll find pictures in there of beautiful millet fields. This is that millet that kept these Hunza people so well. Millet could even be placed near the top as the second or third best starch.

Other Starches I Recommend

Then, of course, we go along to others, and there can be buckwheat. There can be baked potatoes and other starches, even wheat once in a while. Let me bring out the law here now. It isn't what you do once in a while that counts; it's what you do most of the time. Do you understand? You should be able to eat a little wheat without producing a lot of catarrh, but wheat and oatmeal have the greatest gluten base of all starches, and this is what produces the catarrh in the body, so we cut down on them, especially when we are getting well.

When I am taking care of a sick person and things aren't right, I don't want them to repeat the wrong things of the past. That's the secret of my work. Don't do the same thing anymore! Get away from there! Get off the main street! There's another kind of drink. There's another kind of food. There's another kind of thought.

Back to starches. I don't approve of gluten because bronchial troubles, catarrh and mucus are partly due to gluten. These four main starches I've discussed are the best for people with catarrhal and bronchial troubles. If you have to cut down even further, leave only rice and millet in cases of catarrh. I think everybody should have a little bit of starch, however. Also, these four starches don't produce excess glucose and I am convinced that glucose in the body can be responsible for a great deal of catarrh. Have baked, mealy potatoes, and eat the skin, but don't have them too often. Or try baked sweet potatoes and squashes once in a while. Most people get too much wheat — donuts, waffles, pancakes, all baked goods. Wheat is a number one allergy producer.

The mental worker should concentrate on proteins as brain and nerve foods. The physical worker needs more starches. The growing child needs starches. The heavy mental worker can use two protein meals a day; one starch meal. The sturdy man gets along well on starches and

calcium foods. Starches feed the body. The calcium type uses his body. I put bread at the bottom of the list of starches. I don't believe in bread. Most people have bowel problems and it aggravates them.

Balancing a Healthy Diet

Now, in putting these things together you know what a good diet is, and I say it leads to a healthy way to live. Now at the Ranch we have a fruit and cheese diet or nuts and yogurt twice a week in the evening. I think sometimes in the summertime, especially, a little extra fruit is fine when Nature gives us hot days and we don't need as many of the heavy vegetables, the heavy starches, heavy proteins. The meals on these two evenings help to balance things up in the summer.

Overeating Kills Many People

I think overeating kills more people than we realize. It has been the greatest problem in my life and I take a child's portion now more than I ever did. I found, too, that in the beginning, I started cutting my plate in half and I let them throw the other half away. I learned this by sitting with George Bernard Shaw in London. And I remember he said to his housekeeper, "Well, you can't make a garbage can out of my stomach," when she tried to get him to take seconds to finish a dish up. She didn't want to have to throw it out. I'll never forget that. You've got to realize that you must have enough to eat, but the moment to go too fast, too harsh, too much, you find you're killing yourself. The best books that I know of are written by men who lived a long life and they always put temperance as the greatest law. Remember the rule: eat like a prince for breakfast, a king for lunch and a pauper for dinner.

Luigi Cornaro, who wrote the book *How To Live To Be One Hundred,* was given up to die by the age of 49 by seven doctors. At the age of 60 he increased his food because people were telling him how thin he was and they said, "If you don't eat more food, you'll die." He increased his food from 12 ounces to 14 ounces daily along with the usual juice. This amounted to only about two additional tablespoons of food per day, but he was sick for 30 days. He went back to his old way of living again and he went on to live until he was 109. He wrote his best book at the age of 90 without glasses and he buried all seven doctors who gave him up to die. It's something to think about.

Proven Survival Formula

In talking to all the old men I have visited, one of the three rules that they have for long life is never to get overweight, and they're all at the same weight at 153 as they were at 20. They don't vary. They never overeat and they never retire. They never quit working. These things I find definitely in all the old men and all the old people.

Get Rid of Salt and Pepper

A couple of other things I think you should get rid of are black pepper and common table salt. Why? Pepper is 16 times more irritating to the liver than alcohol. For seasoning we use a vegetable broth powder. I don't believe in much salt, and if you use salt make it the evaporated sea salt. Most salt today has been heated to 1,400 degrees and is inorganic. Have dulse on the table for extra iodine; the purple Nova Scotia dulse is also high in manganese — a brain and nerve element for the memory. Get away from other harsh spices and condiments that aren't natural.

God Put It Altogether

God has put a lot of thought into living foods. You can't duplicate it. Man can't make parsley. Man has never been able to duplicate a carrot. The thinking that's gone into that food is superior. And, God has made these foods for man. Man, in order to exist, has to have certain foods. These foods are for man, and man is for these foods.

Remember that 60% of your diet should be raw — from God's garden. Have a large salad with the noon meal and a smaller one with the evening meal. Your diet should also be 80% alkaline and only 20% acid. (Fruits and vegetables are alkaline and starches and proteins are acid-forming.)

I have the greatest misgivings about any foods tampered with by man. God has prepared certain foods for us, and I don't mean to make this religious by any means, but I only ask you to remember that God and Nature were here before man, and we're here because of God. We can't afford to stray from those two things. Nature is the cloak of God. And God is working in parsley, in chive and carrots. A divine architect is putting the nutrients in there for us. We can't ignore this fact.

Foods are almost as wonderfully and fearfully made as people are. There are no duplications, no substitutions and that's why we're trying to get back to Nature. There's a call to come back to Nature these days, and you know what is right. If I put a poison pickle in one hand and a ripe avocado in the other and I asked you which you would eat, there's something inside of you that tells you what is right.

The highest food in iron is the Idaho Black Bing Cherry. If I offered you a handful of iron filings in one hand and delicious bing cherries in the other, you wouldn't hesitate in your choice. I don't know if you have to have your food tested by a laboratory or not, but I will say that the native American Indians watched the birds and if the birds would eat it, they would eat it. And you'll find out by coming close to Nature that you will know what is good for you. That's what I'm trying to teach. Stay close to Nature and to God and you can't lose.

It's Time For A Change

Anyone who is sick knows it is time for a change. One thing we have to change is our eating habits. But food is not an easy problem to tackle because most of us have well-established cooking habits and our past racial habits make it very difficult for us to make changes. While we are getting along in life, we never recognize that there is a relationship between our food and our health. We find it difficult to conceive of an actual relation between the food that goes into our bodies and what happens in our toes or hair or eyes. We have never had a training in this. We do not know that the bloodstream depends upon what we eat. We do not know that what we eat today is going to talk and walk tomorrow. We do not know that what we eat actually becomes the cell structure of the body. This is why if we do not change our faulty ways of eating, we can never expect a permanent turn for the better in our health.

Chapter 3

The vital elements in foods

Dis-ease Destroys Tranquility

I think the spirit is always feeling good, but sometimes we have to get close to the spirit with a good body. I know when you don't geel good and you are sick, you're drawn away from all the good things in life. It is very difficult to be spiritual and to elevate yourself above hardships in life, misery and so forth, when it keeps nagging at you. When you've got a revolution going on in the stomach, it's not easy to have peace of mind. This is the time that people go off. This is the time when mental problems come in and we find out, too, that misery and all of our financial troubles and everything else are caused a good deal because we're not well physically.

I spent time in Italy after the war and saw how they sent over white flour and white sugar to feed all of those starving children. You know, the Italian people are going to build revolutions in their stomachs that are going to come back on us one of these days. People cannot be peaceful unless they have the kinds of foods that make a good body.

Health Is A Serious Business

We're in a business and our body is in a business and we have to consider that to operate a business properly you have to have all the information; you have to have good leadership; you have to have good material to work with. Health is a business of putting together resources, reserves, a good background, good inheritance, but of all the things that we need most, leadership comes first. Someone must be in charge. The car must have a driver. It has to have somebody to give it direction. We must have spiritual things and mental things to know where we are going. Each of us, as a physical body, must talk as a physical body. Few of us know that we're not our physical body. Who is it that says, "my" circulation? Who is it that says, "I feel squeamish?" "I feel like vomiting." There is a normalcy within you that judges and knows everything that is abnormal on the outside.

The Perfect Spirit Is Not Diseased

You were drawn from that normal to the abnormal when you entered into the physical body. As soon as you get into that physical body and become one with it, you are absent from a divine thing or I would say from a place where there is no sickness. I absolutely believe there is no sickness with God. I believe there is absolutely no disease in a perfect Spirit. I do believe the physical body is a servant to your mind; a servant to the direction you take in life. The path you are on is the path you live on. Can you build a good body on coffee and doughnuts? I don't care what kind of training you have had in diet. Don't you know that some foods produce constipation? Do you realize that some foods can produce diarrhea?

The Body Is What It Eats

We mold to the foods we eat. Your body does not know what it is supposed to do. It asks for direction and follows this direction. Therefore, it requires a good leader and a wise man who can do this.

The Chemical Story

One must pick out good foods, good friends, good situations, good environments in order to develop a good body in life. You have a servant in your physical body, but he is never paid. All that is required is a good mind, a spiritual environment and the proper food supply.

God and Love Are Healers

I don't like talking about the spiritual environment. People think of that as a religious thing and that isn't exactly what I am speaking about, because when I talk about love, it should be found in any religion. Any religion which does not incorporate Divine Love in it, is not a religion, because you cannot live without God and Love. These are of a healing nature. We are sculptors, we are here to refine our bodies. From the ages of one to twenty we can repair tissue twice as fast as we can break it down. From twenty to forty-five or even fifty, you can repair tissue about as fast as you can break it down...just even. After the age of fifty, it breaks down faster than you can build it up. Therefore, to assure ourselves of a top performing body in later years we must refine our bodies to make sure that it has reserves that will prevent future development of disease.

Soul and Physical Joy Are Inseparable

The same thing applies to our souls. We must polish our souls in order to develop them. One can see a young soul reaching for things. Yes, the soul can be hungry too. Many people prefer to be alone, and there are those who can't be alone, but realize they must learn to be alone. Some people can't live unless they have their personalities fed well. They have to have a hobby, they must have a change in their lives; some must travel. Those people who travel usually are happy. It's part of their inborn personality. Sometimes giving your wife a trip will make her better and she'll digest her food better; she'll be much happier. You have to be happy to be well and you have to be well to be happy.

Can you see this philosophy working as a unit? Everything you do affects everything you are. When you help the liver, you help the stomach. By helping the stomach, you help the kidneys; helping the kidneys you help the lung structure. Every organ is connected. As you elevate one organ, you elevate your feelings. And, as you elevate your elimination, you elevate your circulation. Every organ in the body responds. It goes through the nervous system, goes through the physical tissues of the body to all parts of the body. When you feel good you're happy. The whole body goes with that joy and that is the reason I put these three things together.

Miracles Do Happen

Some people want to witness a miracle. You know, we had a boy come here named Richard from Hollywood. He was on crutches for 14 years. He wasn't able to control his urine or his bowels. He wore a rubber bag to help, used crutches to get along, but, in one year only, he was off those crutches, did not require the rubber bag, had control of his bowels, control of his urine, for the first time in 14 years. In just a year's time he was well and went back to work as a taxicab driver. One day I said to Dick, "You know, it has taken a whole year to get off your crutches and a whole year to get changed as much as you have. Suppose this all happened in two minutes. What would you say?" He said, "Why, that would have been a miracle!" Well, I want you to know that it was still a miracle. In China I learned one thing, "You don't have to seek a miracle, you are a miracle." That is what the old sage says and you *are* a miracle when you are heading toward a healing or you are going down toward degeneration according to the things that you choose in life. You see, you are now choosing the things you want to do and that's why I say to polish your soul and you become more noble; you become a greater person; you also become a lovelier person in your own heart. These things help to make a better physical body. As I said before, you are a sculptor. In doing these things, you are here to make beautiful skin

and better fingernails. Your hair can be nicer also.

A 75-year-old lady with gray hair went through the healing process in seven months. Her gray hair is now black. I can't say that we can do that for every person, but what a wonderful regeneration to take place in a lady of that age. These are the miracles I see happening.

Every day people tell me that their fingernails are improved, they don't crack as they used to do. They don't peel like they used to and I wonder what has happened. Well, you find that they have taken a new path, they've gone a new way. They have gone the uplifting way.

You Are Your Own Doctor

You are your own healer. Yes, to the extent you are your own doctor. This reminds me of a story about a man who really wanted to get well. He thought, "I'm going to seek the best man possible." And he heard about a Chinese doctor in the mountains. He heard that he was treating people very successfully. He went up to see him and after he sat down, the Chinese doctor asked, "Do you smoke?" He said, "Yes." The doctor asked, "You drink whiskey?" He said, "Yes." "You drink cola?" "Yes." "You have white flour, white sugar? You eat pie?" "Yes, I do these things...I do them all the time." The Chinese doctor got up on his feet and said, "I can't cure damn fool!"

Reaching Above Coffee and Doughnut Consciousness

Are your getting the gist of all this? It is a matter of a way of life, and there isn't any doctor who's going to help a person who doesn't want to live right. He's going to move around symptoms, he's going to kill your pain, but from a healing standpoint, there's nothing he can do. Let's correct it. Let's elevate. Let's put something new in place of the old that will give you satisfactory service. Let's have a body free from toxic material. Let's get rid of the coffee and doughnut state we find ourselves in. Let us raise our consciousness so that we pick out the finest things in life. You deserve the very best, or don't you? This is the beginning of the incentive and the motivation. I taught motivation because after all you need inspiration to get into this new life and you need to be inspired to get started.

Health Depends on You Alone

A man comes in and says, "Well, you're the ninth doctor I've gone to. What do you think you can do for me?" This man needs inspiration to do better things. Or... "I'm here because my wife sent me." Let's do something on our own. I can't help a person who doesn't have the desire to elevate himself, and if you don't want it, then this isn't the place for you. I must tell people to quit smoking, which is not easy. Then I also have to tell you to exercise, get rid of bad habits, and this is not easy. I also have to tell you that finances, marriage, money problems and other irritating things must be released. Learn to work without laboring. Labor will kill you but work will never hurt you. We are designed for work.

Mental, Spiritual, Physical Elevation

When we go back to the Old Testament, which has meant so much in so many religions, we find these pages were written by sages and prophets of the past. They speak of "brass and iron" used in those days. Perhaps they did not realize that calcium was also available. However, there are elements such as iron, calcium, brass, potassium and also iodine. St. Paul said you die daily. This is a physical thing. New skin on the palm of your hand is replaced every twenty-four hours. We must be elevated. From a mental standpoint, we must know better. As Thomas Edison once remarked, "Well...I made 4,000 experiments before the electric light was accomplished." Someone said, "Oh, my goodness, what a waste of time!" Thomas Edison said, "but you know, I know 3,999 things not to do." That's elevation.

Sunshine, Water and Hills

We look at the dust of the earth, look up into the hills and see rocks roll. Then along comes the sunshine, the cool air of the evening; rain comes, which removes all dust from those hills clear down into the valleys. I worked down in these valleys here at Hidden Valley Health Ranch and I've cleared off areas, watered and in four days grass has started to grow. I never planted grass. How did it start? This grass comes from latent seed in dust of the earth.

Today, laboratories have found there is a lot of iron in grass, also potassium. Everything in grass comes from the soil and air. Grass grows at various altitudes, some places have more water, some places there is more sunshine. Where there is excessive heat, grass, in order to protect itself, has a heaver lining on the outside. Cactus contains much water on the inside.

All vegetables really originate from herbs. But, are you aware that all herbs originally came from grass? All of this has been changed. What a tremendous selection of vegetables and fruits and other materials we now have today! So, you see, from the beginning...soil, dust, herbs and grass. Then along comes the grasshopper. He requires grass and we see that he takes what he needs; then comes the chicken. He enjoys the grasshopper; then finally comes the preacher, and he gets the chicken. Out of the dust comes man, minerals, fruits, vegetables, animals, gophers,

grasshoppers, fleas, etc. They are all from the dust of the earth. Earth is really where we come from. So it is often referred to as Mother Earth. You cannot live without this earth, the dust of the earth. Cheeks and lips will never be red unless your body contains iron from the earth...Mother Earth. You'll never have the calcium in your bones unless it can be balanced well from the calcium of the earth. Some foods contain more calcium. We are more in need of calcium when exposed to harsh winds, cold weather, variables in wind, rain, sleet and snow.

Chemical Element Deficiencies Produce Disease

When oats are grown in a good wind, they have more elasticity. Where does elasticity come from? It comes from the silicon that's in it. When veins and arteries have lost their elasticity, I know that you need the dust of the earth to obtain it. Vegetables, fruits, seeds, nuts are what you need. The most important story in the world is the chemical story of human existence. With the proper foods, our bodies heal. By eating properly we can prevent disease and abnormal bodies in this generation.

I have spent some time in Germany where I've seen a foot-and-a-half tall horse developed in nine generations by feeding them certain foods, starting with a horse that was 15 hands high. This can also be accomplished in plant life, fruits and other animals. A lack of certain chemical elements will produce disease.

Calcium: the "Knitter"

Let's get into chemical elements. They all have a story. When you lack calcium, you find you lack tone, energy, power, cannot stand; people push you over. This may be a mental lack. Yes, it is found in the mind as well as the bones. When one has an inferiority complex, you are lacking in calcium. I know that the man who cannot become a success, "I just haven't got the energy to get going..." lacks calcium. Some people who haven't got the stamina nor the guts to get right around the corner are lacking in calcium. When a prolapse occurs in the body there is a lack of calcium. Calcium is often called "the knitter in your body." When a leg ulcer occurs, you are in need of calcium. If a sore does not heal, often calcium is required.

We are just beginning. When all these chemical elements are placed together within a human being, he is bound to be healthy. When there is insufficient calcium in the body, you cannot repair, heal, rebuild, etc. The average 160 pound man has approximately four and one half pounds of calcium in his body. It is most important, especially when growing. If you work late, overwork, become tired, if you are giving out a lot, you must have a continuous intake of calcium. Bleeding, hemorrhages, etc., indicate a lack of calcium.

Suggested Calcium Sources: Where can you get calcium? Natural cereal grains contain the best calcium. The control of calcium is found in greens. Milk contains calcium. Calcium may be mixed with fluoride, fluoride that makes hardness in teeth. If you use pasteurized milk, it makes soft teeth. Calcium is found in cheese, all milk products, grains, cereals, seeds and nuts. They all contain calcium. Practically every food contains calcium. You must have all the chemical elements to remain healthy.

Silicon: the "Magnetic" Element

Silicon is an element found in the nervous system. It is found on the outside of the nerve sheaths in the body and gives that nice slick surface to the ligaments and to the nerves. A message is carried from the brain to different organs in the body by way of silicon. Silicon is called the "magnetic element." A well person is magnetic. Silicon has a reserve in the skin, in the body, in the hair, and in the nails. Lack of silicon creates an unhealthy body.

Silicon carries blood throughout the body. All blood in your body passes through the thyroid gland every hour and a half so it must have the chemical elements to feed the thyroid as it goes through. When we talk of the nervous system, we must have silicon. This is where flexibility comes from. A person who drags his leg, has a nerve depletion, a nervous breakdown, a lack of activity in any organ of the body, has lowered nerve activity.

Every organ in your body is incited to activity through the brain. We need a good nervous system and a good brain. If we do not have these, the stomach is not going to work. Ulcers of the bowel, tension in the bowel, spasms in the bowel are all due to a lack of silicon. Silicon is a magnetic element. Ill people do not have any magnetism in them, whereas a well person does. A sick person cannot wink and mean it.

If you have a lot of music in your soul, you'll still never sing if you don't have silicon in your body. Silicon gives you the feeling of wanting to get with it, to get with life and to get with joy and happiness. To feel all these things, you will realize how necessary silicon is to maintain good health.

When I buy a horse, I feel the hair. I don't want to buy a scraggly-haired old horse. If it cannot run, silicon is needed. I don't want a scraggly old horse, but one that has spirit, has silicon and has a beautiful coat of hair. When I purchase a goat, I feel the hair. It must have a nice coat of hair, because then I know it has the silicon element in its body. Therefore, the milk obtained from the goat will also contain silicon.

When you get married, feel his hair. After all, you don't want an old goat. To be sexually attracted and enjoy your life together, you need silicon. I used to go to a homeopath who gave me a little bottle of extract called Avena Sativa. It is an extract from oat straw. I used this extract to give my body the needed silicon. I worked with V.G. Rocine, one of the greatest chemists who ever lived, from the standpoint of food. He told me that if you consistently give a person oat straw tea, he will get the necessary silicon into his body. His hair will improve. Alfalfa is another of the highest foods in silicon. Grains contain silicon; sprouts, skins and peelings contain silicon. Polishings of rice contain silicon. Take a teaspoon of rice polishings. It will become a part of your reserve blood, hair and nails. You'll have "the skin you love to touch."

Sodium: the "Youth" Element

I had a girl come in who was ten years old. Her mother carried her in, suffering from arthritis. The mother told me that her daughter had had arthritis nearly all of her life. A Mr. Bourne stood up in the audience and said, "I'm 92 years old and I don't have arthritis." Sometimes I wonder why one at ten has arthritis and a man of 92 does not.

We find that calcium enters the picture. One had the calcium out of solution and didn't have enough sodium. This little girl was treated with sodium, morning, noon and night from whey. (Whey contains the highest amount of sodium). In approximately one year the little girl was in ballet classes.

Sodium is known as the "youth element." Arthritis does not have to come with old age. It is a lack of sodium that brings about old age. Sodium can be found in veal joint broth more than anything else. If you wish to rid yourself of arthritis, I would suggest that you fix yourself "veal joint broth." Much gelatin is found in veal joints.

Sodium is also found in goat milk. Goats are much more limber than cows. There is much more sodium in goat milk than in cow milk. Sodium keeps goats young and active. Goats are young; they are active and very limber. Therefore, it is understood that you, as an animal, need sodium to climb, jump, walk, run, and to do the things good joint material lets you do. Each organ in the body has a reserve of one chemical element more than others. It holds certain chemical elements so that it is a unique active organ, different from any other organ.

Dr. Koenig in Germany, in autopsy after autopsy, discovered there is more sodium stored in the stomach than any other organ in the body. When we do not have sufficient sodium stored we get ulcers; that's when we get gastritis; belchy, burpy sensations; we get all those stomach and bowel disturbances. Bicarbonate of soda is not the right sodium to use. It must be biochemical sodium.

Therefore, we stress the use of natural foods, pure and whole. It must come from plant life. Iron cannot come from nails, for instance, it has to come from black cherries. When you get calcium, it must come from green kale, not chalk you use on blackboards. The chalk on the blackboard is the highest thing in calcium, but if the calcium is offered to you in kale and then in green chalk, which one would you eat?

Sodium is necessary to keep the stomach from becoming acid and to digest properly. It's not what you eat that counts, it's what you digest. A tired body cannot digest. A miserable mind cannot digest, a tormented mind cannot eat and digest. A disturbed mind, a miserable marriage, can produce a malfunctioning stomach faster than anything else.

The second highest organ in sodium is the joints. When you get stiff, can't move anymore, Nature's not interested anymore. It's taking you down and you'll finally die like the horse out on the desert when he doesn't have enough sodium. His joints get stiff and he cannot get his food anymore. He can't run, walk or move; that is when nature removes him from the earth. If you can't get goat milk, the highest vegetables in sodium are okra and celery.

Magnesium: the "Relaxer"

Magnesium is known as the relaxing element and it is stored in the bowel. Magnesium is found in greens, all salads and is highest in yellow cornmeal. Some people tell me that they only have yellow cornmeal occasionally. We don't have enough of this kind of magnesium in our bodies. All yellow vegetables, all yellow fruits are high in magnesium. Therefore, we use food magnesium and not milk of magnesia from the store. We must get away from drugs and get closer to the garden. Magnesium is necessary when we have bowel pockets. It is necesary when we're all tied up, nervous, spastic; it's a relaxer to the body.

Manganese: the "Love" Element

When manganese is removed from animals, they will no longer nurse their young. In fact, they sometimes cannibalize their young. Young mothers will in a sense "eat their children," too with resentment, anger. The whole world is eating one another. This is where we need manganese. It has often been called the "love element." It is a brain and nerve element. When you have a poor memory, that's the time to tell you that you can't love either. Because you forgot that possibly the greatest moment in your life was when you could love. Manganese is found highest in black walnuts. Seeds and nuts are high in manganese and they're found high in natural oils. Manganese is found highest in Missouri black walnuts; nuts that remain in shells are very high in manganese. Nuts contain lecithin which is a brain and nerve food.

Potassium: the "Great Alkalizer"

Potassium is an alkalizer in the body. Gayelord Hauser made his name for potassium broth. Potassium alkalizes whenever we produce acids from overwork, running, working too long, sweating, perspiring; then we need to return potassium to the body. Muscular disturbances such as cramps reveal a lack of potassium. Whenever you want to neutralize acids in the body, rheumatic, arthritic or whatever, think of potassium and sodium. We have a potato peeling broth that is the highest potassium broth you can take.

Potato Peeling Broth and Bee Pollen: Everyone has heard of bee pollen. Before the Pope died some years ago, he told me that in his last years he felt bee pollen and potato peeling broth had done so much for him. Therefore, I urge you to use potassium broth or potato peeling broth to help in your elimination process. One woman I knew, who had a great problem in walking up to her second story motel room used two cups of potato peeling broth a day for a month. A month later I received a letter from her telling me that she was able to easily climb the stairs. When you lose potassium in your body, you find that you are dragging, unsteady on your feet, equilibrium is bad, muscle control is not good, you lose your grace in the muscles. You cannot dance well either. All these problems are an indication that the body is lacking in potassium.

Potassium for the Heart: By running sodium salts through a heart you can keep it alive for 15 minutes. If the same process is performed with potassium, the heart will stay alive for three and a half hours. The heart is a potassium organ; that is why one is placed on a sodium-free diet for heart trouble. However, they forget sometimes to include potassium to help rebuild the heart. Chlorophyll can also rebuild a heart. All greens in plants are high in potassium. Potassium is a great healer, a great alkalizer.

Sulphur: the "Heating" Element

Sulphur supplies your body with heat and that is why certain foods in the wintertime are grown because they contain sulphur. Vegetables that resist the cold weather contain a lot of heat. For instance, cabbage, onions, cauliflower, broccoli are all winter vegetables. Fair-haired people usually have a great deal of heat in them along with freckles. This condition suggests an excessive amount of sulphur. Many elements, when combined, work together.

Phosphorus: the "Light Bearer"

There are two kinds of phosphorus. Here is where the vegetarian is confused. There is what we call a brain phosphorus and a bone phosphorus. Phosphorus with a lower vibratory rate works in the bones rather than in the mind. We must get this straightened out. That is why we have to study vibration; also the bones do not vibrate to the same rate as your mind or the mental processes. You may feel if you eat turnip greens, you will have a good mind. But, you need to know it doesn't have the mind elements in it. It doesn't have lecithin, nor the oils. Also, it doesn't have vitamin E, vitamin B-12, nor does it have the RNA factor which is needed in the brain. The higher evolved phosphorus comes from foods in the animal kingdom — fish, eggs, codfish roe. Phosphorus is something that's been a problem with me. By living on fruits and vegetables, you starve the mind and don't exist well. Our essential amino acids and heat are found with phosphorus that has oil with it. Phosphorus is sometimes called the "light bearer." All organs in your body will lag without this wonderful element.

Vibratory Rates of Chemical Elements

These chemical elements have a vibratory rate and there is no need to throw these chemicals away. Urine is made up of chemical elements. When you sweat, sodium salt is being thrown away; you are finished with it. You are finished with these salts and they return to the earth, but when you take it out of live foods, a vibratory rate is there, since these foods have assimilated those mineral elements that the body uses. The influences from these foods makes the difference between dead and live food.

If it were just chemical elements we were using, then possibly we wouldn't be throwing them away as we do, such as the salt, sodium salts from skins, the salts and the chemicals through urine. As they are thrown away, they must be replaced. These elements come from the fruit and vegetable kingdoms to us alive and at a specific vibratory rate. I am certain we live on the vibratory rate more than on the chemical elements themselves which is probably a new study doctors will take up in the future when they explore the role of electromagnetic forces in health more deeply. We must have live foods and this is the vibratory rate that is placed on the chemical elements in transposing the chemicals from the earth and making them biochemical — fit for human consumption and ready for the human body.

You can get calcium other than that from food; however, it is not really fit for human consumption. It must go through our food chain, or we don't call it organic. We call food elements "biochemical." Biochemical substance is fit for human consumption. Actually, chemicals are found in everything you look at. But,

we find that animal phosphorus has a higher vibratory rate than phosphorus from any vegetables. Now of course, I'm not saying that we have to eat meat. I personally do not believe in meat, but I do know I've seen people whose lives have been saved by the intake of meat. I've seen people restored to good health with meat and it seems difficult for me to believe.

Nature As A Last Resort

I can use liver and liver extracts and practically bring a person back from the grave. Sometimes I have to do that; I haven't enough time to bring them back with asparagus juice. I haven't enough time to bring them back with chlorophyll. Some people come here as a last resort when they should have come here first. Many of the cases who have come to me had already made reservations on the other side. It is not always possible to help those who have waited too long before seeking help.

Animal Vibrations Are Highest

When we look to the chemical elements, we find we need the vibration. The highest vibration in phosphorous is found in the egg yolk. Also, it is found in raw goat milk. The vibratory rate, the animal magnetism, the animal fluid that has to do with a vibratory rate in the milk is lost within three hours after the goat is milked. I have seen raw goat milk pull people back from the dead.

Goat Milk Can Perform Wonders

I had a man from Seattle here who was six foot three and weighed only 65 pounds. They couldn't find much wrong with him, but he continued to lose weight. He said to me, "Doctor, I came down here because they didn't know what to do with me. What shall I do? I'll do anything you say." I told him that I wanted him to milk the goat and sit down and drink it immediately. Make friends with the goat, get the animal energies directly from the goat. In less than four months, he gained forty pounds. You could hardly believe it. In six months he gained 50 pounds. When this man went home he had a trailer and in the trailer he had a goat. So, you see why I call it "the wonder milk."

Mahatma Gandhi has been my ideal in life; I feel responsible a good deal for adding something nice to his life by advising him to use goat's milk. He fasted as much as 21 days in order to get a law passed so that the British government would not oppress his people. He fasted so much that he couldn't come back to good health. He was trying to do it on nuts and seeds. So, I suggested he use goat milk. Dr. Faulkner and I wrote to him 45 years ago and discovered that he had added goat milk to his diet, and he recovered his health remarkably well to the extent, that when he traveled, a goat was always taken with him, even on a voyage to England.

Iron: the "Frisky Horse" Element

The one element which attracts oxygen from the air, and without which we cannot exist, is iron. Iron and oxygen are the two "frisky horses" that work in the body. When you have enough iron, you draw oxygen out of the air; otherwise, you don't get enough oxygen and you can breathe and breathe and even take breathing lessons from now to eternity and it will never do any good unless you have sufficient iron in your body. Iron will keep you from becoming anemic. When a person gets tired, it is usually an indication of lack of iron in the body. It is also needed in the metabolism; the activity of the body is dependent upon iron.

There is no iron in white sugar or white pastry flour. These do not have the materials to build a good body. The best iron sources are black cherries, greens and chlorophyll. Also, it is high in blackstrap molasses.

Fluorine: the "Anti-Resistant" Element

Fluorine is called the "resistance" element. Wouldn't you like to resist disease? I'm talking about flu, colds, fevers, bronchial troubles. The newspapers tell us that those who are susceptible to the flu should get shots. I say you do not have enough fluorine. If you do not have enough fluorine, you cannot resist disease. Fluorine is a very unstable gas. Whenever heat is applied, it is destroyed. It separates and is gone. Cooking destroys fluorine in foods. The anti-resistant element is needed to build hardness to our teeth, hardness in our bones. It is also called the beauty element.

We find the highest source in fluorine is the black bass. But, who is going to eat raw black bass to get fluorine? Yes, the Chinese and Japanese eat a great deal of raw fish and are the healthier for it. What do you think has the second highest amount of fluorine? Green quince does. But, who eats green, raw quince? No one except us! I have a good wife who knows how to put the green quince into a liquefier and add pineapple juice. You can also add raisins and some honey. A good supply of fluorine is in greens, tops of vegetables and in nuts and seeds.

The third highest source of fluorine is milk; but who has raw milk? So many people are using pasteurized milk, pasteurized cheeses; so, you don't get your share of fluorine. Goat milk contains ten times as much fluorine as cow milk. A goat can be considered as your best friend. But, when a person doesn't milk these goats properly,

there is a decrease in the amount of milk; sometimes a whole quart is lost. Goats are very sensitive. They live on vibrations and give off good vibrations. The goat can be the "family cow." The "land of milk and honey" in the Bible could very easily have referred to goat milk and raw honey.

Iodine: the "Metabolizer"

The next chemical element which is most important to your body is iodine. Yet, there is no such thing as taking one chemical element and living on it. They must be in combinations. There is no such thing as lacking just one chemical element. Chemical combinations occur in Nature so we can take these elements and whatever compatible elements go along with them.

I know foods, and we're going to learn how to make cocktails; we're going to learn how to make soups; learn to make combinations of foods that are high in sodium. Wouldn't it be nice to know how to make a sodium broth or a potassium broth when you need it? It would also be nice to make an iron cocktail, a nerve cocktail. There are many other elements we can talk about, especially the trace minerals. Iodine is called the metabolizer in the body and it is found in the thyroid gland mostly. We find iodine is difficult to get. Many times because you cook the foods that have iodine in them, the iodine is lost because it is soluble. That is why it is found mostly in the ocean. Water that goes through the mountains or through the valleys ends up in the sea. Turn to the sea for your iodine.

If you are lacking in iodine, it is generally a fact that you don't care for people, you get angry at people, you get mean, irritable; you just want to be alone. Sometimes, if you sit in a room, the doors and windows must be opened or you develop phobias. You find you cannot go up in an elevator; you're squeamish, your hair gets dry, your skin gets dry, nails can get dry, your tongue is dry; you find it can cause constipation. Iodine is necessary when we face many emotional troubles; overworking mentally, a job is too much for you. You're burning out iodine constantly and this is necessary to your body.

Iodine can be found in the egg yolk. Egg yolk has more of the chemical elements than any other food. It is a whole food. It is capable of building a chicken. With the loss of iodine, we can produce goiters, growths. Many of the people of India have goiters. There are a number of people from Switzerland who, because of the high mountains, suffer from goiters. The foods containing iodine is put in the water to keep them from getting goiters. There isn't a trace of goiters in Japan. They use sea food, seaweed. They have over 500 seaweed varieties from which they make candy, soup, milk and other products. You must learn to use Nova Scotia dulse leaves;

soak them and place in your liquefier to obtain some wonderful results. Iodine is a most necessary element.

An actress on the New York stage, became one of the highest paid movie actresses. She stole $4.50 from one of the department stores in New York. Why should she steal? This is a mania — kleptomania. It is from a lack of iodine. It is a physical deficiency and this is why mental and physical doctors have to work together. There is also a mental and spiritual body working together.

Goiters: A Case of Emotions

Let me relate to you another case I had. I was called to San Francisco to see a young girl, 18 years old, with a large goiter. I questioned her regarding this goiter and discovered that she had had it for approximately 6 months and had remained in her room for that length of time. She told me her mother had insisted she drop her boyfriend or she must remain in her room. This was her punishment. While confined, she developed a goiter. Her mother expressed herself by telling me that she would rather the girl be dead than go back to her boyfriend. I told the mother she was doing a good job. However, about three weeks later the mother requested that I come and see her daughter again. I immediately suggested to the girl that she return to her boyfriend. She told me that because of the growth on her neck the boyfriend would not take her back. I contacted the boyfriend, told him from the standpoint of a doctor about her emotional problems and that he should go back with her. He told me that he was now going with someone else. I urged him to go with the two girls, but to definitely return to the first girl for a while. He finally agreed to do this.

He went back to his first girlfriend and would you believe that in six month's time that the girl's goiter disappeared? If the problem comes chemically, it goes out

chemically. If it comes in emotionally, it will also go out emotionally. These two people are now married. They have two children. They are the most beautiful children I have ever seen. This is one marriage that I feel will have a 100% chance of survival.

Emotional Disturbances Relate to the Thyroid

Emotional problems are what causes trouble with the thyroid gland. Don't move into emotional disturbances. Get out of them. Solomon once said, "With all thy getting, get thee understanding." But we have a person who comes along and tells you you're not understanding him too well. Then we need to accept him anyway to have a peace that "passeth all understanding." I tell you that we don't have to love what people do but we have to love them.

Love Can Heal Our Spiritually Anemic World

You must have love, you must love; this is a purity concept. St. Paul said that though we speak with the tongues of angels, but have not love, it's only clanging brass. He said you could be burned at the stake, but if you aren't burned for love, it counts for nothing. He said you can give to charity, but if you don't do it with love, it counts for nothing.

So, I must say to you in putting the chemical story together, that you recognize you are going to fill your body with love, earthly thoughts, heavenly thoughts, sunshine and moonlight. You've been built in the image of God and God travels through so much in life. Don't stop at foods and a glass of carrot juice. Let's encompass the whole spectrum of life.

This old world is spiritually anemic today. It needs love.

Fasting brings a healing crisis much more quickly. The crisis can occur either during the fast or even many months after. Crises develop much faster in the summer than in winter. There are times we need more than one crisis to have a complete body elimination. They may develop one after the other; first in the bronchial tubes, then later in the bowel, then still later in the knees or wherever our problems might have settled.

It is a very interesting thing to watch this body reverse its process of healing, picking up first the problem you had several years ago, then the one you had five or six years ago, and if you continue with proper living habits, even retracing troubles as far back as ten or fifteen years. Again, it shows the wonderful working of the body, and proves that the body works according to law. Without a doubt, we earn the diseases we have, but the wonderful part is that we may also earn our way back to health.

Chapter 4

The physician in your pantry

Aim for the Highest Kingdom

There is some place that we have to draw on for the good of our health. I think you're all aware of the fact that there is the positive and the negative...there's male, there's female. Everything is two in life. Everything is double and we've gotten to the place where it's either Yea Yea or Nay Nay. It's either the place where we are going to go on the right track or we're not. We have to make decisions in life and these decisions are not easy, especially so when we have to give up anything. Most people have the idea that to give up something, we are losing it. But you see...there is nothing lost in God's kingdom. There are no vacuums in God's kingdom. There's no such thing as a nothingness in God's kingdom. There is always something there, and there's no reason why we couldn't pick the higher things and the better things at all times. In the Bible, the people perish for lack of knowledge. Well,... get this knowledge, find out what it is, what to do. Find a path for yourself. It is very, very important.

Depletion and Pollution of Mother Earth

For lack of knowledge, wisdom and guidance, we find that Mother Earth has been depleted, polluted and prostituted. We find that she has gotten to the place where the natural resources are being taken away to such an extent that we are becoming short of many things.

For instance, the topsoil in the Midwest used to be about 80 inches deep when the pioneers first broke the sod there. Now the government tells us that the topsoil is less than six inches, on an average, in the United States. Topsoil is very important. You can't live without topsoil. Our gardens, flowers, fruits, vegetables, everything grows according to the topsoil. Topsoil is made through a natural cycle of life. It's made with leaves, debris...everything that had life must return to the soil again. The secret of the Wheel of Health is the fact that everything that dies goes back to the dust of the earth. We find out that we are always looking forward to perfection. The perfection of the soil is built on the forest floor, where moisture, decay and worms create natural topsoil. Topsoil is made rich in nitrogen from the castings from the worms. This is where the droppings from the birds fall. This is where the feathers drop. This is where insects, birds, animals and microorganisms live and die. This is where the Wheel of Health starts...man begins right there.

When I say "man begins," I mean man is also an organism in the living and/or dying process. To have this life, you have to take care of it. This body is a loaned instrument. It's a very temporary thing, and it's here for maybe a hundred years, maybe two hundred years. It's possible that it could be here 300 years...did you know that? But it depends entirely on what you do with it , and if you find yourself in this Wheel of Health, you can do some lovely things for yourself. You should study the soil a little bit. You're related to the soil. You're related to all the chemical elements that are in the soil.

By the way, your best friends are the worms, in this soil. I don't know whether you know that or not, but worms aerate the soil. They digest leaves and run them through their bodies and pass out castings you have to pay $2.00 a pound for in a nursery, because it's the richest soil you can get. Plant life grows from the castings from worms better than anything else. But you know the criterion that we have of coming back to Nature and finding out what Nature has for us, the storehouse of good health and everything, is to see that each of these worms is a migrator. They move around to find their food. Worms can't live in soil laced with powerful artificial fertilizers. They go...they migrate.

We do the same thing. We try to survive...we dwindle...we suffer disease...our body takes its food, water and air and uses it, but we find out that we cannot make a good body out of polluted materials. You can't make a good body out of foods grown on artificial fertilizer. Nature doesn't like these things. There are many people today who go right into organic gardening and because they don't use any sprays or artificial fertilizer, they think it's perfectly all right. But truly, it takes ten to fifteen years to get the effect of artificial fertilizer out of the soil. People have gone to various parts of the country, trying to develop organic gardens or farms, and we find they've been growing crops on soil that still has artificial fertilizers and sprays in that soil. They get the effects of these for ten years after the previous owners have stopped using them.

Drugs Are A Fatal Enemy

Here we are criticizing how the soil is taken care of; yet, when drugs are taken into the human body, they do not allow for perfect tissue to rejuvenate or grow. Like inorganic chemicals in the soil, drugs pollute the body. The cure is not in the drug. We fight infection; we fight germ life; we fight bugs; we fight these and many other things. We're in a life of fighting. We don't know how to live in a world of growing and bringing in the good things in life.

Deficiencies Encourage Disease

Dr. William Albrecht, former head of the Department of Agriculture at the University of Missouri, has experimented with the various soils and what they could do. If you take a calf and feed it alfalfa grown on depleted soils the calf could end up with a sagging spine, bad teeth and digestion problems. You could almost change this calf into a mutant creature just by cutting out certain elements in the soil.

One of the greatest experiments I know of was where Dr. Albrecht took two pots of soil and put in two sister plants. In one of the pots, Dr. Albrecht removed as much calcium from the soil as he could. Then he took out iron, and let these two plants grow, side by side. In the second soil he made sure all the necessary calcium was there, the nitrogen, potassium, phosphorus, iodine, all the essential elements we've been describing. He made sure the biochemical balance was in the soil.

Both plants grew, and as they grew they entwined with one another. The one growing in the soil without essential minerals, without iron, without calcium and with as little magnesium as possible, was a very light green. It was so anemic looking in the leaves that you could almost look through it. On the healthy plant that had the right minerals, the iron, calcium, silicon and so forth, the foliage was a deep, dark green. This green was entirely different than the "anemic" green of the other plant. And yet the two plants grew. But as they grew, the anemic plant began to show bugs, germ life, viruses and bacteria, and the funny part of it was that none of the bacteria and germ life went over to the dark green healthy plant growing in the soil containing all the right mineral elements.

I asked Dr. Albrecht about this. I said, "This is peculiar. Look at all the germ life that just stays with that light green plant in spite of the fact that it's entwined and touching the dark green plant. You know, I just wonder why the pests don't go on the plant that has all the rich green leaves." He said, "You know, bugs and bacteria are Nature's undertakers. They have to take care of that which is not healthy, that which is degenerating, that which is going back to the earth again. Bug life and bacteria bring it back to the earth. There's a disintegrating process when a plant is dying, and we have to have bugs to break it down and return it to the earth."

And he said, "Doctor, disease prays on an undernourished plant." The simplicty and wisdom of this statement have been so striking to me that I have never forgotten it. We find that it applies equally well to people. The nourishment has to be there. This is what we are talking about. We have to have the right elements...we have to have the biochemical material to work with. Otherwise, disease comes in, when we have a chemically depleted organ in the body. That's when germ life comes in.

Ninety percent of all people have tubercular germs in the throat but that doesn't mean that they have tuberculosis. The germs are ready, willing and able to come in and do their job if we allow our bodies to break down.

When we have toxic settlements in our tissues we attract germlife too. We find out they live on that kind of material. When we talk about using garlic for worms, we find out they don't like that garlic environment...so we can use garlic to get rid of intestinal worms. But we also have to start living correctly so we don't attract them again.

The Body Must be Chemically Balanced

So what we need is life. I would rather talk about life more abundant than I would about health, because we're made of more than biochemical elements. We have to understand, too, that we may need to treat the lung structure with more than chlorine, sodium and iron.

We have what we call a chest brain in the medulla of the brain, and this medulla has to be fed before we can breathe properly. That's one reason people come to the Ranch. They're cold, depleted and run down; they can't breathe well, haven't any energy, circulation is poor, memory is getting bad. We have to feed this brain before the lungs can work right, before the heart can work right; the chest brain is very important to take care of. This chest brain is built with the higher evolved foods of animal origin. It is very difficult it get it through the vegetarian foods.

I'm not saying that the vegetarian life is not good, but we've got to consider that there's a difference between plant calcium and the calcium in animal tissue. There's a difference between types of phosphorus, even depending on where it is used in the same body. The brain needs the highest evolved phosphorus from animal products, the phosphorus with the highest vibratory rate. We find the vibratory rate of animal food is entirely different than the vibratory rate of the vegetarian food. Some people can get by on the vegetarian food, but not all.

The average person has to have two percent phosphorus every day in his diet, but if you're a mental worker, you need five percent. And if you don't have five percent and you use your mind a great deal, you will deplete your brain. Then you'll find out you can't breathe well; you won't have enough power in the chest to breathe in all the oxygen you should have; and it all comes from a mental and nerve standpoint, a nerve depletion.

This is why I feel that unless you get the greater part of life put together, it's hard to be a vegetarian. It's hard to be a vegetarian where lovely fruits don't grow and you can't get ripe fruit right from the tree the moment it should be picked. The supermarket vegetables are not what they should be and fruits aren't either. You don't know how long it's been since they were picked and shipped. You don't know how long they've been in the bin. You're taking a dying food if you aren't picking it right from the tree or taking the vegetables from the ground and eating them when they are fresh and ripe.

We have to consider many things to be a vegetarian, especially if you're doing this day in and day out. If you did it once in a while, probably the good things that you would do would overcome those things that are not right. But how can anyone get these perfect vegetables and fruit? I saw an article one time that the people of Boston have never tasted a ripe blackberry. Many in Los Angeles have not tasted tree or bush ripened fruit either. A lot of people don't know what it is to pick a raspberry right off the vine or a strawberry from the plant or an apple from a tree. When you are sick, when you are depleted, when you haven't everything you need in the body, this is the time when you have to get closer to Nature because Nature is the storehouse for your regeneration.

The Brain: Foremost in Importance

The Number One to think about is that the brain itself is the first thing to take care of because when we haven't got the nerve supply then nothing else works well in the body. Hair won't grow unless the nerves are good. You cannot breathe unless the nerves are good. You cannot digest; you cannot secrete hydrochloric acid unless the nerves are right.

And I might tell you, too, that the sexual system works hand in hand with this nerve supply. The foods that feed the sexual system and the brain and the nervous system are practically the same. Sexual adjustment is necessary because of sexual excess, sexual depletion. We find the sex glands and all other glands must be taken care of, and they are also fed through good thinking, good companionship as much as anything else. The physical feeding can be done through lovely foods—natural, pure and whole foods.

When we get into some of the lovely remedies, we'll see when vitamin E is necessary. We'll see that we've been going through life and have thrown ourselves into a drug approach of handling the change of life for women. They claim that a high percentage of the hysterectomies performed on women are unnecessary. It's hard to believe that we build up to this condition becuase we don't live correctly. Vitamin E is necessary. It's the most prolific vitamin we have to keep the sexual system right, not so that it can work or overwork and do as you please with it because after all, this is meant to be under control too. The sexual energy can be channeled into your spiritual philosophy to be transmuted and to be used more for the mental and spiritual activity that you would like to do in life. But without a good sexual system, you cannot repair and rebuild well. Vitamin E works well with the nervous system.

I bring this out as one of the first things. They say you are as young as your glands. Flabby tissue many times is just a sign that the gland system is depleted, and I'm stressing this because it's important to know.

There's a building side of this, too. First, take care of the brain, the nerves and the glandular system. Nerve force is so important. Nerve force, as I mentioned before, is built up through happiness and joy and by being in the right place and seeking the nicer things in life. This joy and happiness is an electrical thing that works in the body, and you can deplete it by throwing it away. It can be thrown away sexually, too, or you can throw your life away through hate and disturbances. So many people waste their time, waste their energy, living that kind of life. Then, after they've thrown away their life through hate, fears, dissension, jealousy, they come to me and I have to feed back the chemical elements. But there is a time when you have to come to the place in your life where you've got to stop breaking down.

Vegetarianism Is A Way of Life

Vegetarianism is not just a matter of giving up meat. It's a way of life. And this idea that you can just give up meat and not kill animals, but still kill other people with your thinking misses the point.

I say vegetarianism is a way of life because we need to realize it's a hard way to follow. When you've given up certain things, then take up something else, be sure you're going to take it up with enough wisdom to keep yourself well. My worst cases have been vegetarians that don't take care of themselves and don't really know what to do for themselves. I hate to tell you that, but they're easy to take care of if they'll move just a little bit.

Your Brain Directs the Play

We have a directing force in the mind and this directing force comes from the brain to make sure everything works in the body. Diabetes starts in the brain. Wow...that's a hard thing to tell you! We find that epilepsy starts in the brain. High blood pressure starts in the brain. We've got to make sure that that directing force can go to every organ in the body. When you've got cold hands and cold feet the directing force isn't getting the blood down into the feet and the hands and the different parts of your body.

Executive Level: Bony and Muscular Department

Then, of course, we have the executive department in the bones and the muscle structure that follows the orders of the brain, the chief director. And then we have a heating department and a place where all the material is put into fuel to keep you going. Yes, without heat in the body you cannot be well, so we find a good deal of this comes in the brain and the nervous system.

Remedies Headline the Cast

The chemical balance of the body is important. Body chemistry works with good thinking. It works with God, truth, joy, happiness. These are all things that we have to put together. There's a substance that we have to draw on in all of life whether it be from the Father in heaven, the mother in the earth, whether it be the brother in the sun or the sister in the moon . . . do you understand that? These are effects that come, positive and negative, cold and hot, light and dark. We need to know how to draw on all of these—they're all good.

Every food is a remedy, and researchers recently discovered that an extract called "raytheon" from black horseradish cleans up the gall bladder and the liver better than anything else. They just found it out. It was there for a long, long time, however. We use things such as digitalis for the heart that comes from an herb. We have all kinds of herbal derivatives in the pharmaceutical field, but we find out these extracts have to work very harshly in order for them to be scientifically approved.

We don't take the time to gradually "wash" the old material out and to wash in the good, new material. We don't want to take a year. Some of you have arrived at the place where you've got to do something immediately. So the approach is usually this: we go to whatever can work immediately—overnight, if possible. You don't want to fix a cold by preventing a cold in the future. You don't want to get into preventive medicine so that you can be free of sickness and troubles. We tend to wait until it has to be cured, so we're always running for a remedy.

The remedies that I have to share with you aren't worth two cents unless you live correctly. They're for people who want to live correctly and want to do the right thing. These remedies will not come in fast enough for me to say "We'll just take your blood pressure down with one cup of Black Cohosh tea." We can't do that. You've got to start living correctly and we must go back and take care of things we didn't do before making up for biochemical shortages.

Suffering the Sins of the Flesh

I don't like to tell you this, but we suffer the sins of our flesh. You've got to go back and pay for what you didn't do right in the first place. Some of you would like to call it "Karma." Some of you would like to see it in a different light. I can talk Karma, too. I've got it to live out myself. I have a few sins of my flesh that have to be worked out. In fact, I still think there's a little Danish pastry in my left shoulder. And when it comes out, it doesn't come out as nice as it went in! To review my pains and to review my memories of things I haven't done right in the first place isn't a very pleasant thing.

Your favorite flavor ice cream tastes wonderful going down, but when it comes out, it doesn't feel so good. Because it comes out in the form of a crisis, and we're in this reversal process often. This is one of the nicest things I can tell you..you can reverse your troubles. If you can still wait, you find out through right living you can make a change for the better. However, we've got to sometimes be strict about it and the sicker you are the more strict you have to be.

Fruits Have Remedial Secrets

Every food has some effect on the body.

Persimmons are high in sodium and potassium and can be used all year round. Why just have them for the wintertime? We are very fortunate at the Ranch that we can have nice fresh fruits nearly all year round. But we have dried persimmons, too. Do you know how to dry persimmons? You should know. You should know a survival program to take care of yourself all year round. I learned from a Japanese friend that we could dip a persimmon is hot water, take off that skin (which is very bitter, but very high in potassium) and hang the persimmon up to dry on a string. Run a toothpick through the top of the persimmon and tie a string to it. And, if you want to taste the most wonderful substitute for candy, try dried persimmons. The outside turns completely white, and there isn't any powdered sugar sweeter than the natural sugar on the outside of a dried persimmon.

Pomegranates have their effect, too. They're one of the best things to use for genito-urinary problems, kidney troubles, bladder problems.

Apples contain pectin that's wonderful for stopping diarrhea in most instances. Scraped apple can be used many times to regulate the bowel. Apples can be used in an elimination diet. The pectin in apples is also wonderful for arthritis. Malic acid found in apples is also a health booster.

Grapes have cream of tartar that is good for catarrhal conditions. How do you suppose manufacturers get cream of tartar? I've been told they scrape it from the inside of the wine barrels, when you take cream of tartar, it's the greatest thing for breaking down catarrhal conditions.

Cherries have tartaric acid that is beneficial to the liver, as is malic acid.

Apricots are rich in cobalt for blood building. The apricot has about the same amount of water as the human body. Its natural cobalt is wonderful for anemic conditions. A constipated bowel may be regulated by the gentle effect of its laxative properties. It is high is potassium, sodium, magnesium.

Papayas are an excellent digestion aid.

Peelings of certain foods have remedial values. You can use apple peelings for kidney trouble.

Remedial Herbal Teas

You can use peach leaf tea for bladder troubles. You use Disturtian which is high in potassium for the muscle structure. You can use hibiscus flowers or pineapple guava flowers in your salad; you can use lemon grass tea as a stomachic. You can use lemongrass tea and hibiscus to make one of the finest teas for cleaning out the intestinal tract. Red clover tea is great for its blood cleansing ability, blood purifying ability. Do you know these things? This knowledge could save your life. It could make your life a much better one. We find that Hawthorn berry tea is used for strengthening the heart. It's one of the best teas we have for stimulating better circulation in the body. Comfrey and fenugreek tea is an effective combination for draining the catarrh settled in the lungs. Dandelion tea cleanses the liver.

Your Liver Is the Detoxifier

The liver is an iron organ...it needs a lot of iron. Cherry juice (especially black cherry juice) is wonderful for the liver because it's high in iron. The liver must attract oxygen for purification. Your liver is the body's detoxifier. Twenty-five percent of all the blood in your body right now is in your liver. That much blood is in your liver because it is taking out all the toxins, all the garbage your body doesn't need. The liver concentrates it and sends it out in bile, and the bile is heavy and thick and irritable (like some people's mental attitude) but when it touches that intestinal tract, it incites a bowel movement. It's that strong. It's there to stimulate movement. Your body wants to get rid of it, so it starts a peristalic action and things are on their way; but if your liver is not taking out this bile, you don't have good elimination. Bowel movements are dependant upon that liver. Your bowel movements are dependant upon the chemical elements that the liver needs to be in good health.

Variety's Case Is Strong

The liver is as much an iron organ as the stomach is a sodium organ. The stomach needs whey; it needs celery; it needs this variety of sodium foods. It needs ripe fruit; it needs sun fruits because fruits have been taken care of and prepared by the sodium star, the sun. We find out that every organ needs this variety. That's why I teach variety. You can't just have apricots. I don't know any food that's a perfect food. We have to have this variety from vegetables to fruits to seeds, and we go right through the whole story. I'd rather you would stay on this variety idea. I don't want to be responsible for you if you just want to go on peanuts and grapefruit. Your body can only mold from what it is...what it eats and what it doesn't eat.

Soils Make a Tremendous Difference

I don't have to worry about you if you take an apple from Oregon and you take some celery from Salt Lake Valley where there's high sodium. Utah celery is very high in sodium. In fact, it has 30 percent more sodium than celery grown any other place. So if you want a high sodium food, you may have to even think of the soil that it's been grown in. That's why we're made of the dust of the whole earth, not our own backyard, and it's nice to get a variety of foods from a variety of soils, a variety of vegetables, a variety of fruits. Then I'm not going to worry about you because we find out we have a God-given force within us just the same as parsley that can reach out with the roots and take iron, as much as it wants if it's in that soil. Our body can take all the calcium it needs if it is there in our foods. It will take all the iron it needs, but you have to first feed the iron to that body. You have to feed calcium to the body. Probably you understand that Nature cures, but she needs an opportunity. Now you see, too, that God can only do for you what he can do through you. Sometimes the spiritual life has a physical foundation as well as a spiritual foundation. It's just as divine to live righteously physically as it is spiritually. I mean they both work together. So now we're reaching out for the remedies that we can use in various parts of the body.

Nourish Hair from Within

One of the best elements for the hair is silicon. We need silicon. Oh yes, we need pantothenic acid...we need so many things. We need Vitamin E; we need a good nervous system; we need even a good sexual system. They have found today that a man who becomes bald, as a rule, has broken down the male hormones in his body and a woman who becomes bald still doesn't have the male hormones in her body. Today, we're all trying to build up our hair with chemical elements when the glandular system is responsible. This can be an inherent trait.

Women who have excessive hair on their upper lips and too heavily on the arms because they have too much of the male hormones in their body. There are men who don't have any whiskers and they have too much female hormones in the body. The hormones have to be balanced. This can be balanced with the proper amount of seed life, Vitamin E and so forth; but the hair itself is built with the same elements required by the system because we need silicon in the body for both. Alfalfa is one of your highest foods in silicon, and I have found that the hair will respond best to alfalfa. But you must have that blood in the head.

We use the slanting board to get that extra blood back in the head; but of course, if that blood is made of coffee and donuts, then all the blood you get to the brain isn't going to develop good hair. Alfalfa, rice polishings, rice bran syrup—these are wonderful foods. They're remedies. We're going to hit hard on the very part of our body we know is depleted and broken down.

Eyes: Brain and Body Messengers

A surprising number of people have cysts in the eyes; many of them have sties, discharges, signs of inflammation. We are lacking Vitamin A. We are lacking in potassium. We are probably bringing in too much of the toxic materials and we need to have a good liver cleanser.

Every organ in our body is connected with every other organ, and no remedy should go into your body to treat only one organ without treating the whole body along with it. This is why remedies so often fail; because we don't take care of the whole body. You cannot have good eyes without a good liver. You can't have good eyes without a good digestion. So this total body concept of taking care of the total body is necessary. Nowadays, everyone is talking about the wholistic viewpoint. They're talking about *total* health. Why should we go through life and have two good bowel movements a day and no love in our hearts? I mean why shouldn't we have the total viewpoint, the total good that our body needs? If you don't like my exaggerations, I hope you're awakened with them because I'm trying to show you that this life is not all physical. It's just not all chemical. You have to put the whole thing together.

When eyes have these discharges, let's get a lot of Vitamin A in there, let's get on some carrot juice and other juices, let's clean up the liver; let's make sure the bowel is in good order. Then if you want to use something for the eyes when you have these discharges, use linseed oil. Just a drop of this in the eye. But it must be the sanitary king. You can't go down to a paint store and get it. You should get it in a drugstore or a health food store; put a drop in the center of your eye near the nose and the eye will pick it up. It's the greatest thing for "smog eyes"

that I can share with you. It helps that inflammation. Warm milk packs also help the eyes.

There are some people who don't realize that the eyes are an extension of the brain. When we break down the brain and the nervous system, the eyes become depleted right along with them because when you break down the nervous system in one part of your body, the whole nervous system is going along with it. That's why the eyes are one of the greatest barometers among all organs to tell you when your body is going downhill. When your vision is going, then your body is going along too. Something to think about, isn't it? So, if you want to feed the eye structure and it's depleted from a nerve standpoint, it is time you feed the brain and the nervous system. You need to go to the brain and nerve foods.

"Fix" The Brain and Nervous System First

Here we come to brain and nerve foods. The egg yolk is one of the finest nerve foods. Raw goat milk is another food that builds the brain and the nervous system. I've seen the near dead come back to life again with just the brain and nerve foods to bring them back. We need the lecithin foods, iron foods, sulphur foods, foods high in RNA such as Brewer's yeast, sardines, spirulina and chlorella.

When we look to these remedies in all parts of the body, always think of that brain and nervous system first, and remember the eyes are extensions of the brain.

Sinus Trouble Means Catarrhal Conditions

Now we turn to the nasal areas. We've got sinus troubles. "Oh, I've got this drippy nose! What am I going to do?" Listen, it will never be dry until the rest of your body gets well. If you don't digest starches and sugars well with the pancreas and if the pancreas isn't well to start with, that undigested starch will make cattarrh — a runny nose. Why treat your runny nose before we take care of the rest of the body? But in the meantime. . .you'd like a remedy. In the meantime you'd like to have something to take care of that local condition.

Well. . .I'll tell you what, the confidence breath is what I suggest here. Find a place where you can walk seven long strides in one direction, inside or outside. Quick breathing is what it takes. Three sharp inhalations (one with each step) and a slow exhalation in two steps helps the sinuses. Repeat for two minutes or more, holding a handkerchief if necessary. We find out here, too, that garlic oil capsules help to get rid of catarrhal conditions. I used to take patients for walks. and we'd come out and walk in the hills and we'd take some of the sage, rub it in the hands, then breathe it into the nostrils to stimulate the mucous membranes in the nose, the sinuses. Or, we'd take bay leaves and do the same thing; it's stronger, and you'll find out it incites the activity much better. We even used a liquid chlorophyll nasal douche that you can just inhale inside the nose. The same thing can be done with salt and water. Still further, if you want to make those mucous membranes really move, just get a little powdered horseradish, put it on your tongue and take a deep breath. The top of your head will feel like it's going to come right off! Horseradish is really something to make the sinuses move.

Get your proper teas (herb); stop using a lot of wheat (flour products) and oatmeal; use grains like cornmeal, millet and rice that don't produce catarrh. Try to get the whole body in good order.

Tooth and Gum Decay Are Danger Signs

When it comes to the mouth, many people have pyorrhea which is a lot of dead tissue in the gum structures. Let's put in some papaya tablets on each side of the mouth. This breaks down the old material...the old gum material. You can take a handful of papaya tablets and put them on a lamb chop at night and the lamb chop will be practically gone in the morning! Papaya digests dead meat or dead protein, so if you want to get rid of that dead protein that has developed with pyorrhea, just use papaya tablets on each side of the mouth for 10 minutes twice a day then wash the mouth out with a liquid chlorophyll afterwards if you wish. A sore throat also responds wonderfully to a liquid chlorophyll.

Know Your Onion Packs

When we have colds of the chest, onion packs are the best to put on. Chop up the onions really fine; warm them in the skillet; put them in a linen bag. Then place it on the chest, put another dry towel over it and leave it there all night long. You can do the same thing for congestion of the lymphatic glands in the neck.

Ask for Nature's Remedies

I have a book out called *Nature Has A Remedy* that gives all the remedies I've discovered the past fifty years. They're wonderful, but I will admit they aren't worth two cents if you don't live right. It's no use to give you something wonderful for your kidneys and then have you go home and live on beer and pretzels. I can't do any good in these cases; I don't want my remedies wasted in that kind of hands. They just won't do any good under wrong living conditions, and that's why much of this health work has been claimed to be a "fad" thing. It's because it does

not work on those kinds of people. This works if you use it properly, but it belongs in good hands.;

A Supreme Heart Remedy

What we call the Supreme Heart Remedy is made from whole wheat. We grind up fresh whole wheat and take half a cup of fresh ground flour or meal and add it to a cup-and-a-half of hot water in a hot thermos bottle — a wide-mouthed thermos bottle, preheated with boiling water. Then we plug it up with the cork and we leave it all night long. The next morning it has been cooked under low heat and you find it's ready to eat the next morning.

In fact, a good deal of cooking can be done this way. You can grind beans, peas, cornmeal...nuts and if you want to, you can soak them in boiling water this way to make cereal. I am telling you a nice way to do things for yourself at home. You take this every morning for three months. We also use Vitamin E and liquid chlorophyll for heart trouble.

Foods Can Be Your Remedies

There are so many remedies among the wonderful foods and herbs God has created. I've included many of them in my books and they really aren't such secrets, but new ones keep turning up all the time. We should have remedies from our foods and make foods our remedies. Our foods can be our medicine and our medicine should be our food — that's what I'm trying to get across to you.

Bowel Management: Key to Health

I want you to realize that if the intestinal tract is not working right, let's change it. One of the nicest things I know for constipation and for irregularity, chronic, long term problems, is alfalfa tablets. Take four with each meal, crack each one and take them with a little water. This is not an overnight cure, but it will do the job over the long term. Alfalfa has many chemical nutrients, and its scrubbing action tones and strengthens the bowel for better peristaltic action.

There is some chlorophyll in the alfalfa tablet which helps to clean the bowel as you go along. It keeps it sweeter and cleaner and the chlorophyll feeds the beneficial bowel bacteria. Alfalfa tablets are the finest thing I know for all bowel troubles. They're good also for the liver because as you clean the bowel, you take a load off the liver. We use these tablets when we travel. When we go to Europe or to India, we take a bottle of those alfalfa tablets with us. Four tablets are equal to a salad and there are many places you can't get a salad. They come in very handy.

Acidophilus Culture...there's a great thing for changing the intestinal flora. If we have worms, the most effective solution is plain old garlic oil capsules and we find out that garlic is wonderful to cleanse the intestinal tract of pinworms in children. Giving them two or three garlic capsules three or four times daily for three days, then a good laxative, and you know...those worms want to get out of there. "What are you doing to me?" "You aren't giving me a pleasant place to live." So they leave! Very few things would choose to live around garlic. We had one man who went on a garlic diet for one week and what do you suppose he lost? Twenty-five friends!

Acidophilus culture is also wonderful for regaining the proper ratio of "friendly bacteria" in the intestinal tract. Antibiotics, among other things (even chocolate), destroy the acidophilus bacteria and allow the "unfriendly bacteria" to take over. This increases gas and putrefaction in the bowel, so we need to restore the "friendly bacteria" and get rid of the others.

Herb Teas Have Magical Properties

Sage tea...that's a great tea for the lung structure. And we find for the kidney structure you need to have Uva Ursi and cornsilk tea...just the plain old cornsilk at the end of the corncob. You see, the cornsilk was what transmitted light inside and brought all of the vital energies from the sunshine to each kernel in the corn cob. Did you know that? Each one of those little pieces of silk runs alongside a row of corn (kernels) on that cob. And this is what makes corn yellow, in spite of the fact that no sunlight reaches it. The sunshine is brought in through the tassel, the cornsilk. Each of those kernels is reached by the time the tassel has become brown. Cornsilk was used by the Indians for kidney trouble. We know it's very good for gravel, for breaking down stones in the body. Cornsilk is a wonderful kidney eliminant, so we should save it; we should put it away. We should keep a supply during the winter.

More Secrets You Should Know

We use slippery elm for a soothing effect and to get proper chemicalization into the bowel when we have ulcerations.

Beets are one of the finest foods and remedial vegetables that you can put into the body, very good for the liver and gall bladder. It's a laxative. All the natural laxatives seem to have beetroot in them because of its laxative effect. I have read about experiments in Switzerland showing that when beets have been given to laboratory rats with cancers, the cancer stops growing.

Reversal Process by Healing Crises

The body is constantly purifying itself, taking on the new and getting rid of the old. In doing this as you elevate your food life, get more live foods and get better chemicalized foods; your body molds to those foods. It molds to it and becomes stronger, so we go through what we call a "reversal process." This reversal process is just a matter of one "healing crisis" after another—an elimination process that takes place in which mucus is thrown out, catarrh containing the old acids that you don't want, toxic material that the body needs to get rid of.

Never stop a catarrhal discharge. Anytime you stop a catarrhal discharge you're on your way to a chronic disease, so *never* stop a discharge in your body. Instead, become clean so there are no more discharges. Become clean. We allow healing crises to take place until we are clean. It may take years for this to come about, but let us continue to do it until we are clean. This reversal process is more fully explained in my *Doctor-Patient Handbook* dealing with the healing crises and the reversal process.

Now these are not all my own ideas. You'll find out this is related to the work of John Harvey Kellogg, Dr. Tilden, Dr. Shelton. But, many of these men didn't know about the healing crisis. They called it an elimination process. But the oldtime homeopaths knew this very well. There are over 3,000 of them in one organization in Germany, they know if you want to really get well, you just burn out this old waste in the body and put in the new. and that's where this philosophy comes: in taking up the new...get rid of the old! "Cleanse and purify thyself and I'll exalt thee to the throne of power."

From Venous Congestion to Varicose Veins

They have found out just of late that a remedy from the plain old buckwheat called rutin can be used to take care of fragile veins when they break down. When we have venous congestion, we find the energy system of the body begins to break down. The power is not there; the brain energy is not there. Varicose veins set in when you have venous congestion, and we have to return that blood to the head. It's not getting back up from the extremities. Rutin helps, and slantboard exercises and barefoot walks in dewy early morning grass or sand are good for the circulation as well.

Begin Construction of a New Body

One of these days you'll realize as you take this work up, you'll realize that when you have cold feet, your brain isn't being fed with the proper amount of blood — the circulation is poor. It's time to build up this body. We have to work with the feet, the stomach and the whole body.

I have to get everyone who comes to me started doing the right things, living correctly. One lady was telling me recently how she made five pounds of chocolate fudge for her daughter, but her daughter refused to eat it because she had heard about what fudge would do the the body. Do you know what that mother did? She ate it all herself. Then, she came to me to be treated. So you see, I just follow people who eat fudge; I follow people who fudge. I follow people who are full of fudge.

Create a Magic Health Kitchen

If you really want to be well, you have to set up your perfect kitchen. Set up your life so that things are righted, at least nearer the perfect way. In the back of my little book *Creating a Magic Kitchen* we list all the natural foods, but you know there are a lot of foodless foods and I list them also, so you can know the difference, know the devil and can face him. You can spit in his eye because you know the right way to live, and I list them both — the right and the wrong, the good and the bad. It might be nice to get acquainted with these foods. Find out what a good menu is.

You can't be like the lady the other day who said, "I just can't keep my kids out of the donuts." And I said, "Well, where are the donuts?" She said, "They're in my pantry." I said, "They shouldn't be in there!" Have you got that idea? Clean up your kitchen and pantry and put the godly foods in there!

Robust Health Must be Earned

I don't like to promise anything to anyone because I feel that you really deserve what you're going to have in life if you work for it. If people are going to give it to you then you're looking to this world for an easy living. I don't think anything comes to anybody — free. I think you have to work for it. . .you really have to earn it.

You find that people who have money generally manage to keep it. Those who get it without working for it tend to lose it. I have the records of 47 people who have won the Irish Sweepstakes, and there are only 2 out of the 47 who really used the money properly. One of them paid off a $16,000 doctor bill to help his paralyzed child and invested some in a business so they could keep the child busy. There was a good purpose. Another man 70 years of age won it, and he said, "I'm going to put it in the bank; I don't need it because I've got my soil. I work every day and I'm in good health; I'll leave it to my kids."

But the other 45. . .I'm telling you, it was criminal to see what was done. "Well, I owe my friends a good time." So they went out and drank it up. Many of those 45 people died in drunkenness, died in disease, died in suicide. . .none of them seemed to be able to use the money wisely. The worst case I recall was that of a man from Pittsburgh, Pennsylvania, who received $125,000. He had always wanted to have a hotel. Not a bad idea, but in getting the hotel he didn't realize he had to have employees. He had to know how to run a hotel. Wtihout any experience running a hotel, he hired people. He made a large down payment on the hotel. He didn't pay it all because the government took one-half of his winnings. After one year's time this man went out and shot himself because he couldn't handle what he'd gotten into. He hadn't earned that position in life. He tried to have something that didn't belong to him. The man started with six cents. When he got $125,000, he had a good job and a moving van.

Another "winner" got the money and went out and spent it on a beautiful high powered sportscar. Four days later, he ran into a telephone pole and killed himself, going 125 miles an hour. I mean. . .what foolishness we can have.

We only keep what we earn, in health or anything else. I've earned the knowledge I've been sharing with you here. I have paid dearly for it. . .I have crawled for it. I've gone to the Sahara Desert. I have traveled to Germany walking in the Kneipp baths over there. I've been to Lourdes, France. I've visited the psychic surgeons. I've been with faith healers. I've talked to Sai Baba. . .I have been with the Masters of the Far East, as they are described. I know what Eskimos live on. I've been there. I know that in Africa one tribe lives on little else but milk and blood. They have perfect teeth at the age of 65. They don't live a long life, but they've got good health while they're alive.

I have never met a vegetarian who lived a very long life. This is a great disappointment in my life, because I believe in vegetarianism so much. I find that the meat-eaters have had as good health as the vegetarians. I don't believe that meat produces disease, but I do believe there is diseased meat. We have to be cautious of the meat used in the diet if it is used at all. So we get to the place now that I feel the body is the greatest thing we have. It can mold to any situation. It can mold to seeds and nuts. It can mold to grapefruit and peanuts and it can *get you by*, so to speak, but don't you want to see how much more there is to life than getting by?

A Good Life Lived Is Long Enough

This is the thing that I would like to bring out: It's more important, much more important, to be happy than to be well. It is much more important to be close to God than it is to be with the devil. It's much better to be close to the Garden of Eden than the drug store, closer to your garden than the supermarket. It's much more important to be close to natural food than the can-opener. All right. . .if you don't see this, you don't know the importance of life. A long life lived isn't always good enough, but a *good* life lived is always long enough.

In St. Louis a man got on the speaker's platform before a large audience and he said, "Today I'm 75 years old, and at the age of 16, I was in a wheelchair with arthritis. Tonight I don't have complete use of my hands, but five years ago I was able to get out of this wheelchair. Now I can walk. I'm not completely well, but I can tell you that at the age of 70, getting out of this wheelchair, that I'd been in most of my life was a tremendous thrill. I can even sign a check now. This is from following Dr. Jensen's teaching, I'm going to tell you something else...tomorrow for the first time in my life, I'm going to go to work!" Think of that! At the age of 75!

Nature's Health Highway

Maybe it's time for you to go to work; but you have to be well in order to work, don't you? This whole thing can be put together very beautifully. Just think now that life is made up of deficiencies. Take care of your deficiencies! Many of you are bankrupt in terms of health. You'll find out that you've overused..you've abused, but let's not go through life starving to death as we are because disease is definitely a form of starvation. Maybe your body has begun to degenerate a little. All I can tell you is...let's get on this thing! Stay close to God; stay close to Nature! Let's get away from the doctor's office and get out on Nature's highway. Find out where good health is. We're interested in building good health, not feeding disease. You've been going the wrong way long enough. It's time to get on the high road. You've been running after a cure until you're tired out—you're weary. Get in and start doing the right thing for yourself. Balance your day. Look to these nice foods because here is where the remedy is. Here is where your health is.

To Live Well, Use Seeds and Sprouts

High on the list of the finest foods to help us live well are seeds and sprouts, two items we should always have in our diet. There are times when it is impossible to get foods supplying the value of seeds and sprouts. That problem is overcome by learning how to sprout seeds: alfalfa, rice, oats and wheat, as well as many others. When it is difficult to get fresh raw salads, sprouts will take their place. Seed cereals, like millet seeds, are one of the finest cereals you can have. When you turn to seeds, you are getting "whole" food. They never lose their value. Wheat seeds taken from the Pyramids, and oat seeds from King Tut's tomb, 3,000 years old, grew when planted. Three thousand years did not destroy the life in them. As long as we keep seeds intact, all the nutritional material remains perfect. A tree grows from the seed: its trunk, bark, leaves are all represented in that seed—and, though the tree may warp or even eventually die, all that it ever was came from the seed.

In much the same way, taking seeds into our bodies is beneficial. They contain the elements we need for the digestive system, the liver, glands, nerves— everything. Wonderful food, seeds! The sesame seed, for example, is used in a variety of pleasantly palatable ways. The following is an excellent seed drink:

To 1/2 cup of sesame seeds in your liquefier, add 1-1/2 cup of water. Blend for a few minutes then strain off the hulls through a couple of layers of cheesecloth. This, in itself, is a marvelous drink, but you can elaborate upon it almost without end. You can add dates, soymilk or goat's milk; if you want flavoring, try a banana, maple syrup or carob.

Sesame seed is rich in calcium, and there is no better substitute for milk, if for any reason you must leave milk out of your diet. It contains a natural oil that brings out the oil of your skin. The famous sesame seed oil made in Arabia, called Tahini, is much in demand by those with dry skin.

Chapter 5

Food facts for your body

Knowledge Is Our Greatest Wealth

There is one thing we should remember in life: that our search on this path of enlightenment should be guided by the fact that we need knowledge first. Knowledge is the most powerful thing in the world. The man who knows is the man who feels secure in what he is doing. Knowledge brings security. We find out knowledge is not everything, however. We find out knowledge is only in realizing how things are put together, how you can take them apart. Wisdom lies in putting knowledge to work in living, creating, developing, progressing.

Success Has Many Disguises

In years past a man came to my office with shaking hands and he said, "What do you think you can do with these hands?" I said, "I don't know. We'll see what we can do working with diet and with chiropractic adjustments over a period of three months." In three month's time his hands were as straight as a die. I thought this was wonderful. Well, he thought it was wonderful, too. In fact, he paid his bill and even gave me $25 extra. Of course, I felt very good.

I had almost forgotten this man when about six months later I saw in a newspaper: MR. NORWALK ROBS A BANK. Now, this was the man I had helped. I couldn't believe that I had assisted a man who would rob a bank! On the right hand column in the article it said that the secret of this man's success was due to a steady hand. There I was, almost a partner to that crime! I had helped him get that steady hand!

All Paths Should Lead Upward

It is difficult when you wake up to the fact that you are doing things in life that aren't of the best. What I teach in my spiritual lectures is to identify yourself with the highest things in life, the best things in life, because if you associate with the higher and the better things in life, what you are actually able to attain in life, you've got good helpers. A good helper may be just a good thought.

A good helper may be a friend; you find you've got to pick good friends. And you have to pick out good associates...you have to pick out good books to read. There are some people who are living on misinformation.

Some people are going to have to unlearn what they have learned, and this is the biggest problem that I face. A lot of people have gone to school, but of all the old men I have visited throughout the world — none of them ever went to school. If you want to live long, don't go to school because you might find that what you learn may cause you trouble, worry and loss of peace of mind. We have to go to school, but we may have to unlearn some of what we learned.

Wisdom Is A Child of Guidance

The second thing that comes out is wisdom, as I have mentioned. It's wisdom. You've got to be wise enough to know when to try something new and when to avoid it like the plague. In other words, wisdom must go along with knowledge. If you want to get out of your troubles, knowledge helps and wisdom helps and then you find you need guidance.

We all have a little heavenly angel on our shoulder. We all look upward in life and know of a higher level that we are attracted to. I was almost going to say a divine image. Something bigger than ourselves, something really worth doing or being. It's just the opposite end of the stick. You find out that if you can go that truth way and reach for those lovelier things in life that have been offered long before the body was formed, then you may attract a power that can guide you into a much better path than you're walking today. Now, some of you who are advanced souls will understand what I say. Some of you are not sure where you are yet — you're lost but you'll still find out there's a lot of guidance in life and there is a lot that you could depend upon beyond yourself. There's something more to life than meets the physical eye, if you know what I mean.

Humanity Deserves No Excuses

I hear this all the time..."People make mistakes"..."I'm only human." You need to get out of this business of making excuses. Obviously, at the human level we make mistakes. Yet, at the Divine level there are absolutely no mistakes. Truth is. God is. And what is, is and what ain't, ain't.

You'll have to find out what is good, but not from a personality standpoint. On the higher path we find that *what* is right is most important, not *who* is right. And this stands by in coming to Nature and coming to God in our work because we want to do the right thing. Some of you had better get on that path. Some of you are ailing. Some of you are sick. Some of you have attached yourself to negative influences for too long. Some of you have too much white flour in the right knee. And some of you have too much junk food in the stomach tissue and kidneys. You're going to have to take a new path.

I received a letter the other day saying, "I'm enclosing 25 cents. Please send me your cure for psoriasis." Well, I can't give out such information. You're not going to get a cure anywhere for twenty five cents. *You* earn it. You work for it. Another lady wrote in her letter, "Every time I take a drink of soda pop, I get stomach trouble. Tell me why." And did I tell her!

Could I come out and tell you that doctors make a living from ignorant people? Did you know that? I mean it's time for us to get wised up. There's enough wisdom around so you don't really have to have all the sickness we have today. It is said in this country that 92 percent of the people are sick. There's a reason for that.

Malnourishment from Processed Foods

A short time ago one of our U.S. Senators stood up in Congress and announced that something had to change in the processed breakfast cereal business "because there is more nourishment in the boxes than in what's inside them." That's a serious statement to make! He may be telling a little more truth than we'd like to admit because when we get our breakfast in a box, we get it devitalized, roasted, preserved, salted and sugared until it's no longer really a food. Do you think you're going to build a good body on that kind of food? It's an impossibility.

You Can't Get Well on Cream Puffs

Once a man in my sanitarium in Altadena, California had a systolic blood pressure of 210. I was taking the blood pressure every third or fourth day, and it stayed right at 210. At the end of the month when it was time for him to go home he said, "You know, I don't feel any better." I couldn't believe that my work hadn't done anything for him because I believed in my work.

Three months later I was walking in town and I passed by the bakery. A lady came running out of the bakery and she said, "Don't you have the Nature's Retreat up there in Altadena?" And I said, "Yes." She said, "Then you owe me $96.!" I said, "$96.?...How do you figure that?" She said, "A man from your place has been charging two dozen cream puffs every day for thirty days!" That was the same man I just mentioned. He was more cream puff than anything else; and you can't get well from anything on cream puffs! I paid the $96.

Emphysema Case Becomes A Tennis Champ

Another man, who came down to the Ranch from Washington some time ago, had emphysema. Doctors had given up on him and they told him he couldn't get well. It was supposed to be an incurable disease. It was the last degree—the last degree of having lung and bronchial disturbances, and he could hardly get his breath. Two years later, we went to Washington to lecture and do you know, this man was the Northwest tennis champ that year.

This is what happens. I mean, this is what can be done in changing this body, so I'm trying to get you to the place where you realize you can change your life. But you have to change it through foods, nutrition, right living and reaching for the very best there is in life...the very, very best there is in life.

Prevention Is the Answer

We don't cure disease. We're trying to develop new tissue in place of the old or to prevent disease if we don't have one. What a wonderful thing you can do to keep yourself well! But, try to talk to a person who feels good on a junk food diet and try to tell them they should change their diet and you're in trouble! The average person doesn't want to listen to this. The average person refuses to listen until he has become ill.

One Step Short of Dying

I feel that sometimes people have to be scared to take their health seriously. I told one man that he had to go into town to see another doctor because I couldn't help him. He wouldn't quit smoking. And do you know what the other doctor did? He came in and looked him over and said, "Do you smoke?" The man said, "Yes." The doctor said, "Well, you've got to quit." The man said, "I can't quit." The doctor said, "Then die!" and he walked out... Well, the kid quit. I mean, do we have to scare people to death before they will learn to live right?

A lady came to the Ranch one day and said, "I have bronchial troubles, and I'd like to get over them, but my doctor said I'd have to quit smoking. I suppose you'll do the same." I said, "Well, I certainly don't believe in smoking," and I continued with my iridology analysis, thinking about what I could say to her.

When I was done, I said, "I'll tell you what, darling. I'm not going to tell you to quit smoking...How many cigarettes do you smoke?" She said, "Two packs a day." I said, "I'll tell you what. Why don't you smoke four packs a day?" She said, "You're crazy! Why do you want me to smoke four packs a day?" I said, "If you smoke four packs a day, you'll get cancer a lot quicker. Then you'll be able to have your operation when you're younger and you'll be able to go through it better." Later, I found out she quit smoking. We have to think about these things. The mind does strange things with habits.

First Prize at the County Fair

Most of what I know has been learned through experience. We've had over 350,000 patients in the last fifty years, and you realize that people respond to food just like animals do. If you want the animal you take to the county fair in top condition, you have to feed it right. You want a nice glossy coat of fur; that's one that takes the first prize. You want a lovely duck, a lively duck. You want a spirited horse. You want your animals to look their best. I feel we can do this now with our own bodies. We have to eat right and exercise right if we want to be winners.

The World of Biochemical Elements

Our food should supply all the biochemical elements the body needs. Calcium foods are necessary. Silicon foods are necessary. We find that silicon is one of the greatest things to clear up diabetes. The pancreas is a silicon organ. And we need zinc, one of the main ingredients of insulin. All diabetics are short of zinc. When we have bone disturbances we have to think of calcium . . . or when there are menstrual problems. When we need oxygen in the body, we may have to take more iron foods. When the liver is causing trouble, there's a possibility that more iron is needed to cleanse it, and we can do it with greens. There's a possibility, too, that when a person becomes unfriendly and mean, you will find he needs iron . . . he needs a better liver.

A person with hepatitis isn't a friendly person to live with. Joy and happiness in your personality at this very moment depends upon good health. Now, we find that foods have an effect upon the body and the mind. Foods found in Nature always have a definite remedial effect. There are certain things in each food that can be attracted to each organ. Iodine from iodine foods can go to the thyroid gland, and maybe you need it very much.

Eggs Should Have a Tough Shell

I remember the time I was foreman of the Lucerne Creamery in Oakland, California. I had about 140 truck drivers. I was a young man at the time. In fact, I was the youngest chiropractor in California and I worked my way through college at this creamery. But, do you know, these heavy truck drivers with their brawny arms had to deliver eggs along with everything else. And, they shoveled these boxes of eggs into the stores, and we had more breakage!

I could hardly stand to see all these eggs broken by manhandling. And I had to account for them. But, a thought came to me.

I found there was a place you could buy eggs where the shells wouldn't break. That was in Petaluma, California. It's called the egg center of the world. They were sending eggs to Australia, New Zealand, different parts of the world, and they arrived unbroken. They didn't have any problem with breakage. I thought, "This is a wonderful thing. I'm going up there to see what they're doing."

I was surprised when I found out they were feeding their chickens green kale. Green kale is the highest vegetable in calcium, so I began feeding the chickens differently at my place and I found out when you give greens to chickens, they give a dark orange yolk. If they don't get greens, the yolk stays a light yellow. You can change the condition of that yolk just by feeding them greens. It's hard to believe, but do you know I cut the breakage down so much that I received a sizeable raise!

Food Isn't the Entire Solution

A lot of people are breaking down. A lot of people don't realize that we have to put all this together to have a good body. Before I discuss the rest of the foods that we're going to get into, I want you to realize that food is not everything.

We have climate to consider; we have humidity, altitude, electric energy in the air. There are qualities in the air when you can't put milk out. There's a quality in the air sometimes when we don't feel right. There can be electrical tension. Brainwork can break down this whole body. Loss of sleep can affect every organ in the body. Worry, disappointment, passion, jealousy, unfavorable emotions . . . all of these have an effect upon the body. We've got to know, too, that barley is a rich food and heats the blood. Rice eaters can become lazy and indolent without other things in the diet. They become feeble and lose their quickness. Rice isn't a stimulating food. Eating red meat raises the blood pressure; it's stimulating to the body. Using fruit to a high degree in the diet can lead to nerve starvation, because the nerves are fed by protein. Proteins are a brain and nerve food. Each food has its effect on the body. There's no reason in the world why you shouldn't know about these biochemical elements and what they do for the body.

We've got to realize that these biochemical elements do special things for the body. Sulphur brings heat to the body, and heat is needed in the extremities. Possibly a little sulphur food could help you. When you need the brain and nerve elements, always have sulphur foods with the brain foods. It will drive them to the brain.

Chlorine gas was used during WWI by the Germans. Of every hundred American boys who were killed or wounded, 30 were casualties of gas. But, chlorine is the greatest cleanser when it comes in food form. Chlorine is a wonderful cleanser.

Which Chemical Type Are You?

We are all chemical types, as people. Chlorine makes certain types of people. Too much calcium makes a certain type of person. We have silicon people who love to be happy and to dance. We have sodium people, and sodium is the "youth element." I'm a sodium type and I hope to always be youthful. My joints are soft and pliant, and very few people can push their joints back like I can. When a person comes in, I take the hands and feel their fingers and I can tell when arthritis is settling in and calcium is coming out of solution into the joints.

We have different types of people we have to treat. There are people we call the hydropheric type. They tend to retain water easily. We have chlorine types of people. The Chinese are chlorine types, very clean, very water-oriented.

The calcium person or race, such as the Russian and German people, has an entirely different outlook in life. It's hard to get a calcium person aware of spiritual things in life. He is as stolid as the earth from which he has attracted the calcium elements in the form of foods. He makes a good real estate man; he makes a good contractor. He pours concrete and works on steel girders; he is close to the earth. People can migrate to certain jobs depending on their chemical type. And, certain types don't like certain work.

Why am I bringing this out? Because if you know who you are and can put this together, knowing the type of food you need and how to live properly, and how to get the right philosophy — if you can put all of these things together, this is the system they call Bromognosis.

Discover the Healthy Way of Life

A healthy way of living is something we all need. Very few people know what a healthy way of life is as far as nutrition is concerned. We should know about changing to a better way of life. A healthy diet is one that is half building and half eliminating. On this you don't have to fast so much. You wouldn't have to fast for elimination. It's going to take you a year to see results, though.

You can't get well in 30 days. In a year 98 percent of your body changes. They say that in one year ten percent of the brain is disintegrated. So in ten years you'd have no brain structure if you don't rebuild it.

There is more to life than the physical realm. We are meant to live a whole life — mental, physical and spiritual. . .the higher path. If you haven't lived enough to know that coffee and donuts aren't going to give you a good skin structure, good eyes, good hair, then you haven't lived. You haven't been thinking. If you don't know that cigarettes, alcohol, coffee and chocolate are destructive to the body, then you haven't graduated from first grade yet. You need to use that brain before it atrophies too soon.

Every person has some weakness, whether acquired or interited. You must get acquainted with these weaknesses and take care of them. The strong organs take care of themselves. It is possible that you should know about certain types of foods, a certain way of living to help a depleted nervous system or to renew broken down bronchials.

You have to recognize that what goes into this body will eventually become your tissue, your bone, your eyes, nails and hair. It isn't what we eat that counts; sometimes it's what we *don't* eat. White flour is deficient in calcium. If you eat white bread, you're going to go bankrupt one of these days in calcium. And white sugar is the biggest calcium leach in the body. Add it all up! Eat that processed white stuff and you're in the red; you lose.

Sometimes we break down our bodies faster than we can build them up. Strain and stress need rebuilding faster than we give our bodies time for. Let the good life flow through those tissues. Find out what the good life is. Live it. The body repairs and rebuilds best when it is in a peaceful occupation; we need a peaceful outlook, a harmonious attitude. This is when repair and rebuilding takes place the fastest.

If you're like most people, when you're well you see how far you can strain the body. Then, when we have a tired body, we can't eliminate, we can't assimilate, we can't repair. All sick people are tired. There is more to life than just food. We have to take care of our bodies in all departments — mental, spiritual and physical.

Mahatma Gandhi once said, "There is more to life than increasing its speed." We are getting into troubled waters with our speed of living, our stress and strains, fears and hates, processed and convenience "fast" foods. We're living in the fast lane, where speed kills.

Whole Foods Are Our Remedies

Herbs are among the finest healing remedies we have. We have herbs for the kidneys; we have herbs for bronchial troubles. There are herbs for the liver like dandelion. Oat straw tea and shavegrass tea have a lot of silicon. We'll be getting into some of these herbs that you can use for various parts of the body. Our drinks should be natural. When we have our drinks at the Ranch, we have health drinks for breakfast, lunch and the evening meal. What is a health drink? We should think in terms of herb teas, juices, nut milk drinks.

Even milk is a remedy. Every food — if it's natural, pure and whole — is a remedy. Pasteurized milk doesn't fill the qualifications, but raw milk is a good health drink. Soup is a good health drink; carrot juice is an excellent health drink, rich in vitamin A. One of the best nerve tonics is an egg yolk in black cherry juice. Whey can be a good drink, or clabbered milk.

We have our vegetable salads. There are many different wonderful salad vegetables. Some people don't realize you can use raw spinach in a salad. Some people don't know that you can use raw peas in a salad — if they're tender. We can add grated carrots, grated beets, grated turnips, grated parsnips — all raw. This brings us to one of our most important food laws. We should have at least sixty percent of our food raw every day. Sixty percent.

You should know about cold-pressed oils. They should not be heated. We never cook anything in oil or grease. Our oils should be cold-pressed if at all possible. Heated oils are a deadly kitchen enemy.

Reconstituting Dried Fruit

You can get raw food in dried fruits, too. Our dried fruits haven't been cooked. We bring them to a boil in water the night before, turn off the flame and let them stand all night. We start from cold, so it heats to a boil and kills all the germ life, the bugs, the insect eggs that can be in the dried fruits. Then, cut off the flame and let it soak there all night long. Don't eat dried fruit out of the bag. This is why I have to treat a lot of intestinal disturbances.

Apprehend the Three Kitchen Robbers

I'd like to bring out here, also, that cooking is something to think about. There are three robbers in the kitchens. These three robbers are first, cooking with a lot of water. That takes all the nice soluble salts and vitamins out of your foods. The second robber is exposure to air, which kills more of the nutrient values. Use stainless steel cookware with tight lids. It would be best to cook with a vacuum where no air at all could get to the vegetables. The third robber is high heat. Again, you can cook in stainless steel, low heat cooking utensils. Use them to prepare your cereal grains. If wheat is cooked right with low heat, you can plant it in the ground after it is cooked, and it will grow.

Live Foods Contain Vital Vibrations

The average cooked food is so destroyed and broken down that we find it no longer has life in it, and what we're trying to do is get live, not "dead" food. These live foods have the essential vibratory rates in them that we need for healing and optimum well being.

Sulphur has a vibratory rate. Silicon has its vibratory rate. Every organ works to a certain vibration. Disease has its own vibratory rate. All organs can't work like the brain. Some have to go slow sometimes. We find that we have different vibratory rates in the different structures of the body.

Easy, Economical Parchment Paper Cooking

There are various ways you can cook and if you only had one or two in your family, it might be nice to get acquainted with parchment paper cooking. There is a parchment paper about 18 inches square or so that you can use and if you want to cut it up and have it smaller, do that.

You can wrap some vegetables in it, bring it to the pot and put a string around it (or one of those little wire twisters they put around plastic vegetable bags). Soak the parchment paper first so it's nice, soft and pliable; then cut your carrots, beans and beets and put them inside this parchment paper in separate bags. Get all the air out; and now you're going to put them in boiling water; you can put the separate bags in the same vessel if you want to. And you can put onions in another bag. You can put fish in another one. Fish will take you 20 minutes to cook, the onions 15 minutes, carrots 12 minutes, beets 13 minutes. You can know the time, and by the way, it's all scheduled in writing on the wrapper. First put in the one that has to cook the longest, then the next and the next, so you can take it all out at the same time and serve it.

Where do you get parchment paper? Look for it at your local health food store. It is advertised in leading health magazines.

One advantage is this: the heat will never be higher than 212 degrees F, the temperature of boiling water. The second thing: There's no air to get in it. And the third thing is: there's no water used directly in the cooking. You cook without water. You'll find out that the water doesn't get into your food. You lose none of the food value when you cook with parchment paper. If you open up the package with asparagus in it, you'll smell wonderful asparagus all over the house! It's all there, even the odor.

Have you ever walked down the street and smelled cabbage cooking in somebody's home? Why, of course. Don't you think these aromatic gases are vital to your body? Yes, they are. These gases get into vital parts of your body that even blood can't get into, and that's why we have to save all of the trace minerals.

When you cut these foods, never cut them crosswise; you always cut lengthwise. Why? Because the fibers are aligned this way. If you cut them crosswise, they'll "bleed" and much of the juices are lost. The same is true with carrots or beets; they should be cut the long way. Otherwise, they'll bleed, and you'll lose juice. Do the same with string beans. I mean, you should know these things.

If you can lock these vital juices in, you'll find they're much better for the person who is eating them.

You can cook onions right in this parchment paper in the water right next to the fish or asparagus, and the odors will not mingle. They will not taint or touch one another.

America's Raging Sugar "Addiction"

In 1900, by the way, we averaged 10 pounds of sugar a year per person in the United States. Today, we average about 130 pounds of sugar per person! That's each year. Can you see the increase in the acidity we're developing in the body? Sugar is a calcium leach. It sucks out the calcium in the body, and I don't like to tell you to cut out sugar because I was raised on Danish pastry until I nearly died on it. And I tell you, we all have to make changes, but with all of that sugar now, we have to understand we must leave this out. . . we must leave it out!

Seeds and Nuts Are Superior Supplements

Now, of course, there are seeds that we should think about in our diet. I think people should have seeds every day and I would like to mention here the four supplements that you should have in your diet every day which I think are wonderful nutrients. I want to make up for what you haven't had in years past.

I see people every day who have had just "a little too much" of the white flour products. They have had just a little bit too much of the white sugar products. It shows. We can do better than that.

Seeds are one of the things that we should have as a food supplement. I think we should have flaked seeds, seed milk, seed butter or seed meal every day. That's one of the supplements I feel we should all have. A tablespoon every day. Why? First of all, raw seeds are a whole food. Roasting seeds and nuts destroys the lovely oils in there, and they are salted, so they're really no longer a *natural* food. These natural seeds and the seed butters are necessary; or, we can use nuts.

Almonds in the form of almond butter, almond milk or in flaked or meal form, are absolutely wonderful. This is a supplement everyone can have every day. It's going to supply some of the things that I know you need because it's a *whole* food. I'm building whole bodies; do you understand that? I have to have the *whole* food — the seeds, skin, the inside, the vitamin E, the lecithin oils — we have to have the *whole* thing to get well and stay well.

Flaxseed is the second supplement. . . flaxseed meal. It has vitamin E; it has vitamin F. It's very good for the

intestinal tract. It corrects inflammation of the bowel, helps ulcers, stomach disturbances, gastritis. This flaxseed is one of the most wonderful supplements. It is slightly laxative. I don't like to use it when people have diarrhea, but the very thing they don't have is the thing they should have because here's where we need the Vitamin F; so we use flaxseed. Many children have constipation. They haven't been taught that they should have natural bowel movements, but to have a tablespoon of this flaxseed meal mixed right in the cereal every morning will help to bring natural bowel movements.

NOVA SCOTIA DULSE is the third thing to have because it is high in iodine, and most people are cooking so much these days they don't get enough iodine for the thyroid gland.

Rice Polishings are the other supplement. Rice polishings are the highest food in silicon, and I have never met a person who wasn't short of silicon. It's one of the best elements for getting rid of catarrh, and catarrh appears at the beginning of every disease. So, I want you to have the silicon you lack. I've looked for a healthy person, but I've never been able to find one. There's no such thing as a hundred percent well person, but you find out that people are not even ninety percent. They're usually down to forty percent, thirty percent. But, I can tell you that I can take that forty percent person and add silicon to increase his health level.

Rice polishings. . . I use them, because their value was discovered in one of the first experiments to find out about Vitamin B in the body. Researchers found out that by giving chickens and pigeons polished white rice, in four day's time they flap backwards and are on the verge of collapse. In the Philippines they fed chickens white rice and they developed droop-wing. When they started giving them the *whole* rice, the chickens recovered. When the pigeons were at the point of dying, they were given rice polishings and that brought them back. It cured a disease in birds that was comparable to beriberi in humans.

It was a nerve problem caused by vitamin deficiency. Do you know, I have some very interesting birds come to the Ranch, too. Some can't hold their wings up. Others have fatigue problems. None of them can fly very far or very high. Rice polishings help a great deal.

So, here we have the nuts and the seeds. I believe sick people should use the nut butters and the seed butters. Many a vegetarian I've met was starving to death because he wasn't getting enough heat in his body; the circulation was poor, the digestion underactive. Often they can't break down the nuts that they chew. It takes ten hours to soak nuts thoroughly enough so they can be digested and assimilated to get the good out of them. The stomach doesn't have any teeth in it. You must grind nuts and seeds fine before they get to the stomach, and if you have to break them down into a liquified form, do that. Make nut and seed milk drinks. [See recipe chapter.]

Nature Takes Her Healing Time

Now what are you going to do with these supplements? It's not a matter of having them one day and saying, "Well, my hair isn't any better." You can't take silicon for two weeks and say, "I don't see any change in my nails yet." You're going to have to do this for as long as one year. You must understand, these supplements build up slowly in the body. You'll need to keep taking these supplements for up to a year to see results. I want you to wash your tissues with the chemical elements, build them back in, gradually develop a reserve, and you do this much to break down the body...a little at a time. You cheated your body out of the calcium it needed with "a little" pastry, "a little" white sugar. You cheated your body out of the food value in the vegetable and fruit peelings. It takes ten, fifteen, twenty years to develop a disease in the body — with diligent effort. Now we're going to need to slowly add to the body all the things it needs, and we know that good health will come eventually.

You need an entire year to rebuild your body. Take a year out of your life and make the change to better health.

Orange Juice Every Day??

One of the nice things I know, is that there are three things I'd take away from everyone when a person wants to get well. I have learned my diet work through an apprenticeship that very few doctors go through. I used to make all my patients write down their diets for an average week and give it to me. And do you know one of the things I learned? What do you suppose people have every morning for breakfast? Orange juice...Don't you know there are other juices besides orange juice?

We find most of the oranges are picked green. I live in a citrus growing community, and I know they pick those oranges 2 months before they're ripe enough to eat and that's what goes to the supermarket and juice companies. I hear arthiritis patients complain of increasing pain, because they make it worse with green citric acid. They have too much citric acid. When you have stomach troubles, orange juice makes them worse. When you have excess acidity in the body or acid formations in the joints or in any part of the body, you stir it up and make it worse with this green citric acid. My patients often have acid joints. Many are an acid mess...with acid stomachs. Fruits, especially green citrus fruit, stir these acids up.

You're often not able to get rid of the acids you stir up in the body because the elimination channels are so underactive. I work on these elimination channels, so I know they are underactive. After you've worked on them a while, you'll be able to get rid of your acids through the elimination channels; but until then, we go to the vegetable kingdom more. The vegetables carry off the acids. Fruits

stir them up faster than the body can carry them off. So I cut out citrus fruit with almost everybody who comes to me. I used to sell carloads of citrus fruit, but I didn't know any better at the time. If you must have oranges, I think you should have them cut in sections, not in juice form. Never have orange and grapefruit in juice form. You need the nutrients and bulk in the membranes. The calcium control of the citric acid is in the pulp, and we find that pulp is a wonderful bowel bulk. The white has the pectin in it, and this is especially good for the bowel. Just to have this in juice form is not giving us the *whole* fruit for our body.

Never Head for the Head Lettuce

Now what do you suppose is the second thing I found when I looked at all these people's diets? Head lettuce! Everybody uses head lettuce in salad. They dress their meals with head lettuce. Yet, leaf lettuce has a hundred times more iron in it than head lettuce. In fact, head lettuce has no nourishment in it whatsoever. It's leached out. It doesn't even have chlorophyll in its "anemic" leaves.

Furthermore, head lettuce has a chemical in it related to cocaine that slows down digestion, and probably your digestion is too slow now; why slow them down still more? We find that lettuce juice acts as a tranquilizer. It's capable of putting you to sleep. That's what lettuce juice will do for us. So much for head lettuce...it's one of the greatest gas producers in the body also.

Bread Dependency Has To Go

The third thing these people write down on their diet is bread for breakfast, bread for lunch and bread for dinner. At breakfast the bread was in the form of toast or muffins or waffles or hot cakes; for lunch they had sandwiches; many people form their meals around bread. Now, white bread is constipating, and I had noticed the bowel problems, the hypoactivity and the bowel pockets (diverticula) from analyzing the eyes and wondered how to take care of these problems. I found I did more good for people's bowels by cutting out bread than anything else. I'm very sorry to tell you this, because I'm a man who would rather have a nice sandwich for lunch as much as anyone else, because I was brought up that way. But, I have had to break away from it. When you get into iridology, you'll find how healing is speeded up by getting rid of those three things I've just told you.

Wheat and Milk Saturation

I also ask my patients to cut out wheat and oatmeal. I'm not totally against bread, because there is good bread if you have to have it. I'm not an extremist or complete purist on these things. It isn't what you do once in a while that counts; it's what you do most of the time. You see, when you take orange juice, head lettuce and bread (among other things) for twenty years, I've got a patient. And, aren't you reading this to find out how to keep away from that trouble?

Let's go a step further. The government tells us that twenty-five percent of the American diet is made up of wheat products. They tell us that twenty-five percent of the American diet is made up of milk products. Now that's fifty percent of the American diet... wheat and milk products! When you look outside at God's Garden, do you think that is anything like an appropriate diet? When you look at all the fruits, vegetables, seeds, nuts and other foods we have there, shouldn't we be getting more variety? Wheat and milk products should be about six percent, maybe four percent, each.

Do you know the reason I say this? Ask any allergist, and you'll find there are two foods that cause more allergies than any other food products... and that's wheat and milk. Most Americans are wheat logged, milk logged. Allergy sufferers have too much of these products. The body is rebelling, loaded with too much catarrh. By having an overloading of those two foods, we produce that excess amount of catarrh. You can get catarrh from other things as well, but you'll find out by just cutting out wheat and milk you will be greatly cleansed and purified. You can wipe out all that milk in your knee in a year's time; you can wipe out all that wheat in your liver in eleven month's time. It becomes clean and pure and new again, but if you want to do it with different material and have the best health, cut out the wheat and milk for a while. We don't serve much of it at the Ranch. This is where the nut and seed milk or soy milk substitutes come in. They aren't catarrh forming.

Alternatives for Enjoyable Dining

I'm doing this work from a corrective standpoint. You're learning, that's all. You're reading this to learn, aren't you? I know... because I've done it for so many years. My patients have been my textbooks and my guinea pigs. I've learned from them experimented with them, but I tell you now after fifty years of practicing... I said *practicing*... now I know a little and I'm not practicing so much.

You get to the place where you say, "I don't know what to have for lunch if I can't have sandwiches." Find a way of having a midday meal without bread. You can have a bigger salad. You can have a protein. You could have a nice rice pudding instead of wheat.

Now, I don't cut out the grains when I cut out bread. I believe in cereals. But preparing hot cereals does not destroy the oils, the vitamins, and lecithin like we do when we bake bread. That's one of the main reasons I don't ap-prove of baked goods. I'm taking this from a health standpoint, strictly from getting well. Now you can eat as you please, but you can go along a better way, too. Just try this and see what a wonderful thing will happen. You can always go back to your old method again. Remember: Everything you eat will find its way into the skin, the hair, the joints, the cartilage, the brain, the bones. Wouldn't you rather get off the foodless foods and wrong diets and get into a healthy way of life to build a good body?

Nutrition is very important. It can be underestimated. We feed our brains through the foods we eat. Good sight and good hearing depend on good nutrition. Many diets leave you short. Many people are on reducing diets, elimination diets. We need to get away from diets.

Delicious Natural Ice Creams

There is a natural ice cream you can make. We have it here occasionally. On Sundays we may have a nice apricot whipped ice cream. It isn't difficult to make. Take any of the dried fruits or any of the fresh fruits and freeze them. For instance, many times we have frozen fruits such as mulberries or persimmons or others... frozen peaches, frozen apricots — and run them through a juicer or a liquifier and puree them. Freeze the liquifier vessel first in the refrigerator; add ice cubes if you want to. But, you don't have to use ice cubes and you can make the most lovely ice cream this way.

Clabbered Milk or Yogurt??

When we stop and think about the milk products, we find the greatest of all is clabbered milk culture. Now that's different from yogurt. Yogurt has been heated, but clabbered milk is simply soured and coagulated at normal temperature. We put a towel over the vessel and let it sit all night long. I never realized the value of clabbered milk until I traveled in search of secrets of longevity. All the oldest men I met, many over 100 years of age, used clabbered milk. I believe it is one of the main secrets of keeping youth well into old age.

Don't Undersell Whey

I'm going to give you another secret of the oldest people on earth. The whey that comes from clabbered milk is a special food that they always give the old men. Have I mentioned what the highest source of sodium is? (Sodium keeps the joints young and active, keeps us limber and pliable.) Whey. This is the whey that comes from coagulated milk or from cheese — the drippings from cheese making; and it's the highest youth food element you can find. Here we mean the food sodium, not table salt.

Sprouts Are for Survival

We should get to know our foods and what they can do for the body. I think one of the best whole foods is sprouts. Sprouts are a wonderful food from a bulk standpoint for the bowel. Sprouts are pure, whole, natural — and one of the highest foods in silicon. I consider them a survival food in this age where so many foods are potentially or actually contaminated.

Cocktails to Toast Good Health

When we come to making up interesting and lovely food supplements for our bodies, there are cocktails... and there are cocktails. There are drinks we can make; there are tonics we can use. You should know a good nerve tonic — an egg yolk and cherry juice, or egg yolk and prune juice. Prunes have the most nerve salts of practically all our dried fruits. A lot of people are bothered when they take fats and oils. It helps to have a green juice with it. You can put an egg yolk in your fresh green juice and find that the green juice will help the egg lipids go through the liver without trouble. This is how we think to create these cocktails.

Soups and Broths for Everyone

There are wonderful soups we can make. There are sodium broths for the joints, potassium broth to bring us back from fatigue and serious illness. There are certain chemical elements we need in our bodies, and we must use them constantly. If you need silicon for catarrhal trouble, then anytime you liquify foods in the liquifier, don't use straight water in the liquifier, use oat straw tea. And if you need something to help the kidneys and you still need the silicon, put Shavegrass tea in the liquifier. This is the art of using foods for healing, something very few doctors know anything about. I just bless the day I met Dr. V.G. Rocine, a homeopath who knew how to use the biochemical elements in foods and who knew how to use food as medicine.

I use basic multipurpose remedies in my work. For instance, I use vegetable broth and put lecithin in it, a wonderful tonic for arthritis. We can add many things to a basic broth. And then you find that cherry juice is wonderful for the liver and for arthritis, too. Beets are a good liver cleanser. Chlorophyll in greens is necessary for blood building and cleansing, good for the bowel flora as well. Have watercress often...it is a high potassium food for alkalization and heart support. Apricots, rich in cobalt, are for blood building. Seeds are high in Vitamin E. Pomegranate juice (with the seeds liquified) is a tonic for kidneys and bladder. Carrots are a fine source of Vitamin A; papayas are for digestion; and apples are high in potassium.

These illustrations show how food variety can help us stay healthy. The right foods help prevent disease. Disease can't invade the healthy body, one that has good health built into it. God intended us to live the natural, pure and whole food life, and it is the only road to good health. Good health is a gift you earn...nobody can give it to you — *but* you.

Why Should Natural Foods Cost More??

Now, foods were once really cheap in their natural form, but you can't get them in their natural state these days unless you pay more for them. I can't understand why raw milk should cost more than pasteurized milk. I can't understand why raw sugar should cost more than white sugar, but you see when they sanitize these processed, refined foods, they do it in such massive amounts that production and marketing costs are lower. It takes a lot of handling comparably speaking, to prepare the sugar that people buy in the health food stores. Furthermore, raw foods do not keep well. We find that whole wheat doesn't keep like refined white flour products do.

Animals Prefer Organic Foods

I used to put out a brand of bread called "The Bread of Life," and it was made of the whole grains, tomato juice instead of water and avocado for leavening. I'm telling you when we sold this bread, I had more complaints that it couldn't be kept long in the store because overnight the rats and mice would get at that bread. But they would never touch the white bread, the long "shelf life" kind.

I had a cousin in Kansas City who was paid to put out rat and mice traps around the storage bins of the white flour and the whole wheat flour. Rats and mice do not go after white flour. They know better. They have an instinct for self-preservation. They don't go for those things, and the craziest thing is that they've never been to my lectures, so I don't know how they know it!

But, there is something. Animals will go for organic foods first. I wish I could tell you some of the experiments to prove that they go for the organic food, grown from naturally composted soil foods. They stay away from artificially fertilized foods to the very last. They have to almost be starving to death before they'll touch it.

Geographical Factors Affect Draft Physicals

During World War II 49 percent of the draftees called up failed to pass the physical examination. But there was a place in the Midwest where 89 percent of the boys were passing the draft examinations...not 51 percent...89 percent! They didn't have fallen arches, bad backs, trick knees, asthma or congenital heart defects. This was from the mid-part of Kansas into northern Texas.

A government committee went there to find out why. And I tell you, it will surprise you that in that area, particularly around Deaf Smith County in northern Texas, they had the finest high-calcium wheat that you could get. Dr. George Hurd, a dentist friend of mine down there, told me he'd never pulled a tooth in the thirty years he'd practiced there. And, we find that when people have a healthy food supply, nothing much goes wrong with them. Deaf Smith County wheat is famous.

Researchers decided to do a little experiment to check this good wheat further. They put two grain bins in a livestock yard with cattle and their calves, and in one bin they put wheat and corn from farther north in Illinois and Ohio, while in the other they put corn from Kansas and wheat from Texas. Can you guess which one the cattle preferred? You know, those animals chose the corn and wheat from Deaf Smith County and Mid-Kansas, the areas those boys came from with the good draft physical records. Isn't that something to think about? These animals didn't touch the grain that came from the North.

When you consider the cost of foods, consider the quality, too. What is good health worth? Find out what's best and pay for it, even if it costs more.

Secrets You Should Shop By

When you go to the store, you need to know how to buy your foods. This is a thing we should think about seriously. When you get into the market, find out what days the greens come in and come in that day to buy yours. They don't deliver them every day. In our own area it's hard to get greens every day. But I'm telling you, on the days they come in, they're beautiful. Greens should be eaten the day they come in. Watercress should be eaten the day it comes in. You should know about such things. The solid vegetables like carrots and parsnips can wait a few days if necessary. You buy them at the same time you buy greens, but remember, greens have to be taken care of first.

When you buy fresh, whole pineapples, pull the top, and if you can pull it out easily, you'll know the pineapple has taken everything it can from the top to become fully sweet and ripe. It is the top of that pineapple that brings down the sunshine element for that yellow inner fruit. When you buy an apple, look into the bottom of it where the flower was. If it's still green, it's not ripe, even though the rest of the apple may be red. It wasn't finished by Nature. When you buy a melon of the female variety you are getting the sweetest melon. The stem end is indented and also the flower end. And if you run your fingernail over the top of the melon and the green chlorophyll runs up your fingernail, then you know it's ripe on the inside. That watermelon has taken everything from the outside it can.

In getting the best out of peas, for instance, you should use the Chinese peas so you can use the pods and get the *whole* food. Cantaloupe and cucumbers follow the same principle as the watermelon; the ends are indented in the female and in the male they come to a point. When you pick cucumbers, you should have rubber gloves on. You can make your cucumbers bitter if you pick them when the hand touches the vine. There are a lot of things we need to learn about foods.

Seven Spiritual Thoughts: The seven best spiritual thoughts that I think we can get into are to believe first and then demonstration will come along. Most people want to see a demonstration and then they'll believe. If you will believe some of these things a demonstration will come to you. Most people keep away from some of the lovely things. Most people don't know that they were created for joy. Did you know that? A loving Father doesn't want you to live in misery and disease. You've got to learn to serve. You've got to be an uplifter in life and love. These are the seven that I thought you ought to get started in and think about.

Seven Best Mental Aphorisms: The seven best mental aphorisms: Fear is faith working in reverse. What you are seeking is also seeking you. Time is here to stay; it's we that go. We must love people, but we don't have to agree with what they do. Right rights itself. We are meant to work, so we might as well work with joy. We have mind over matter, also mind over platter. These are mental aphorisms.

Seven Soups: There are seven good soups that you should learn about. One of the finest calcium soups is green kale and barley. If you have a growing child that has trouble with his or her teeth and hasn't got the calcium in the body, give him green kale and barley soup. Potato peeling soup is the best crisis soup, the best soup for strengthening those who are weak and bedridden. Learn about making soup with a liquifier. Make raw soup. Cut up fresh corn, put it in the liquifier and make a nice yellow corn soup with a little warm cream or milk. Add a pat of butter in it if you wish; flavor it with seasoning — broth powder — and you have a wonderful soup. You can use raw asparagus, raw beets and other vegetables. Veal joint broth is a great soup for sodium, for helping get calcium deposits back in solution.

All right, the seven best starches. . . I went over those.

Seven Seeds: Seven best seeds. . . I think alfalfa seeds are probably the best. Alfalfa seeds are the most wonderful thing I know for arthritic joints, taking a tablespoon to a pint of water. Bring it to a boil, let it sit for a couple of hours, strain it, and use that tea or broth. It's the most wonderful thing for joint troubles. Sunflower seeds are wonderful for calcium and for balancing cholesterol; use the sunflower seed butter or make a seed milk drink with them in a blender. Sesame seeds can be taken the same way. Wild rice is one of the best of the seeds. Fenugreek along with comfrey makes a good tea to get rid of catarrhal problems in the body. Flaxseed tea is high in vitamin E. Boil, or let a fourth cup of flaxseed soak in one quart of boiling water overnight. Never use the seeds twice. Ground flaxseed on top of cereal or salad is good for the bowel. Watermelon seeds can be ground in a blender for a fine kidney drink. Chia and pumpkin seeds have useful remedial values.

Seven Basic Teas: We might consider fenugreek more in the tea category. Number one is a peppermint or spearmint tea. Number 2 is the oat straw tea and number 3 is comfrey; you can mix them if you wish. There are also shavegrass, hawthorne berry, camomile and cleaver tea. Cleaver tea is a fine diuretic for those who gain weight by picking up water easily.

One of the secrets of nutrition is variety. You can't live on potatoes every day. You can't have tomatoes all the time as the only vegetable you cook or have raw. You must have variety. You can't have prunes all the time. You'd be full of prunes. Some people depend on these foods, and they become one-sided with them.

Seven Bad Habits to Break: Eating too often. Eating too much. Talking about sickness, losses and diseases. Fried foods. Smoking. Worrying about what is yet to come. Can you understand there are seven times seven?

Healing Crisis Notes: There are seven things to expect from what I have been telling you...the ups and downs. You're not going to have steady good health. You're not going to go steadily into well-being. Your body is going to go through elimination processes, and we call them *Healing Crises*. Another thing you're going to find out is that when you go this way, you're going to be alone in life. You'll find very few people will go with you on it. You may even have to leave some of your relatives behind. You don't have to worry about leaving them...they'll leave you. You have to have the approval of the Wise Ones in what you're living on. You can expect a longer life, more beauty and abundance. You can expect freedom from disease and worry. And one of the nice things, you'll be polishing your soul. You'll be ennobling the Great Within.

Some Foods I Don't Approve Of

The two foods I especially don't believe in are rhubarb and cranberries. These two are high in oxalic acid which will cause joint disturbances and lead to arthritis, especially when you cook them. (Who eats raw cranberries...who eats raw rhubarb?)

If you'll find an Indian and follow him, he will only eat the things the birds eat and the birds will not eat cranberries or rhubarb. When you eat it you have to sweeten it a lot, and we've talked against all this sweetening. However, you can have rhubarb and cranberries at Thanksgiving or Christmas...and only then.

A Valuable Lesson from New Zealand

I had one of my great lessons down in New Zealand. I visited some of the lovely springs there, and at one of them were fish, good-sized fellows about 30 inches long. In one beautiful pool there must have been at least 500 of these fish, and when they fed them the fish almost went crazy after the food. There was one fish in the pool that people called Harvey, a fish half yellow and half brown. In the frenzy of competing for food, Harvey's body turned all brown. It was an amazing thing to see. Can you understand that? The body of this big fish actually changed color in the stress and anxiety of fighting with other fish for food. I know that anxiety changes our whole body. The Bible says, "In nothing be anxious."

Our Physical, Mental and Spiritual Home

There is much I could say...physically, mentally and spiritually. Let us try to balance our lives. Balance is what we need. A person who is sick is going the unbalanced way. A person who is all spiritual has gone the extreme way, "to the edges" as they say in London. We meet people who go to the extremes in diet and we find out that the body is not an extreme building. It is a temple of all the good that you can think. It's a temple of all the dust of the earth. It's a temple of all the loving things that you can put into it, and you must take loving care of it. This is the Temple of the Living Soul. We find as we look to this Temple, you have rooms in it just like your home. You have a living room. Yes, you live in it. You have a hobby room where you enjoy. You have a basement where you store things. You have a fence around your house. You have a draft system in your home. You have a heat circulation in your system, and you have heat circulating in your home. But you have still more. You have furniture in that home. It has doors that are open to allow your friends in. You have the warmth of good feelings. Yes, it's all in your home, and you are built as a home. But remember, too, that we have to furnish it with love. You have to furnish it with some of the lovelier things in life, like *peace* and *joy* and *happiness*.

Chapter 6

The brain: your navigator

What Does the Brain Have to do with Nutrition?

If we were to pick the most important organ in the body, it would have to be the brain. All the brain activities, every expression of thought and action, every physiological action of every organ, is dependent upon the brain. Basically, the brain has to be fed properly so that it is working efficiently with the body tissues. It has to be repaired, rebuilt, rejuvenated from day to day. We use many of our examples in this book as inspirations for you to take better care of your body. Why? Inspiration is breath for the brain, life for it.

Inspiration to keep the body in good health is neglected. Many people only care for the body after they have lost their health. A new system of education must be introduced. We need to be reminded that we have many God-given qualities enabling us to harvest a better childhood, harvest a better marriage, harvest a better and more successful life. Health is the first consideration. Through ignorance we lose that health only to begin a series of quests, a search after a solution to physical pain and misery. In too many cases, the search ensues after we are "lost."

Know Thy Soul to Know Thyself

A lot of people ask me questions, and a lot of the questions are very questionable. When I stop and think a little bit about the things I am asked, I am reminded of how little we really know about life and health. We have so much to learn. People ask about chelated minerals...about yeast and vitamin B complex. You ask these questions because you want correction; you want to add something to your life; you want to do something good for yourself and you're seeking.

I think the thing that we should seek is our soul. If you'll look into the soul faculties of a man, it's these soul faculties that develop the brain potentials, and it's the brain that keeps everything else working in the body. We have never gotten to the very beginning of life, the beginning of how we really put a body together. A lot of you are hungry, and soul-wise you may have a health center in the brain, but it has never been taken care of. We have centers in the brain that should be nourished. We have personalities that should be nourished. We all have weaknesses in the body, but seldom do we sit down and study how we can take care of ourselves.

For instance, some months ago a little lady — a schoolteacher — was telling me about all the troubles she had. She'd been with me for about a month, but when she first came, she was a nervous wreck. She was a nervous wreck because she allowed so many things to take her over. She allowed the school classes to take her over; she allowed the children to take her over. She was a receptacle for everything that came at her. She didn't know herself. She didn't know how to control situations. She didn't know how to take care of things. I told her that there was a way of controlling those classes for her good. She had an idea that she had to serve. She felt she had to do something for those classes, but she made herself a wreck by the way she was trying to serve. I said, "No class should ever start until you set yourself up in good order and know what you're going to do in the next hour. If that class has to do any arithmetic, if they're going to do English, if they're going to work in any of the curricula that they have in the schools today, first of all you should get those children ready to learn. What bothers you with these children?"

She said, "They're noisy and fidgety. They will not listen. They talk in the back of the room. I'm trying to teach and I find that two chilren are way off in another world."

I said, "Well, why don't you gather them all together?"

She said, "What do you mean, gather them together?"

I said, "The first thing you need to do is to establish that you're not going to give anything until you have absolute quiet and attention." I learned this long ago from a lecturer named Krishnamurti, I told her.

Krishnamurti was a man who would stand before an audience of a thousand to five thousand people and he would not talk if it took them 15 minutes to quiet down. He wouldn't talk until you could hear a pin drop. I mean...he wouldn't talk until you were ready to listen. Now, this woman was making herself a wreck, because she was under time pressure. Time was her tyrant. She had to accomplish so much; she was thinking about the examinations that were coming up.

I said, "Get absolute quiet. Demand absolute quiet and show them there isn't going to be any talking. There isn't going to be anything done until absolute quiet prevails in that room."

And then I said, "Besides talking about arithmetic, English or the subject of that period, take the first two or three minutes and talk on a new subject every day.

Something that has meant an awfully lot to you. First day, talk on beauty and talk about the beauty that you met that day and impart it to these children.

She gave it a try. It went over well the first day when she talked about beauty. The next day she spoke to them about joy and what it meant to her. She said, "You should be joyous, too. One of these days when you have learned your arithmetic and you have learned English and you have learned all your subjects, it will be joyous for you. It should bring you a lot of happiness. Now, these are the things that we're going to study today."

She developed such control over that class that other teachers wanted a meeting to know how she could control her children the way she did. I mean...this is something to think about. You can demand quietness that you can't bring any other way, and we find that kids in greneral are very unruly today. They abuse the privilege of education. You find our schools are in very serious trouble. Now I'm only bringing this thing out to show that you need to find yourself before you can go through life and take care of yourself properly. You must learn to put not only the classroom in order, but to put yourself in order first.

You are a classroom as well. You have a lot of faculties in your mind. I don't know whether you know, but you have a joy center in the mind, a happiness center. And did you know that many kinds of love, all different, reside in the brain? Our love for a friend is much different from the love of a flower or love for a dog or love for a lover. These faculties are all different, and I would like to tell you that all of these faculties demand a different food supply. Each one of them has to have a different vibratory element coming to feed it.

The Brain Keeps Law and Order

The brain is really the directing principle of your life. We find the liver will not work unless the brain is in good order. They have worked it out and, you know, you can cut the nerve to the muscles of the arm and those muscles will not work. So those nerves are the first thing to be taken care of. You cannot see right unless the brain is in good order. The eyes are extensions of the brain. The olfactory nerves are extensions of the brain. The auditory nerves are extensions of the brain. You taste with the brain. You find out that the brain is the faculty where everything is known in your body, including the past stored in your memory...you see? And you'll find out that the memory of flowers, the memory of a good time, the memories of life — the memory is diffused throughout the brain. All our memories are stored along with the feelings that went with them, just as we experienced particular events at the time.

If life is a school (and it is), the brain is really the principal's office, and you must take care of that brain —

otherwise you'll find that weaknesses will result. Ulcerated colitis can come in, but it comes because of a brain faculty that is broken down. Ulcers in the stomach are developed because the vagus nerve, the pneumogastric nerve, is broken down. They have severed certain nerves involved in high blood pressure, and they find the people no longer have a high blood pressure. But, you'll find also that degeneration begins in other parts of the body when they do these things. You have to learn to take responsibility for these brain faculties that rule the body. We find an over-motivated person can make that liver overwork. It can degenerate. Many times you think that livers degenerate just through excessive drinking of alcohol. It can also degenerate through mind abuse as well. We don't usually realize that we can get drunk on our own ideas. Many times we can become emotionally unfit to make this human body work properly. You'll have to put your brain in good order. Now we find the liver has a center in the brain that directs its function. Diabetes starts with a pancreas that isn't working properly, but the pancreas is either underactive or overactive according to the brain faculties.

Don't Overload the Brain and Nervous System

A person who is critical, a person who is serious, a person who is analytical and exact can make a success out of his life. He has to have those faculties to make a success; but the overuse of those faculties will break down the very brain faculties that have made him a success. There is a limit to those things.

This is why I have as many hobbies as I do. This is why I get to determine when I want my time off. You can't talk to me then. I won't see you. I won't hear you. I can't use my nerves anymore for that purpose. I have heard enough complaints through the nerves of my ears until they just can't take anymore. You've heard about the straw that broke the camel's back.

You need a diet which is two percent phosphorus to nourish the brain and nervous system; but you know through being resentful, through being bad tempered, through working against other people's ideas and activities, you could burn out five percent of the phosphorus in your body and then certain mental faculties become over-developed and other mental faculties become broken down because you've overworked the brain faculties.

Your toes wiggle because of your brain. A person can have a nervous breakdown lecturing too much. We find that the left side of the brain controls the right side of the body and vice versa. If you have a stroke, for instance, your tongue will always go to one side and it does that because this tongue is dependent upon the brain and upon the nerves that go from the brain to the tongue. One eye can go out of alignment with the other. It's because the brain faculty is not controlling the muscle properly. Many times nerve weakness in the muscles leading to the eye can cause cross-eyedness; or many of these conditions can be caused from the brain itself.

Right or Left Handed?

Many people are left handed; and the mother and father often insist upon that child using his right hand all the time. We find out that a person whose mentality and brain faculties are designed to use the right side of the brain so that the left side of his body is successful — and we have what we call "southpaw" or left-handed baseball pitchers, batters that hit best left handed. But, manufacturers do not make much left handed equipment or tools. They are making more left handed sports equipment now. I knew a golfer who was left handed. I made him left handed golf clubs and he became a champion in the Los Angeles Open Tournament.

I used to be ambidextrous, but I always use my right hand now and I never use my left hand at all. I suppose I have only developed one side of my brain. The right side of my brain wasn't developed because I wasn't using it. We find out that the eye we use most is the same side as the hand we use. But if you have a weak right eye and you're always using it, you're using the left side of the brain to help make the right side of the body become stronger. Some children end up stuttering and stammering...they're trying to use a part of the brain that is not yet successfully developed. These are important things to find out.

Faculties Depend on Brain Control

If you have a weakness in the lung structure you should think about taking care of medulla in the brain; you even swallow from the brain. Some people have a problem with the faculties of swallowing. Singing comes from the brain. There's hardly a thing you can mention that doesn't have to originate in the brain force behind it.

Some people come into this life to sing, but if you don't have the physical faculties to go along with it, you're not going to sing. You're only going to sing soul-wise. Some of you have music in your heart. Some have a soul for music that should be expressed, and it's a shame for them to go through life not doing the things they love to do. Most of us are artists, but we don't use all our talents — usually only one at best. I have seven talents and I know where they are, but we find that some people don't know their talents.

Know Thyself and Heal Thyself

We have some people who are calcium types — earthy. You can't pry an invitation out of these people.

And then we have some people who are mental types; they can become wonderful spiritual people, but they are mechanical idiots. They can't find success in another direction.

So what am I leading to? Learn to "know thyself." When you know yourself you can develop yourself more in the right direction. You won't be having to chase healing anymore. You won't have to go after chelated minerals and so forth. You'll find out that you'll chelate those minerals naturally in your own body. We have been doing it for a long time. Nature chelates all these minerals and elements right for us. Without the proper amount of silicon, you can't keep Vitamin B in the body. That's why we find that rice polishings, the highest food in silicon, but not the highest in Vitamin B, works very well. Vitamin B goes with silicon more than anything else. The two work together; silicon is for the nervous system and Vitamin B is for the nervous system. You can take Vitamin B from now on to feed this nervous system, but if you don't put silicon and a few other chemical elements back in there, you'll never hold it.

You'll never be able to rebuild a nervous system on Vitamin B alone. The funny part of it is, that's what you get in yeast. You don't get silicon, but it's one of the highest foods we have in Vitamin B. We're going to go back and study where Vitamin B is in Nature. Yeast is a man-made food. Rice polishings are not a man-made food. God put these elements together beautifully and, when I say beautifully, we can consider cholesterol in eggs. We always need lecithin to use cholesterol properly, and we find out that while eggs are a high cholesterol food, they are also high in lecithin; God combines these foods in perfect proportion for you, and you'll never have to worry about it.

Calcium and Silicon Are the Stars

If we were meant to get out and study all that we can find in Nature, we would die frustrated, miserable, and ignorant; you cannot find out all these things. So many of Nature's secrets are hidden that it's an impossibility. But if you would look around and see all the different chemical types of people, we would learn about Nature from man. One of these days we will find that silicon even helps to control the calcium in the body. Silicon and calcium are very likely two of the most important elements to put in the body. I find these two elements are lacking in everyone who comes to me. Also, sodium and iodine are nearly always lacking.

Seek the Beautiful and You Shall Find It

Many of those who come to the Ranch are broken down from a mental and a nerve standpoint, and they've done this because they don't know their own faculties. They don't know how to love and take care of the life they've been given. They don't know how to bring out the best in life. Your father and mother hated people, so you may do it, too. You inherited that capacity to hate or you *think* you did...you think you did. Do you understand what I mean? You find out you've never really touched the lovely part of life, the lovely gifts.

Now our eyes are meant to see light, but you find out you can close your eyes and you can still see, or can you...? What do you see with them? You can still see with the mind, the brain. The brain is the greatest faculty we have; we should cultivate the brain. That brain knows about the secret place of the Most High. The brain knows how beautiful things are generated in the body. The brain knows these things.

Never Neglect Brain and Nerve Foods

The brain also knows that when you eat certain foods that you have to have phosphorus and sulphur together in order to make lecithin in the body which is a brain and nerve food. All of you vegetarians need lecithin more than anything else. You're eating dry nuts that have come from soft shells, paper-thin shells. You're eating these dry almonds, these paper-shell pecans and peanuts. Do you think you're getting lecithin? You should be getting it from hard-shelled nuts like the Missouri black wanuts and macadamia nuts. You should get the Brazil nut you have to dig into. You know the oil you find when you dig into those nuts? That oil is a brain and nerve food. Is it any wonder we don't develop and bring out all the lovely faculties in life?

Life Needs Expression

Why is it so many people are born to be musicians and are not physically able? They don't have enough coordination in their fingers. We find many a person who would make a beautiful pianist but he doesn't have the brain faculties developed — physically and mentally. And then a person goes through life sick. I say mentally because, after all, playing music is sometimes the one thing that would keep that person really alive. A person comes alive when you touch these faculties he loves to work with.

Take any course in salesmanship. "Talk about the customer's hobby first," they tell you. "Talk about fishing first. Find out what he likes to hunt. Find out what he does in his spare time. And then talk about your experiences and lower the boom when he isn't thinking." I know salesmanship. I've taken the courses, and you'll find out salesmanship is an art where we take people unaware. You shouldn't be subjected to that. You should be aware of all these mental faculties, and they should all be usable.

Many a person goes through life and never knows true expression. Each person has something wonderful on the inside, because we're wonderfully and fearfully made. What we usually experience is nothing compared to the brain faculties we have and that we should develop. We are meant to be happy, not slaphappy. No! We are meant for joy. We should be able to jump for joy, but very few people have joy enough that they can jump with it. We don't have the physical body to jump for joy. Well, you see kids jump for joy when you take them to the circus. You just have to tell them about going to the circus and then watch them respond!

People need to be touched. Do you understand that? There's a way of touching and you can do this by word of mouth. You don't just have to slap a person on the back and tell a person you like him. You find feelings can be detected in the tone of your voice. People can tell when resentment creeps into your voice. It can be discerned by the tone, and that tone can destroy you, too. Did you know that? You have to have a good tone in your voice. The vibratory rate that goes out of your body can destroy certain chemical elements that have been put together by the brain. You're a very finely tuned instrument, you know.

Asthma Can Be Emotional

Once I took care of a lady who had lost her husband and also a man who had lost his wife. They were attracted to one another by loneliness and were married. The man developed asthma after the marriage. He couldn't understand why he developed asthma. And I asked him, "Have you ever had it before?" He said, "No, I've had bronchial trouble; I've had some wheezing at times, but since I married this lady I have terrible asthma attacks. You don't mean to tell me that I would be allergic to the woman I love?"

And I said, "Well, there's something in that homelife that isn't good, and we ought to find what it is." I asked him if he had any resentment. "Is there any reason you don't feel good at home? Is there anything you're possibly fighting?" The man was a mental worker and he had just gone a little too far, too hard. I saw the medulla faculty breaking down in the iris of the eye. Something was breaking him down.

He said, "Well...doctor...I'd like to confess something. I'm the only one who knows this, but you know, her children have never taken me in. When I come home it would be nice to have these kids greet me or have these kids look for me. But they don't want to have anything to do with me. They avoid me; they even try to take her away from me. They try to steal her affections, and whenever there's any affection between the two of us, they come right between us. You know, I'm getting to the point where I dislike the kids, and I don't mean to. I love this woman very much."

I said, "There's a possibility that you're not clicking someplace. Maybe you have to do something for these children." He said, "I'd like to do something for them, but I don't know what." I said, "Maybe I can do something. I'll come over for a visit and see what the score is."

We went over to his house. Those kids were all likable, but you have to like kids their way. As we sat there, I wondered what it would take to win them over. Finally, I asked them to go outside with me.

I said, "Is there anything you kids would like to do more than anything else in the world?"

They said, "We'd like to go to the circus!"

I said, "How about me taking you to the circus?" and they said, "Gee, we'd love to!" I was trying to find if we could really win these kids over. So, we went to the circus and had a great time. While we were there I saw how they admired the little ponies.

I didn't say anything about it, but when we returned I told the man, "Listen, do you want to solve this situation? Just buy each of those kids a pony. You'll find you won't have any more asthma."

He got together with those kids and said, "You know, I missed going with you to the circus today. What did you see?" All they could talk about was the ponies. He said, "It would be nice if we could get a pony, wouldn't it?" Well, those kids forgot all about the jealousy thing with their mother. They were only interested in one thing and that was a pony. He told them, "Let's go out shopping for ponies and find out which kind is the best." He had more fun taking these kids looking for ponies, and they bought one.

Do you understand the salesmanship that goes on here? You've got to touch these kids where they live. These kids received the pony, and he got rid of his asthma. This is the way to touch a person through mental faculties. You have to do this. These are many ways of doing this.

We have faculties for motion in our bodies, but we have to have motivation — some people don't move at all. We have sexual faculties, but these faculties are no good unless there is communication. Why do people get divorced?..."I hate that person...they're cold...uncaring...frigid...impotent." They have no sexual activity any more. But, we find that with the right person there's a spark that makes those things move, and that spark is essential. Mental faculties come alive when they're touched with the good life.

Build Health Within Your Soul

Many of our mental faculties are soul faculties. Often we live on memories of the past. I don't like to tell you how much "past" we already have at the time we were born, but many of you are a little older than others. Some of you don't have to learn the same lessons that others do; but this is where the soul has you. You are your soul. These soul faculties should be developed. You should know how to go back inside — you should start learning how to enoble the Great Within you have and start developing your soul.

The reason I speak about this is because everybody is chasing a cure. Everybody is looking to green clay or to chelated minerals for a cure. Everybody is looking at Vitamin B tablets. We should learn how to live life so that we don't need these things. Now, I'm bringing this out because the clay treatments wouldn't be necessary if we treated the mind first. That's what I'm trying to bring out.

Get acquainted with yourself. If you have music within you, don't sit and fix watches all day! Get away from it. There's another time piece that we have to take care of and it's the timing within ourselves." There's a balance; there's a time to be quiet. At night you should learn to relax and let go. The beginning of the day is when we should exercise and go into our physical living.

We have to get acquainted with the soil. We find that in topsoil there are millions of worms to every acre; without worms we could not be alive. We have to depend upon these worms. These little worms take in the leaves and debris and mix it together to be thrown out in the form of castings. This builds topsoil. All we need in my valley is topsoil. I spent $35,000 in truckloads of manure compost to put on topsoil out here. I wanted the topsoil to be the very best. When you have good topsoil, you have good vegetables, you have good fruits; this is the reason for these things. How many people study the soil? Did you ever follow a plow? Have you smelled that new mowed hay? Have you stood in a newly plowed field? There's something about the odor that invigorates us, harmonizes us, directs us toward what is fulfilling in life.

Cultivate A Satisfied Mind

Many people don't eat properly because they don't develop their minds to put food in the right perspective. Many people crave sweets because they have no love in their life. Wow! This is hard to believe. If we're going to be pleased and we need sympathy, we're going to do something for ourselves. "Can't get it this way; I'll get it another way." So we shift our pleasure-seeking to another channel. We had a lady here who ate a chicken every night before she went to bed, but she'd never let her husband see it! "I don't want to feel guilty about my husband knowing," she said. But, she *ought* to feel guilty from eating a chicken every night before going to bed!

We take up abnormal behavior by not knowing how to balance our life. I'm bringing these faculties out because we should turn a lot of our energies within and try to see how we can make a better person of ourself. We should go inside so we can learn to become a stronger person. We need to get to the place where nothing of an inferior nature disturbs us on the outside.

We can look at the stars and feel something wonderful from them. Many people have lived under the stars all their lives and never really looked at them. I was moved one night when I took my ten-year-old son walking out under the stars. David said, "Dad, how many stars do you think are up there?" I answered, "I don't know, David." He said, "Well, you ought to know — you're my daddy!" And I began to think...well, maybe I ought to know. I had never studied it; it's beyond calculation. I said, "David, I just don't know how many stars there are." He said, "I'll bet the last number is up there." I wish I had thought of that one! How many stop to think about it? I mean...that's getting into thinking about it!

Live According To Good Vibrations

How many of you have gotten into music far enough to realize how many chords there are? How many vibrations are going from the lowest note to the highest note? Some of you don't even know that there are more vibrations going on in your life than you can hear.

I blew a high frequency whistle one night and my dog heard it and barked outside, but none of us could hear it. We don't have the ears to hear above a certain frequency threshold. But the dog can hear higher frequencies, and they used this type of whistle to train the dogs during World War II.

There are endless vibrations beyond those we can detect with the senses. You only know what your own body shows you on the outside. You look in the mirror and you say, "There I am." That's not you at all...and that's the same as doubting Thomas coming to the Christ. He said, "You talk so much about the Father; why don't you show Him to us?" Christ said, "If you see me, you see the Father." And doubting Thomas went away scratching his head. He came back the next day and said, "I still don't see the Father." The Christ said, in effect, "If you see me, do you see a man...?" We are built in the image of Divinity, the image of all the Godly laws. We've been built in the image of God and we need to get acquainted with ourselves.

Feed the Soul First

The reason we take chelated minerals is because we are not living the mental way we were meant to live in. We are beautiful creatures; we are beautiful human beings. Today we hear talk of being beautiful. But some women think they have to put on a new dress to be beautiful. Some men think they have to get a good suntan. I don't think about your dress or suntan at all. You're all beautiful now. When an atheist was buried, they had to put him in a tuxedo and a beautiful coffin and lowered him into the ground. Over his grave they put a gravestone that said;

HERE LIES AN ATHEIST, ALL DRESSED UP WITH NO PLACE TO GO.

We're looking at the physical body. We're not looking at the soul...you see? The soul is very important... to polish our soul is very important. We have to learn about these things.

Noise, Climate and Altitude

We should learn about climate along with the soil. We should know that we can go to the hills for regeneration. That is, you go to a higher altitude, and there you build up your blood count. My wife can take all the iron you could possibly give her without being able to build up her blood count. But if I take her to a higher altitude, she can build a high blood count. In the Andes, people live at 10,000 and 12,000 feet. They have a blood count of seven million five hundred thousand. The highest blood count you can get at sea level is five million. If you have a degenerative disease, if you have chlorosis, if you have conditions in the body where the thyroid isn't working right, metabolizing and making the body move right, you'd benefit from moving to the mountains. This is taking care of your physical body. More people should go to the mountains to get well.

To get out of the city may be your best move. The noise in the city can cause deafness. But, also, to resent a person, to not want to listen to whatever they say, can cause deafness. Ask a psychologist. He'll tell you we can learn to turn a "deaf ear" to those we don't want to hear. Finally, you'll block things off. Deafness may come when a man has a nagging wife. I mean...these things happen; they exist. What are we going to do? You're going to get some chelated calcium to cure the ear trouble. Once a man who couldn't sleep went to the doctor to get some sleeping pills. When he got home he gave them to his wife and got a good night's sleep.

Create A Harmonious Life-Style

People need to know, first of all, how to get along with other people. If you can't get along with people, you'll find out that you can't be well. I absolutely believe that people can cause more disease in one another than anything else. "Dis-ease." Did you catch that?...Disease...a lack of ease. Many times it's our own fault that the lack of ease exists.

It's very difficult for us to live with just anybody, and this is why, when we marry, we hope we have a balanced wife or a balanced husband who can help us in all the faculties of our life. But it doesn't always happen that way. That's why many of you have to have a hobby. That's why you have to have spare time. That's why you have to go bowling. I could sit home and knit with my wife if I wanted to, but you find out we all have to do some of the things we love to do. Married couples can't all do the same things at all times. It's an impossibility. We are different, but the one thing we have to learn — this is important — is to get along with one another.

It is so important to get along with one another that if we don't, we may become sick. You've heard people say; "You make me sick to my stomach!" "You give me a pain in the neck!" Have you ever heard these things? Certainly you have! You find out that people go through life and deliberately — I don't even like to say this — but some people deliberately cause disturbances with other people. Some people like to fight. Some people only feel good if they bring the worst out of you. Did you know that? Some people bring the worst out in others and they like to agitate and they like to irritate. We have people who have those tendencies. We find people who have destructive faculties developed in the mind. There are some people who have seductive faculties. We find people who are sadistic.

Evolve To The Good Life

There's a story about a lady from England who said she would believe in God if seven trees would grow up from her grave. And seven trees did grow from her grave, but. . . it was a little late.

I remember another story about a man who was all humped over, bent into a deformed shape. While he was near death, they started making a coffin to fit his body — an almost U-shaped coffin to fit his deformed body. But, after he died, he straightened out! You figure that out! What was keeping him bent over while he was alive?

While we are living many of us are crippled. Do you understand that? Many of us are looking for crutches. Many of us are looking for something to live on and to hold on to, something that would be good for us. I think it's necessary to know how to get along with people. We all have different soul faculties, different mental faculties, and we aren't meant to harmonize with everybody.

As you evolve, you begin to live with people who are going to do you the greatest amount of good. It is very necessary. As I evolve, I have to go on to new people, not the same kind of people I knew 20 years ago. Some people I knew 20 years ago never study now. They're all finished. But I never finished studying. So I have to talk to somebody new who can bring out some of the things that I'm talking about or reading about every day.

The Wise Man Walks Alone

Sometimes I think I'm very much alone because I can't talk about some of the things I've learned. Many others haven't studied, so I can't communicate with them.

This is where we go on alone many times. And this is one thing that I've learned, too, when you get into health work and you develop the body, develop the mind, you start picking out wiser people. Mother used to say that the more truth you get, the more alone you go, and there is a lot of loneliness in this world. A lot of lonely people, too. The wise man is a lonely man.

I've met many remarkable men. I've been with the Masters in India and have seen men who lived on white rice and dung tea. One man had lived on it for forty years and was 110 years of age! But I'll tell you what, I think first of all these men knew how to control their bodies and minds. When I came to them I wanted to know the answer to a certain question, one man said, "Sit down, son." And I sat down cross-legged, lotus leaf position. I sat there for six hours! I got so tired sitting there that I got to the place where I couldn't feel my body anymore. I pinched my skin. The feeling was gone. Finally, I said, "Did you hear my question?" He said, "Yes, I heard your question." I sat there for another half hour. Finally I asked, "Are you going to *answer* my question?" He said, "You sit there long enough and you'll get the answer from the same place I do."

I had to leave. I had to go back to America and I didn't know when that question was going to be answered. But, I remember looking at this man during that six hours. The only thing he moved in his body in six hours was his upper eyelids, four times. That's all he moved in six hours! That man didn't need any food; that man never wore out his body enough to need food. Do you understand that?

Nourish Your Brain And Body

I'm telling you a few things now because some of you are wearing yourselves out faster than you can build up. But, if you could get back to this mental faculty idea and get acquainted with yourself and know how to take care of yourself, you would never burn out the oils in your body. This is the most useful secret I can tell the vegetarian who still has resentment in the body and cannot love completely. He'll burn out the oils in his life. He cannot be a vegetarian because he can't get the brain and nerve foods from a lettuce leaf. The oils aren't there, and we find that many a person today is starving to death on these different diets, and we have to feed these different faculties different foods.

Always Include Brain Food

There are two foods that will feed most of the mental faculties most successfully — egg yolk and goat milk — *raw* goat milk. I believe these will feed the mental faculties better than anything else. Missouri black walnuts are the highest manganese food for feeding the memory faculty. We need that, but the memory faculty is also fed by raw goat milk and egg yolk.

But there isn't any brain food in lettuce. Did you know that? Or in turnips, turnip greens, or in carrots; all the fruits, all the vegetables have nothing for the brain. The brain faculties have to be fed by certain vibratory foods that you don't find in the low vibratory rates of the vegetables and fruits. Foods that feed the brain and nerves have to go through an evolvement.

Your brain faculties know intrinsically what nutrients to select from the blood stream to nourish themselves. Nutrients from goat milk have been organized and evolved for use through the brain, nervous system and glandular system.

Goat milk is wonderful because it comes from an animal that moves nimble and makes a good pet. Goats love people and respond to affection. A goat needs the human touch more than a cow does, and milk from a goat has a chemical balance exactly like mother's milk. There is a rapport that develops between the goat and the milker. That's one reason why goat milk is so good for human beings. The biblical land of "Milk and Honey" refers to goat milk. It wasn't cow's milk. We find out that goats can be treated as part of your own family, and they will respond. Goats increase their milk output when music is played in the barn where they are milked. You'll find out, too, that if you put a stranger in with that goat and that goat doesn't want that stranger to milk her, she'll drop down to one-half of the milk supply she will normally give. Just through resentment. . . just through resistance. The goat has these mental faculties just like a human being does. We find that the milk of human kindness is broken down in our associations with one another.

The Quest For Human Love

Yes, the milk of human kindness can be destroyed. People don't give well unless they're wanted. You've got to go where you're wanted. You've got to go where you're loved, but you've got to love so you'll be loved. I mean it's another story. It comes from within us. I'm bringing these things out because these mental faculties are very important to develop. . .to take with this Great Within and to see what we're made up of. If it is music, if it is charity, if it is loveliness, develop them and make them greater than ever. We start eliminating junk thought and emotions as well as junk foods that feed the lower natures of the body.

We start building the body with good food, and the principle in reaching for the higher things in life, going the higher way and the higher road will get you there. Going the negative way will only bring destruction. You can't get anything but anemia out of pickles and ice cream. There isn't anything else there. Nor can you build a good blood stream from the frying pan! An impossibility!

The Highest Path Should Be Your Choice

So, we have to take this higher road, and we find God in his wonderful wisdom gave us the capacity to choose the higher road. But you have to learn to reach for the higher things. Man can be more than human. He can reach for these higher things. Train yourself to reach for the higher life, the higher things in life.

If I put a poison pickle here in one hand and a ripe apricot in the other hand, which would you choose? Don't tell me. You know you deserve the finest. So, seek out people, who give you the nicer things in life, who want you to be well, who are interested in your song, who are interested in bringing out the lovely things that you have within your soul, your mind.

Most of us are stifled; most of us are stuck; most of us have everything repressed on the inside. No chance to get it out. Some of you need nicer people around you. You may need a trip. Some of you need to work in more harmony. You need more peaceful surroundings. Some of you have to recognize that cold air isn't good for you. Some of you have to recognize that a foggy, clammy day doesn't make you happy. There are some who need a lot more sunshine than others. Some people can live in the fog and feel very good. There are others who don't know that when you get into very dry air, it can produce constipation. Your body molds to these things. Your body molds to the climate; it molds to the air you breathe; it molds to the pollutants that you take in. All of these things your body molds to, and you can have a much better life and body by knowing yourself, knowing that you are a certain kind of person who needs a certain kind of life.

You may be a mental-motive person, a silicon person, or a desmogenic type like I am. I move. If I had to walk up to my house tonight, I wouldn't walk all the way around; I'd jump the fence and go right over. That's my body and you find out, you have to have the foods that feed that kind of body. I'm a sodium type. All of you need certain kinds of foods.

The Whole Path Is the Right Path

When that hair starts to fall what are you going to reach for? Are you going to reach for a salve? Are you going to reach for a shampoo? Or are you going to look for a remedy for the outside of the body? I'm going to tell you to reach for something for the inside; find out what's causing the trouble emotionally. There may be something on the inside of your body that's causing all the trouble. I've seen baldheaded men produced through emotional upsets. It's possible, and we find that our body works as a whole. You're looking at an army of organs and tissues, but the directing general is the brain. I'm stressing this brain more than anything else because you're not going to do it on diet. You're only going to do it on a Healthy

Way of Life. You're going to do it when you get the animal proteins in your diet. It's almost an impossibility to live on nuts which are much higher evolved than many other foods, but we find out they still can't "talk." They still can't work in this mental realm.

The nervous system potential that's found in the egg yolk is going to build your nerves, your nervous system. Many people's nervous systems could be quickened by adding an egg yolk to their diet every day. I bring this out because you don't have to be an extremist. I do not teach extremism in my work. I want you to go down the middle path.

Now...if you could take the right climate, if you could take the right attitude, the right altitude; if you could be married 100 percent and if you could wear fewer clothes and live down around the equator; and if you could walk barefooted most of your life and if you could do all these things that bring on a perfect body, I believe then that you could skimp a little bit on foods and wouldn't have to have animal products whatsoever. But you have to have a certain amount of heat. You don't get any stimulation from lettuce and fruit. You can thin the blood too much. People with cold, clammy hands need silicon. I tell you that goat milk can make them over. So, we find that this food and feeding is for the mind, for the brain. This food and feeding is for the knee, but it's also for the brain faculty that moves the knee. It can't feed the knee alone without feeding the brain. Lots of you have good knees, but you haven't got the brains to make them move. A lot of you have joy, but you can't jump with that joy. Can you understand that? Now we find out that you have to work in all directions to make a whole person.

You really are wonderfully and fearfully made. Stop and think about it.

Chelated Minerals Are In Natural Foods

The chelated minerals are put together so the body can absorb and take care of them, but you find out that natural foods were made that way, too. So man is trying to take certain parts of foods to feed certain parts of the body that are broken down. The body, under the direction of the brain, is able to select from the bloodstream the nutrients it needs. You just give it all the natural things it needs, and you'll find that if the body gets an excess of any of these natural foods, it will throw it off; but it will take what it needs.

That's why we have the law of variety in our diet work. We must have a variety of foods. There are chelated minerals in nuts; there are chelated minerals in an apple. There are chelated minerals in all Nature's foods. Chelated minerals are in all foods if they are natural, pure and whole. Did you get that? Not in as concentrated a form as you can get in a bottle. I will say this: it is possible that

mineral tablets from a bottle will not do you as much good as the chelated minerals in foods that we have today.

Some people using chelated minerals are producing such a dissolving effect with the calcium that's settled in their body that the calcium itself is floating around in the blood stream and will deposit someplace. They have found that people using various treatments to dissolve the calcium in parts of their body are experiencing unanticipated side effects, even to the place of causing invalidism or causing clots that settle in the heart or in the lung structure, sometimes fatal. It's better to go Nature's way. It may take you more time Nature's way, but in one year's time you're younger than you are today, and if in two years, you're better than you were today, take the time out. You're going to live a longer life. You don't need to worry when you live with Nature and the natural things in life. You're going to live a better life for doing it.

Solutions Are Within Us

I want you to think about the brain activity. It's so important...stop breaking down...stop breaking down ...so you don't have to chase a cure. I believe that 90 percent of the cure for every disease is found within ourselves. It's not found in trying to overcome what you have done, but it's in stopping breaking down. It's in living as we were meant to live...breathing as we were meant to breathe ...and associating with people we were meant to associate with.

Minerals Are The Building Blocks

So, we go through life a little wiser for knowing each other and knowing about these things...knowing that silicon holds Vitamin B, and finding that unless you have some mineral that holds Vitamin E, then E will not do you a lot of good either. We do not build bodies on vitamins. Vitamins are like gasoline in an automobile. They are necessary to run the automobile, but they don't build it. It takes minerals, chemical elements to build it.

Minerals are the building blocks. When you look at skin we know that it needs Vitamin B; we know it needs E; we know it needs certain vitamins, but it needs the minerals first. Go for the minerals. We've been built of the dust of the earth and we will return to the dust of the earth. We in this cycle of dust to dust, living beings sculptured out of dust...Mother Earth! Let's go back to Mother Earth and get our nutrients there.

Clays With Healing Properties

Now we have clay...I don't care if it's green, yellow, blue or pink! Green clay has certain properties, and we find out because it's a green clay, it's different from pink clay. We, too, have the different properties or faculties. We have a love memory for animals. We have a love memory for people. We have a love faculty for a woman or for a man or for flowers and they're all different. Now green clay is a little different than pink clay, and we find the different function of that vibratory action may be needed for different people. Wouldn't it be nice to say, "I need green clay today instead of pink clay?" Wouldn't it be nice to know how each clay has a different activity in the body...and it does. I know it does! But on the other hand, I know that clay, most of it, has properties a good deal like Bentonite, which is an active absorptive agent that draws impurities from the tissues. You can use it to tighten up the skin because it is an absorptive agent. It draws out and it dries up. You can use it for face packs if you wish. You can use it on wrinkles. There are many things you can use it for. In Germany they have what they call "lubos mud" and they get it out of mines. Right in Palm Springs, California, they have mines where they get Bentonite. It comes out like a slate and is ground up into a clay. It's the most wonderful thing I know of for sores. Whether the clay we use is green or pink, it has different properties. For healing, green is one of the finest, but I know, too, that when water begins to dissolve this clay there are many trace minerals in it.

Apples from the state of Washington have an entirely different makeup than the apples that are grown in the Salinas Valley. Celery that grows in Utah or Battle Creek, Michigan has much more sodium than celery that grows in New York. There's nearly 20 percent less sodium in New York celery than there is in celery from Michigan or Utah. Utah celery is high in sodium because of the great Salt Lake flats up there. If you want to grow food that has a lot of sodium, you can grow it best up in Utah. We don't grow high-sodium celery here, and, many times I see what they call Utah celery; it's not.

So we need these various biochemical elements, and I believe we can get trace minerals from this clay, and in some places they eat it and they use it for colitis or for rectal troubles. Indians had rectal troubles, but they knew to sit in the mud, and we find out that a dog will do the same thing. He'll get clay, he'll get mud on a sore on his body. I believe that clay has healing qualities; I think it has vibrational properties; I think it has magnetic qualities, and while I don't know which clay would fit a particular disease best or a particular person best, I believe there is a particular best solution for each problem. I think the day will come when we're going to have instruments that will know these things. I think the day will come when we'll know more than we do now in this "hash-house" way of doing things.

Science Can't Rival Nature

But in the meantime...I'm waiting for science to catch up to Nature and to find out what's in Nature. I think it's best to come right back to Nature because there are a lot of things about the chelated minerals that we don't know yet, and there is much to learn. There are a lot of things we don't know about Vitamin B yet, and you know, we now have something like 27 vitamins. I didn't know 27 vitamins existed 15 years ago! The alphabet may not be long enough to name all the vitamins in Nature. Nature has more. I'll bet the last vitamin is in Nature, and I'll bet man hasn't found it yet. Can you understand that? And I'll bet the last star's radiation is found in some of these minerals and trace elements.

Look to Nature First — Not Last

Once I went to see a doctor about a bad cough that hung on for months. I thought for sure I had a cancer. Since I kept clearing my throat constantly for almost six months, I couldn't believe I had to clear my throat so much. So, I thought...well, I'll take the chance and go down and see if I have cancer. So I went in to this doctor and had him examine my throat. He looked at it, and after about five minutes he stood up. He walked around and said, "Why do you clear your throat all the time?" And, I said "I don't know." He said, "Then stop it please: That will be ten dollars." You know, I haven't used that method of clearing my throat any more. As long as that doctor couldn't find a cancer, I wasn't going to make one...I quit!

All of you ought to quit your bad habits. You ought to quit the path you're on. We ought to have learned better by now. Learn about the brain faculties...your brain faculties. Work on your relationships. Understand that it's not necessary to talk about our troubles when we're with one another. We're not really together when we do that. Talk about things that are very lovely...very wonderful. We should train ourselves to talk about positive things. I have trained myself; when I see people, I say, "I feel wonderful." I don't ask people how they are anymore, because they tell me and I don't like it! You have to get over that. I don't let people talk about their troubles to me anymore. So, let us find a better way of doing things. things.

Have you heard the story about the man who had halitosis? He spent $3,000 going to doctors to cure it. He finally got rid of it, and found that nobody wanted him around anyway! The important change to make is on the inside.

Knowledge Without Wisdom Is Useless

Now, there are many hungers for which the brain must care for. There are personality factors that we must care for; there are food factors that we must feed the brain with...there's the love center...there's a soul hunger...and we have to take care of these things.

I wish I could point to one book or one thing that you should study, but you get a little here...a little there and you have to put it all together. What I've presented here is a gathering of many things. But the most important thing is to take care of your brain...take care of knowledge...get all the knowledge you can...get all the wisdom. Wisdom comes from the "wise domain." Live in this wise domain, but don't foreget it comes through the brain. A wise philosopher has said, "Knowledge is proud that it knows so much. Wisdom is humble that it knows so little."

Tropical Delicacies

You ought to visit the West Indies and see the people downing the big white grubs found in the pith of palm trees. That's a sight! They spit 'em on a sliver of palm, toast 'em over hot coals. The nasty looking things swell up and pop open like roasted chestnuts. In Mexico (as Verrill relates) no wedding feast is complete without a dish of honey ants.

The egg mass of the water beetle is also considered a real delicacy and is gathered and marketed in vast quantities.

In Brazil and Guiana, the big queens of the vicious umbrella ants grace the epicurean tables. Traveling in the jungle, the carriers throw down their loads when they discover a big ant's nest with myriads of insects swarming about their big-winged queen. Heedless of the bites from these warrior-ants, with blood streaming down their legs from the punctures made by the insects, the men scramble over to the nests, gathering the queens by the handsful. Then, brushing off the biting ants, they retire to a safe distance, squat down and munch the queens with as much enjoyment as children eating candy. These ant queens are half an inch long with bodies distended with gooey eggs and taste like condensed milk. Folks down there also eat with gusto the big fat brown sphinx-moth caterpillars; they drop them in boiling grease. They puff up and brown and look like fritters.

Breast-Fed Babies

We are inclined to think that we can make a substitute on nature at any time in our growing pattern that we wish. It is impossible to start the baby out on any formula or any substitute for mother's milk that can equal that which the mother can furnish the baby. We have a lot of knowledge today that is not too good for us and when we try to substitute the sweetness found naturally in the mother's milk by using saccharine, a coal tar product or Karo syrup or any other abnormal substitute sweetening products used in the formulas, we only harm the baby. We use pasteurized or homogenized milk and the vitamin C content which is found in the regular milk has been so destroyed and is so negligible that it is practically nonexistent. Vitamin C is the vitamin that protects us from colds and helps the body in cases of catarrhal discharges. A baby fed on a milk formula is depleted of the vitamin C and this lack is one of the causes of many colds for the baby.

II
Nature does the curing

"Nature does the curing; but She needs an opportunity."

The word "physician" originally referred to a health teacher. The term has drifted far from this initial meaning today, now generally describing one who administers drugs or treatments to suppress localized symptoms. In fact, little is known about the basis and cause of disease or poor health symptoms. Thus we find that no permanent restoration of health is obtained through the method of symptom suppression.

Lucille Steele, author of *Food Science, Nature's Supreme Healing Art*, sums up the work of Nature — the greatest physician and the true healer — by writing, "It is Nature alone who can assemble usable material to rebuild an organ or any part of the body." We find that drugs cannot rejuvenate or rebuild tissue.

She continues, "In her process of recuperation, or rebuilding worn out tissues Nature uses no drugs or chemicals — except those sytetically prepared by action of the sun and soil through growing plant life...It is obvious that foodstuff and oxygen alone, contribute in many ways to tissue building within the body."

There is a definite obligation on the doctor's part to see that his patient is taken care of properly. The obligation in the future is to recognize that there is a preventive medicine way and it may be in our foods; it may be in our kitchens, in our pantries. The new age doctor has an obligation to his patient to see that he or she is knowledgable — that the material is placed before the patient.

The doctor cannot make a patient do what has to be done. We find that the wise man waits for the student and as soon as the student is ready and wants to learn, *ALL* good things will be revealed to him. It is not a matter of any secrets in life. All of this is for you the moment you are ready. We feel that the greatest obligation of anyone learning this Nature healing work, or wanting even to keep well in these disasterous days of sickness, hardship and misery, is to reach for the higher things that will make better body tissues, to rise above the main street foods of the "coffee and doughnut" stage, the "pickle and ice cream" consciousness. For the person who wants to get out of this state of being there is a way and it will be revealed to him or her. There are no secrets in Nature.

The new age doctor should be ready to refer the proper information and material to that person who wants to live correctly. We are living in an age where we expect "George" to do everything for us. We are living in an age of treatments, pills and drugs. We are our own best nurse; we are our own doctor to a great extent. And it is necessary to recognize that our kitchen is the place for the making of the new tissue that is coming into the body this next week — two weeks — that is responsible and basic in respect to building new brain substance, new cartilage, new kidney tissue or a better digestive tract or a feeling of well-being as we go through these things. Our mind, our body and all our endeavors in life are dependent on how well or how healthy we are. The few moments, or few hours, that you take to learn to use this book properly will mean the difference between having the best health or just mediocre health or no health at all.

The wise man picks out his friends; he chooses his environment; he selects his food also. This is the value that we are trying to impart to you. There is a new-day consciousness arriving, and it's one found not only in the doctor, but in the patient of the new age. We're going to have to have a new conciousness in the patient we handle. A new breed of doctors are coming into existence. Many are going to learn to work with Nature and natural healing methods because they need it themselves. They're going to live right and impart how their patients should live from what they have learned in their personal experience. After all, doctors have children and families as well as anyone else, and this is for the family.

We realize also that there must be a new breed of patients in the near future. It is too difficult for a doctor to help a patient get well who doesn't live right. I am positive without a shadow of a doubt that 50 percent of the hospital cases could be cut out by following a sound basic diet such as the one I advise. I am convinced that we can prevent at least 50 percent of the arthritic conditions as found in this country. I am convinced that 25 percent of the mental cases could be removed from the mental hospitals and kept out by following this nutrition regimen. I am convinced, too, that the diabetes we are treating today — while we may control it with insulin and pancreatin maneuvering — could be prevented or taken care of by proper diet measures. I am convinced that 75 percent of the asthma cases would never happen if they knew this particular diet work we are teaching. I'm convinced that 50 percent of the most frequently used drugs would be found unnecessary from the standpoint of treating allergies, infections in the body, bowel disorders, heart troubles and so forth. Laxatives could be dispensed with entirely if a good dietary regimen was followed. Epidemics would be cut out or at least greatly reduced. But this new breed of doctor — new age wholistic doctor — will undertake a new system of healing — one of teaching the patient how to live correctly.

The new day doctor is going to have to spend a certain amount of time writing, lecturing, teaching and setting up health facilities for public good health. He's going to have to get in and work for humanity's good in his spare time. He's going to have to realize that there's a dedication to the health and welfare of his patients. The knowledge that this doctor has will help him educate his patients, to make them better patients.

The patient must realize that there must be a place where he can get the right information and training for better health Nature's way. As doctors see the dawning of a new day, their colleges and universities will teach nutrition. The patient won't have the trouble finding a good doctor as he or she may have in the past. The new day is dawning.

DID YOU KNOW THAT...

"Nutrition" is the sum of the processes concerned with growth, maintenance and resistance to disease?

The life cycle is 5 times the age of maturity?

If we can help our body cells by supplying them with the chemicals they need in our foods, we can make old age wait?

Lately there has been an increase in the bulk and yield in crops and animal foods, but a loss in protein value and an increase in carbohydrate and fat content? So, we are becoming overstuffed, but undernourished.

88 million people are suffering from chronic conditions?

Most people are consuming 5 ounces of saturated fats a day, when only 1/2 ounce is needed?

Sodium nitrite (a commonly used preservative) prevents hemoglobin from picking up oxygen?

Children 1 to 14 years of age have the highest cancer death rate?

One person in three will develop cancer?

Cigarettes are sold at the rate of 3,500 per capita each year?

During a day, the body requires 2-1/2 pounds of food, 4 pounds of water and 30 pounds of air?

Experiments with laboratory animals show that the rate of cancer can be reduced by feeding them yeast and liver? A lower intake of starches, sugars and fats brings about a reduction. In the tumor stage, the cancer subsides.

With a vitamin C deficiency, we bruise easily, gums bleed, teeth loosen? These days, we need extra vitamin C because so much is used up counteracting poisonous chemicals.

People who have weaknesses of the glands should look to the glandular foods such as sesame seed, squash seed, sunflower and flaxseeds, raw peanuts, raw whole wheat? As a matter of fact, any live food is a glandular food. Remember sprouts. Any sprouts are good, but particularly alfalfa. Raw turnips, raw radishes and tops should be included.

Chapter 7

Life, light, color and vibrations

We should always know what our thoughts will do
In bringing us hate or love;
For thoughts are things
And their airy wings
Are as swift as a carrier dove.
They follow the law of the universe—
Each thing must produce its kind;
And they speed o'er the track
And bring us back
Whatever went out from our mind
(Unknown author)

Nature Is the True Physician

Food is not everything we have to watch for. Man has gotten off on the wrong foot today, in most of his thinking. He wants to have his cake and eat it, too, so to speak. He wants to live on the worst possible foods and then take something for alkalinizing his stomach, for the headache that may result or the constipation that may come later He is constantly fixing things up, while if he did the right thing in the beginning he wouldn't have that trouble. We find that there are other things that are coming in the future and science is running away with us. They have to realize that Nature could keep us in control and keep us well.

Scientists Are Developing Weapons

In the past 16 years 3 trillion dollars have been spent in developing weapons to kill our fellowmen, says the Arms Control Association of the International Peace Research Institute and other research organizations. Nearly $25 billion is spent each year in the world for military research. THIS IS ROUGHLY 4 TIMES WHAT IS SPENT IN HEALTH RESEARCH. It is said that a recent year's world military budget was nearly $30 billion.

A Synthetic Heaven on Earth??

Americans consume enough barbiturates, amphetamines and tranquilizers to administer 65 doses of these drugs to virtually every man, woman and child in the country according to "Today's Health."March 1974.
Man is becoming progressively more materialistic and egocentric, essentially promising a synthetic paradise on earth. Alcohol, however, is the most widely exploited and abused drug in the U.S. today. Over nine million Americans are alcoholics and it is claimed that over 50 percent of our crimes are alcohol related.

We will enumerate a few of the drugs currently under research and consideration. A fertility control pill is being devised to render one infertile for 20 years. New chemical aphrodisiacs are being investigated to increase sexual appetite, potency, etc. A hibernation drug is being contemplated which will induce human hibernation in case of famine. Appetite appeasement pills will chemically ease hunger pangs. A drug is being considered to combat boredom, sloth, melancholy, despair and other depressions. Mind-expanding drugs will carry man to mystical heights never before experienced. Intelligence quotient pills will be able to raise I.Q. levels, to improve memory, enhance talents *and* control intellects. Also, research is underway constantly and feverishly to increase longevity. The question arises, what do we want mind expansion for?? What are the good and evil consequences accompanying such undertakings? Science may be able to create such marvels, but does that mean we should use them?

What Will Life Be Like in the 21st Century?

Man is increasingly leaving his life to science. Mother Nature is seldom consulted, but is she ever misrepresented!

Some of the predictions for the quality and manifestation of life in the future are incredible, but not to some doctors and scientists. It is believed by the scientific communtiy that drugs will cure mental illness, raise the I.Q. level, reverse the progress of cancer and allow people to grow new limbs. In addition a chemical substitute for human blood — the life stream — is being worked on. These disclosures were made in a new study by McGraw-Hill Publishing Company from the predictions of 131 of America's top doctors and scientists.

"Electronic prosthesis — the replacement of lost arms and legs with electronic limbs that will function better than the originals—will be widely available," said Douglas Greenwald, who led the study.
new limbs early in the next century — possibly by the year 2050."

He continued, "By the 1990's we'll see the widespread use of drugs to permanently raise the intelligence of people. A few years later, we'll have chemical control of aging — and total elimination of senility with drugs by 1995."

"Also, before the end of this century, we expect to find chemical substitutes for blood," Greenwald added, "eliminating the need for blood banks, and putting an end to deaths due to lack of blood supplies."

The researcher emphasized that the advances depended on the funding of medical and scientific research.

We don't know what this means to the quality and sacredness of life as the Creator originally intended. Why should so many of these scientific and medical interventions be necessary? Didn't the concept of life include natural health and vital strength from harmony with the laws of Nature and the Universe? How many of those laws are we breaking? How many will we have to answer for ultimately?

Mind Is Stronger than Matter

The visible realm is composed of force and matter. Of course, matter is what we call rock substances which we can feel and taste and see. We do not realize that this matter comes out of the invisible. There is more in the invisible that makes up the construction of matter than we realize. From the invisible to the visible is the order of material existence without a single exception in the Universe. We know that there are many substances that exist which we cannot see. For instance, we have never seen the wind. There are many substances too subtle to be capable of making any perceptible impression upon the brain cells. We walk through streams of wind and never see them, but we see the cyclones and extreme wind storms and the destruction they leave in their wake. Wind certainly is real and we cannot deny that it does exist. There are many objects in the air that we cannot see. They are very finite. If you walked through a fog with your eyes closed you wouldn't even know it was present. I have flown through clouds many times in our plane trips and I often wonder how we can do this without any perceptible knowledge on our senses. Yet a congealment of this fine mist can form mighty floods with enough power to destroy man-made bridges and buildings.

Mind Organizes Matter

There is much to realize when we stop and consider that we have so many of the bio-chemical elements in our bodies. Probably one of the greatest statements to make and yet a lot of people wouldn't realize it, is that the working of our mind is central to the proper directing of the bio-chemical food elements that makes up our bodies. We find out that hard thoughts, angry thoughts, hating thoughts can't possibly put this bio-chemical matter in the right place.

The World Beyond the Five Senses

The day is coming when we realize that there is something to mind power and it will be mind over matter. Many of the things we see, hear, feel and smell are simply mental states. We find that the brain does not see; the optic nerve does not see, nor does the eye. The function of sight arises as a result of the light vibrations striking upon the optic nerve terminals in the retina of the eye. We live in a world of light vibrations and we depend upon this vibration. We have to have sufficient strength in these vibrations to make an impression on the brain cells. Otherwise, the mental condition of sight is not produced.

The Unseen World of Vibrations

We have to recognize that there are different levels of vibration and possibly many more than the brain may even be aware of, at least those that can come to our perceptions, recognition and conscious awareness. There is a definite limit to human powers, especially among those who insist that matter is all we have. When we stop to think about it, oxygen, hydrogen and nitrogen have never been seen, and yet they make up 85 percent of the human body. Oxygen makes up half of the entire substance composing the earth. Rocks are almost 50 percent oxygen.

Can Animals Predict Earthquakes

Accurate predictions of earthquakes are at least 10 years away, say most experts. But while man is searching for the answers animals may have always had them. Chinese and other Eastern seismologists believe that certain animals are natural earthquake barometers. They seem to have an innate sense of impending quakes and change their behavior patterns accordingly. Some of the creatures they speak of are pigs, dogs, chickens and fish.

Two UCLA researchers have been awarded a research grant of $23,000 from the U.S. Geological Survey to see if animals are indeed capable of forecasting earthquakes when humans can't. The research, by geophysicist Dr. Durward Skiles and biologist Dr. Rogert Lindberg, began with seven pocket mice and 20 kangaroo rats as draftees. The scientists chose these rodents because they are native to the area and are burrowing animals naturally close to the earth. Also both species have predictable behavior patterns. Unofficial reports say that animals usually become hyperactive before a quake, but some may huddle together in inactivity. These observations lack scientific backing, however. The make-shift laboratory is situated in San Bernardino County on the southern edge of the Palmdale Bulge.

Maybe animals sense a vibration too sensitive for human faculties to comprehend. After all, dogs can hear higher frequency sounds than humans can detect. But at this point all is speculation. If the scientists prove that animals sense upcoming quakes, then they must try to determine how this is possible. Geophysicists now associate impending earthquake periods with foreshocks, magnetic field variations and the release of gases from rocks and ground water. The scientific community hopes to duplicate this animal talent with instruments or to set up the animals as monitoring stations to warn of coming tremors. Chinese and Japanese earthquake authorities have claimed for centuries that animals behave strangely before an earthquake, but American scientists have not acknowledged such assertions. In October of 1976 a Geophysical Survey Conference opened the subject of animal kingdom earthquake predictions and the research is still in its infancy. But, it is something for us to think about.

Perhaps the unseen is more real than we realize.

Science Can't Duplicate the "Human Machine"

The difference between a man-made machine and the machine that God created is that man is self-starting, self-building, self-operating, self-governing, self-adjusting, self-repairing, self-regenerating. We find that the substance and parts of the man-made machine are entirely different from the tissues of the human body. No one can make human tissues — no physician, no chemist, no biologist. With all his learning and skill, today's scientist is far from making the simplest part or particle of the human machine. Nor can he explain even the simplest of its processes.

Does the Physical Body Possess Life?

There has been much said from the scientist's standpoint and from many a person in humanistic studies, and they're all asking, "What is life?" When we look around us we see people, animals and plants, and they are all living. But the life that makes up the unseen part of our environment is more multitudenous and universal and influential on our lives than that which is seen. Another question is one of profound mysteries in our science. They have explored human tissue down to the single cell and its process, but exactly what makes that cell alive is not known. The power of unfolding any physical thing that we may see is found in the Vital Force that operates in the plant, the animal or the man, and it is that force which

vitalizes the seed and causes it to sprout and to grow. Force is invisible; its presence is known only by its effects. Life Force is always a prerequisite to doing work in any material form. This force must be intellingently and persistently applied.

I like the thought of this little poem:

The law which molds the tear,
And bids it trickle from its source,
That law preserves the earth, a sphere,
And guides the planets in their course.

It is natural law that keeps us in the shape we are in. By working with this universal force we can make changes through the matter, the food, the sunshine we live in and the good habits we keep. There is a Hidden Artist who performs this art of the making of man. And it has been said by Drummond, "The Artist who operates upon matter in this subtle way and carries out his law, is life."

It is hard to give a definition of life. But it is said very well in the Good Book: "It is the spirit that quickeneth; the flesh profiteth nothing." It is the spirit that quickens the flesh and though it may be quickened by life, it is physically still flesh made from the dust of the ground. Life is not the function of the body; it is the source of the function; life is the builder, the Hidden Artist. When we have seen a person inactive — even many pronounced dead — we find out that the signs of life are not there although the body has changed very little certainly, we can't detect any physical changes that have taken place at death — only fuctional changes. Yes, we know the heart stopped beating, the brainwaves fell quiet; but why?

It isn't through a greater microscope to aid our human vision that gravitation will be revealed to us; neither will it reveal life. We cannot see the force that holds us on the earth. We cannot see the force that animates our form. Life is the invisible force that moves. Matter is the visible form that is moved. We have an idea that when we see matter moving we say it is alive and it moves by the virtue of its own power; but this is not true; it is not truth. We know that the unknown is understood by its law. For instance, we see the ray of light passing invisibly through space and we only see its colors as it passes through some object like the prism or reflects from the things of this earth. Life passes invisibly through space, permeating and penetrating all things down into the deepest recesses of the earth. It is truly well-said that, "In Him we live and move and have our being." Even going further, "The Father that dwelleth in me, He doeth the works."

We can ask the question, "Can the open eye of a dead man see?" If the eye itself is possessed of the power of sight then the eye of the dead man could see equally well as the eye of the living man. For what is lacking in death that is not lacking in life? We say that in death the life of the man has gone out of him — a thing you cannot feel, you cannot discover by any of the human senses, but is of the greatest reality in this world. Only faith can deal with this. The things that are seen are temporal; the things that are not seen are eternal. The eye of itself has no more capacity to see than has a glass eye lying in a jewelry store. The eye is made up of many chemical elements, and for Life Force to make that eye anew it has to have all the elements to work with and must know where to put them. It is this God-given force within us that needs a good environment, that needs everything to work with. And you find that all things can be made new by this Life Force that is within you asking to be fed, to be taken care of, to be given all that it needs, through the dust of the earth. The same applies to every organ in the body and the brain itself, which possibly we think "sees" more than the eye itself. Yet, again, in its physical condition it must have the elements for the building of the temple of the body and when that temple has deteriorated, it needs the right elements for rebuilding. That's the key for the building of a good body, the goal you are seeking.

We have to look at this body as a temple of the Living God; it is simply a house that is built with mineral materials. We recognize that with this Life Force we can build this body beautiful with all sensations working well, knowing and having every one of the senses working in good condition by just making sure that we put to the Life Force all that it needs to make this new body. When we look at this we can almost come to the conclusion that all sensation resides in life itself and not in the physical body that you think is you.

The Body's Vital Force

To have a better definition of life, science holds onto the idea that life is a manifestation of electric energies, magnetic energies and chemical activities of the physical, material elements composing the living organism. It was Dewey who said that the head is the powerhouse of the human plant, and we find that the dynamo or the brain is the source of every possible human energy. Dewey pointed out that through the power of the brain we are able to carry on all the activities of life — physical, mental and vital. Disease is cured through the power evolving and emanating from the brain. An exhibition of the physical energy flowing from the Vital Force is called strength.

Sunshine Is A "Doctor," Too

During the spring and summer months when the child gets plenty of sunshine he grows, but he practically stands still through the winter. This is the reason that in the tropics where the sunlight is so prolific that man reaches maturity by his 14th year. man responds the same as

flowers to the sun and is influenced by the sun. If man is deprived of sunlight he withers and dies.

Go back and see where Zoroaster of Persia, Hippocrates of Greece and many others of the past have looked to the sun as the life-giving energy source we have to look to. They considered it a god and a force that man needed to live. Sunshine in the future may be considered not in terms of how it destroys germ life in our cities but in terms of how it raises the resistance of our bodies to overcome germ life.

There was a health officer at one time in England by the name of Dr. J. Bell Furgeson. He had a schoolroom glazed with a form of quartz glass that permitted some 50 to 60 percent of the ultraviolet rays of the sun to pass through. He had another room the same size and with the same exposure that was glazed with ordinary lead glass. children were put in these rooms in the school where they studied under these two different types of glass and Dr. Furgeson found that those who were in the quartz glass room gained an average of an inch more in height and three and one-fourth pounds more in weight than the children under ordinary glass.

If we watch the animals in sunshine we find that they avoid the heat and seek the shade when it grows hot. The heat is depressing and enervating. We find that with a sufficient amount of sunshine and ultraviolet rays, the blood corpuscles can be built up in the blood. Those people who live in large cities in tenement houses have the greatest infant mortality rate and, of course, we also know it is the chief breeding place of calcium deficiencies, bowleggedness and tuberculosis. The milk from cows that live in lots of sunshine sustains their young calves very well. But those cows that live out of the sun, fed on fodder, will not sustain the life of their young ones as well. This is according to the research of Dr. Hess of Columbia University.

Mules used in underground mines have considerably more eye trouble than the mules working out in the sunshine above the ground.

The World Beyond Five Senses

In talking about vibration we might just mention that man lives in his own little five-sense world. He doesn't live beyond and in the vast unknown. Without the five sense organs man would be as unconscious of his own existence as a stone. We find that the vibratory rate can be felt through our senses and is found so in plant and animal life as well. It has well been said that man without the special sense organs would be as one buried in a dark silent tomb, not unlike a corpse in the grave. He would be blind and deaf without the ability to taste touch or smell. He would be destitute of feeling, insensible to cold and heat, to odors and sound, to bitter and sweet, to light and darkness.

Vision occurs within the brain; we sometimes think

we see in front of us or outside of us. We say that the sun rises in the East and sets in the West, but yet, again, it is the rotation of the earth on its axis. So you see, we are deceived by our senses. You think the earth is motionless; you sit and relax and everything is serene; yet the earth is whirling through space faster than a bullet and turning on its axis at the same time. Thus, we are deceived by our senses. We see various colors, and they come to us as various waves of vibration. You actually can run your hands through them. And we find this high vibration — ranging from low [red] to a high [violet] in the color realm — and it is only felt in the brain which is capable of registering.

We think we hear the sounds of horns, violins and so forth. These instruments produce vibrations that agitate the atmosphere causing it to strike against the tympanic membrane of the ear. It is here that the vibrations are carried by the auditory nerve to the brain. A Mr. Kellogg in Central California used a certain note and a certain sound and could put out a lit bunsen burner at some distance. In fact, over a radio station, he was able to produce this sound and through the radio waves received by a receiver set (and the sound) was able to put out a bunsen burner 500 miles away. The vibrations give off no sound; we are not conscious of the sound until the vibrations reach the brain where they are translated into a mental state called sound.

Every cell has a vibration because of the chemical balance within it. The vibration rate of calcium is different from that of silicon. The sum total of the vibratory rates of all chemical elements in the cells and interstitial fluid between them gives the vibratory rate to organs. This is why we have health vibratory rates and disease vibratory rates.

Raising our Vibratory Rate

The chemistry of the body builds up the vital forces in the body; it builds up the vibratory rate of expression that we have, the power to visualize, to take on challenge, to run or to jump and it is this that gives us the will and the resistive power deep within ourselves to take on the power to prevent disease. The vital force in our body called life force, magnetism and many other different names is actually the universal "medicine" in our body. This is well when the chemistry of the body is kept in top order. It is the vibratory force in the body that is important to attract and direct the chemical elements, and this comes before anything else. But the body is kept in good running order by the foods we eat. I sometimes think this vital force comes from breathing, inspiration, from sunlight, from motivation, from being satisfied, relieved, feeling secure. All these things enter into the body's vital force or vital energy.

More About "Dr's Light and Sunshine"

Exposure to fluorescent lighting robs the body of Vitamin A — especially the eyes. Some authorities have stated that we can't have good eyesight and good hair when exposed to a lot of fluorescent lighting. Others believe they affect reproduction and cause tooth decay. Sun glasses block part of the sun's full spectrum of light. They shouldn't be used and glasses should have plastic lenses that let the full spectrum of light into the eye. Plastic lenses only block 15% of the ultraviolet light and glass lenses block 85%.

Sunlight is invaluable for producing Vitamin D — the "sunshine" vitamin in the body. When the skin receives ultraviolet light from the sun it changes a skin sterol into Vitamin D, and this is slowly absorbed back into the body. But we find the oily substance on the skin called 7-dehydrocholesterol comes from a diet of fats, especially the unsaturated fatty acids and sterols. Washing the skin before sunbathing or less than six hours after removes these body oils and Vitamin D before the body can absorb it.

It was John Ott who wrote in the book, *Health and Light*, that his arthritis improved when he got rid of his sunglasses and spent lots of time outdoors in sunshine. The new science called phototherapy is being noticed more these days, even using light to treat jaundice in premature infants and malignant tumors.

What is full spectrum light? Natural sunlight in a continuous spectrum that starts in the invisible infrared, peaks in blue-green, and has its end in the ultra-violet wave lengths. The earth's ozone belt has a lot to do with light rays. The ozone belt protects the earth from harmful short ultra-violet light rays. You may recall that the supersonic transport (SST) was opposed by some scientists who said its exhaust fumes would let more harmful ultra-violet rays reach the earth by lessening the ozone in the atmosphere. And we find out that the spray cans containing fluorocarbons have been said to harm the ozone layer.

However, we have to consider the new high rise office buildings that have all artificial light and some of them *no* windows at all. What effects do they have on health? The lighting is either fluorescent or incandescent. What about the people who wear glasses or contacts all the time and those who don't step outside without sunglasses? And there are car windshields, X-rays, television sets and nightlife events.

An experiment with rats kept under fluorescent lights should make us think about some of the effects. The rats became irritable, and if the males weren't removed at the time babies were born they were likely to turn cannibalistic! The fathers kept under full spectrum light were loving and helped care for the young.

In another case at a zoo, the birds wouldn't mate unless they were kept under full spectrum light. And poultry raisers find that egg production is increased under light. It does this by passing through the eye of the chicken and stimulating the pituitary gland.

Another study by the Russians says ultra-violet light raises concentration, increases attention and improves brain functioning. Still another U.S. finding was that there is less tooth decay under full spectrum lighting.

We absorb light in two ways according to MIT scientist, Dr. Richard J. Wurtman. The direct way is through the skin and the indirect way is through the eyes to the endocrine system. The pineal gland above the pituitary is known to intercept light impulses from the optic nerves.

Dr. Albert Schweitzer found that in working with Africans they didn't have much cancer until they began wearing sunglasses. It sounds unbelievable, doesn't it? But if we stop and think about it we know so very little about the finer forces in life and in Nature perhaps we should study them more.

What can you and I do to get the most from full spectrum and natural sunshine? Throw away your sunglasses. Get plastic lens glasses and go with out them often in the daylight and open air. Ask your optometrist about full spectrum glasses and plastic lenses. Look into the new full spectrum lighting that is available. It is best not to use glass covers on lights.

Is Gene Splicing Another Pandora's Box?

A battle within the scientific community rages over the moral and scientific possibilities of the new research that recombines genes of differing organisms to make entirely new forms of life. The real question is whether the box that has been opened will prove good or evil. Has science "fooled Mother Nature" in a way that will prove detrimental to life on earth?

We find that until this new recombinant DNA research breached a genetic barrier, unlike species of organisms were unable to mate and reproduce due to genetic differences specifically *insured* by Nature. Does science have the moral and technical right to tamper with the very essence of life? The favorite guinea pig of the laboratories in this testing is the Escherichia coli, (E. coli) a laboratory strain from the human intestinal tract. This bacteria contains some three to four thousand genes that have been identified. But we find that humans contain hundreds of thousands of genes in 46 human chromosomes. At the present time scientists across the nation are recombining genes of E. coli DNA with the DNA of plants and animals and bacteria. This may result in new forms of life that have never existed before on earth.

Questions have been raised in Congress, the White House and the Health Education & Welfare Department concerning the need for federal and local regulations controlling such unprecedented scientific experiments. Congress is preparing legislation for federal controls now. The National Institute of Health (NIH) has formed guidelines for research using highly controlled environments with decontamination chambers, sealed and airlocked containers and so forth. Universities and institutes across the nation are building similar though less security oriented facilities.

One of the proposed security measures is to develop a defective strain of E. coli that could not survive out of the controlled environment of the laboratory, and without materials supplied by the scientists. However, you will recall that a bacteria has developed a resistance to penicillin treatment recently. The same principle, that of different plastids, smaller closed loops of DNA that are made up of only a few genes, pass from one bacteria to another during reproduction. When cell division, or reproduction takes place the new hybrid plastids become part of the new carbon copy. Researchers say they have perfected a defective E. coli that is safe for experimental use.

It was about five years ago that scientists in California first successfully combined genes from different organisms. By adding only one or two new genes a hybrid was produced that was strictly contrary to the genetic laws of nature and evolution.

A temporary ban was requested in April 1974 on certain recombinant DNA research that involved animal tumor viruses and viruses that increased drug resistence or toxicity. In the summer of 1976 the NIH set guidelines of safety according to the danger level of experiments and their risks from high-security to normal laboratory precautions.

Those that favor the "paved road to the promised land" of this new research say that it can lead to cures for cancer, diabetes, hemophilia and other diseases, pollution control; improved agriculture without fertilizers; new antibiotics and vaccines; and even improved human beings! On the other hand, those who oppose it say it could lead to new diseases and epidemics that we are unable to control. It could destroy the balance and harmony of Nature's and God's domain.

Nobel Prize-winning scientist, George Wald said society could fight cancer more effectively by taking carcinogens out of the enviroment than by looking for the cause of cancer through genetic research and recombinant DNA testing.

The DNA factor can be altered by splicing genes in the laboratory test tubes any way the scientist chooses. They can produce humped over people, people with less vertibrae in the spine; they can produce abnormal bone structures; they can produce three eyes or one eye in a person if they want to. And I believe we have to be very careful of leaving our lives and our future in the hands of the scientist. They are beginning to recognize that this probably can be a very dangerous thing. They've already been able through electronic control of seeds to produce a destruction of the gene life that results in the most unusual and atrocious looking flowers, buds, trees and so forth. And now they are thinking about trying this in the human being and in test-tube babies.

One of the main things we can learn from the gene-splicing issue is just how much of our lives we have trusted to scientists. We have left our foods to science for many decades. We have canned our foods, preserved our foods, according to their guidelines. We have found scientific ways of killing germ life in the foods. But we have also destroyed a lot of other useful things. For instance, the enzymes, natural digestive aids, aren't present in foods that are "dead" due to preservatives, salting, pickling, additives, etc. This destroys the biochemical balance of the body. We are scientific-minded today and if science says it we follow. But we have to back up a little bit and keep science from taking "over the hill," so to speak. There has to be a line between what belongs to science and what is Nature's.

One of the greatest potential dangers, if man gets the opportunity, is controlling our weather. Scientists have arrived at the place now where they're able to seed the clouds to bring rain. and this is only the beginning of one thing used in controlling our weather. We find out that the nuclear bomb tests over the years and even the aerosol gases from pressurized spray cans that have been banned are changing our atmosphere. In changing our atomosphere, we're changing the weather. If we are going to try to control our weather, we may encounter changes we didn't foresee, changes that require us to have a different lung capacity, a different lung structure, a different body entirely. We may even have to alter the medulla of the brain to redirect or reprogram our respiratory and cardiovascular functions. So, man is gettng mixed up with scientific progress, and all I can say is that we must be very careful in our next steps.

We find that throughout the world racial decline and racial degeneration is coming about. The nations of the world today no longer live that natural life they lived in the past. The cultures are gone. Science has moved in— new plows, new tractors; new technology. The horse is beginning to leave. A well known hotel chain has moved into the land of the Hunzas, even. We find out that we have made a change with progress and technology as our guide. I'm sure it's going to be profitable, but I wonder if it's going to be healthy. How long can we survive in this scientific and synthetic world?

In experimenting with test-tube organisms what are scientists doing to humanity? We will get into trouble with genes and test tube babies because the mother transfers an aura of feeling and surrounds the child with it before birth, at birth and even after birth. We are developing a hard-hearted race to contend with. Everybody is a number. There are few deep feelings anymore. Test-tube babies will be able to adjust to any environment — a police state, military state, state of greed, anything. Yet, right now there are people who wonder where the next dollar will come from, where energy will come from ,where food will come from. We are in survival times now, friends, and we must think about what the world is coming to.

Foods and Color Healing

We must have beauty and color in our foods. Yellow fruits and vegetables are laxitive. Black berries are used to stop diarrhea; black is an astringent color. The greatest rejuvenators are the greens. Chlorophyll is one of the greatest blood builders you can put into the body. All the black berries, give you iron. Every sick person needs this. We can't have all brown, fried foods — brown steak, brown fried potatoes. They're monocolored, limited, and you'll find they can't build a good body. Cod liver oil and castor oil are laxatives by color. Some of the blood building foods are dark red cherries and beets; green foods are body mineralizers.

Here is a more complete list of the colors in foods:

Red:	Yellow:
apples	bananas
beets	corn
red cabbage	eggs
cayenne pepper	figs
cherries	lemons
radishes	olive oil
strawberries	castor oil
tomatoes	pineapple
raspberries	prunes
red currants	yams
red plums	yellow squash
watermelon	parsnips
black cherries (deep red)	peaches, etc.

Green:	Orange:
avocado	apricots
cucumber	cantaloupe
beans	carrots
broccoli	mangos
green pepper	persimmons
asparagus	tangarines
spinach	nectarines
peas	pumpkin, etc.
beet greens	
okra	
chives	**Blue:**
leaf lettuce	
vegetable greens	blueberries
wheat grass juice	blue plum
parsley, etc.	grapes, etc.

Indigo:

included foods under
blue and violet.

Violet:

blackberries (deep red)
eggplant
purple grapes, etc.

We know that health depends partly on a variety of color foods in the food program. [Refer to *Journey Into Color* by Dr. Jensen for more on color and its effect through vibration.]

Natural Remedies

Let us use Nature's remedies. We are so in the habit of expecting to get rid of things in a hurry that the doctor who can erase symptoms overnight is considered the best man. But getting rid of these troubles in a hurry is not always the best way. It takes time to repair tissue. It takes 24 hours to make new tissue in the palm of your hands, and anyone who is trying to make a new stomach overnight and thinks he has done it by coating it with some artificial food preparation or drug isn't working with Nature. If you really want to get rid of leg ulcers, you will find that chlorophyll salve (made with liquid chlorophyll in lanolin, a sheet fat that will hold the chlorophyll) is quite a wonderful ointment. Garlic oil is a wonderful healer. Mix garlic oil with lanolin. This makes an effective ointment for rashes and other breaking out of the skin.

Make sure that you use teas for the weaknesses in your body. Everyone should find the tea that best fits his weakness. If you have weak kidneys, try cornsilk tea. (When you are buying corn, save the tassels or the silk at the ends; dry it and use it for a tea.) Parsley tea is also excellent for the kidneys. Use papaya tea for a weak digestion, flaxseed for the bowels, oatstraw for skin and hair beauty, valerian to help you sleep. There is no reason why we shouldn't know our foods well enough to use them for healing.

When buying corn, always make sure it is the yellow type. Yellow corn has 4% phosphates, while white corn only has 2%. You need these phosphates in your body for the brain and nervous system. I've never found anyone too alert. I've never found anyone with a memory that was too good for them. I've never found anyone with a mind which couldn't be improved. So let us all have more phosphates as found in yellow corn. The best way to use yellow corn for the greatest health benefit possible is as a liquefied soup. Learn how to make it.

RAW CORN SOUP. Liquefy the corn (fresh corn-off-the-cob preferred) in a little hot water, add soymilk or some sweet raw cream, and for seasoning, add vegetable broth powder. This makes the most nutritious raw creamed corn soup that you would ever want to eat. And I know it is 100% good food. For a smoother "bland" soup, sieve out the corn hulls after blending.

Yellow corn has been used by whole countries: Guatamala, Mexico and the countries of South America. It is considered one of the finest foods you can get to keep you well. It is almost a whole food. If I were to tell you one of the finest oils for your kitchen shelf, it wouldn't just be wheat germ oil, it would be corn germ oil. This corn germ oil is just as important in taking care of your heart, to give tone in the arteries, and to keep cholesterol from being deposited in the body as wheat germ oil. In fact, one half of each is a wonderful mixture for energy building and vitality.

Chapter 8

The neglected "bio"-chemical story

"We are made from the dust of the Earth."

This is merely an introduction to the chemical effects of foods in the human body. The full story is told in my book *The Chemistry of Man*. The biochemical elements found in foods are necessary in every cell, every organ, every ligament, every muscle, every tendon, every gland and hormone in the body. You find that sulphur or iron, for example, are found in a multitude of locations. The function of the body depends on the presence and balance of these bio-chemical elements.

Dr. V.G. Rocine was the greatest teacher I have studied under. He was an Norwegian homeopath who used foods as a basis for correcting biochemical deficiencies in the body. Dr. Rocine is responsible for developing the 16 chemical types of man through their relationship to the biochemical elements from the "dust of the earth."

Everyone Should Digest The Chemical Story

Our major difficulty today is in finding natural, pure and whole foods — unadulterated and uncontaminated. Anyone who handles food should read and understand the basics of the biochemical story and its implication to the health of the human organism.

Sodium, necessary for supple joints, is present to a higher degree in certain foods. We must learn what these foods are. It is one of the best elements for improving digestion. The stomach must be fed sodium for perfect digestion. Merely neutralizing acids with baking soda or bicarbonate of soda doesn't solve anything. It only masks the symptoms.

Too many today employ relief measures that neglect the body underneath. Relief measures only strengthen the condition through suppression, allowing it to return tomorrow — be it constipation, headache, stomachache and so forth.

Diseases Begin In The Diet

One day man will recognize that the greatest source of disease is in detrimental eating habits and the absence of proper biochemical elements in our foods. We exist on foods that should furnish the bricks and the building materials to rebuild the body from the breakdown through everyday bodily activity. Every 24 hours new skin grows in the palm of the hand. If we depend on coffee and doughnuts, hamburgers and soda pop, or pickles and ice cream we can't expect good health and strong bodies. The food we eat builds tissue and bones for tomorrow.

Proper diet is the most healing agent in the quest for good health. In discussing the biochemical elements, we find that they have magnetic qualities; they have electrical qualities. They attract and repel; they stimulate and sedate; they have color qualities. They have building colors, laxitive colors, repairing colors, rejuvenating colors, repelling qualities, heating and cooking properties — to heat the blood in winter and cool it in the summer. They are capable of keeping the body in good health and operating at peak performance and maximum efficiency.

We recognize that a low sodium diet leads to stomach trouble, that a high sodium diet could lead to heart disturbances; a low iron diet leads to anemia, and yet inorganic iron can produce constipation. A low calcium diet can produce tuberculosis, exhaustion, extreme sweating and can prevent bones from mending or "knitting" properly. Certain one-sided diet programs can bring on old age symptoms within a matter of months. These same symptoms disappear as a result of the right diet for rejuvenation. Old age and senility aren't something we have to take as normal and unavoidable. We can be young in old age or old in a few years through our nutritional habits. The key is in balancing the elements of the body correctly and catching up with deficiency hangovers from past years.

Specific food excesses and deficiencies are responsible for many ailments and so-called "dis-eases." Declining health, disturbed mental symptoms, kidney problems, heart irregularities, blotchy skin, boils, pimples and rashes can take over the body when the diet is deficient in certain elements. Youthfulness, vigor, beauty, clear complexion, a magnetic life — one full of energy — with the nerve force necessary to feel good and enjoy the expression of life in the normal manner depends on supplying the necessary biochemical elements in the diet. Possessing a good clean blood stream is the beginning of building a healthy body. To build a good blood stream we must first have the best foods. Wrong diets result in defective secretions, faulty elimination, acidity, flatulence, auto-intoxication, headaches, nervousness, stomach troubles and thousands of other ailments and diseases described in the medical texts and scientific journals.

Through the correction of deficiences, rather than the

treatment of specific ailments, we allow the body to heal itself. Nature does the curing if we give her the opportunity.

If we know how to use foods as medicine, we can change the body chemistry and improve health tremendously. We are meant to enjoy good health, not suffer in sickness and misery.

Calcium — The "Knitter"

Calcium oxide (lime) is essential for bone building, bone oxidation, contraction of the skeletal muscles, for sinew cohesion, strength of bone and sinew, for teeth building, for tissue repair, gelatinization, heart and pulse vigor, alkalization of bone and for numerous other purposes. It is of the greatest importance to the pregnant mother in building the baby, in preventing or healing rickets, tuberculosis, bone softening, osteoporosis, etc. Without calcium we would be a shapeless mass of jelly; we could not walk. Scars and bone fractures don't heal without calcium. It soothes the nerves, promotes proper cell function, resists germs, guards against hay fever, asthma and heals ulcers.

Symptoms Calling For A High Calcium Diet

When will-power is lacking, so is calcium. Fears, wear and care, fear of future, indecision, lack of strength, bone softening, pus formation, nose bleeds, crumbling teeth, lung trouble, swelling glands, fractures failing to heal, flabby flesh, rickets, noises in ears, thin blood, earache, sensitiveness to moisture — all call for a high calcium diet. Food lime is in demand when the calves of the legs are crampy, bones ache, chest is sunken, pulse is tremulous, spine is curved, tired feeling upon slight exertion, nose is stuffed, limbs weary, blood is sluggish, coughing tendency, tremulous pulse, bronchitis and when there is a consumptive tendency.

On the other hand, when calcium is in excess in bones, blood, secretions, on canal walls and not enough sodium is present to keep it in solution, there is danger of lime hardening, gout, dull hearing, poor eyesight, growth of bone spurs. The lips crack, joints become rusty, walking difficult, tendons are stiff, short, perhaps painful, the ears seem stopped up.

Highest Calcium Foods

Goat milk, cheeses, chlorophyll greens are high in calcium. Kale, nettles, swiss chard, turnip greens, collard leaves, dandelion greens, mustard greens, watercress, beet greens — sesame seeds, dulse, almonds, soy bean (dried), parsley, horseradish, filbert, Brazilnut, cottage cheese,

sunflower seeds, dried figs, ripe olives, broccoli, okra, sprouted mung beans, soy beans, lentils, chickpeas and dry red chili (hot) contain calcium. Also cow milk and skimmed milk, egg yolk, gelatin dishes, agar, celery, leaf lettuce, cauliflower, bone broth, eggshell broth and solid white fish have calcium.

Silicon — The "Magnetic Element"

Silicon is protective to the skin and body. It is an insulation agent, helping to keep and retain our own generated heat and muscular electricity. A lack of silicon makes one feel cold in warm weather. It increases hair and nail growth; the hair weakens and falls when silicon and sulphur are deficient. It is found in the enamel of teeth — teeth decay and crumble when silicon, fluorine, calcium and magnesium are lacking. Silicon enters into hair, nails, teeth, membraneous tissue, resistive tissue, ligaments, arterial and throat walls, linings of organs, walls of alimentary tract and skin. It stimulates the physical brain and the sexual system, is a powerful antiseptic, gives body resistence, increases working energy, sexual power, endurance, vigor, brain power, makes flesh firmer, joints more elastic, veins stronger.

Symptoms Calling For A High Silicon Diet

Food silicon is beneficial for sexual weakness, self-abuse, hair growth, nail ailments, varicose veins, firm flesh, brain work, ulceration, throat ailments, sores, wounds, cuts, neurasthenia, weakened canal wall linings. It acts favorably upon the sexual system.

A high silicon diet is of value when one is like a broken down machine. Morbid vigilance, alternating sleeplessness and sleepiness, disease fear, morbid imagination, tender spine, tossing wakefulness, nervous dyspepsia, skin or tissue numbness for hours or days, low body temperature, twitching eyelids, mental strain, weakened physical powers, menstrual colic, gloom, fatigue, timidity, old age ailments, husky voice, odorless gas in stomach, sore thighs, light amber urine, weak lower limbs, involuntary urination, sweating fingertips, gristling joints, heart pressure, stiff neck, kidney pain, falling hair, loose lax flesh, scars that do not heal, skin blotches, pus ailments, low healing power, running sores, neurosis, gurgling in joints, thirst after midnight, germ growth, scabby lips, itch and soreness between toes.

There is no danger of an excessive silicon diet.

Highest Silicon Foods

Asparagus, parsnips, dandelion greens, rice bran, barley, leaf lettuce, horseradish, cucumbers, dry onions, spinach, strawberries, leeks, artichokes, swiss chard, celery, pumpkin, cauliflower, cherries, fresh apricot, dried figs, beets, ripe tomatoes, oat straw tea, alfalfa, rice, mustard greens, apples, carrots, watermelon, and sunflower seeds have silicon. Also barley foods, marjoram, steel cut oats, alfalfa broth, wheat bran, Italian onions, whole rice flour, cooked whole rice, wild rice, wild strawberries, rice broth, rice bran and oat muffins, are known for silicon content.

Why Everyone Needs More Silicon

V.G. Rocine always said we needed a high percentage of silicon because the body stores many reserves in various parts. It is found in the skin, nails and hair. We need it for the nervous system — it is crucial to the proper functioning of the nerves. If it is lacking the hair grows slowly and hair loss is often noted; teeth beauty fades; agility and elasticity of tissues decreases; brain vigor, pep, sexual ability and motor energy fails. It is also necessary in fighting the invasion of germs and bacteria. If it is in short supply catarrh, discharges, pus, mucus — all of which attract bacteria — develop. Only about 1.5 ounces of silicon are found in the body, but we need it daily throughout the body. It carries messages from the brain to different organs and structures; it is needed in every movement and every thought. The magnetic element is crucial for the liberty of man — for his every activity and function. The life force itself depends on silicon; it controls our vibratory rate.

We find that food processing removes silicon; it is not in refined grains and cereal products. It is high in rice polishings, oat straw tea and is found in the peelings and outer covering of grains, nuts and seeds. The person lacking silicon needs two to four high silicon foods daily to pay back the loss the body has suffered for many years. In some cases the silicon reserve is almost entirely depleted and without reserves we cannot get well.

Generous Silicon Menus

Cooked whole rice (brown) with prunes, steamed parsnips, strawberries or strawberry sherbet, veal joint jelly, oatmeal muffins made with unrefined oats is rich in silicon.

Barley muffins, asparagus tips, steamed Italian onions, veal joint jelly, or broth, wild strawberries with well beaten egg white, marjoram tea as a drink is another good silicon menu.

Cucumber, dandelion, leek or onion salad with well beaten egg white and finely cut up dill as a dressing, veal joint jelly or broth, steamed savoy cabbage, barley bread, mulberry sherbet.

Other foods high in silicon are Jerusalem artichokes, steel cut oats, horseradish, rich bran muffins, chard,

spinach, steamed parsnips, collards, celery, cauliflower, millet, sweet potato (with skin), dried prunes, figs and apricots, fresh apples and ripe tomatoes.

Sodium — The "Youth" Element

Food sodium is active in the lymph and in the blood. Food sodium, iron and chlorine make the blood a salty liquid. This favors the generation and conduction of heat and electrical magnetism within the body. Sodium keeps calcium and magnesium in solution. Lack of sodium results in hardening, stiffness, rheumatism, gout, gallstones, and bladder ailments. It helps keep casein in solution and prevents dangerous blood clotting that could easily cause paralysis and congestion.

It plays an important part in salivation, bile action, pancreatic functioning and in the emulsification of fat. A deficiency results in dyspepsia, gas generation, bloating, constipation. Food sodium acts upon the brain, secretions, mucous and serous membranes, throat, alimentary canal, secretory glands, synovial membranes, stomach, intestines, spleen, pancreas and on albumin metabolism. It helps increase osmosis and helps to hold calcium, albumin and fibrin in solution. The spleen contains twice as much sodium as the liver.

In fact, sodium is needed almost all over the body. It works with potassium in the nerves to conduct nerve impulses. It excites the stomach and the bowels to greater action. With sulphur it acts upon the liver. All tissue should be bathed in an alkaline medium every hour. It counteracts acidity by neutralizing such organic acids as acetic, butyric, lactic and others. The ingestion of fatty foods drains the system of its sodium resulting in stomach trouble, fermentation, prostration. A fatty starchy diet demands sodium in abundance, or fermentation takes place. In times of calcic gout, arthritis, stomach trouble, constipation, acidity, etc., a high sodium diet is of great value.

Symptoms Calling For A High Sodium Diet

Sodium is never in excess in man, woman or child. It is always deficient. Almost all people suffer from sodium hunger. Sodium hunger symptoms are calcic gout, delayed digestion, vomiting of infants, frontal headaches, bloating, dim eyesight, difficulty in reading small print, mental confusion, catarrh, arthritis, constipation. The tongue and skin are dry. Some cases note sleepy days and wakeful nights. Other symptoms are heavy feeling in a warm room, cracking joints, stiff tendons, bruised feeling, bad breath odor, lack of saliva, great thirst after meals, difficulty in digesting starches, sweets and fat, slow digestion and gas, restless nerves, weariness and lax muscles.

Highest Sodium Foods

Although these foods are high in sodium, they are low because the soil in much of America lacks sodium. Highest sodium foods are goat milk and whey, okra, celery, dulse, Irish moss, ripe olives, Swiss chard, beet greens, dry hot red peper, spinach, beets, whole sesame seed, carrots, parsley, artichoke, dried figs, mustard greens; dried peas, chickpeas and lentils; dried and fresh apples, goat buttermilk, collards, unpolished rice, fish broths, romaine lettuce, strawberries, Swiss and Roquefort cheeses, dried apricots, raisins, red cabbage, horseradish, dandelion greens, kelp, kale, watercress. Also celery, cabbage, fish roe, wild strawberries, brown cheese, rice bran muffins, New Zealand spinach, have sodium.

Iron — The "Frisky Horse" Element

Iron is absorbed by the duodenum and small intestines and deposited in the liver, spleen and bone marrow. Iron content is highest at birth and during youth and lowest in old age. Iron in grains is lost in milling processes. Magnetism, cerebellum, breathing processes, oxidation, all require iron. Iron (hematin) in the hemoglobin is the oxygen carrier. It promotes the function of blood oxidation and magnetic induction. Rosy delicate cheeks and beauty depend on a high iron diet, not drug iron. Iron in the blood attracts oxygen and increases blood pressure, arterial elasticity, greater functional energy, circulatory power and the free excretion of urea. Blood pressure is below normal when iron is lacking; all functions are at a lower rate; one only half lives, becoming either obese or emaciated.

An excess of iron in the blood makes the whole person heavy in mind, senses, hearing, blood and functions. Brain and blood pressure become excessive. Seldom does anyone suffer from iron excess.

Symptoms Requiring A High Iron Diet

When the heart palpitates from slight effort, iron is in demand. A one sided face flush, peevish disposition, crying spells, mind confusion, great fatigue, hazy mind, alternate pains in kidneys and spleen, old age, pregnancy, hemorrhages, tumor, great craving for coffee or stimulants, sneezing, hacking cough, tired legs, cold feet, itching and bloating are all deficiency symptoms. Others are tightness somewhere, dim eyesight, tingling in ears, asthma, head colds, anemia, aching shoulder blades and neck, husky voice, hay fever, painful lungs, restless sleep, tired nerves, faded cheeks, acid stomach, sensitiveness to pressure, obesity, or emaciation, night sweats or frequent urination, weak ankles, fussiness, hot head and cold spells, lax muscles and a craze for fresh air and the hills.

Highest Iron Foods

Highest iron sources include dulse, kelp, rice bran, rice polishings, wheat bran, whole sesame seed, wheat germ, sunflower seed, leeks, collards, kale, egg yolk, dandelion, blackberry juice, leaf lettuce, okra, strawberries, prunes, radishes, asparagus, artichokes, mustard greens, salsify, parsley, dried apricots, almonds, millet; dried lentils, red beans, pinto beans, chickpeas, soy beans, limas, mung beans and peas; dried peaches, wild rice, Irish moss, butternut, dried hot red pepper, goat milk and whey, sorrel, rye meal, cherry juice and steamed onions. Also containing iron is dewberry juice, bone broth, wilted spinach, black radishes, rice bran muffins, ;whole rice, wild strawberry juice, rye meal bread and muffins and wild cherry juice.

Magnesium — The "Relaxer"

Food magnesium or its compounds is essential for solid bones and teeth. Our lungs, brain, nerves, muscles require it for normal functioning. It promotes cell building in nerve matter and lung substances, promotes excretion, blood fluidity, osmotic pressure and helps to maintain normal blood pressure. Lack of magnesium leads to chronic constipation and auto-intoxication. It makes body fluid alkaline, tissues more elastic, joints more flexible, acts upon glands, upon serous and mucous membranes, nerves of excretion, secretion and elimination. Magnesium foods are laxative, nerve calming and sleep inducing. It counteracts body gases, toxins, acids and auto-intoxication products. It helps prevent phosphatic deposits from forming in joints and solid structures. It subdues nerve pain, relaxes the brain, cools the liver, prevents certain cramps, reduces temper, relieves pain, destroys many germ species, neutralizes certain acids and toxins or rushes them out of the body.

Symptoms Indicating A High Magnesium Diet

When the bowels are in a state of putrefaction and indican and urates appear in the urine, magnesium food is needed. Headache in the lower forehead, aching in the body, stasis in the colon, burning feet, constipation, bloating, sleeplessness, terrific excitement and passion, hot blood, fever, great nervousness, burning urine, cramp, colic, nerve pain, nervous disorder, neuritis, neuralgia, nerve block, nerve congestion, itching pimples, liver hardening, acid ulcers, heart palpitation, eye catarrh, alternating food hunger and disgust, gastric acidity, jerky nerves, spring ailments, sleeplessness, nerve strain and shock, stammering and headache after menstruation are a few states indicating a lack of magnesium. An earthy taste in the mouth, fainting, over-heated blood, stiff shoulder and neck muscles, great forgetfulness, late and scanty menstruation, yellow in whites of eyes, sore calves and legs, sleepiness after meals, nausea at meals, leg fatigue, motion sickness, fondness for tart foods, tender scalp, dizziness and a tendency to ulcer are all magnesium hunger signs.

There is no danger of disturbing health by an excessive magnesium diet. There are few high magnesium foods.

Highest Magnesium Foods

Relatively high magnesium foods include yellow cornmeal, dulse, wheat germ, kelp, almonds, cashews, black walnuts, sesame seed, filberts, millet, pecans, bananas (dried), dates, dried apricots, dried figs, brown rice, rye grain, beet greens, wild rice, gelatin, mustard greens, barley food, sorrel, pomegranates, savoy cabbage, wheat, Brazilnut; dried limas, peas, white beans, red beans, coconut meat, lentils, soy bean, cowpeas; dried peaches, sweet corn, avocado, sunflower seed, raisins, and turnip greens. Also it is found in whey, garbanzos, plums, rice bran muffins, wild rice, whiting, veal joint broth, chicken bone broth, barley soup and gelatin.

Phosphorus — The "Light Bearer"

Food phosphorus, or its compounds, acts in bone and brain mainly, but also in muscular tissue. Phosphorus aids in the formation of the complex lecithins and phospholipids. The brain thinks through phosphorus. Normal growth in bone and muscle is impossible without phosphorus. Lack of phosphorus and lecithin in the brain leads to brain fag. It is present in the fluid and solid tissue as a potassium phosphate; in bones as a calcium phosphate. It improves nutrition of nerve matter; acts upon nerve matter, brain matter, bone, ganglia, nerve nets and especially upon the heart nerves. It stimulates the sexual functions and the higher intellectual functions. It vitalizes the brain, nerves and bones. Vegetable phosphorus feeds the bones mainly; animal phosphorus feeds the brain and nervous system mainly. Lack of phosphorus makes the bones soft. Phosphorus affects blood production, improves tissue nutrition, acts upon mucous surfaces, and without it the brain decays and intelligence fades.

Seldom is there an excess of phosphorus in the body. But if there is an excess, it results in fatty degeneration of the muscles, heart, kidneys, intestines and stomach glands, progressive emaciation, degenerative changes in connective tissue, trouble with the under jaw, and so on.

Symptoms Indicating Phosphorus Hunger

Neuralgia calls for a high phosphorus diet. This is the case with brain softening, debility, impotence, a bloodless face, lassitude, dislike for exertion, wakefulness at night, sleepiness towards morning, a desire for stimulant, gloom or when something is undermining life and the person is a victim of his own imagination. He dreads the future. The following symptoms call for a high phosphorus diet — gnawing, throbbing sensations, specks before the eyes, nightly discharges, numbness of the skin, or of some finger, arm, leg or tendon; twitching eyelids, great timidity, aversion to society or to the opposite sex, brain fatigue, dislike of brain work, pain in the small of the back, waxy skin; numb or weak joints and hands; deep cough, crumbling teeth, small bones; tongue blisters, bleeding piles, shallow breathing, water drinking craze, chills, chest cramps, ulcer, chronic stomach and bowel trouble, trouble with the bones, brain, nerves, spine, liver and sexual system — all call for phosphorus foods.

Highest Phosphorus Foods

Some high phosphorus foods include raw egg yolk, rice and wheat bran, wheat germ, rice polishings, sunflower and sesame seed, pumpkin and squash seed, barley, raw goat milk, black and English walnuts, Brazilnut, almonds, rye, cashew nuts, hard winter wheat and soft winter wheat, fish roe, bone broth; dried soy beans, pinto beans, white beans, red beans, broadbeans, lima beans, lentils, mung beans, peas and chick peas; wild rice, filbert, pinon nut, pistachio nut, brown rice, garlic, dulse, pecans, millet and hot red pepper (dried). Also it is found in raw cow milk, white fish, yellow cornmeal, fish broth, mustard greens, Swiss and Roquefort cheeses, trout, sole, bass, blue and black fish, pumpkins, raisins, garbanzos, and concord grapes.

Potassium — The "Great Alkalizer"

Potassium as a potassium phosphate enters into and supports the entire muscular system, both of voluntary and involuntary muscles, as well as all muscular fibers and cells throughout the body. It plays a vital part in the formation of glycogen from glucose (sugar), in the digestion of fats and proteins, in the manufacture of red blood corpuscles, in brain functioning, in the normal processes of heart and liver and in synthetic processes of chemical combinations of organic life. If food potassium is lacking in the blood or heart tissue, the heart valves shrink.

It has a great deal to do with blood and tissue alkalinity. Heat generation is greater in the muscles when potassium is abundant. Healing power is greater as is resistance. The metabolism of albumin, casein, fibrin, is more perfect; constructive power is better. Injuries, cuts and bruises heal more quickly due to calcium and potassium. It has to do with the rest processes of the nervous system, with internal oxidation, with heat distribution, cell life, alkalination of the blood and especially of the urine, nerve conductivity, muscular coordination, hair growth, hair life. Due to its intense affinity to oxygen, potassium increases tissue oxidation.

High And Low Potassium Diets

If there is an excess of food potassium in the blood and in the tissues, it has a bad effect on balance, health, sexuality, function, tissue, heart, circulation, arterial pressure, bladder and stomach. It results in sudden flatulence, and sodium and chlorine elements are alarmingly precipitated. It may result in exhaustion, depressed breathing, vomiting, purging, jaundice, convulsion, stringy secretions, chilliness and other ailments.

Conversely, when there is a deficiency of potassium in the body, there is danger of sickness and ailments of a different kind, such as falling tendencies, throbbing, periodic headaches, lusterless eyes, perspiration, chills with thirst, muscular atrophy, numbness, valvular ailments, inward fever, itch, blisters, angry ulcers, gnawing in the stomach, jerky muscles, fallen stomach and uterus, diarrhea, muscular anemia, spasm, gagging, hallucination, and muscular fatigue.

Highest Potassium Foods

Relatively high potassium foods are dulse, kelp, Irish moss, wheat and rice bran, dried banana; dried soy beans, lima beans, white beans, mung beans, cowpeas, peas, pinto beans, red beans, chick pea, chestnuts, lentils and lychee; dried hot red pepper, apricots, peaches, prunes, raisins, dates and figs; Jerusalem artichokes, asparagus, red and yellow beets, broccoli, garlic; cabbage: red and savoy; celery, cucumbers, endive, yellow corn, parsley, parsnips, dried olives, potato peeling broth, romaine lettuce, green spinach, Swiss chard, yellow tomatoes, walnuts, rye, cashews, potato with skin, kale, sunflower seed, sesame seed (whole), peanuts, coconut and avocados. Also it is found in dried apples, dried pears, rye bread and muffins, wild black cherries, beaten egg white, wild cherry juice, watercress and dandelion greens.

Manganese — The "Love" Element

Food manganese seems to act upon nerve cells, brain cells, heart linings, uterine linings, biliary passages, linings of the larynx and the excretory duct. It makes nerve and brain matter more alkaline; it increases the ability to notice objects at greater distances. It makes the mind highly impressive, intellectual and emotional; makes the senses more acute, the person and his mind is more alive; the brain, soul and emotions are keyed up to a high tension.

Food manganese is never in excess in anyone, as it is not found in many foods.

Manganese Deficiency Signals

When a pain stays in one spot for years and is always worse when sitting still and at night — manganese food is in demand. A person cannot bear to be touched. Pains run from above down; perspiration is burning and profuse; waves like warm water seem to pass through the body associated with shivers of the spine; hot foggy weather is unbearable; mind and senses are dull in the open air; food aggravates; drink produces toothache; a rushing sound is heard in the ears; fingers and toes are warm in between; knees are weak; headache from laughing, talking, dancing, walking; there is wind in the stomach and the bowels are lax; cold drinks and foods produce a crampy dention in the abdomen; the ears itch and sting; there is a greasy taste in the mouth; the skin has a fetid odor; the skin is shriveled, nose tip sore, facial bones neuralgic, eyesight poor in strong light; the world and objects seem to move; reading at night produces pain in eyes, and headache next day; there are angry silent moods; there is a rushing, ringing sound in the ears with a strong tendency to sneezing; there is a contraction in the legs during menstruation from acid and from a lack of food iron; there is a cracking in the joints; the shoulders are bruised; there is an intense dislike for moisture whether hot or cold; terrible pain sensation from gout in the bone linings at night but no other time; some suffer from terrible nightmares. All these moods, sensations, symptoms cry for food manganese.

Highest Manganese Foods

No food contains manganese except in traces. Almond nuts, walnuts, especially the Missouri Black walnut, contain manganese to a greater extent. Other foods which contain manganese are acorns, black-eyed peas, breadfruit, cardemon, chestnuts, French beans, hickory nuts, marjoram, rye bran muffins, rye bread, pumpernickel bread, rye cereal and preparations, almost all nuts, steel cut oats and muffins.

Chlorine — The "Cleanser"

Chlorine is the chemical element that helps cleanse the body tissues and keeps secretions flowing well in the body. Most foods are chlorine free or very low in chlorine. Only on rare occasions is there an excess in the body; almost always the reverse is the case. This element is called for throughout the body in proportions up to 15 times the quota of other elements such as magnesium, manganese, iron, silicon, fluorine and iodine. The blood uses great quantities of chlorine for the liver, bile, gastric secretions, stomach secretions, intestinal secretions, joints, muscles, tear glands, membranes, brain, lungs and bones. Every hour of the day these body components call for great quantities of chlorine. Strong emotions also require large amounts — such as passions. The sexual system, lymphatic system and heart couldn't function without it. Albumin can't be digested or assimilated without the presence of chlorine. Brain fibers can't be reconstructed without it. We find that chlorine is exceedingly important in a hundred different ways.

Hyperchlorhydria is a state of excess chlorine; excess hydrochloric acid in the stomach; when the stomach burns like a furnace, a chlorine free diet is indicated. The stomach should never be empty; hot chlorine drinks and most drinks in general should be avoided. Beaten egg white is high in chlorine, but should be taken to give the excess chlorine in the stomach work to do; it absorbs poisonous gases in the stomach.

High Chlorine Foods

Some of the relatively high chlorine foods are ripe tomatoes, celery, fish, lentils, cabbage, coconuts, spinach, beans, lettuce, dried figs, dates, beans, radishes, milk and carrots. Even these don't have very large percentages of chlorine. Other sources are black beets, wild blackberries, parsnips, watercress, Swiss chard, sweet potatoes. Considering the daily quota the body needs these are extremely low.

High Chlorine Menus

Concentrated chicken bone broth, broiled rockfish, raw celery juice, gelatin with beaten egg yolk and Florida orange juice dressing, whole wheat bread, and a glass of goat milk is a high chlorine menu.

Imported Swiss cheese, bran muffins, goat butter, salad made of kale, lemons, goat cream, celery heart and a slice of veal joint jelly, a glass of goat milk, orange and lemon sherbet is another example.

Baked cabbage with goat milk, broiled fish, crisp celery, on half glass goat cream and milk, wheat bran muffins, cream of onion soup is also a good chlorine meal.

Try cottage cheese (goat), with Florida orange, egg-shell broth, finely chopped leaf lettuce, celery heart, goat cream and lemon juice combined to suit your taste; eat with whole rye bread and goat butter and a glass of raw goat milk.

Make a broth of fish bones and have with the above menus.

Increased Oxygen Means Better Health

Oxygen combines with many other elements. Our health depends on a generous supply of oxygen.

1. A diet that supplies iron to our blood.
2. A diet that charges and recharges our blood with sodium phosphate.
3. Strong light, because it increases free oxygen consumption and oxidation.
4. Deep, slow breathing (4 to 10 breaths per minute), because it favors the force of the blood stream, and the oxygen supply in the lungs.
5. Mountain air that is fresh, pure and rare, because it is less loaded with impurities, gases, carbon dioxide, smoke, vapors and fumes.
6. Physical exercise, though exercises call for more air, and forms more tissue waste.
7. Optimism, because it favors oxidation.
8. A low carbohydrate, protein, fat and sulphur diet with heavy meals lowers oxidation.
9. A great deal of oxygen, because it stirs every cell, function, passion, thought and emotion to greater action.
10. To avoid heat and sultriness, because heat and sultriness lower the oxygen function.
11. Frosty air, because it stimulates every cell, function, thought and emotion.
12. A high altitude, because it increases the demand for oxygen and makes appetite pungent.
13. Oxygen in abundance, because oxygen hunger, or lack of oxygen in the system results in great indifference, sleepiness, poor memory, fatigue.
14. Oxygen, and more oxygen, because upon a heavy sugary, starchy, fatty and protein diet our system is filled with pus, catarrh, mucus, waste matter, tumors, soil disease, toxins, gases, impurity. Thus, disease is often mainly a lack of oxygen. Health requires fresh oxygen, frosty oxygen, in abundance.
15. Oxygen in abundance, because lack of oxygen results in constipation, stomach trouble, and many disorders, which we have proven to ourselves in hundreds of ways and instances.
16. Oxygen, because if we don't obtain sufficient quantities of oxygen as we are growing older, we appear old, and we may appear old even in youth. It should be remembered that age decreases oxygen consumption and that youth increases it.

17. Deep breathing, because it is important for oxidation, though an iron and sodium diet is even more important.
18. A diet that supplies iodine and fluorine, because both of those elements have a tendency to increase the demand for oxygen, and promote the oxidation of blood and oxidation of tissues.

Known Essential Elements
For The Adequate Nutrition of Man

Air Elements
Carbon
Oxygen
Hydrogen
Nitrogen

Twelve Major Mineral Elements

Chlorine	Calcium	Magnesium
Fluorine	Iron	Manganese
Sodium	Phosphorus	Sulphur
Silicon	Potassium	Iodine

Trace Mineral Elements

Cobalt	Boron
Aluminum	Nickel
Zinc	Lithium
Tin	Rubidium
Arsenic	Cesium
Vanadium	Barium
Selenium	Strontium
Beryllium	Titanium
Silver	Copper
Gold	Zirconium
Cadmium	Cerium
Mercury	Antimony
Germanium	Bismuth
Lead	Chromium
Bromine	

Alkalinity Enemies in the Human Body

Most alkaline foods contain sodium, iron, magnesium, potassium and calcium. Alkaline foods, however, are not always alkaline in the human system. The human laboratory can react differently. Acids, germs, impurities, gases, secretions and emotions must also be considered. The chemist and lmanufacturer's laboratory often fail to consider such variables. Favorable emotions make tissues, secretions, the entire body more alkaline. Pessimistic or unfavorable passions are invariably destructive to alkalinity or alkalinization of the blood, tissues and secretions. Hatred, fear, ill will, temper, jealousy always encourage acidity in the stomach and secretions. No such passions are at work in the chemist's laboratory. Free oxygen has an effect on alkalinity and alkalinization. Work, heat, cold, work habits and many other factors and conditions enter the activity. Moreover, soil is almost depleted of alkaline salts in many localities so that the foods grown there don't contain sufficient calcium, sodium, magnesium, iron and potassium.

Such observations form the basis of taking care of a patient mentally, physically and spiritually. In many cases the person may produce more acids mentally than all the alkaline broths will ever neutralize. Nutritionists must remember that it is not what we eat that counts, it is what we digest and assimilate. It is the manner in which the various elements are arranged in the human laboratory that makes the difference in good or poor health in many cases. The body and stomach must be prepared — mentally, physically and spiritually for the food it receives.

What Is The Body Composed Of?

We have said over and over that we are the dust of the earth. And here is a look at what the body is made of in biochemical elements: (There are many other trace elements not mentioned.)

Element	Percentage
1. Oxygen	72.00
2. Carbon	13.50
3. Hydrogen	9.10
4. Nitrogen	2.50
5. Calcium	1.30
6. Phophorus	1.15
7. Sulphur	0.1476
8. Sodium	0.10
9. Chlorine	0.085
10. Fluorine	0.080
11. Potassium	0.026
12. Magnesium	0.012
13. Iron	0.010
14. Silicon	0.0002
15. Iodine, copper, lead, aluminum	0.(trace)

TOTAL 100 Percent

Rocks are made of chemical compounds that produce certain colors; they have been organized to produce certain characteristics. They maintain a predetermined hardness or a softness, an affinity for other chemical elements. We have the same principles existing within our own body. We have hard teeth, a soft colon, a tough tendon, malleable fingernails, a red heart, yellow bile, a visual purple in the eye.

Carbon: The Foundation Of Organic Chemistry

Organic chemistry deals with carbon and the compounds it forms. Carbon combines with oxygen to form carbon dioxide. Plant life is made up of carbon with the addition of hydrogen and oxygen. Some of the best known of the products are sugars, starches and cellulose. We find that the animal kingdom adds nitrogen to the elements hydrogen, oxygen and carbon to form such proteins as fibrin, casein, albumin, and the various amino acid combinations.

Carbon is abundant in the atmosphere in the well-known form of carbon dioxide. It is common in the earth as corbonates such as marble, chalk and limestone. Diamonds are in the form of free carbon and so is graphite.

Carbon Dioxide — It is one of the most common products of natural life processes; all animals, including man, exhale it in breathing. Also, it is a product of combustion of all carbon-bearing compounds. Decay produces it from both animal and plant matter.

Plants absorb the carbon dioxide from the air and convert it to food materials in the process of photosynthesis, using chlorophyll, water, mineral salts and sunlight. The plant must have sunlight acting on its chlorophyll to make carbohydrates. So the making of food material by plants, beginning with carbon, is a basis of life. Without this process animal life could not exist.

Carbon Monoxide — It is a by-product of burning a carbon-containing substance or compound in the presence of sufficient air. The blue flame you see in the embers of a coal fire is burning carbon monoxide. Carbon monoxide gas is very poisonous and accounts for many deaths a year since it is odorless, colorless and tasteless.

Nitrogen — While it is used in explosives, nitrogen is very necessary in life processes. Protoplasm, a jellylike substance that is part of plant and animal cells, is often termed the physical basis of life. It is made up of many complex chemical compounds and the principal elements include nitrogen, carbon, oxygen and hydrogen.

Nitrogen is found in all tissues of animal life and in all the body substances. The following are a few of the nitrogen compounds.

Alkaloids, or narcotics, many of them very poisonous, are found in or derived from plants. Some of the more important are cocaine and obromine (present in cocoa); nicotine, a lethal poison, found along with malic acid in tobacco leaves; morphine and narcotine the powerful alkaloids in opium, which comes from poppies; caffiene, a deadly poison, is from the seeds of the Nux Vomica.

Organic acids — These acids are also made up of carbon, hydrogen and oxygen. Formic acid is the simplest type and you find it in the sting of nettles or the bite of red ants; it blisters the skin. Acetic acid and water forms common vinegar. Apple cider vinegar aged in wood is superior to the common method, but it is more expensive. Fatty acids combine with glycerine (a complex alcohol in fats); these fatty acids treated with alkaloids at a certain temperature make soap.

Organic acids not classified as fatty acids include oxalic acid (found in plants such as spinach, rhubarb, and cranberries chard). Oxalic acid is an active poison and should be limited in the diet. Other non-fatty acids are lactic acid in sour milk and malic acid found in fruit. Tartaric acid comes from cream of tartar found as the white substance in wine casks. Citric acid occurs in citrus fruit. (Avoid when green).

Carbohydrates, chemically speaking, are compounds of carbon, hydrogen and oxygen. They may be divided into three classes: monosacharides, disaccharides and polysaccharides. Included in the monosacharides are pentoses, glucose (grape sugar), levulose, (fruit sugar) galactose. Disaccharides are sucrose, (cane sugar) lactose (milk sugar), maltose (starch sugar that is converted to glucose). Polysaccharides are made up of starch (cereals and other vegetable sources), insulin (closely related to starch), glycogen (complex carbohydrate similar to starch), gums (complex carbohydrates), pectins (fruit source), cellulose (for peristalsis).

Fats and oils are found in plant and animal products; they contain carbon, hydrogen and oxygen. Fats are produced by the combination of fatty acids and glycerine (an alcohol). Some of the common fatty acids are stearic acid and its compound tristearin; palmitic acid and tripalmitin; oleic acid and triolein; butyric acid and tributyrin.

Ordinary animal fats are made up mostly of tristearin, triolein and a mixture of the two. Triolein is liquid at room temperature; tristearin is solid. Triolein is also fairly high in olive oil, cottonseed oil and other vegetable oils. Tributyrin is found in butter, but not in margarines. Heated fats are common, though detrimental to health.

Proteins are the building and repairing blocks of the body. Simple proteins are made up of nitrogen, carbon, hydrogen and oxygen; also, some have sulfur. Proteins include albumin, found in egg whites, milk and blood; globulins found in egg yolk and blood. Casein (phosphoprotein) is the valuable substance in milk; it's the curd of clabbered milk. (A similar form is found in peas and beans.) Proteosis and peptones are derived by the digestion of more complex proteins. Ptomaines are nitrogen waste products of bacteria that cause food poisoning.

Chemical elements are the simplest building materials of substances. If they are further divided they lose their individual properties. Some are known as free elements in Nature because they are found alone as well as in compounds; common metals are free elements. More common is the existence of elements in compounds because they combine readily with other elements. Water is a compound of hydrogen and oxygen, for example. The process of changing a substance to one of a different composition is called a chemical change. We find out that the souring of milk or the process of digestion are examples.

What causes these chemical changes? They are due to the force of attraction that binds elements together.

Following is a list of some of the most common elements in Nature (over 100 are known) and their common "short-hand" symbols.

Aluminum - Al	Gold - Au	Oxygen - O
Arsenic - As	Hydrogen - H	Phosphorus - P
Boron - B	Iodine - I	Platinum - Pt
Bromine - Br	Iron - Fe	Potassium - K
Calcium - Ca	Lead - Pb	Silicon - Si
Carbon - C	Magnesium - Mg	Silver - Ag
Chlorine - Cl	Manganese - Mn	Sodium - Na
Chromium - Cr	Mercury Hg	Sulfur - S
Copper - Cu	Nickel - Ni	Tin - Sn
Fluorine - F	Nitrogen - N	Zinc — Zn

Atoms are the simplest building blocks of the elements; they are chemically indestructible by ordinary means. Atoms of different elements combine to form various compounds. A chemical compound is simple to represent using the "short-hand" form of element names and the numbers of their atoms. Water, for instance, is H_2O. There are two atoms of hydrogen to one atom of oxygen. Air is chiefly made up of oxygen and nitrogen. Oxygen must be present for combustion (burning). Air also has other substances present such as carbon dioxide and water vapor. We find that oxygen is the most abundant element in Nature. It makes up 89% of water and 20% of the earth's atmosphere; the earth's crust is 50% oxygen.

A slow decomposition takes place in plant and animal life with the aid of oxygen. The function of oxygen is extremely important in the body. Every three or four minutes, with the aid of the beating heart, the body's blood goes through the lungs. The blood stream carries carbonic acid waste to the lungs to be oxidized by the oxygen and exhaled. Oxidation produces heat. By this fact it is possible to burn foods in a laboratory to determine tha amount of heat (calories) it produces. The same amount of heat is generated in the human body through oxidation.

The human body is up to 70% water; it is high in all living organisms. Water from falling rain is the purist source available, although it can pick up impurities as it passes through the air.

Hydrogen, the lightest substance known, makes up one ninth of the weight of water. Plant and animal life contains hydrogen in compounds with many other elements.

The "fiz" in carbonated drinks comes from its content of a dissolved gas, usually carbon dioxide. The gas begins to escape in tiny bubbles from the effervescent waters when the beverage is exposed to the open air.

Nitrogen unites with oxygen to form the air. It is a common element found in all forms of life, in compounds such as potassium nitrate (saltpeter) and other nitrates.

Chlorine is widely distributed in Nature, but not generously. It is commonly in combination with sodium in the form sodium chloride (common table salt).

Fluorine is a volatile gas; iodine is a purple solid, for instance, as found in dulse; bromine is a thick red liquid. Yet the chemical properties of these elements are much like those of chlorine. They form acids when united with hydrogen. Chlorine for example, when united with hydrogen forms hydrochloric acid (HCl). Tissue salts from the acids are found in the body.

All substances, or compounds, are bases, acids or neutral, depending on the hydrogen ion liberated. Any substance that bears a positive hydrogen ion is an acid. Bases liberate a negative hydrogen/oxygen combination called a hydroxyl ion. (For example, calcium hydroxide [lime].) When an acid and a base are placed together in solution both compounds lose their original properties to form a salt compound and water.

Litmus dye, often in the form of litmus paper, is commonly used in determining acid or base properties. Litmus turns blue in basic solutions and red when exposed to acids. If a substance causes a change in color of litmus from blue to red, the test substance is acidic; a change in color from red to blue means basic. A neutral substance produces no change in color. Hydrochloric acid (in gastric juice) is an acid important to nutrition and the base calcium hydroxide (lime) is also very important. Calcium phosphate is the bone mineral.

We are the dust of the earth. I want to bring out that we come from these different chemicals and compounds, as found in different minerals, rocks, granite, amythest, turquoise and so forth. We are made up with the elements of turquoise; we have it in various combinations with other elements in the body. Everything that is on the face of the earth is in our body because we are that dust and all the compounds of that dust as well. So these minerals that make up the human body each have a different story to tell. We give this idea throughout the course of my work; these elements all have functions in the body. We must never lose sight of this fact. And we have to depend upon the plant and animal kingdoms to convert these elements to a usable food form.

While fruits are not rich in iron generally, the apricot has been found useful in anemia cases. It is high in iron and also cobalt. The iron found in apricots, apples, bananas, cherries and peaches is easily assimilated by the body; so is the iron in carrots and celery. Black cherries are a good iron source and blackstrap molasses can be good for children added to milk, which is low in iron. Soybeans are rich in iron and about 80% of it reaches the bloodstream. Greens have a good supply of iron; the egg yolk is a good iron source, also. Women need more iron and so are often anemic due to the monthly loss of blood from menstruation.

Red blood corpuscles have a life span of about 120 days before they are worn-out and excreted. Enzymes break them down in the liver and spleen for elimination; they are excreted in the bile. The non-iron part of the corpuscles is excreted and 85% of the iron is recycled in the blood; the other 15% is excreted.

We find out that life and health depend upon a good oxygen supply to every cell to remove waste and carbon dioxide. Hemoglobin is responsible for these functions. The normal blood count according to experts is four and one half million per cubic millimeter for women and girls and five and one half million for men and boys. Hemoglobin is 14 grams per 100 cc. in the female and 16 grams in the male. The percent of hemoglobin is 80-100 in the female and 100% in males.

The recommended minimum daily allowances of iron are as follows:

	Milligrams of iron
Children	
Under 1 year	6
1-3 years	7
4-6 years	8
7-9 years	10
10-12 years	12
Boys and girls over 12	15
Men	12
Women	12

A calcium deficiency often goes unnoticed for some time except for possible tooth decay. Bones become rarified before stunting of growth takes place.

Calcium is necessary for the nerve impulses that travel between the brain and nervous system and for regulating the body processes. Nerves are tense, jumpy, irritable, and we are short-tempered when calcium is lacking. Children lacking calcium are over-sensitive and cry with little reason. They are very nervous and have frequent temper tantrums, chew their fingernails and display bad dispositions. The adult who is deficient in calcium often shows nervousness, quick temper, restlessness and insomnia and nervous little habits like foot tapping and the inability to relax quietly. He complains of not being able to fall asleep easily.

Cramping of all kinds in the muscles and organs is another sign. Growing children complaining of leg cramps lack calcium. Girls and women notice stomach cramps and trouble with the menstrual cycle and severe cramping around that monthly time. Calcium is extremely important to the heart muscle; the correct heart beat is about 72 times per minute. If calcium is in short supply the heart can't relax and rest properly, and the pulse can become too rapid. Experiments have shown that a living animal heart can be kept beating many years if it is kept in a solution supplying all the necessary minerals found in the blood.

Good posture depends on enough calcium in the body; it gives tone to the muscles. The muscles should be like elastic bands poised for action at all times. Without calcium they become soft and flabby. A lack of calcium can be noted in the protruding stomach, a head carried forward and rounded shoulders rather than square. Rickets is a calcium and vitamin D deficiency.

Blood clotting depends on a good calcium supply and reserve in the body. If a person bleeds easily from small cuts, calcium may be deficient. Coagulation or clotting of the blood can mean the difference in life or death in case of an accident. If calcium is not in good supply it is dissolved from the spine, thigh bones, jaws and other bones. Dental trouble and loss of teeth through decay can cause great difficulty and result in large dental expenses.

If Vitamin D isn't in good supply along with calcium, much of the calcium can be lost through the colon. Also, if the stomach secretes an undersupply of hydrochloric acid, calcium may not be assimilated. Calcium has to pass through the intestinal walls into the blood stream to be used by the body. Hydrochloric acid also helps in the assimilation of other nutrients and minerals such as phosphorus, iron, magnesium. When vitamin B-complex is deficient calcium assimilation is indirectly harmed through poor nerves that affect digestion and secretion of HCl. Vitamin D (sunshine vitamin) helps make sure the calcium and phosphorus are absorbed through the intestinal walls. The digested food must be acid to be absorbed readily. Sugar foods, especially refined, leach calcium out of the body because the bowel contents are changed to alkaline which prevents absorption of calcium.

Calcium must be held in reserve in the body. Much of it is stored in the bones along with phosphorus. The stores, or reserve, of calcium are called on when enough calcium is not obtained in the diet. What happens when this reserve is exhausted? Calcium is drawn from the bones and the teeth causing decalcification and bone rarification, along with tooth decay. When all the possible calcium is robbed from these sources the calcium blood level finally drops.

Normally, the calcium blood level is about twice that of the phosphorus present. The two minerals work together and if one is lacking the other is lowered in efficiency. Vitamin D is thought necessary to calcium absorption and is known to be used in phosphorus assimilation.

The best animal sources of calcium are raw milk products. Greens, especially green kale, are high in calcium. Sesame seed (whole), dulse, almonds, parsley, watercress, carrots, agar and Irish moss and kelp have good supplies of calcium. Other nuts and dried beans contain fair supplies of calcium, such as soybeans, filberts, Brazil nuts and chickpeas.

Phosphorus, the companion of calcium, is rich in rice polishings, wheat germ, egg yolk, sunflower and sesame seeds, Brazil nuts, black walnuts, dried soybeans. It is also found in fair supply in lentils, wild rice, millet, barley, pinto beans and dulse.

Vitamin D comes from the sunshine and also some foods, such as cod liver oil.

An adult can safely use a gram of calcium a day (1,000 milligrams). 800 milligrams are the recommended daily requirement. Growing children and pregnant women need more than the average adult.

The Whole Body Must Have Calcium

According to J.T. Irving, in his book, *Calcium Metabolism,* there is hardly any activity that goes on inside your body that doesn't involve calcium. It is the mineral which makes up the greater part of bones and teeth. Ninety-nine percent of the body's calcium is concentrated in the bony skeleton. Persons of any age need a generous supply of calcium in their daily diet. It must be replaced continuously. Calcium is also necessary for muscular health. Extreme calcium deficiency results in severe muscular cramps. The heart is a muscle and depends on a diet adequate in calcium. Nerves, too, depend on a plentiful calcium supply; restlessness, "nervousness," pain and other symptoms related to nerve function demand food calcium.

Calcium is essential for proper clotting of the blood — to protect against strokes and hemorrhages, for example. It protects the cell walls and prevents invasion by unwanted and harmful substances by maintaining permeability.

Along with Vitamin C, calcium is responsible for the cementing substance that holds body cells together. Cells are held together in bones, nerves, muscles, cartilage and so on. We would "fall apart" without this cementing. This is the case with severe cases of scurvy — bones and tissue deteriorate.

As Dr. Irving sees it, the single most important attribute of calcium is its ability to combine with proteins forming compounds occurring all through the body. This accounts for the need of calcium in almost every bodily function and activity.

Calcium acts with phosphorus in many processes. If the diet is deficient in calcium as compared to phosphorus, a certain amount of both minerals will be lost. In general, the American diet is lacking more in calcium than phosphorus, due to heavy meat and cereal consumption. The most plentiful source of calcium is milk.

Vitamin D is derived from the sun's rays acting on a steroid substance in the skin to produce the vitamin. Lack of vitamin D is known to cause rickets in babies;

(Rickets is a disease characterized by soft, deformed bones.)

A normal balanced diet does not contain either too much or too little fat to harm calcium metabolism. However, either an excess or deficiency of fat in the diet can cause a waste of calcium. The average fat intake, according to some researchers is about 20%.

J.D. Drummond and Anne Wilbraham in the book titled *The Englishman's Food,* described 15th Century diets which contained as much as one-fourth pound of cheese daily, or 1 pint of (raw) milk, a pint of whey and two ounces of cheese. A sailor's diet in 1615 consisted of a half-pound of cheese daily, one pound of wholemeal bread and three ounces of wholemeal oatmeal. (And a gallon of beer.) Such a diet would not produce calcium deficiency.

Dr. Roger J. Williams, University of Texas, has researched "biochemical individuality" quite extensively. He points out that in laboratory test animals bred to be as similar as possible, wide differences in the animals' calcium requirements exist. He maintains, "There is considerable evidence to indicate that health and longevity are conditioned by an adequate continuous supply of this element."

So the individual calcium requirements vary greatly as illustrated by an experiment Dr. Williams cites. Nineteen healthy young men were found to require calcium varying from 222 milligrams to 1018 milligrams per day, a large difference.

Recommended Daily Allowances

The National Research Council's "Recommended Daily Allowances" of calcium are as follows:

	Milligrams of Calcium needed per day
Men	800
Women	800
Pregnant women	1500
Lactating women	2000
Children 1-9	1000
Children 10-12	1200
Boys 13-19	1400
Girls 13-19	1300

These figures are intended to cover "normal persons as they live in this country under usual environmental stress," they state.

Charting Your Calcium Intake

Here are some figures to check your normal intake of calcium against the recommended allowances. Keep tabs for a week or longer. These foods form the basis for calcium content in foods.

Food	Milligrams of Calcium
1 cup whole milk	285
1 cup whole powdered milk	968
1 cup non-fat powdered milk	1040
1 cup half-and-half	259
1 one-inch cube cheddar cheese	133
1 cup grated cheddar cheese	874
1 cup creamed cottage cheese	207
1 cup baked custard	278
1 cup yogurt	295
1 whole egg	27
3 ounces canned mackerel	221
1 cup oyster stew	269
3 ounces canned salmon (with bones)	159
3 ounces sardines	367
3 ounces shrimp	98
1 cup shelled almonds	332
1 cup brazil nuts	260
1 cup peanuts	104
1 cup broccoli spears	195
1 cup cooked collards	473
1 cup dandelion greens, cooked	337
1 cup cooked mustard greens	308
1 cup cooked turnip greens	376

As stated in a United States Department of Agriculture publication, "...the chief fault of many American diets is that they provide too little of the essential minerals and vitamins."

Organic or Inorganic?

We find out that inorganic substances, generally speaking, have not been transformed or changed to organic or biochemical form. There is much confusion today in what the difference really is. In the evolution of matter from the soil to plants to animals and man, it must be remembered that we cannot assimilate the earth elements as food without the plant kingdom to convert them to biochemical form. Plants can assimilate inorganic matter, but animals, including man, cannot; we must have organic substances.

The Difference Between Chemical and Biochemical

Few of us are really living the good life, the happy and joyful life that depends on good health for its existence. If things aren't right it's time for changes — changes in thinking, relationships, even diet and the air we breathe. You can get along only 6-8 minutes without air. You can survive about 2 weeks without water. But, according to some figures, 95% of the U.S. water supply is polluted. Some people have been known to go 60-90 days without food and survived nicely. But today's foods, air and water leave a lot to be desired.

Foods that aren't biochemical — life-giving — have an accumulated effect in the body. There is calcium in chalk and calcium in wood; but the best source of calcium occurs naturally in foods. It is biochemical. Unfortunately, many people don't know that green kale is a better source of calcium than chalk. A 160 pound man has iron equal to a 10-penny nail in his body. But the iron in nails isn't food iron. Liver is high in iron. Bing or black cherries are high in iron. Wouldn't you rather get iron for your body from foods? One is biological, biochemical — that is, life-giving (bio means "life"). Both the iron in nails and that in food are chemicals, minerals; only one is fit for human consumption.

The drugless profession and the medical profession will never marry. Aspirin, for example, has many side effects, some of them cumulative. Some of the effects are anemia, circulatory problems, hemorrhaging and bowel troubles of all kinds.

Iridology can reveal these accumulated effects, showing that the drugs do not belong in the body because they are not biological, they are not biochemical — they are not life-sustaining. When we look in the iris of the eye, we can't tell if a person is eating apricots or spinach in his diet; but we *can* tell if a person is using coal-tar products.

If I give you the choice of a sweet, ripe apricot or a poisoned pickle you should know which one to choose — which is the right food to promote good health. You must always remember that this body is a servant to the mind and the spirit, and only does the bidding of the master. And unless you can use the mind and spirit to direct your body to follow the right path, eat the right foods, you will never be well.

Today we are suffering from the ill effects, the accumulated effects, of drugs. We have some 3,000 food additives at the present time. People actually think they are eating well on packaged foods; they think they are living well on them. But, they are actually dying from them. A massive reform has come in the food industry. The health-minded people of today will aid in this reform. The chiropractor of the future will counsel about nutrition.

Unfortunately, the nutrition that should be taught isn't being taught in many colleges. The chiropractic colleges are initiating this move; the medical colleges haven't sufficiently turned to this direction. In the average medical college, it is taught that we can take calcium from any source. Iridology shows that the source does make a difference.

100% Natural, Pure and Whole

The word health comes from the old Teutonic language and means "your salvation." The word implies that your salvation will come from the natural, the pure, the whole. This is the basis of my diet work. Everything must be natural, pure and whole. If foods don't measure up to these standards, they shouldn't be eaten. The laws of Nature and the Creator must be obeyed. How can we expect good health if we constantly break this universal order?

Man's mind is dangerous, especially today. Even man's education is dangerous. Unless we consider one another's health and welfare, and unless we go to the foods that can repair, rebuild and replace old tissue, then we're not eating for the right reasons. We aren't building optimum health.

What Does Potassium Mean to the Body?

We find that potassium is the most common electrolyte in the cells of the body—in blood and tissues, especially cartilage and muscles. (The heart muscle is a potassium organ.) Potassium is called for in normal heart beat, other muscle contractions, normal nerve functions, glycogen formation (stored carbohydrate energy), normal pituitary function, among many other uses. Using ACTH or Cortisone depletes the potassium level in the body.

A few of the common symptoms of potassium deficiency are: muscular weakness, hypertension, rapid respiration, dull muscle and abdominal aches, dry mouth, low gastric acidity, constipation, dehydration, depression, etc.

The importance of potassium has been stated as follows: "Potassium is essential for normal heart rhythm and nerve activity. Deficiencies result in decreasing pituitary and adrenal function along with tachycardia, hypertension, rapid respiration, gastrointestinal toxicity and constipation." (Journal of Medical-Physical Research, Vol XXII, NO. 2.) And, "Potassium and magnesium deficiencies result in cardiac, liver and kidney lesions." (Selye, Hans, *Chemical Prevention of Cardiac Necroses*.)

Support for the Value of Magnesium

We find that magnesium is the "relaxer" in the body that promotes good elimination and removes toxins from the system. Here are some recent supports for the vital place of magnesium in the chemically well balanced and healthy person, from scientific data.

"In cirrhosis of the liver, magnesium is low throughout the body tissues... while retention in the liver is abnormally high." (Min, H.K., *Chem. Abs.*, 57:7808)

"In normal or diabetic persons the metabolism of glucose is aided by magnesium. In non-diabetics copper and zinc are also helpful." (Haugaard, E.S., et al, *J. Biol. Chem.*, 240:1495, 1965)

"Alcoholics with withdrawal symptoms have low blood levels of magnesium." (Mendelson, J.H., *Metabolism*, 4:88, 1965)

"Irritability, dizziness, poor muscle coordination and muscular weakness were observed in hypomagnesia [low]." (*Lancet*, 2:172, 1960)

"Manifestations of magnesium deficiency included profuse sweating, tachycardia, anxiety." (*Modern Medicine*)

"Muscle contraction depends in part upon the availability of both calcium and magnesium. The calcium requirements are about the same in smooth and skeletal muscles, but for smooth muscle contraction ten times the concentration of magnesium is needed — thus indicating that magnesium plays some regulatory role in the activity of smooth muscles." (Filo, R.S., and Bohr, D.I., *Science,* 147:1581, 1964)

"Rats deficient in magnesium showed myocardial necrosis, calcification, fibrosis, swelling and vacuolization of sarcosomes, along with fragmentation of myofibrils." (Heggveit, H.A., et al, *Am. J. Pathology*, 45:757, 1964)

"Increasing magnesium content of diet eight times (from 24 mg% to 192 mg%) prevented atherosclerosis and kidney lesions," (Vitale, J.J., Meeting Am. Soc. Exp. Biol.)

Lecithin: A Phosphorized Fat

Lecithin burns in the brain like an oil lamp. If the brain becomes de-lecithinized it results in brain trouble. Lecithin is a phosphorized fat of a highly evolved origin — not as we find it in soy beans, avocados and other vegetable kingdom sources. The body takes lecithin and evolves it to the next stage of development (evolution) by transforming it into a brain and nerve fat. It is beneficial to include it generously in the diet. When a person experiences brain fag (fatigue), depletion of brain and nerve functions, it is a sign that lecithin and phosphorus are lacking.

Sodium Aids Potassium Combustion

Sodium is necessary for the combustion of potassium; this is the basis for feeding foods with higher sodium content than potash (potassium). Potatoes carry 26 parts of potassium to one part of sodium. Valuable sodium foods are celery, spinach, beet greens, Swiss chard and red beets. Strawberries lead the fruits. They should be of the sweet variety to have the most sodium from sun ripening — ripened on the plant. Otherwise, an irritating acid may be present.

All Structures Need Phosphorus

No physical structure — namely the brain and nerve centers — could remain healthy without phosphorus. It is essential to the mental worker; the nervous type must have it liberally. Neurotic and neurasthenic types are always suffering from a shortage of sodium. Their personality or nature demands sodium or their body becomes over-acid.

Phosphorus is vital to the sexual system. It also increases calcium and iron utilization or assimilation. Insanity could be halted in many cases by generous food phosphorus. Its lack causes hair to turn prematurely grey. Studious types are known to grey younger than most. Their tremendous draw on mental faculties drains phosphorus from the body.

Phosphorus is a chemical constituent of proteins. The largest source is in dairy products, all kinds of cheeses and fresh fish from the sea. Meats are high in phosphorus — turkey and mutton leading. Egg yolks have a good supply of this element. Vegetables such as cucumbers (leading), cauliflower, asparagus, lettuce, celery, cabbage and spinach furnish a fair source. Fruits are low in phosphorus because they have very little protein.

Iron for Improved Oxidation

Low-blood pressure individuals, and a few with high blood pressure, suffer anemia and a lack of food iron. Iron is important in forming the red blood corpuscles to a great extent; these absorb oxygen through the lungs and carry it to the body's cells. Body warmth is raised by more efficient oxidation and imparts a health blush to the skin and especially the cheeks. It improves skin tone and encourages creative pursuits and personal magnetism.

Magnesium for Sound Sleep

Food magnesium is the laxative element — the relaxer of the body. It encourages natural, healthful sleep through good bowel elimination. The following foods are most generous in magnesium: Tomatoes, spinach, carrots, lettuce (leaf), Swiss chard, celery, kale and string beans in the vegetable family. It is in citrus fruits, apples and blackberries of the fruit kingdom. Yellow cornmeal is a valuable source.

The Solid Calcium Type

Calcium makes for fixed ideas with an iron grip, so to speak. Such individuals are slow and plodding — earthy and determined — but they get there in the end. They don't know the meaning of "give up." They make good marriage partners because they marry for keeps; they don't usually make use of the divorce courts.

The pioneering spirit is born in the calcium type; they love the earth, Nature and the outdoor life. Home means

much to them, and they find pleasure there. Society life, pomp and ceremony mean little to the calcium type.

Chest ailments and digestive difficulties bother the calcium type. Calcium is used liberally by Nature to heal tubercular ulcers among many other ills. If it is not generously supplied, healing can't take place properly. If Nature is also short of sodium, calcium types tend toward arthritis, rheumatism and hardening of the arteries. They marry successfully with one of their own type or the opposite — potassium or oxygen types.

The Active Sodium Type

Sodium types live an intense and very active life; they are extremists in all things; yet their standards of life don't stand as tall as with some other chemical types. Their restless nature needs many "isms" and they are eager to accept ancient and Oriental philosophies because it allows them additional freedom and expansion or change. They love to follow their own inclinations and to justify such tendencies and actions through philosophy.

For this reason they do not mate well in marriage with the calcium type who is fixed and unyielding in ideals and lifestyle. Calciums are unable to relate to the sodium type. The ideal mate for the sodium type is one of the potassium or oxygen types—easygoing and good natured.

Trace Minerals

Manganese. The greatest amounts have been found in the liver, pancreas and suprarenals and have to do with metabolism regulation. The *Food and Life* Yearbook of Agriculture (1939) of the U.S. Department of Agriculture says, "Experimental rats deprived of manganese show sterility in the males and lack of maternal instinct in the female. During pregnancy manganese passes into the bloodstream of the unborn child, and the fecal discharge of the newborn infant contains a remarkable amount. The recent discovery that leg-bone deformity in chickens, known as perosis, is accompanied by manganese deficiency has suggested the possibly necessity of this element for normal bone development. Studies indicate that as little as one ounce of manganese taken over a period of twelve or fifteen years will furnish an adequate amount for children."

Cobalt. "This element has been found in extremely small amounts in most of the organs of the human body except in the pancreas. Cobalt is known to increase the number of red corpuscles in the blood, and there is evidence that it may be beneficial in certain types of anemia. Some persistent human nutritional anemias refuse to clear up completely with the usual iron treatment, and the partial cure effected by iron compounds in such cases is now believed to be due to the traces of cobalt which these salts have been found to carry as impurities." (U.S.D.A.)

Copper. It is believed that copper is essential to plant and animal life.

"The copper present in the human body, estimated at 100 to 150 milligrams, or 0.10 to 0.15 gram, is almost all contained in the muscles, bones, and liver with only a small amount...in the blood. Since the animal body is not able to form red blood cells and hemoglobin in the absence of copper or at best can form them only at a very slow rate, both iron and copper must be administered before the anemia will be cured." (U.S.D.A.)

Iron. Cobalt and copper have to do with the assimilation of iron; they are co-workers. Iron must come from a food source for body assimilation. If the soil in a certain location is short of iron, the foods grown on it and the people who eat those foods will lack iron. This is why a greater deficiency of iron is found in some people's blood. Many researchers have suggested that the intake of iron for women during child-bearing years should be between 17 and 20 milligrams daily. (U.S.D.A.) Anemia is much more common in women than in men. The liver is an iron organ, and iron is also found in other glandular tissues and in the red bone marrow.

Iodine. Research by the U.S.D.A. found that 1.0 to 2.0 milligrams of iodine is needed daily. A deficiency of iodine causes goiter. This affliction is common in Switzerland where iodine is extremely scarce, but we find that the Japanese in their homeland rarely develop goiters because their sea food and sea vegetation diet is so rich in iodine. Inorganic iodine in the drinking water or iodized table salt should not be depended on for a source of iodine. Nova Scotia dulse, kelp and sea fish (white fish with fins and scales) are some of the best food sources of iodine. The thyroid is the iodine gland.

Fluorine. It is known to be essential to the body, especially for the hardness of tooth enamel and bones. University of Rochester scientists found that the occurrance of cavities is proportionate to the amount of fluorine in the enamel. The fluorine in drinking water is inorganic and has in past instances caused brown mottled teeth if oversupplied even minutely. Food fluorine doesn't have any adverse effects. (We go back to the basic difference between organic and inorganic again.) Fluoridated water supplies may not be the boon the experts believe.

Magnesium. It is a known essential mineral to good health. It was found that with less than two parts per million of magnesium test animals sickened and finally died. It is needed for good bowel elimination and to relax the body. It is also believed to have to do with fat metabolism.

Zinc. "For a period of more than fifteen years there has been considerable interest in the possible necessity of zinc in the diet. It is always present in human tissues, the greatest concentration having been found in the sex organs and thyroid. The liver of an infant contains more than three times as much zinc as the liver of the adult. This suggests a storage of zinc in the child before birth, as is known to occur in the case of copper and iron. Human milk, as well as that of cows and ewes, contains zinc; in each case the amount in the milk is greatest immediately after birth of the young. For a period of ten to fifteen days there is a sharp drop in the amount of zinc found; thereafter it remains the same. After repeated attempts by several investigators, a zinc deficiency in experimental animals was finally produced in 1935. While this work demonstrated the necessity for zinc for normal development, the exact action of this element in animal nutrition still remains obscure." (U.S.D.A.)

Tin. "Since the great use of tin is in the canning industry, considerable attention has been focused on the tin content of canned foods and its ultimate effect in the body. There appears to be no danger of harmful effects to those ingesting the quantities of this metal found either in canned or natural foodstuffs. (This includes inorganic and organic sources alike.) Tin has been noted in many of the human tissues; it seems to be concentrated in the suprarenal glands and occurs in considerable amounts in the liver, brain, spleen and thyroid gland. One investigator found exceedingly large amounts of tin in the mucous membrane of the tongue." (U.S.D.A.) The organic form is in the safe form.

Arsenic. The inorganic form of arsenic is a widely-known poison. But we find out that it is essential to nutrition in food form. Traces of arsenic are found throughout the body, and it is concentrated more in the liver. The liver seems to store this element and release it in the bloodstream when called for. It is released to the blood during menstruation and the fifth and sixth months of pregnancy; and also in cases of cancer. "Here, then is an element that seems closely associated with the physiology of man. In just what manner it acts is a question that remains unanswered." (U.S.D.A.)

Bromine. A lot is not known about bromine at the present time. . . ."in certain mental conditions known as manic-depressive psychoses, the normal blood bromine is reduced to about half and remains low until there is an improvement in the pathological condition. The bromine content of the blood is changed also during menstruation. The growth-regulating portion of the pituitary gland contains concentrations 7 to 10 times greater than that of any other organ. There is also considerable variation in bromine content of the tissues with age; after 45 the amount begins to fall and at 75 years of age only a trace, if any, remains. All of these facts suggest many important questions regarding the action of bromine which need investigating." (U.S.D.A.)

Aluminum. It is found in many parts of the human body and the bodies of animals. Its necessity to health has not been determined. However, the aluminum that comes from inorganic sources such as the absorption from cooking utensils could be harmful. If it is in the body by Nature's placement it is natural organic.

Boron. It is known to be an essential part of nutrition for plant growth. In experiments it was found that plants could not grow without boron in the soil even if everything else was present. It is thought to have to do with the utilization of calcium by plants. Since boron is found universally in the soil and in plant life, it is recognized as

essential to animal nutrition; but for what purposes is yet undetermined. (U.S.D.A.)

Nickel. "Nickel has been found more widely distributed than cobalt in the human tissues and is particularly concentrated in the pancreas. Thus far nothing is known of its physiological function." (U.S.D.A.)

Other Trace Minerals. Lithium, rubium, strontium, beryllium, silver, gold, cadmium, titanium, germanium and traces of nearly all other metals have been found in human tissues. Their role in human nutrition is not yet known in many cases. Much more research and testing is needed; however, more and more is being discovered all the time to link them to human health. Don't underestimate the importance of these and all other minerals in the diet. Make sure they are from organic (food) sources.

MORE ABOUT CATARRH

When a person has a catarrhal condition, how much milk should that person use? Well, I thought I could spend a whole chapter on that question alone, but here are a few salient things I'd like to bring out.

Firstly, I don't think that milk is the only thing that produces catarrh. Don't run away with the idea that dairy products are the only things that do it. I think starches can produce catarrh. I believe wrong combinations of foods can produce it. I believe an enervated body can produce catarrh on the best foods in the world. Catarrh and acids are the beginning of every disease. Now, how much milk should be cut out? I do believe cutting out the dairy products often helps eliminate catarrh. I say this because, many times, our body has been so loaded with dairy products in the past that cutting them out and using other foods changes the chemical balance, and this should be done.

Asthma is considered a catarrhal disease. It is a heavy catarrhal condition of the bronchial tubes, the lung structures, etc. Yet, you know I have put asthma patients on goat's milk and they have gotten well—absolutely well. Now why should they get well on goat's milk and not cow's milk? They are both milk. But I believe in goat's milk much more than I do in cow's milk. What I usually do is cut out milk and other dairy products for one solid month. That means butter, cheese, buttermilk, yogurt—everything but the cow! I use soy products for a while, soymilk products, soy powder, soy chocolate, all the soybean products. You can use sunflower seeds for a good protein. I think meat is a good protein, if you haven't given it up entirely. Meat is considered one of the best proteins we have from a protein standpoint. I did not say that you had to use it. But if you have been using it, it will not produce catarrh. I'm convinced of this; however, I know that meat can cause other troubles and we have to be a little careful of it.

Chapter 9

Landmark natural food experiments

Where Is Humanity's Health Interest?

No secret has ever been made of the experiments and findings presented in this chapter. Millions must have read them. They are described in countless books of travel and health work. Many have happened in America — on our back doorsteps. Yet few laymen and professionals have taken heed, even among those in the medical profession, who should be health crusaders. Government officials and agencies should also lead efforts to improve the state of our national health. Action should have been taken long before now.

McCarrison's findings could be amplified, expanded and enlarged through new research avenues. It is not up to the general public to instigate health research. Government agencies should undertake studies. The medical profession should be interested in such experiments. Rats, other animals and human volunteer groups should be studied. Diets from various localities and regions should be compared. The health and dietary states of countries and races should be studied, findings documented and the results used for the benefit of the entire world. Such studies and research are not difficult. Think of the tremendous cost of cancer research and research on other degenerative diseases right now.

Countless documented experiments undoubtedly link food to health — both physically and psychologically. What more needs to be said?

Columbus' Sick Sailors Recover in Tropics

A number of Christopher Columbus' sailors became extremely ill during his New World voyage. The cases were diagnosed as hopeless. So when a lush green island came into view, the men asked to be set ashore to die there. After the ships set sail without them, the men began to eat the strange tropical fruit of the island — and to their own surprise and delight, they rapidly began to recover. Several months later Columbus returned. Imagine his astonishment at being hailed by men he thought were long dead! Strong, healthy and very much alive, they came back aboard, and the island was named Curacao, the Portuguese word for "cure."

Natives Give Cartier a Scurvy Remedy

French explorer Jacques Cartier sailed for Newfoundland in 1535. A number of his crew members fell seriously ill with scurvy, which often proved fatal at that time. The Newfoundland Indians gave the men a tonic made from spruce tree needles, and they miraculously recovered. Cartier was said to have reported, "All the doctors of Montpellier and Louvain could not have done so much in a year as that tree did in six days."

Captain Cook Conquers Scurvy in Hawaii

Why didn't the experiences of Columbus and Cartier make an impression on the world so that the devastating attacks of scurvy were eliminated? British Captain and colonizer James Cook, the discoverer and colonizer of Hawaii, faced scurvy again 200 years later. If it were not for the Hawaiian natives giving his men tropical fruits and their juices, many of them would have died.

Not until years later would the British Navy make limes a mandatory ration of sea voyages. (Lemons were at that time called limes.) Scurvy was not yet linked to a deficiency of vitamin C.

Advent of the British "Limey"

In 1740 Lord Anson set sail from England to the New World. His well prepared and equipped expedition numbered 961 men — all the strongest seamen — and six sturdy ships. The rations consisted mainly of salt-cured meat and biscuits. Typical of the times, they brought no fresh vegetables or fruits because they were so perishable. In six months time Lord Anson lost two-thirds of his once healthy crew and was forced to leave three empty ships adrift in the ocean. By the end of a year he was compelled to abandon two more ships due to many more deaths. What was this "dread disease?" It was the same scurvy described in our previous accounts — vitamin C deficiency.

Lord Anson returned to England three-and-a-half years later in a single ship with a pitiful skeleton crew of less than one-fifth of the original 961 sailors.

In 1757 Lind proved that lemons (called limes) could prevent scurvy, and, at long last, the British Navy added "lime juice" to the sailors' rations. From this time on, British sailors were nicknamed "limeys".

Birth of the Science of Nutrition

The science of nutrition was actually ushered in by a young Dutch scientist named Christiaan Eykman, who discovered that the cause and cure of beriberi were in the diet. Closely following his lead were Casimir Funk a Polish chemist and Sir Frederick Gowland Hopkins, of Great Britain. Eykman (to be explained elsewhere), was sent to investigate an epidemic in Java — among prisoners and Dutch officials.

Casimir Funk, carrying the pioneering experiments of Eijkman further, discovered that yeast, along with rice bran or polishings, corrected beriberi. He is responsible for coining the word "vitamins."

Hopkins proved that carbohydrates, fats and proteins — even with the addition of minerals — do not form a balanced diet. He began the quest for "accessory food factors," which turned out to be vitamins.

Today the vitamin alphabet is growing by leaps and bounds. Knowledge of vitamins and their effect on health is becoming voluminous. However, we must remember that although vitamins are essentially the "gasoline" for running the engine, minerals build the machine. Consider the use of vitamins in conjunction with the minerals — the "dust of the earth." It is of little value to isolate specific nutrients without considering the wholistic view of their use in the human machine. They must work with countless other "accessory food factors," minerals and so forth.

Enter the Mystery Dis-ease: Beriberi

The Norwegian Mercantile Marine didn't suffer from the "disease" beriberi until 1894. Why? Well-meaning humanitarian crusaders compelled the ship masters to stock up with white bread in place of the usual whole grain bread to soften the harsh conditions of the deck hands' life at sea. Consequently, beriberi broke out. One captain who insisted on whole grain and rye bread for himself didn't get the beriberi that afflicted his crew. When his ill sailors were given whole grain bread, their symptoms left rapidly. Thus, both the cause and the cure for the disease were discovered at the same time, although the basic mechanism was not understood.

The dictionary defines beriberi as "A thiamine deficiency disease characterized by partial paralysis, emaciation and anemia." The disease is believed to be closely related to scurvy, pellagra, neuritis and pernicious anemia. A diet rich in fresh fruits, vegetables and unrefined grains along with complete proteins prevents any of these deficiency dis-eases.

Nevertheless, it took over 200 years for this proven method of prevention to be introduced — and then by laymen — into the British Navy and 300 years for induction into the mercantile marine.

Another instance pointing to the value of whole grain bread was during the Siege of Kut. British soldiers contracted beriberi while Indian soldiers who had to eat the cheaper whole grain bread never developed a case. After the white flour ran out, the British had to make their bread from the Indians' whole grain flour, and the beriberi symptoms vanished.

Beriberi and the Japanese Navy

The latter 1800s were beriberi years for the Japanese Navy. From 20 to 40 percent of its 5,000 men were afflicted yearly. A navy medical officer. Dr. Takaki, received permission to run a nutritional experiment on one of the ships. The tour of duty was nine months, covering many foreign ports, and Japanese seafarers' diet was primarily white (refined) rice. About 169 cases of beriberi and 25 deaths were recorded. On a similar voyage, more barley, with the addition of vegetables, some meat and condensed milk were the provisions. White rice was decreased. As a result, only 14 men came down with beriberi, all of whom had neglected to eat what had been recommended. The Japanese Navy, recognizing the significance of the experiment reduced the use of white rice. After that, beriberi cases became rare. (Later, B-1 was the original "Vitamin B" to be identified — now commonly called thiamine.)

Eijkman Solves the Mystery Disease

During the 1890s when Dutch missionaries, army personnel and colonial managers took over Java, an epidemic hit them. Among scientists sent to control the "plague" was young Dr. Christiaan Eykman, who returned for a second time. Using chickens as test animals, Eykman innoculated them with the blood of beriberi victims. He was mystified that they didn't catch the "dis-ease." One day he noted his test chickens beginning to show beriberi symptoms. The oddity was that *both* vaccinated *and* nonvaccinated poultry had it.

The key to the mystery was in the feeding of the fowls. They'd been given relatively expensive white rice due to a temporary shortage of their regular, cheap brown rice. Eykman observed them closely when their diet of unpolished rice was restored and came to the conclusion that a diet restricted to white rice produced beriberi. He found that the afflicted chickens recovered at the last moment on unpolished rice.

Unfortunately for humanity, Eykman's findings were largely ignored for many years.

Dr. Funk Finds the "Anti-Beriberi" Factor

Dr. Casimir Funk, a Polish chemist, was inspired by the findings of Eykman to conduct further investigations. He ground unpolished natural rice, took the rice bran from it and fed the bran to pigeons crippled by beriberi. Only very small amounts were used. Within hours, they miraculously recovered. In 1912, Dr. Funk published his findings, stating that a substance in unpolished rice, vital to health, was removed in the milling process. Combining the Latin word for life ("vita") with the word "amine" (a nitrogen compound) he coined the word "vitamine," calling it the "anti-beriberi" vitamine.

As usual, Funk's tremendous discovery was ignored by his contemporaries.

Dr. Goldberger and Pellagra in the South

Dr. Joe Goldberger of the U.S. Public Health department traveled through the South where he noticed pellagra was commonplace among the very poor people who didn't have vegetable gardens, cows or chickens. He also discovered pellagra in hospitals where patients were given inferior foods; the better-fed staff members didn't have it. Dr. Goldberger wanted final proof, so he persuaded a governor to offer a pardon to prison inmates who would agree to eat the foods the very poor lived on. The diet was made up of fat pork, cornbread, corn syrup, dried beans and peas, sweet potatoes and yams. Although they could eat all they wanted, the volunteers developed pellagra in a few months, severe in many cases. The dietary deficiency was cured by the addition of greens, yeast and liver.

Pellagra is defined as " A chronic niacin deficiency disease, marked by skin eruptions and digestive and nervous disturbances."

Faulty Food Disease Manifestations

Around the turn of the century, few laymen believed that food had any effect on health — good or detrimental. And I believe fewer still would have faced the possibility that mashed potatoes, white bread, margarine, pasteurized milk and milk products, salt, pepper, vinegar, tea, coffee and alcohol are destructive to the body. The following account shows what can happen to healthy men on an inferior diet. It is from Alfred McCann's work, *The Science of Eating.*

The Kronprinz Wilhelm "Poison Squad"

"The Kronprinz Wilhelm, converted German cruiser, left Hoboken August 3, 1914, and roamed the seas for 255 days, subsisting upon supplies taken from British and French merchantmen before she sent them to the bottom. [During World War I.]

"During the time she touched at no port, depending entirely for coal and provisions upon her raiding ability and her speed in escaping from enemy warships bent upon her destruction.

"She was fairly busy during these 255 days. She sank 14 steamers and seized vast supplies of fine white American and Argentine flour, millions of pounds of the finest of fresh beef, enough to give every one of her crew of five hundred men, three pounds every day for a year — a considerable quantity of fresh pork, hams and bacon, potatoes, canned vegetables, dried peas and beans, sugar cakes, coffee, sugar and condensed milk.

"In January the increasing pallor of the members of her crew was noticed by the chief surgeon, also the dilation of the pupils of their eyes and marked shortness of breath; but these symptoms were not considered significant, nor did anybody dream of connecting them in any way with the "high grade diet" upon which the men were living, it being in every way equal to that eaten daily by the "best people" of the United States; and the men went merrily along, drawing their typical American meals of fresh beef, with occasional rations of ham and bacon, potatoes, canned vegetables cooked in the juices that stood in the can, cheese, fine [refined] white bread, oleomargarine, coffee, tea, condensed milk and fine granulated sugar, three times every day, with sugar cakes, champagne and beer thrown in between meals.

"In February, the Kronprinz Wilhelm sank a steamer loaded with a cargo of wheat — whole, unground wheat. The germ and bran of that wheat would have been worth more to the rapidly succumbing Germans than its weight in precious stones, but they did not know that they were sick, nor how badly they needed that whole wheat, with its alkalin calcium and potassium salts. Almost every week they added to their store of red meats, potatoes, canned vegetables and oleomargarine. But little fruit was found upon any of the destroyed vessels, not more than enough to last the crew one day; so that was confined to the officers' mess; and be it noted, none of the officers were prostrated with the disease that followed.

" Also, in February, many of the crew complained of swollen ankles, pain in legs and arms. But they continued eating freely of the refined foods of high caloric value, now so extensively relied upon throughout the United States.

"In March alarming conditions developed; symptoms of paralysis, dilated heart, atrophy of muscles, and pain on pressure over the nerves, with anemia and constipation, were marked. Fifty of the men could not stand, and they were dropping at an average rate of two a day.

"On April 11, 1915, she made a dash into James River, and anchored off Newport News, (Virginia) a floating hospital, with 500 sick men on board, 110 of them in bed, and the rest coming down at the rate of 4 every day.

"We find out that no medical doctor was able to diagnose the cause of the malady, though many were consulted. Finally Alfred McCann appeared on the scene, a representative of the *New York Globe*, and a Nature student. He didn't even need to see the men or examine them to know where the sickness came from. He knew the men suffered from the wrong diet because they had lived on cooked, denatured, "dead" foods, without raw fruits and vegetables. The "disease" he also knew was not "contagious."

"The ship's surgeon, Dr. Perrenon, because he had tried all else, and science had failed, agreed to try a simple diet (the same as in Genesis 1:11 and 29) of natural foods. What were the results? We find that within 10 days of the beginning of the diet, 47 of the sick men were discharged from "sick bay" and no more came down with the "disease."

"Dr. Perrenon made the following statement to Alfred McCann about his experience during the seige of illness:

"We had many cases of pneumonia, pleurisy, and rheumatism among the men. They seemed to lose all resistance long before the epidemic broke out. We had superficial wounds, cuts, to deal with. They usually refused to heal for a long time. We had much hemorrhage. There were a number of accidents aboard, fractures, and dislocations. The broken bones were slow to mend. Nature was not doing her duty. Food is indeed the cause of much disease. In nine months we can learn much that is not found in the [medical] textbooks."

(*Science of Eating,* p. 213)

Many would say that Nature was not doing her duty. She is held responsible for the troubles and diseases. But we find that the fault lies not with Nature, but with man. We must be willing to meet Nature half-way, and wonderful results can take place.

Menu of the German Kronprinz Wilhelm

Alfred McCann gives the menu of the German sailors aboard the Wilhelm. We find that he has the following to say about the diet and illnesses, according to his book, *Science of Eating*.

"From the ship's cook, with the chief surgeon's assistance, I obtained the following chart, showing just what each meal consisted of, prior to the breaking out of the disease described by scientific men as 'beri-beri.' The chart...tells just what was behind the beri-beri, acidosis, neuritis, jail edema, trench edema, war nephritis, pellagra, or whatever term is adopted to describe the sufferings of the men."

MONDAY

Breakfast:
Cheese, oatmeal, condensed milk, white bread, butter (oleo), coffee, sugar.

Dinner:
Pea soup, canned vegetables served in juice that stood in cans, roast beef, boiled potatoes, white bread, coffee, condensed milk, sugar.

TUESDAY

Breakfast:
Sausage, white bread, butter (oleo), fried potatoes, coffee, condensed milk, sugar.

Dinner:
Potato soup, canned vegetables served in juice that stood in cans, pot roast of beef, boiled potatoes, white bread, butter (oleo), coffee, condensed milk, sugar.

WEDNESDAY

Breakfast:
Corned beef, white bread, butter (oleo), fried potatoes, coffee, condensed milk, sugar.

Dinner:
Beef soup, roast beef, boiled potatoes, white bread, butter (oleo), coffee, condensed milk, sugar.

THURSDAY

Breakfast:
Smoked ham, cheese, white bread, butter (oleo), condensed milk, sugar.

Dinner:
Lentil soup, fried steak, fried potatoes, white bread, butter (oleo), coffee, condensed milk, sugar.

FRIDAY

Breakfast:
Boiled rice, cheese, white bread, butter (oleo), fried beef, coffee, condensed milk, sugar.

Dinner:
Pea soup, salt fish and pot roast, boiled potatoes, canned vegetables served in juice that stood in cans, white bread, butter (oleo), coffee, condensed milk, sugar.

SATURDAY

Breakfast:
Corned beef, cheese, fried potatoes, white bread, butter (oleo), coffee, condensed milk, sugar.

Dinner:
Potato soup, roast beef, boiled potatoes, white bread, butter (oleo), coffee, condensed milk, sugar.

SUNDAY

Breakfast:
Beef stew, cheese, fried potatoes, white bread, butter (oleo), coffee, condensed milk, sugar.

Dinner:
Beef soup, pot roast, canned vegetables served in juice that stood in cans, boiled potatoes, white bread, butter (oleo).

"At four o'clock every afternoon the men were served a plate of Huntley & Palmer's fancy biscuits or sweet cakes with coffee, condensed milk, and sugar."

Supper:

"Evening meal either of fried steak, cold roast beef, corned beef, as beef stew with potatoes or cold roast beef with white bread, butter (oleo), coffee, condensed milk, and sugar."

Does the menu sound familiar to you? It probably does because it is the diet civilized and affluent societies and countries generally consider necessary for "good health." The same menus are found in hotels, restaurants, airplanes and luxury liners. The sailors didn't dream of connecting their failing vitality and illness with what they ate. How many today even think of the foods they eat as possible detrimental health causes? Alfred McCann added this thought later in the book:

"The raids never resulted in any large quantity of fresh vegetables or fruits. If such fresh vegetables and fresh fruits as were confiscated, had been divided among the crew, they would not have suffered for more than one day. In consequence, they were reserved for the officers table, which they managed to provide with fair quantities from one raid to another.

"All the officers showed symptoms of anemia and mild acidosis, but none of them was prostrated. From their tissues and blood the lime, iron, and potassium had not been robbed to the degree suffered by the tissues and blood of the men."

Not one of the officers fell ill to the extent suffered by the crew members. Why? We note that they received small quantities of fresh vegetables and fruits. This small ration was just enough to save them from the sickness of the crew. Do you see the wonderful building material found in natural foods — fruits and vegetables? Meet Nature half-way, and she can do the rest. It is no credit to civilization that such a diet is common today. Where will it lead us? The prognosis is not encouraging.

Denmark's Wartime Diet

The story of the fate of the German sailors aboard the Kronprinz Wilhelm may not have reached the consciousness of everyone. It plainly shows what the disasters of heavy meat-eating and a generally poor diet lacking fresh fruits and vegetables can be. The body is truly the "temple of the living God" and should be treated with care.

Denmark was forced to carry out a nutrition experiment during the first World War because the food supply was so limited and threatened. Under the direction of a physician, Dr. Hindhede, four-fifths of the hogs and about 34 percent of the cattle were killed. The food that had gone to this livestock population now went to the people. It is noted that Dr. Hindhede was not a supporter of meat-eating . The whole grain and the bran, not just the pure starch, was now used in bread making. The rest of the diet consisted of vegetables, some fruit, limited dairy products, no tea, coffee or alcoholic beverages. At the end of the first year of rationing, the death rate had dropped by 17 percent to a mortality rate of only 10.4 per thousand. We find that this is the lowest death rate ever reported by a civilized country. Strangely enough, all around the Danes the death rate of other countries was rising tremendously in such countries such as Sweden, Spain, Norway, Holland, Switzerland. Spain had the greatest increase — 46 percent!

Dr. Hindhede reported the results and their underlying reasons as follows:

"...we reduced our cows 34 percent, and withheld the wheat bran from the cows and incorporated it in our coarse rye bread. We thus obtained a bread that not only contained all the rye bran, but 12 percent of wheat bran extra. It was, indeed, the coarsest bread ever seen. Moreover, we forebade the production of spirits for consumption, and the English deprived us of coffee and tea. We thus arrived at an impossible diet, according to the old theory, but an ideal one according to the new theory...

"What was the relation of health to this extremely Spartan diet? It was so remarkable that the mortality for the whole country in the first full rationing year, October 1, 1917 to October 1, 1918, fell 17 percent. We came down to a mortality of 10.4 per thousand, the lowest death rate ever seen in any country.

"In the last three months of 1918, however, influenza appeared, which quite disturbed the mortality figures. But it is striking to note that Denmark was the only European country which had no higher mortality in 1918 than in the years preceeding the war."

"There is no reason to doubt that, under normal conditions, influenza — which raged injuriously in our midst — would have put up the death-rate in Denmark to the same extent as in the neighboring countries. But we seem to have saved this 25 percent by our rationing.

"What were the active factors? This cannot be answered definitely. But it is safe to say that a diet consisting mainly of dairy produce, coarse bread, barley porridge and potatoes, and coffee substitute, was a healthy diet for the old people; but that it was less fortunate that, when rationing was abandoned, they returned to a heavier meat diet, with ordinary white bread and genuine mocha coffee.

"I have worked for many years to induce my countrymen to return to the simple peasant's diet, which they lived on in the country 50 years ago. I have maintained that this diet . . . was most healthy besides being by far the cheapest. During the period of rationing I had the opportunity of helping to introduce the old diet of the peasant's again; and the results quite came up to expectations."

— *The Practitioner,* London, Mar. 1926.

It is well known that many condemn dairy products —especially milk—and also eggs. But, according to the experience in Denmark they are much less "harmful" than meat. (You will note that in our diet work we favor goat milk, its raw dairy products and egg yolks.) We find that the national health held up very well under the influenza epidemic; this is something more to think about. While the mean increase of mortality was 30 percent in the non-warring countries, Denmark showed a *decrease* of two percent from what it was before the war.

The idea first taken from the Dane's experiment is that this is the ideal diet. This is not the case. But we find it more importantly shows the destructive qualities of meat in the diet, along with devitalized, refined and denatured foods — namely the grains. And it shows that if given even half a chance, the body can build health through the help of Nature.

If we look back at history we find out that grains and modern vegetables aren't the original food for man, or the natural food. Primitive man didn't use these feeds; they were not known to him. They evolved through the ages

from simple grass seeds and plant roots. The Aryans left the first record of cereals and grains at about 2,000 B.C., in southeastern Europe. They brought these along with the plow and metals of gold, bronze and silver. The grains included rye, barley and wheat according to some historians.

Eating largely cooked grains and flour products can cause mucus and clogging of the body's lymphatic system. Overeating tuber starch vegetables can add earthy deposits that harden the joints, tissues and organs. This condition is called "old age."

A case in point is that of the Trappist Monks, who live entirely on tubers, cereals, lentils, beans and peas. They are entirely against flesh eating, but show extreme cases of hardening of the tissues and blood vessels, even to the kidneys, liver and intestines, because of the high starch diet.

The Staff of Life Is Overly Starchy

All grains, such as rye, oats, wheat, barley, etc., are nearly entirely starch. We find that all starchy foods are acid-forming and starch-acidosis is the cause of a great deal of our stomach and bowel disorders. Unfortunately, many a vegetarian believes he is taking the right path by replacing meat-eating with a heavy starch diet. But they soon become physically sick and weakened. Why? The elements cereals contain, if taken in large quantities, especially refined, irritate the nervous system.

Hindhede also gives much credit to the change in the bread from fine meal bread and whole meal to whole meal with extra bran. He gave the proportions as 67% rye, 21% oats and 12% bran. The entire diet of the Danish people consisted of wholemeal bread with added bran, green vegetables, potatoes, other root vegetables, fruit, milk and butter; meat was not a constant part of the diet, with fewer cattle and pigs to slaughter. There was much less alcohol consumed.

Hindhede is correct in assuming that this was a superior diet. It produced the record low death-rate in Europe in a relatively short time. It is noted that this diet was similar to that of the Hunzas and Sikhs in West Pakistan and India. The Hunzas and Sikhs depend on whole grains, vegetables, fruit, lots of milk, butter and limited meat and alcohol.

The Hunzas differ from most groups in the manner in which they grind their bread flours. Most of the grain is left visible in the flour; it is coarsely ground. The bread they make from this grain is whole meal bread like the Kleibrot bread, Professor Hindhede described that he used with the Danes. It has its own bran.

The Westerners grind their flour to fine white powder, leaving out the valuable parts of the grain. McCarrison termed the Hunza diet the "unsophisticated foods of Nature," foods not artificially processed for the consumer. A "sophist" is defined in the English Encyclopedia Dictionary as "a cunning and skillful man, a teacher of arts and sciences for money." This is not part of the Hunza culture. (Or at least was not before civilization invaded the land of the Hunzas.)

Staff of Death in the Wilderness

In the June 2, 1929 issue of "Philosophy of Health," a story tells about a northern trapper who died on a diet of principally white flour. His body was discovered by two other trappers in the vast wilderness. The cause of Hogarth's death was scurvy. When his brother undertook an investigation, he found a diary of the tragedy. Hogarth had set out in latter July, 1924 with his dogs and adequate provisions.

The first diary entry was August 12: "Landed at headquarters shack about 4 p.m. Everything O.K." From the entries, his diet consisted of white flour, sugar, tea, tobacco with fresh meat and fish at intervals. On Christmas Day he wrote, "Around camp, feeding on the pig" so that it was assumed that he brought a live pig with him. He made frequent hunting trips to get food for his dogs.

On February 16 he wrote, "In camp with sore teeth," the first mention of sickness. The end followed swiftly.

"February 17 — In camp; ulcerated teeth.

February 18 — In camp sick.

February 24 — Went up the river hunting dog feed. Dogs have had nothing in four days. If I can't get anything for the poor devils will have to shoot them tomorrow.

February 25 — Feeling real tough. Mouth all swollen up and legs and neck swollen. Spat about a pint of blood this morning. Went out for a little while this afternoon and got some dog feed."

Later, on March 13, the condition was fast worsening as he wrote, "Can just walk. Can hardly get up when I fall down. Was around a little today. Will try to bake tomorrow, have been eating boiled flour the last two days.

March 15 — Will try to make Blank's tomorrow. [The only neighbor; a day away.] Bread never raised an inch but I baked it. It is hard as lead.

March 16 — Tried to make Blank's today; went through the ice. Got both feet wet.

March 18 — Legs turning blue. Shot one of the dogs today. No feed for them.

March 19 — Legs and mouth all swollen up. Can't walk. When I get up to walk I fall down. There doesn't seem to be any strength in my legs. If someone doesn't come along here pretty soon, don't know what will happen. I have only about 30 pounds of flour left and three pounds of barley. I have not got enough for my dogs. Feeling darn sick and weak. — "

The officers who buried him set March 19 as the date of death. The saddest part of this depressing tragedy is that it was senseless; it was entirely preventable. If Hogarth had only known that white, refined flour would not support health while whole grain flour would have restored him, he would have survived. It took only about 30 days from the first danger symptom for the unfortunate man to die. He didn't die of starvation in the way we usually think about, and yet he died on the same flour that is used to make our modern society's valued and favorite breads, biscuits and pastries. The wheat berry had been robbed of its minerals and most vitamins by milling. It is an even greater pity that it cannot be said that he died so that others might learn, and live. Good health is our greatest and most priceless gift, our birthright. Why don't we guard it loyally even fiercely, if necessary?

Deficient Diets Are Deadly

Harter says of one experiment:

"Three pigeons fed upon white bread and casein lived 13, 25, and 29 days respectively. Two dogs fed upon soaked meat, fat, sugar, and white bread were at the point of death at the end of the 26th and 36th day respectively. Two other dogs, completely deprived of food, were comparitively active at the end of 40 and 60 days respectively...One dog fed upon bread made from bleached flour, died in 15 days; another fed upon bread made from ordinary white flour, died in 24 days..."

Dr. Sansum's High Blood Pressure Tests

W.D. Sansum, M.D., had this to say in "Food Facts" about wrong diets and their detrimental effects on test animals:

"Four years ago we began a series of experiments on rabbits to ascertain whether the blood vessel and kidney damage which is responsible for high blood pressure could be produced in such animals by unbalance diets. These preliminary experiments have been successful.

For our control we chose twelve healthy, young rabbits. These rabbits were given a balanced diet consisting of grain and alfalfa hay. The grain has an acid-ash and the alfalfa hay has a alkaline-ash. During the two years of this experiment, these rabbits, with the exception of one which died from pneumonia, remained in excellent health. Their blood pressures were taken each month and remained essentially normal. Their urines were slightly alkaline. There was no retention of waste products in the blood. When these animals were killed and the tissue carefully studied microscopically, there was no evidence of the type of blood vessel or kidney disease which is the cause of high blood pressure.

The second group of twelve healthy, young rabbits was given a diet consisting of grain, having a acid-ash, together with minor additions to prevent the so-called deficiency diseases. These rabbits did not grow well. Seven of them died during the course of the two year experiment. Every rabbit that lived longer than a period of eight months developed high blood pressure, and Bright's disease with albumin in the urine and retention of sewage products in the blood. The remaining five were killed and the tissues have since been studied, together with the tissues of all those that died earlier in the course of the experiment. Depending upon the length of life, the blood vessels show increasing degrees of the same type of blood vessel damage which is seen in human beings afflicted with high blood pressure. The kidneys show the same type of kidney disease which is seen in patients dying from this type of disease.

The third group of twelve healthy, young rabbits was started later. They were given a diet consisting essentially of grains and meat. For this experiment liver was used and was baked, dried and ground with the grains. Minor additions were made to the diet to prevent the so-called deficiency disease. During the course of this shorter experiment of fourteen and one-half months, eleven rabbits died. Increases of blood pressure were noted at the end of the third month. The blood pressures were much higher, averaging nearly 100 percent above normal. The sewage retention in the blood was much higher. The care of the rabbits was very difficult for many of them were sick the greater part of the time. Gross and microscopic findings were even more marked than in the grain series.

Many people believe that blood vessel disease is due to overconsumption of protein foods. The above unbalanced diets were high in protein foods, and to prove that high protein in itself is not the cause of blood vessel disease, we started a fourth group of twelve healthy, young rabbits on high protein, excessively alkaline diet, consisting essentially of ground soya beans. These diets were as excessively alkaline as the other diets were excessively acid. The rabbits developed serious Bright's disease and all of them died during the twenty months of the experiment. The gross and microscopic findings showed no evidence of the type of blood vessel disease which is associated with high blood pressure."

The Underfed Live Longer

Dr. Clive McCay, of Cornell University tested rats on low vs. high calorie diets. One group of rats was allowed to eat all they wanted of a balanced diet; the other group received small meals that kept them slightly hungry, but with plenty of necessary vitamins and minerals. The overfed group lived an average of 600 days; the underfed group lived an average of 1068 days and remained youthful looking until late life. According to the Cornell scientist, the 600 days would equal about 60 years in human life and the 1068 days 107 years!! That's quite a difference.

Calcium Is Linked to Height

Studies have shown that the tallest people of the world have eaten the most high calcium foods. The Scandinavians and Bulgarians have a diet that includes about eight times the amount of calcium as the common American diet. These people are noted for being tall.

The Oriental races such as the Japanese and Chinese have diets low in calcium and are known for being small-boned and short. But we find out that second-generation Chinese and Japanese children raised in America, with a higher calcium intake than in their native countries, are about three or four inches taller than the parents. It is found that the same is the case with American-born immigrants of Russian-Jewish heritage.

Another interesting fact is that as diets improve through the generations, taller and larger boned people are produced. Bones all over the body are larger, and the chest cavity measures larger. The human body contains up to about four pounds of calcium and somewhat over 95% goes to the skeletal structure; the rest is in the nerves, brain and other parts of the body.

McCarrison's Rats and the Diets of India

A young English physician, Dr. Robert McCarrison, observed that the peoples of certain areas in Northern India enjoyed better health than their counterparts. Among these hearty northern groups, arthritis, heart disease, polio, cancer and diabetes were almost unheard of. He vowed at an early age to discover why they were so healthy — both physiologically and psychologically — as compared to their neighbors. McCarrison strongly suspected that the differences were due largely to their superior dietary program. He noted that in the North the quality of fats, the mineral content and the food balance was as a whole far above that found in any other location — East, West or South.

In the North, where some of the finest races of men dwell, whole wheat is the main staple; next comes fresh milk and its products (unpasteurized, of course); following are pulses; then come fresh fruits and vegetables. Meat is sparingly eaten, except by the Pathans.

In the East, West and South rice is the principal food. It is milled and polished, boiled, washed in many water changes; very few milk and milk products are available; vegetables and fruits are scarce.

Years later, Dr. McCarrison became director of the government laboratory at Coonooor, India. In 1927 he was named head of Nutrition Research under the Research Fund Association of the Indian Medical Service. Here was the chance he had dreamed of many years earlier.

McCarrison raised 1,189 white rats on a diet patterned after that of the healthy Northern Indians. The rats were subjected to the experiment for the equivalent of about 50 years in human life. Then he autopsied each rat, finding that there were almost no afflictions or diseases. He reported, "Disease and death have been excluded, almost completely."

Then Dr. McCarrison put 2,243 rats on the inferior diet of the other regions and Indian groups, with opposite results. The list of diseases was lengthy and similar to the diseases listed in medical texts. Some of the maladies he noted were eye diseases, sinus trouble, lung diseases, kidney stones and kidney and urinary diseases, gastrointestinal diseases, sexual system afflicitons in males and females, hair loss, anemia, nervous system disorders, endocrine gland deseases, skin ailments and endless other abnormalities. He proved that faulty diets are the basis for the development of disease. "I know of nothing so potent in maintaining good health in laboratory animals as perfectly constituted food," Dr. McCarrison maintained. "Is man an exception to a rule so universally applicable...?"

The thorough researcher wasn't finished by any means. Isolated test groups of rats were fed the diet of the healthy Northern Indian group and the inadequate diets of other areas; each groups held 20 rats. The poor diet was made up of white bread, jam, margarine, heavily sugared tea, little milk, boiled vegetables and canned meat once a week.

The first groups (good diet) got along joyfully together. They grew rapidly and were generally hardy. The second group grew poorly and did not gain weight properly; they were stunted and their bodies ill-formed; their coats lacked sheen. They were "nervous" and vicious toward the attendants; they were unhappy, began to quarrel and fight and turned cannibal toward the weaker members of the community.

The Doctor concluded his evidence as such: "The newer knowledge of nutrition has revealed, and reveals the more with every addition to it, that the chief cause of the physiological decay of organs and tissues of the body is faulty food, wherein deficiencies of some essentials are often combined with excess of others. It is reasonable, then, to assume that dietetic malnutrition is a chief cause of many degenerative diseases of mankind."

He often quoted the passage: "Harken diligently unto me, and eat ye that which is good." (Isaiah 55:2)

The McCarrison findings are on record for anyone to study. The conclusions he drew, any serious, intelligent student of Nature and health will support. The essence is: food is the greatest single factor in producing bad health if it is of the wrong "nature."

The doctor was insistant that he could produce symptoms of dysentery, diarrhea, dyspepsia, gastric dilations, gastric and duodenal ulcers, colitis, intussusception and failure of the bowels to move properly (colonic failure), simply with a faulty diet.

Peptic ulcers are a great concern, even today. Dr. McCarrison was asked to undertake an experiment with his Coonoor rats to see what could be learned about the ulcers common among the poorer classes of southern Travancore. He placed rats on the identical diet of those people for 675 days; at the end of the test period he found peptic ulcers in more than one-fourth of the rats.

Stefansson and the Arctic Diet

Arctic explorer, Vilhjalmur Stefansson, discovered some significant facts regarding a raw meat diet. He observed that the Eskimos enjoyed excellent health on a diet of raw meat — blood, liver and bone marrow — from seal, fish and walrus chiefly. He lead a group of healthy young men into the Arctic climate. Stefansson put the party on a diet of raw meat finding that they remained warm, strong and healthy. A few weeks were required for the men to become accustomed to the strange diet; many at first were nauseated. However, they soon came to like the diet and were free from constipation and indigestion. Upon cooking the meat or adding salt the men complained of severe indigestion. It is well known that raw meat is heating and stimulating; these properties are essential for survival in extreme Northern latitudes.

Further study disclosed that the urine of those on the raw meat diet was free of the putrefactive acids of protein indigestion.

Pottenger's Extensive Cat Experiments

Dr. Francis Pottenger, Jr. carried out extensive and in depth studies to prove the disadvantages of cooked animal protein. He used cats, natural carnivores, as the test animals. When their diet was raw protein alone their health was excellent. Dr. Pottenger used 109 cats in a five year study to arrive at his conclusions. He found that not one cat or offspring of the raw protein diet group developed diseases. They lived to an old age.

However, the group placed on the diet of cooked animal proteins all developed ailments and diseases similar to those found in humans — loss of teeth, hair, pyorrhea, arthritis, bone rarification, gastritis, cirrhosis and atrophy of the liver; also, they showed degeneration in the brain and spinal cord. We find that pasteurized milk was part of the cooked protein diet.

It is unfortunate that most people are unaware of his classic findings, and the medical profession chooses to generally ignore his conclusive evidence. Here are a few of his outstanding conclusions: (Note the special significance of the final point.)

1. Cats kept on the raw protein diet stayed healthy; cats on cooked protein (including pasteurized milk) developed diseases.
2. After the cats suffered health damage due to the cooked animal protein diets, they could not fully regain the good health they once possessed.
3. Liver dysfunction was progressive on the cooked diet; the bile eventually became so toxic that the felines' excretions used as fertilizer would not support even the growth of weeds.
4. The first generation of kittens showed abnormalities; the second was often born dead or diseased; there *was no third generation* because the females had become sterile!

It is important to note that the milk used was pasteurized, along with its pasteurized products — cheese, ice cream, buttermilk, canned and dried milk — cooked eggs, fried, roasted or boiled meats and salted and heat-dried meats. Dr. Pottenger's findings are something for all of us to think about seriously.

Hardening of the Arteries in Young America

Korean War physicians found that the American soldiers often showed large deposits of cholesterol (athero-sclerosis) in the arteries. Autopsies of young Chinese and Korean men revealed almost no signs of atherosclerosis.

Since that time many further studies and comparisons have been made. It has been discovered that the Japanese in their homeland display very low levels of cholesterol deposits; their diet contains very little fatty foods. The Hawaiian-Japanese eat more fat and show more athero-sclerosis accordingly. California-based Japanese, "enjoying" the typical American diet, show the same rate of cholesterol corrosion as Causasian Americans.

New Zealand School Lunch Experiment

A noteworthy school lunch study was conducted in New Zealand. Two hundred and fifty children were provided with nutritious lunches such as whole wheat sandwiches, vegetable salads and fruit for dessert. Parents were amazed at the behavioral changes in their children. Such observations as the following were made. "Our children no longer suffer from constipation; they don't have skin troubles; they aren't so ornery and obstreperous any longer; they are more calm and less hyperactive and nervous."

Letters stated that colds were reduced or eliminated. A group of dentists and dental technicians observed a strongly marked decrease in tooth decay over several years. If U.S. officials could recognize that the foods coming to school children are devitalized and broken down, nutritionally inferior and loaded with harmful additives, perhaps a positive change could be made. Someone has to make the recommendations. The health of our future generations depends on our action today.

Diet and Delinquency

Can diet cut juvenile delinquency? A survey of 17 maladjusted or delinquent girls between the ages of 11 and 15 in a Salvation Army hotel here seems to prove it can. Previously the girls lived on the poorest possible type of meal: white bread and margarine, cheap jams, lots of sweet tea, tinned and processed meats. Fish and chips had been one of their most nutritious meals.

A year ago their diet was changed to raw fruit, nuts, vegetables, salads, whole wheat bread, dates, prunes, honey, cheese, meat, fish, eggs, crushed wheat and oatmeal.

This is what happened: They quickly became less aggressive and less quarrelsome, bad habits seemed to disappear. "Problem children" became less of a problem and the bored ones lost their boredom. Physically, they improved almost beyond recognition. A spokesman said: "It is amazing to see the difference in their complexions, general brightness and poise. But the difference in their behavior is most significant." He continued, "The part diet has played in their personalities is undeniable."

Chapter 10

Crusaders who shared their knowledge

"We only have what we give."

Many Crusaders Deserve a Tribute

It has been difficult over the years with so many techniques, so many new ideas in the healing art. Necessary biochemical elements don't always come from strict vegetarian diets. At times I have had to resort to protomorphogens, meat extracts, glandular extracts, though they were against the principles I would like to uphold. Working with chemical elements and the V.G. Rocine doctrine, I was able to do the greatest amount of healing work. Through the years I have stood fast to this philosophy and doctrine with great success. Chemicals and various essences, tonics, food preparations of a healthful nature are used in my healing work.

Dr. Henry Lindlahr, Dr. John Tilden, John Harvey Kellogg, Ralph Benner of Bircher-Benner Sanitarium in Zurich, Switzerland, Dr. George Weger, of Redlands, California and countless others have been instrumental in giving me a solid foundation in nutritional principles to help my patients.

Dr. W.A. Albrecht, University of Missouri Agricultural Department, has taught me much in the respect of feeding animals, to see the effects of deficient soils on plants and animals.

Dr. W.A. Sansum, of Santa Barbara, fed test animals certain kinds of foods and produced specific diseases and ailments. These foods lacked proper chemical elements — minerals — and also other nutrients. He produced diabetes in animals by feeding them degenerated, devitalized foods; he produced hemorrhoids in animals by giving them coffee and other products their bodies considered toxic.

We consider disease an altered state of body chemistry. Disease preys on an undernourished body, as Dr. Albrecht found in plant and animal experiments. A little voice in Nature whispers to us, saying that this balance is not correct when our body is in a state of revolt — not working — properly. I consider myself extremely fortunate to have had the privilege of working with patients, people who have gone through hard times, made harsh sacrifices, suffered through elimination processes, reversal processes and the healing crises to such an extent that I have felt at times "the cure is worse than the disease," as it is said. But cleansing, purification and elimination has to take place; when the body chemistry is sufficiently built up, when reserves are replaced, the body undergoes a cleansing and rebuilding procedure. New tissue takes the place of old. Nature does the curing; she just needs the opportunity.

Many experiments support what these Nature cure crusaders believe and teach. This text is coming from an experimental station, so to speak, where nutrition has been used as the foundation to regain good health. It was worked out on my Ranch where patients come to live with "their doctor" so he could teach them to live correctly. I was able to watch their progress, chart it and keep track of their subsequent check-ups after they had returned home to follow the programs laid down specifically for them. There must be a foundation to live properly. Most of these ideas are supported and developed by work with over 300,000 patients taken care of in the past 50 years of my practice. By experimenting with diet, certain foods were found to have unfavorable effects upon specific patients. Some foods disturb a delicate, nervous, convalescent person; the same foods may be easily tolerated by the robust, healthy, muscular person who could "digest nails," so to phrase it. Some foods produce bloating and discomfort, headaches and other ailments in the delicate digestive system. This is the reason behind the development of nut milk drinks, behind the finer foods.

I believe the future will see more healing done through education, teaching patients to live properly. More will be accomplished in this manner than in doctors' offices where pills, treatments, supplements, potions, vaccinations and other drugs are so widely used.

Dr. V.G. Rocine —

I consider Dr. V.G. Rocine, one of the greatest biochemists in his day, my greatest professor and teacher. While he drew many of his experiments, results and conclusions from other scientists and chemists throughout Europe, he brought it all together and, through further development, study and experimenting on human beings, developed a system of healing that I feel is the greatest that any man has produced. Dr. Rocine was more complete in his reasoning. He looked to all sides of life. If you were a good student, you were kept on your mental toes constantly. He never opened his mouth without giving me something to think about. He helped me see that every man is unique. There are no duplicates — not even a twin exists. Health and happiness depend on many factors — the earth, the sun, the sky, plants, feelings, the shape and type of each person, and how that type is developed over a period of generations from Nature's biochemical laboratory. Dr. Rocine's development of the temperament types and chemical types of people opened up a whole new world to me.

One time I sat with Dr. Rocine while he interviewed a patient. The lady said, "I'm 5 months pregnant and I would like to start living right so I might have a healthy child." "My dear," Rocine answered, "you should have started 20 years ago."

Once this came flashing through: "Some day you may want to correct a disease thinking of it hypothetically. Let us start now so we will not have to correct it."

Rocine brought out that our relationships and attitudes toward life depend on our temperament "type" development; we can only draw from life according to the type we are, and to understand these things brings greater understanding with one another.

We understand things according to our chemical type. I could tell you some things you would not understand if you are a different chemical type from me. Importance of some things done in life is dependent upon your ancestors and the chemical balance in your body derived from them. The chemical elements make up your glands, your feelings, mental attitudes, etc. I know why you don't understand because I'm a quick sodium type — I like to jump over the fence. Some of you couldn't jump a fence and you may think I'm an oddball for wanting to get there before you.

The Chinese is a chlorine person. Chlorine is the cleanser, and we find the Chinese are among the cleanest people in the world, always working around water. The Russians are calcium types — like to work with the land. They really enjoy working with the earth.

Dr. Tom Spies

Dr. Tom Spies, M.D. was recognized by the American Medical Association in 1957 for his great contributions to the healing art through his work with foods. He summed up his philosophy as follows:

"All diseases are caused by chemicals. All diseases can be cured by chemicals. All the chemicals used by the body except for the oxygen which we breathe and the water which we drink are taken in through food. If we only knew enough, all diseases could be prevented and could be cured through proper nutrition.

"As tissues become damaged, they lack the chemicals for good nutrition. They tend to become old. They lack what I call 'tissue integrity.' There are people of 40 whose brains and arteries are senile. If we could help the tissues repair themselves by correcting nutritional deficiencies, we can make old age wait."

Dr. Spies is one of the few medical doctors who works with a food routine. The above statements were delivered before the annual meeting of the A.M.A., where he was honored for his healing art contributions.

Dr. John H. Tilden

The generation of an unlimited supply of human energy is not possible. A good deal of our energy is consumed in bad habits, and our batteries can run low. Our metabolisms drop down a few notches when enervation or tiredness comes in. Dr. Tilden brought this out in so much of his work, that enervation is the beginning of every disease. Organic function is impaired. In a state of lowered nerve force, we cannot build a good body. We deplete ourselves through physical, mental and emotional work and through over-eating, over-stimulation, over-clothing, lack of clothing and through excess and dissipation of all kinds, through worry, fear, anger, self-pity, exercise, jealousy and starvation from light. We find that bad habits will really kill us. There is only one way we can get rid of the toxemias in our body, and that is through cleansing of the body and through good eating and right living.

Dr. Tilden wrote,

"The strongest organ may be broken down by the strain and stress of toxemia. When organs are over-worked and undernourished from nerve starvation, congestion takes place, leading to acute or chronic inflammation and eventually to degeneration... Toxemia is an accumulation of acid and body waste, uneliminated from lack of nerve energy. One authority has remarked that overweight is a sign of approaching disease. This is true because the body's functioning is lessened in a heavy toxic medium... Toxemia or disease may localize itself in any part of the body, producing there a manifestation, locally named, and considered by the average person a disease entity affecting only that particular area."

Professor Ivan P. Pavlov

Pavlov, the Russian scientist, conducted experiments that proved concentrated starches and animal proteins shouldn't be combined at the same meals. For instance, meat and potatoes are not advisable. The mixture caused fermentation, improper digestion and the production of "unfriendly bacteria" in the intestinal tract. A further finding was that the unhealthy mixture slowed down the transit time of food in the large intestine (colon) — resulting in constipation.

Dr. Melvin E. Page

Melvin E. Page, D.D.S. says in his book *Degeneration — Regeneration* that, "I believe sugar to be the most disasterous substance of civilization not only because it is a deficiency food but because through its use we impose undue hardship upon the sugar-converting glands. The reason it does so is this. Our bodies were originally made to manufacture glucose, a simple sugar from natural foods. Our bodies are the same mechanical contrivances that they were one thousand or ten thousand years ago and they are still capable of turning 68 percent of our food into glucose, that percentage of our food which must be used for energy and heat. In the process of digestion, carbohydrates, fat, starches, etc., are converted into glucose so slowly that a small but nearly continuous supply is made. It is like pouring a bucket of water on the top step of a long flight of stairs. It takes quite a time to collect the water at the bottom step. On the other hand, if we pour the water on the next-to-last step it all reaches the bottom step in a hurry."

Dr. Page says of disease, "It would appear that the greatest handicap in the solution of these diseases has been in the study of the diseases themselves. The cancer men have studied the cancer tissue, they have implanted it in other animals, they have tried drugs and chemicals to inhibit its growth. The arthritis men studied arthritis, what happened in the joints in a person so afflicted. The dentists have studied the teeth and their surrounding tissue. All have studied from these angles, but the complete answer does not lie in the study of these diseases; it lies in the study of the host of these diseases."

Dr. Clive McCay

Dr. Clive McCay of Cornell University studied nutrition and its relationship to aging for many years. Here are some of his conclusions from "Chemical Aspects of Aging and the Effect of Diet Upon Aging."

". . . the requirement for calcium rises in old age and may exceed the amount needed at any other period in life. Likewise the need for vitamins and protein seems just as high in old age as in middle life.

"The second great hazard in later life is the temptation to consume foods that provide little beside energy. The two that create the greatest danger are alcohol and sugar. The next two in order of importance are cooking fats and white flour. With the exception of alcohol these substances all offer the additional temptation of being cheap sources of energy. They are not cheap if they lead to years of ill health in later life. . .

"Since the old person may be dependent upon foods ready to eat he should give special attention to basic products such as bread. Bread can be made from excellent formulas containing milk, wheat germ, soy flour and yeast, or it can be made very poorly of white flour with few additions. What is true for bread is also true for breakfast cereals and sweet baked goods.

"The older person can help his own diet by mixing dry skim milk or dry yeast into his foods. He can keep a sugar or dry yeast into his foods. . . Milk is probably the best food for later life. Tests with animals have indicated that they can be reared and kept for the whole of life upon no other food than fresh milk. Older as well as younger people can profit by the use of more milk. . .

"Nutrition during later life requires regular study by every individual to insure sound food habits and avoid the pitfalls of alcohol, sugar and fat." [We advise goat milk in our work, in limited amounts.]

Dr. N.S. Painter

N.S. Painter, senior surgeon at London's Manor House hospital authored a paper called "Diverticular Disease of the Colon, a Disease of this Century" in 1969. In his view diverticular disease is a deficiency due to a lack of roughage in the diet. He said he had seen it increasingly among those who lived on refined diets (such as white sugar and flour) that lacked natural fiber. Dr. Painter added that a diet with more bran and fiber "would achieve more than all our surgical endeavors and show that diverticular disease, like scurvy, is preventable."

Dr. Denis P. Burkitt

It was Denis P. Burkitt, F.R.S., in a paper called "Related Disease — Related Cause?" who said: "Appendicitis, diverticular disease, adenomatous polyps [small glandular tumors], and bowel carcinoma [cancer growing on the mucous membrane] appear to be directly related to a Western way of life." He added that cancer of the colon and rectum in England was second only to lung cancer. Most diseases, he said, are caused by environment and not genetics and inheritance. In concluding he said, "If a relationship can be established between dietary habits and disease patterns, it should not be necessary to await an understanding of the mechanism whereby benign or malignant disease is produced before attempting prevention."

Lancet carried a paper by Mr. Burkitt, "Relationship as a Clue to Causation" the next year. In essence he described how milling of white flour and white sugar removed indigestible fiber and led to the diet of excessive refined carbohydrates and low residue. He linked England's increased consumption of refined carbohydrates in the 50's and 60's to increasing obesity, diabetes, diverticulitis, appendicitis and even atherosclerosis. We find he also mentioned that "refined carbohydrate is believed to alter the bacterial flora of the feces," and said we get to the place where the intestinal flora is changed and harmful substances are produced that could lead to tumors in the bowel.

Dr. E.V. McCollum

Dr. E.V. McCollum of Johns Hopkins University believes we should stop thinking of nutrition in terms of merely preventing deficiencies. He points out that there is a health-building side also. He stresses the difference between adequate nutrition and optimal nutrition. His idea of the optimal diet promotes the following conditions:

1. Encourages good growth
2. Allows the highest fertility rate in the female and the highest virility in the male
3. Makes the highest level of success in rearing healthy offspring a reality
4. Adds the most years to the life span
5. Guards youth and delays old age and senility longest.

Dr. McCollum points out that China and other parts of the Orient known to include a generous supply of green, leafy vegetables in the common diet are relatively free from rickets in children. It is almost never found. Rickets is found often in Europe and America due to the habit of the average family to use a larger percentage of refined cereals, milled grains, meat, legumes and tuber or root vegetables. He adds that raw, green and leafy vegetables are vital additions to the typical American diet of meat, potatoes and bread. If we want good health, don't neglect them.

Dr. Roger J. Williams

Dr. Roger J. Williams, University of Texas biochemist, placed 64 rats of four different strains on a diet of white bread, "enriched" as it has been for nearly forty years with [synthetic] niacin, iron, riboflavin and B1 (thiamine). An additional sixty-four rats of four different strains were placed on an "improved" bread made of flour with these nutritional supplements: "magnesium oxide, copper sulphate, manganese sulphate, calcium phosphate, folic acid, vitamins A and E, cobalamine, pantothenic acid, pyridoxine and the amino acid lysine which is a vital link in the protein chain." These nutrients added little cost and weren't intended to make the best possible bread. "After ninety days on the commercial bread," [group one] observed Dr. Williams, "two thirds of the animals were dead of malnutrition, and the survivors were severely stunted, whereas practically all the other animals [group two] on the improved bread were alive and growing." It is worth noting that Dr. Williams pointed out that the "improved" bread would raise the cost of a loaf of bread about three cents. He expressed regret that the milling in-

dustry and the FDA allowed bread to be "nutritionally far below" what it could easily be. He laid the blame for this lack of knowledge and action on "the apathy, if not antagonism, exhibited by classical medical education toward nutrition," and also on the fact that "medical science has generally failed to take nutrition seriously as a part of the cause of disease."

Tooth Decay is Linked to "Civilized" Diets

The teeth as well as the rest of the body are made of the dust of the earth, and we find that they need nourishment; a well nourished tooth never decays. We must have good circulation. We must make sure that all the biochemical elements are there in order to build good teeth. In the Museum of Natural History in Washington, D.C. is a collection of Indian skulls representing all ages of life picked up on the Pacific Coast of the two Americas about 200 years ago. Of the thousands of teeth in these skulls, only one shows signs of dental caries.

Taking care of the teeth by brushing is not the complete answer. In fact, we find that teeth are built from within. A healthy mouth is a clean mouth and an unhealthy mouth cannot be kept clean no matter how much brushing we may use. This is the same with any orifice of the body. Some have to brush their teeth more often than others, and this is because of the bodily condition. I believe that pyorrhea, and various bad mouth conditions, are an expression of many dietetic errors of malnutrition. I am convinced that the hardness of the tooth comes from within first and I believe that decay comes from within, also.

It is Dr. Percy Howe who said that in Forsythe they have produced — within a period of six weeks — all the classic symptoms of acute pyorrhea by drastic diet deficiencies and then cured them completely in ten days by balancing the diet.

Good Teeth

Infants fed on formulas tend to develop poor and decaying teeth. The same is true of diets that don't require chewing of hard foods, with accompanying tooth and jaw exercises. Hard, fibrous foods exercise the teeth and jaws as well as cleansing the teeth. Our current refined, artificial diets also leave the teeth and mouth coated, or dirty.

Calcium shortage is a chief factor in tooth decay, among many other deficiencies. Dr. E.V. McCollum, of Johns Hopkins University says:

"It is not possible at this time to name any one deficiency which specifically causes dental or oral disease; it would appear to be that any slight variations in the American diet, which always so dangerously approaches the level of dietary

101

deficiency, might become active to start decay at any period of lowered resistance or of physical or nervous distress."

According to Dr. Melvin E. Page, dentist and nutritional research scientist, "Dentin, the bony structure of the teeth, depends for its well being upon its nourishment. If it is not well nourished, it is soft; if it is well nourished, it is hard and dense and resistant to bacterial invasion. Not only does the dentin depend upon its nourishment for the internal factors which inhibit disease, but the external environment is affected as well by the state of well-being of the body as a whole. These external environmental factors include the buffer action of the saliva, which in turn results from the state of efficiency of the internal factors. The buffer action of the saliva is dependent upon the mineral content which is derived from the blood. Thus the blood levels of calcium and phosphorus determine resistance to decay from both the internal and external standpoint."

Dr. Weston A. Price

Dr. Weston A. Price, of the American Dental Association Research Commission, spent many years traveling among and investigating the worlds' primitive peoples. Among the races and peoples he studied were the Swiss, Gaelics, Eskimos, North American Indians, Melanesians, Polynesians, African tribes, Australian Aborigines, New Zealand Maoris, and Peruvian Indians. The evidence is documented in his book *Nutrition and Physical Degeneration.* He compared the primitive people in natural settings to those who took up the ways of civilization and to this he added the comparison to the civilized races of the world.

Dr. Price compared the teeth of villagers in isolated Swiss Alp areas with their "civilized" city dwelling kin. He studied the Alaskan Eskimos and the Indians of North and South America; the pattern was the same the world over. He found the isolated, primitive groups living on natural foods almost free from dental caries. They didn't need dentists, doctors, medications and toothbrushes. Their diets were made up of fruits, vegetables, grains and meat they killed or raised themselves.

He noted cavities in the people who moved to the cities and took up the diet of so-called affluent societies. This consisted of white sugar and white flour products, polished rice, soda pop, candy, pastries, cakes and ice cream.

In studying skulls of the Florida Seminole Indians, he found no tooth decay in several hundred specimens. When he researched the Seminoles of today's generation living in the isolated swamps, he found that they were still highly immune to tooth decay. Four teeth in every 100 examined showed tooth decay. In comparing their "tourist attraction" relatives, 40 out of every 100 teeth showed

signs of dental decay. These Seminoles have taken to the diet of the civilized American society. The diet of highly refined carbohydrates had taken its toll. Clearly, this illustrates that good teeth and health depend on natural, pure and whole foods.

Dr. Price Praises "Primitive" Diets

Dr. Price found no scurvy among the primitive tribes, even in the Yukon of Alaska where no fruit could grow. They told him they knew better than to buy the white man's white sugar and flour. Their teeth were free from caries, and the general health was excellent in these isolated peoples of the world, whether they were in Alaska or New Zealand or anywhere in between. Their diets of natural, unrefined and unsugared foods were the key to their excellent physical conditions, Dr. Price concluded. Degeneration was observed in one generation after they left the "primitive" ways for "civilization."

Ellen G. White

Ellen G. White wrote the following about fats close to a century ago, before we became seriously concerned about the fats in our diets, especially high serum cholesterol: "Nut foods are coming largely into use to take the place of flesh meats...When properly prepared, olives, like nuts, supply the place of butter and flesh meats. The oil, as eaten in the olive, is far preferable to animal oil or fat."

In 1915 white flour was becoming a big part of the American milling operations and food supply. Nutritional authorities were not rising against its use like today's nutritionists are. Mrs. White wrote: "For use in breadmaking, the superfine white flour is not the best. Its use is neither healthful nor economical. Fine-flour bread is lacking in nutritive elements to be found in bread made from the whole wheat."

We realize the value of food combining and the dangers of overeating and obesity today. Ellen G. White wrote, "There should not be a great variety at any one meal, for this encourages overeating and causes indigestion. . . . Abstemiousness in diet is rewarded with mental and moral vigor; it also aids in the control of the passions. Overeating is especially harmful to those who are sluggish in temperament; these should eat sparingly, and take plenty of physical exercise. . . . At each meal take only two kinds of simple food, and eat no more than is required to satisfy hunger."

Mrs. White also warned against the practice of gourmet dining already common during her lifetime. "In the entertainment of guests there should be greater simplicity. . . . We should not provide for the Sabbath a more liberal supply or a greater variety of food than for other days. Instead of this the food should be more simple, and less should be eaten in order that the mind may be clear and vigorous to comprehend spiritual things. . . . There is a large class who will reject any reform movement, however reasonable, if it lays a restriction upon the appetite."

And, again: "We know yeast is preferable to baking powder in baking. Inorganic salt is also detrimental to the body. . . . The use of soda or baking powder in breadmaking is harmful and unnecessary. . . . Do not eat largely of salt."

Studies of Vitamin A and Infection

It was "Drug Therapy" that carried the thought that skin diseases are a sign of low vitamin A blood levels. They said this is especially true with acne or ulcers.

Dr. Sherman, of Columbia University says about Vitamin A, "We now have good reason to believe that surplus vitamin A in the body is not simply a passive reserve asset to be used at some future time but also actively increases the vigor and the ability of the body to resist disease."

The minimum daily requirement of Vitamin A is set at 5,000 units but 8,000 I.U. are needed to prevent night blindness alone. When infections invade the body and during illness, much more Vitamin A is needed. That stored supply is quickly used. We find that below normal levels are found in the blood of ill persons. It is especially low in cases of colitis, tuberculosis, pneumonia, liver and kidney diseases.

Note: Pure, whole, natural cod liver oil is the best if you need a source of Vitamins A and D, especially during the winter months. If ergosterol is irradiated for too long a time, it becomes toxic, due to the formation of a poisonous substance. Other natural forms of the vitamin have never been noted to be toxic.

National Cancer Institute researchers say they have protected hamsters from lung cnacer after exposing them to carcinogenic substances by using Vitamin A. (Medical World News, April 5, 1976)

Dr. George Wolf of the Massachusetts Institute of Technology says a deficiency of Vitamin A is noted in 30 percent of the U.S. people and that with a lack of it there is a danger of being vulnerable to cancer-causing substances.

Vitamin A is found in vegetables [high in carrots], some fruits and dairy products, cod liver oil, and other foods; it is an extremely vital nutrient to general nutrition. Dr. Frank Chytill, Vanderbilt University, says deficiencies of Vitamin A make susceptible body areas less able to resist cancer. He says the vitamin can help prevent cancer.

We find there is new evidence that cancer and air pollution effects can be partly neutralized by Vitamins A, C, and E. And there is scientific evidence that Vitamin C can protect against cold viruses to some extent. These findings come from the National Institute of Health, Stanford University and the Albert Einstein College of Medicine.

Vitamin A Fights Infection

Vitamin A has a definite influence on infections in the body; its undersupply can result in noncontagious illnesses. Dr. Tistall of the University of Toronto ran tests on vitamin A deficiency using rats. He had two groups; one was given plenty of vitamin A and the other group was lacking it. Then both groups were fed bacteria that cause rat typhoid. We find that only 20% of the well-fed rats died and 76% of the vitamin-A-deficient rats died.

Xerophthalmia, an infection of the eyes due to a lack of Vitamin A, has been common in the Orient for centuries. The eyelids swell and become sore, and the surface of the eye is dry. It can eventually result in blindness. This eye disease broke out in Denmark during World War I among the poorer Danes because they sold their butter and milk products and gave their children skim milk and margarine. Many children consequently became blind. Butter and cod-liver oil saved the sight of the others. Xerophthalmia is still found among the poor people of Egypt, China and India where the diet is mostly cereals.

Foods high in Vitamin A are mentioned in an Egyptian medical record written about 1600 B.C. Translated it reads, "A treatment for the eyes: liver of ox roasted and pressed, give for it; very excellent." Hippocrates, the Greek physician honored as the Father of Medicine, born 460 B.C., prescribed ox liver in honey for eye disease. Countless other early references are made to eye diseases, especially in late winter. The herb eyebright, similar to parsley, was suggested as a remedy.

Nutritional Deficiencies and Mental Disturbances

Pellagra, caused by niacin deficiency was the first mental disorder linked to nutritional deficiencies. The symptoms of pellagra are irritability, apprehension, memory loss and confusion that can lead to delirium.

It was Professor Linus Pauling who said a deficiency of B-1, nicotinic acid, B-6, B-12, biotin, C and folic acid are responsible for brain disorders — mental illness — and nervous system troubles. Professor Pauling is a Nobel Prize-winning chemist of the University of California.

We might add that the ability of the body to assimilate and use B-complex vitamins depends on silicon reserves. When we take B-complex, silicon should be taken at the same time.

In "The New Psychiatry," Dr. Masor gives examples of treating mental symptoms with vitamins, even schizophrenia, and the dosage was high with no adverse effects or the need to return to psychotherapy.

We find that in "Lancet" (1969) it was said that "Occult vitamin B-12 deficiency is a commoner cause of mental illness than is generally believed." And it recommended a closer study of pernicious anemia in mental patients.

And it was in the "British Medical Journal" (March 1966) that doctors wrote: "It is true that vitamin B-12 deficiency may cause severe psychotic symptoms which may vary in severity from mild disorders of mood...[to] paranoid behavior."

Dr. Rosenfeld, a U.S. doctor, believes that nutritional deficiencies are the cause of thousands of divorces a year, rather than blaming them on emotional problems. This is something to think about.

We agree that improper diets can have much to do with bad tempers, irritability, hostility and even crimes. The basic common diet of "advanced" societies consisting of white bread and white flour products, white sugar, refined carbohydrates, carbonated drinks and processed foods are partly the cause of mental and social troubles today. In the book *Natural Health, Sugar and the Criminal Mind,* J. I. Rodale says, "The best place to solve the problem of juvenile delinquency is in the cooking pots of the homes."

We find that violence in the schools is on the upswing all over the world. In New York City more than 100 teachers had been stabbed, robbed or threatened with violence in less than three months in one year. They were forced to ask for protection and threatened to go on strike if it wasn't given.

"The Times" has stated that juvenile crime is rising in almost every European country and the biggest increase is in the most developed technological nations. Is this the price of "progress?"

It is a medical fact that a lack of Vitamin B-1 can produce swelling of the adrenal glands; this makes them excrete too much adrenalin — the "fight or flight" syndrome. Too much adrenalin makes for over-aggression.

A test conducted by the Mayo Clinic shows what effects a lack of Vitamin B-1 has on disposition and behavior. Volunteers went on the common diet of the American family— processed carbohydrates, skim milk [pasteurized], butter, cheese, egg white, canned vegetables and fruits, coffee, tea, etc. To make the diet balanced in all but B-1, brewer's yeast was given but with the B-1 taken out. Cod liver oil supplied Vitamins A and E; and iron, calcium and phosphorus were also given. (This diet was better than the average American diet.) All volunteers soon showed personality changes, such as irritability, depression, quarreling, lack of cooperation. Among the physical symptoms was a lack of hydrochloric acid flow in the stomach. By the end of the twenty-first week, symptoms were so severe that the experiment had to be ended. When B-1 was reinstated to the diet, they became happy and agreeable within a few hours! It was about 12 days before the hydrochloric acid began to flow normally again, but the mental symptoms were gone much sooner.

Dr. Price's World Behavior Patterns Findings

We find that during the course of Dr. Price's travels and studies of world peoples, including fourteen primitive tribes, he made interesting observations about social and mental behavior in addition to physical degeneration. In spite of the diversified races and customs, he found that the primitive tribes lived in harmony with one another and violence was relatively unknown. However, changes were noted as soon as they came into contact with civilized foods [processed], refined white sugar, white flour, carbonated drinks, etc. The first generation reared on these foods showed changes in behavior from happy contentment to fighting, depression, quarreling and dissatisfaction. In view of the rise of crime today, this is something we should think about.

The Behavior of McCarrisons' India Rats

Sir Robert McCarrison fed rats the diets of various Indian races and showed that they [rats] developed the same physical symptoms of good health or disease according to the diet. They tended to behave consistently with human characteristics. And McCarrison also fed a group of rats the typical "poor European diet" of white bread, oleomargarine, sugared tea, cheap jam, canned meat and few vegetables. The young produced by these rats showed poor bone structure, skin disorders and other symptoms strangely like those of people on the same diets. But we find out that the behavioral patterns were surprisingly similar, too; the rats became foul-tempered, fought among themselves, bit the attendants and finally started to kill one another — turning cannibal against the weaker members.

Other Notes on Nutrition-Behavior Links

Sugar and sugared foods cause the deficiency of B-1 — called the "morale" vitamin [thiamine]. The state of depression produced by this shortage can get to the place where suicidal tendencies appear. Is this part of the reason pep pills and other "high" producing drugs are more and more common? Professor Rene Dubos, ecologist and author of *Man Adapting* said: "A society that depends on sedatives and stimulants cannot achieve the resilience necessary for survival, let alone growth."

Darwin's Evolution Observation

Soil and climate differ all over the world. Through Darwin's law of survival of the fittest, plants develop to meet the environmental conditions in their area. Over many generations these characteristics become fixed. For example the palm tree can exist only in certain climates, and the cactus has its suitable climate. The same laws apply to animals, humans included. Certain diets fit the characteristics developed by many generations; certain altitudes and climates are conducive to the best health of various types. Species or individual types become extinct if they cannot change fast enough to adapt to changing environments. We often fail to realize that the same applies to the human race. We are as bound to the laws of Nature as other animals. As a result, size, height, color and race differ.

Evolution of the Shetland Pony

It is said that many centuries ago the Shetland Islands were uninhabited by horses of any breed until some swam ashore from a wrecked ship. The horses increased in numbers, but the limited vegetation forced them to eat seaweed. The seaweed was a good food except for the lack of sufficient calcium. Since calcium is necessary for bone growth, the horses through the generations had to compensate for the deficiency. Today Shetland ponies are noted for their small size, inbred smaller and smaller over the generations, partly due to this lack of calcium. After many later generations had been fed on calcium-rich food, their stature changed little. Their characteristics seem fixed in the new species size they were forced to adapt in order to survive.

Evidence of Devolution in Reduced Height

The average brain capacity of modern man, that science believes has reached the utmost in human development, is about 20 percent smaller than that of Cro-Magnon man. This specimen lived 25,000 years ago or more and his average height was thought to be well over six feet.

A picture in a newspaper of June 6, 1931 showed a giant skull now in the museum of Keswick, Cumberland County, England. In Ripley's "Believe It or Not," he says that by measurement of the skull "the stature of the giant must have been in excess of ten feet, or about the height of the Philistine Goliath," ["whose height was six cubits and a span" — about eleven feet and a half — (I Sam. 17:4)].

Today's advanced science does not accept the belief that any man in history has ever been nearly twelve feet tall. In a publication of March 9, 1931, Ripley said that Jan Van Albert of Holland was nine feet, three-and-one-half inches tall; that Fedor Machnow, the Russian giant of Charkow, said to be the tallest man of modern times, was nine feete, three inches tall at age 23; he weighed 360 pounds; his middle finger was 12 inches long.

In the press of July 27, 1930, Ripley tells us that Angoulaffre, the Saracen giant who lived in the 8th century A.D., was twelve feet tall; his middle finger was 11 inches long. It is written that he was slain by Roland a nephew of Charlemagne, who stood eight feet tall at Fronsac.

Ripley published a picture of a skull in the Witlen Museum, Amsterdam, that was 12 inches wide at the temples, and 20 inches from the chin to the crown of the head. This is interpreted to mean the height was over thirteen feet tall.

The following was in the press of November 17, 1933: "A Persian with a long name, Siah Ibn Kashmir Khan, standing 11 feet three inches tall in his socks, believes that he is the tallest man in the world. And who can dispute it? When he made a trip to Europe recently, he had to be lifted aboard ship by crane because of the difficulty of getting him on the gangway from a small boat in a choppy sea."

Dr. R.M. Johnson, in the *Chiropractic Record* of 1926 said: "Man has degenerated from a normal time of existence of some hundreds of years, to the present average duration of less than two score years, and from a race of giants to the modern dwarf and cretin.

"As late as the 18th century may be found examples of primitive physical perfection. In 1830 there was exhibited at Rouen a living man 18 feet in height. A few years later, near the same city, was found a human skeleton 19 feet long. Three human skeletons unearthed near Palermo measured 21, 30, and 34 feet in length respectively.

"During the year 1566 a native of Bengal died at the age of 370 years; during the 18th century a South American slave died at the age of 175 years; Mrs. Keith of Gloucester, lived 173 years; Raparth of San Salvadore 180 years; and in Caledonia, Wisconsin, Joseph Creola died at the age of 142 years."

Is There a Land of the Giants?

In the summer of 1929 a ship sailed from Sydney, Australia under Captain C.N. Olsen with five adventurers on board. The Captain was to take these brave and curious souls into unknown waters in search of a South Sea island they had heard so many tales about. No map showed the tiny island located in the Gilbert group called "Tarawa." After much difficulty and good fortune they sighted the island.

The group had to drop anchor half a mile from shore and take small boats, wading the last 200 feet to shore. In the captain's own words this is what they saw:

"To our amazement we found the island densely populated with a race of as handsome a people as I ever saw. They appeared to be a mixture of Malaysian and Polynesian.

"The men were giants in stature. They were modeled like Greek gods, standing well over six feet, and well proportioned and developed.

"The women were tall, too, and as graceful as nymphs are said to be. Their half-clothed bodies are bronzed and unblemished, and every one of these strange people seem filled with immense vitality, even though the temperature of their island home seldom drops below 90 degrees."

The island, the account says, was only four feet above sea level and some of it under water at high tide. The only fruit or vegetable tree was the coconut. The islanders' diet was a mush of coconut meat and fish.

Captain Olsen went on to say:

"At meal time, each family gathers around a huge sea shell filled with about 10 gallons of this thick concoction made of fish and coconut meats, which does not taste nearly so bad as might be supposed. On the contrary, the island's sole dish is very pleasant to the palate and rich in nourishment.

"What impressed us most, was the great stature of the people, their rugged health and great vitality."

This simple and physically superior people had probably lived on this diet for centuries, and yet we find them giants as compared to civilized man and more healthy.

Basic Study Finding of RNA

Dr. Benjamin Frank says, "The initial studies were done with a mixture of metabolites or nutrients containing ribonucleic acid (RNA), dioxyribonucleic acid (DNA) and sources of amino acids, B-complex vitamins, minerals, phosphates, glucose and lipids (fats). This mixture, conceived as a basic enzyme-forming and activating cellular fuel leading to increased cellular function, produced the following effects in man and rodents:

"1) Marked increase in 'energy' or activity; 2) Antianoxia action; 3) A large increase in ability to tolerate low temperatures, especially with high nucleic acid dosages; 4) Growth inhibition of young mice and rats; 5) Antiaging effects, among them a notable decrease in skin wrinkling and increase in elasticity; 6) An apparently increased mental function; 7) An antiviral action (anticoryza)."

Dr. Frank mentions that Darwin found a century ago that the remedy for altitude sickness by the Andes Indians was the onion. And we find that they are high in nucleic acids. He adds that possibly where other foods (sardines) effect anoxia-related conditions, the same case is true.

A Theory of Why We Age

If the price we pay for living longer is illness and disease what have we gained? Isn't the quality of life actually more important than the quantity? After all, a good life lived is long enough, but a long life lived may not be good enough. If we could delay the aging process and live our last years in health, that would be a great accomplishment.

The theory of aging held by Dr. Frank is that DNA decays or breaks down under the attack of destructive enzymes due to breakdown of Lysosomal membranes. Other causes of this breakdown can include different radiations such as cosmic rays. When DNA decays, abnormal RNA

messengers are programmed. And since RNA is responsible for the formation of enzymes the body must have, enzyme function can be abnormally altered. They may even be absent. It is believed that by giving RNA and associated nutrients, denatured DNA may be repaired. Through this repair the proper enzyme synthesis can be restored and aging can be reversed.

Experimental Case Findings

A group of 21-month-old mice were given injections of the "anti-tumor formula" including the nucleic acids, triphosphates, amino acids, various B-complex factors, sugars and minerals with outstanding results.

Dr. Frank states, "Not only did the activity of these mice increase considerably, but their dry and matted hair became more soft and their general and obviously old appearance became more youthful. These changes occurred without change in diet or maintenance conditions."

An easy test for aging skin is pinching the skin on the back of the hand and seeing how long it takes to return to normal. Using an oral formula on patients after 3-4 months of treatment the skin returned to normal quicker in the majority of patients. An improvement of 30 to 40 percent was noted in 15 patients for age 40 to 71.

Two old male dogs, 14 and 16 years old were put on an RNA regimen. The younger dog was a 24 pound mongrel nad the older an 18 pound chihuahua. Their eyesight was nearly gone and the hair was brittle and dry and below normal thickness. They showed arthritis to a degree that interfered with movement. A veterinarian affirmed that both had severe myocardial weakness. The dogs both had little life left, it appeared.

The younger dog was given 8 gr. daily of RNA and the older dog 4 gr. each day; each got a B-complex vitamin and ½ tsp. cod liver oil daily. By the end of the first month they both showed marked improvement, both in looks and behavioral activity. Their hair became softer and the coat thickness increased. At the end of 6 years of therapy, the younger dog was killed by a car and the older died at age 23 of a severe case of intestinal worms. Both animals were in excellent condition before their deaths.

An Interesting "Old Wives' Tale"

The nucleic acid-rich diet has an interesting relationship to an old wives' tale that says sardines and other fish and seafood make heart patients feel better. They were correct, though they didn't know the scientific basis for the fact. It is likely, Dr. Frank observes, that the good results with heart disease are due to the high content of nucleic acids in these foods. (The general scientific opinion would tend to be that it is due to the high unsaturated fat content of fish.)

Dr. Frank mentions that there is about 10 times the amount of ribonucleic acid [RNA] in small sardines while yeast was generally considered the highest RNA source in the past.

Sardines — an Elixer of Youth?
Dr. Benjamin Frank & His No-Aging Diet

Dr. Benjamin Frank, in his *No-Aging Diet* book lists sardines as an important anti-aging diet staple.He also suggests beets, asparagus, and beans to help energize fatigued cells. "Nucleic acids are the missing links in our nutrition," he says. His theory is that the trillions of body cells we each possess must have nucleic acids to build cells and repair cell walls. As we age, cells begin to lose energy. The diet, says Dr. Frank, is effective in acne, arthritis and degenerative diseases.

Other foods rich in nucleic acids (RNA and DNA) are anchovies, salmon, other fish and seafood, liver, dried peas, nuts, beets, radishes, leafy vegetables. His diet also emphasizes fluids. He suggests skim milk, fruit juice and a quart of water daily to flush the system. Dr. Frank describes the improvements in appearance as a smoothing out of wrinkles and tightening and moistening of skin within a few months. He believes that doctors in the near future will change their opinion of diet and its effect on physical health.

DNA is the cell blueprint, so to speak, and RNA is the messenger that carries the information where it is needed. The two have been termed the keys to life. RNA is responsible for renewing faulty or failing cells due to a decrease in cell energy. This failing energy is said to be the cause of aging; or it at least leads and contributes to aging. RNA therapy and diets supply more messenger RNA for the genes controlling cell growth and reproduction. With added age cell energy levels drop; this starts the cycle of aging.

Improvements To Look Forward To

Signs of improved youthfulness, Dr. Frank says, are smoothing of forehead wrinkles, lightening of "crow's feet" in eye corners and softening of the deep lines from nostrils to the corner of the mouth. He says the elbows and back of hands are smoother in about four months, and foot calluses begin to disappear. Skin shows new moistness and glows with color and health; the whites of the eyes take on a sparkle. For young people with skin troubles, it dries up oily skin and improves the acne condition. Patients at 70 or 80 can look 10 to 15 years younger; the 60-year-old can go back 10 years; the 30 to 50 age group can look 5 years younger. For others in good health the diet is great prevention.

The Theory Applied to Diet

"The heart of my theory," explains Dr. Frank, "is this: There are natural direct and indirect sources of high-quality RNA and DNA that can be supplied from outside the body to nourish our cells and return them to a healthy state.

"Nucleic acids in the diet increase production of ATP, (adenosine triphosphate) the body's main energy-storing molecule, and step up the energy of the electron transport chain in the cell even after some parts of it are damaged.

"This energy repairs damage in old cells, causing them to function like younger ones. I have shown this anti-aging effect of nucleic acids time and again with my patients. My no-aging diet is essentially simple.

"You have fish seven times a week, sardines four times, salmon once, seafood once." He adds such foods as liver, beets, beet juice, lentils, peas, lima beans, soybeans, asparagus, radishes, onions, scallions, mushrooms, spinach, cauliflower, celery. Muscle meats are not recommended; neither are sugar and starches, alcohol (cocktails, beer and wine); very little vinegar, salt and other seasonings. Skim milk, fruit and vegetable juices and at least four glasses of water a day should be included. Dr. Frank also advises a good multi-vitamin supplement with each meal. Small sardines are better that the larger herring; sardines and other fish have little cholesterol. One to two grams of nucleic acid a day is needed. He cautions to undertake this or any diet under the supervision of your physician.

For the vegetarian he suggests combinations of grains and milk products; legumes with grains; nuts and seeds with legumes (beans); also asparagus, mushrooms, beets, beet juice or borscht (beet soup), collard greens cauliflower, spinach, soybean sprouts, turnip greens; add fruit and vegetable juices, skim milk, four glasses of water a day and a good multi-vitamin supplement, at least with the main meal.

Raw Vs. Cooked Foods

Today there are very few in the world who are not sick. I have searched the world to find a completely well person without success. The average person is operating with lower than 50 percent efficiency. Science can't full understand and explain why there is so much disease and suffering today. Could part of the disease be caused by civilized living's denial of the Garden of Eden diet? I believe wrong living accounts for most of the problems. Our bodies can't function, and we can't be mentally and spiritually sound unless we feed the body properly. The diet God gave Adam and Eve in the Garden of Eden was organically grown and unrefined; it was natural, pure and whole. The Good Book contains no "cooking" instructions for the Garden of Eden. They were taught not to build a fire to roast nuts and seeds, and they were not told to eat meat. The Bible says:

"Behold I have given you every herb bearing seed, which is upon the face of all the earth, and every tree, in which is the fruit of a tree yielding seed. To you it shall be for meat."

— Genesis 1:29

Permission to eat meat was not granted until after the flood in the time of Noah and the ark.

Disease is rampant in every nation of the world, especially the so-called civilized countries. In spite of lengthened life spans, degenerative diseases are on the rise. Man has perverted his taste. Multitudes have ruined their health — physical, mental and spiritual — by uncontrolled appetites and civilized foods (refined, processed, adulterated).

Adam and Eve could be called "fruitarians" because they ate the natural pure and whole fruits, herbs and seeds in their own garden. Today most of us buy our foods from the market and most, if not all, has residues of pesticides and chemical sprays. You will be far ahead in the long run if you make every effort to get organically grown produce. The best solution is to live where you can grow your own. As soon as produce is picked (often in the "green" or unripe state for trucking to market) it begins to lose its life force. Raw food is the most "living" food we have, and cooked food is dead food.

More experts are finding out that uncooked or unheated foods offer the best way to overcome disease and poor health. Live on raw foods that are organically grown, give strength and endurance to the body and add intellectual ability to the mind.

The University of Oregon conducted an experiment in the early 1950s using cooked vs. raw foods. Their human subjects on raw food reported that they felt better than those on the cooked diet and also were pleased to find out that they cut their food bill by ⅓ or more.

There is no way to overemphasize the advantages of eating fresh vegetables and fruits from your own organic garden. There is no better way to get the natural minerals, vitamins and enzymes than from fresh, raw foods. Wait to pick them just before using. It is believed by many that organic raw foods can lengthen the life span and make it healthier and happier; it can save us much pain and suffering and discomfort.

Cooking doesn't improve the value of food. Rather in most cases it destroys part of its value, especially vitamins, enzymes and minerals lost by exposure to heat, water and air. All fresh, raw vegetables, nuts, fruits and seeds are basic foods; many seeds can be sprouted for the best nutritional value and many hard grains also sprout well. To these raw foods we would add raw goat milk and raw egg yolks. These products provide the animal magnetism and heating protein the body often needs.

Dr. H.M. Shelton said the following of raw foods: "Can you think of more delicious foods than peaches, apricots, nectarines, plums, cherries, dewberries, strawberries, raspberries, watermelons, muskmelons, cantaloupes, honeydew melons, casaba melons, avocados, mangoes, papayas, persimmons, bananas, pineapple, sweet lettuce, pecans, walnuts, hazel nuts, Brazil nuts, almonds, paradise nuts, apples, pears, grapes, oranges, tangelos, grapefruit, tomatoes, cucumbers, and even tender young carrots?"

Notice what wonderful variety nature offers us.

Advantages of Raw Foods

There are many advantages to eating raw foods. For one thing, as we have said before, cooking destroys vitamins, minerals and enzymes. Hot food, moreover, is not good for the stomach (nor are cold foods such as ice cream). Chewing raw foods produces healthy teeth and gums, promotes salivation and better digestion and helps avoid overeating. Raw foods don't ferment as rapidly in the body as cooked foods, and eating them saves a good deal of kitchen work. By eating raw foods, we not only get more nutritional value for our money but we get the bulk and fiber that has been shown to reduce heart disease by bringing down blood levels of cholesterol and triglycerides. Bulk and fiber promote bowel tone and are considered to be effective in preventing colon cancer. Overeating is far less likely when we eat raw foods.

The Cases Against Excessive Cooked Foods

It was Dr. P. Kouchakoff who discovered the abnormal rise in the number of white cells when food heated to 83-87 degrees centigrade was consumed.

The European nutritionist, Professor Ziegelmeyer, is convinced of many deleterious effects from cooked foods. He says, "The more the food energies are maintained in their intimate compound and correlation, the greater the total effect and the higher the efficiency."

We find that cooked starches are most likely to cause digestive fermentation; raw food does not tend to ferment. Hyperacidity is common in Bengal, where cooked rice is the chief staple. Cooked foods remain longer in the intestines than raw and this encourages putrefaction and fermentation — believed to be a prime cause of disease.

Metchnikoff was convinced that such putrefaction is a source of poison and the major cause of senility. He believed longevity is not possible without the presence of a larger ratio of 'friendly bacteria" in the intestinal tract. (The ratio is said to be best at 85 percent friendly and 15 percent other bacteria; in most people the reverse is likely the case.) It is well known that intestinal putrefaction rapidly diminishes with raw foods, bowel movements being rapid and the feces almost free from odor.

Raw Vegetables: A Miracle Diet??

Ralph Benner of the famous Bircher-Benner Sanitarium, founded in 1897, says that "raw vegetable food is the most potent healing factor existing." He terms raw food "sunshine food." Success at this sanitarium has been so dramatic that patients flock there from all parts of the world.

Juices contain the life essence of the plant, chemical elements in their most potent, most easily assimilated form.

In Germany, Dr. Evers has reported success with 600 multiple sclerosis cases using a raw food therapy.

Raw food programs have overcome cirrhosis of the liver, according to Dr. Friedrich Peters of Munich, Germany.

Case History of Arrested Cancer

Dr. Kristine Nolfi, M.D., founder of Denmark's Humlegaarden Sanitarium, tells of arresting cancer of the breast in herself by use of an exclusively raw diet. In *My Experiences with Living Food* she relates the story in her own words, "In the spring of 1941, I discovered, quite accidentally, a small tumor in my right breast. In spite of my fatigue, I disregarded it. Five weeks later this tumor had grown to the size of an egg and had grown into the skin. Only cancer acts this way.

"I started immediately, going to a small island, where I lived in a tent, ate raw vegetables exclusively and sunbathed from four to five hours a day. When I felt too warm, I plunged into the sea."

Dr. Nolfi describes how fatigue continued for two months and then the recovery began and the tumor grew smaller. She followed the 100 percent raw fruit and vegetable diet for about one year. Upon a return to a diet of 50 to 75 percent raw vegetables the cancer became active again. Once again she turned to the 100 percent raw diet, and the cancer was brought under control.

Due to extensive publicity, the doctor was suspended from medical practice permanently in Denmark. At this time she and her husband began plans for opening Humlegaarden Sanitarium. Since its founding, writes Dr. Nolfi, treatment of patients by natural methods has had profound and wonderful results.

In January, 1948, due to disbelief by physicians that she actually had had cancer, the crusader underwent a biopsy of tissue for cancer. The biopsy was positive. She states, "There were cancer cells in the scar tissue in the skin on my breast, but it was the most benign form in existence, the one called scirrhus. My rapidly growing and previously virulent cancerous tumor had been converted under the influence of raw vegetables and fruits into the most benign form in existence."

The operation caused the cancer to once again become active, but in six months it was again under control and has remained so, Dr. Nolfi testifies.

It is the belief of this physician that cancer is the result of many years' suffering from gastric catarrh and constipation. Cancer is the final stage in an overacid and degenerative organism. "If cancer is discovered at an early stage, consistent consumption of raw vegetables and fruits may in many cases keep it in check, even for a considerable number of years. I am a case in point myself. Many researchers believe cancer is a blood disease; once you have it, you have it for a lifetime. The induration is a local manifestation," Dr. Nolfi concludes.

While I am not an extremist, I believe raw food diets are necessary at times. After the disease has reached advanced stages, time is valuable and extreme measures sometimes have to be taken. We must then do the perfect things.

Dr. William A. Albrecht

William A. Albrecht, of the University of Missouri, has carried out extensive research on the relation of soil to plants as they derive their nutrition directly from mineral elements in the soil. He showed sulfur to be necessary to chlorophyll development. [Chlorophyll is the plant "blood" stream.] Phosphorus is believed essential for strong and healthy roots and stems and possibly an aid to enzyme functions. Potassium helps both plants and animals "digest" food well and it has been found that it also has to do with cell division [reproduction] and early growth. Magnesium and iron are found to be involved in the production of chlorophyll; the iron is more an enzyme or catalyst and magnesium becomes part of the chlorophyll molecule. Calcium is very important in many jobs; it aids food transportation throughout the plant and reinforces or strengthens cell walls. Many other "trace" elements are found to be necessary beyond a doubt, such as boron.

Vitamins are also needed in animals and are the products of plants. They are most commonly associated with enzymes to aid digestion and assimilation of nutrients.

The Relation of Food, Soil and Health

To quote Dr. Albrecht, "It is obvious that plants must depend upon the available supply of minerals in the soil in which they are growing for the elements essential to their lives; that man and his domestic animals in turn must depend upon the plants for these nutrients. Complicated as these relationships are between the plant and the soil, they are direct. These relationships are further simplified by the fact that the plant stays in the one spot where it is growing. Animals, on the other hand, move about and get their nutritive requirements from many parts of the country and a great variety of soils. In addition, irrigation waters and drinking water for the animals may bring, from deep-seated rock formation in distant areas, mineral nutrients which may or may not be already available in the local area.

"With the intensification of growing populations, animals become more and more restricted to an ever narrowing range of soil types. As a consequence, soils in certain areas were recognized as being incapable of sustaining the health of certain species of domestic animals or of wildlife while proving quite satisfactory to other unrelated species. The fact that certain animals thrived while others in the area developed specific disorders and the further observations that the sick animals recovered if moved to another region focused attention on the relationship of soil deficiency to disease. This was the beginning of *The Geography of Disease.*"

He continues, "Investigations of the last 30 years extending to many lands have shown that such disorders are, in fact, nutritional deficiencies resulting from an inability of the local soils to furnish the essential mineral needs of these animals in adequate amounts or in proper proportions.

"It has been shown further that these disorders may be caused by too much as well as too little of the trace elements from the soil. .... All of these factors are primarily a reflection of soil contents in which the plants which the animal eats have been grown.

"The effects of nutrients on infectious diseases and health of plants is the same, in principle, as in animals.... The effect on the plant of the nutrient depends on relative amounts of the other elements.

".... As with animal and human diseases, so with plant diseases. The impact of the favorable factors and the unfavorable factors gives a happy balance or an aggravation of the disease."

Dr. Albrecht stresses the following, "The relationship between soils, plants, and animals is unquestionably of increasing practical importance to our health and that of our animals as our Society becomes urbanized and our agriculture industrialized. Its complexity, however, extends beyond mere qualitative and quantitative differences between plants and animals or within the variety of plants and animals or within the individual plant or animal and their requirements for a particular trace element. It involves as well the inter-reaction of one trace element with another and with the major elements in the field as a result of differences in soil composition and the kind and amount of fertilizers and manures which have been applied. For instance, soil differences may influence the sulphur content of the plant. This in turn may have a profound effect upon the molybdenum metabolism and through the molybdenum upon the utilization of copper by the animal."

Biological Properties of Foods

"Quality in a food," Dr. Albrecht states, "is the sum of its biochemical properties and these may be listed as external features, suitability, and nutritive values. Since protein is the stuff of which life is made and all other essential substances are auxiliary to it, the ability of a food stuff to furnish all of the building blocks (amino acids) for replacement of worn out proteins in the cells of our bodies becomes of the greatest importance. Any food therefore will be limited in its capacity to support growth, reproduction, and repair of our bodies by that particular amino acid which is present in the least amount. Since vegetable proteins are the major source of protein intake of our domestic animals and in the unsophisticated diets of the bulk of the world's population, the plant proteins and especially their amino acid content become of major importance."

Conclusions That Can't Be Denied

Dr. Albrecht concluded from his findings that the concentration of trace elements in plants, the most important source, for quantity in man and animal food depends on the following:
1. The variety and species of the plant;
2. The nature of the soil they were grown in;
3. The climate, season, amount of sun;
4. The stage of growth the plant is harvested and eaten;
5. The method, character and content of the fertilizing material.

The Doukhobors: "God's People"

The right to migrate to Canada's wild frontier was "won" by the Doukhobors' courageous refusal to bear arms in their native Russia. The long voyage of these hardy Christian vegetarians began at the port of Batoum in Southern Russia in December 1888. The untamed Canadian wilds offered them religious freedom and military exemptment. The cold wilds of Canada did not discourage these brave people, who had faced persecution in Russia in the forms of torture, death and imprisonment and never weakened.

The name "Doukhobors" in Russian means "spiritual wrestlers," a name tagged on them derogatorily by Archbishop Ambrosi back in 1785 because of their refusal to follow the Russian Orthodox Church. For decades before this time they were called "God's people." Unlike members of the Orthodox Church, they refused to bow down before ikons or observe church rituals. The church was unable to force them into orthodox participation — even through torture, imprisonment, banishment to Siberia and death.

Many Doukhobors were banished to the wild Caucasus Mountains and left to survive among primitive, war-like tribes. The czar's officials were confident that these gentle people would perish there, but they prospered and grew stronger. Many Doukhobors who didn't migrate to Canada still live in the Caucasus in southwest Soviet territory.

When the czar ordered compulsory military service throughout the land, the Doukhobors burned weapons to demonstrate their pacifism in 1895. By this time the "spiritual wrestlers" had gained worldwide publicity that so annoyed and embarrassed the Soviet government that they agreed to allow the Doukhobors to emigrate to Canada.

The immigrants settled in Saskatchewan and organized a communal way of life, holding all possessions in common. Their society was named the "Christian Community of Universal Brotherhood." In the difficult beginning, fields were often prepared by a dozen women hitched to a plow! In 1902 Peter Verigan was released from Siberian exile and allowed to come to Canada. His strong leadership unified the people in their attempt to make a new life in the wilderness.

In 1903 trouble struck. The Canadian government enforced the Homestead Act of Canada, requiring would-be settlers to declare support of the British crown. The Doukhobors refused to acknowledge individual ownership of property and allegiance to any political ruler or country. As a result, the government confiscated 256,000 acres of their land. The loss was estimated at $11 million.

Some 6,000 Christian Community members moved to British Columbia, where they purchased land without an oath of allegiance. They began with 15,320 acres, pushing back the stubborn forest to plant fruit trees, build villages, roads and sawmills. Soon other crops — small fruits such as strawberries and raspberries — were cultivated. A brick molding factory was set up along with fruit canning and preserving factories. Then came a wooden pipe factory and other works, including a flour mill.

Tomato canning plants sprang up as well as other industry endeavors, including the greatly successful K-C brand preserves factory. In spite of years of outside strife and resulting set-backs from the government over military service and public school practices, their industries prospered. When the depression of the 30's swept the continent, terrorists began to attack and vandalize their businesses. Then bankruptcy struck a cruel blow. The British Columbia government took over their holdings. Later many of the Doukhobors were able to purchase land and rebuild.

In spite of repeated tragedies and hardships through the years, this peaceful vegetarian group has held fast to their religious faith and has remained forgiving and peace-loving toward all. Their motto then and now is "Pride in toil and peaceful life."

Pasteur's fame, like that of Cock and Jenner with vaccines, is slowly fading as science is finding that pasteurized milk is not the boon to civilization it was first thought. We find that it harms health by leaching vitamins from the body. Pasteurized milk putrefies in the intestinal tract in spite of any measures to prevent it. Other foods cannot counteract this process, and neither can sterilization or homogenization. The human digestive system is congested and constipation is promoted. Healthy digestion and normal peristalsis require a diet of natural, pure and whole foods. Pasteurized milk is no longer considered a whole or natural food for man or animals, as experiments have shown. (See Chapter 11 experiments by Dr. Pottenger.)

Lactic bacteria — capable of souring milk — are an excellent food addition. They naturally destroy "unfriendly bacteria" in the intestinal tract. Clabbered milk, largely because it is not altered by heating, builds health by feeding the friendly bacteria and destroying the harmful variety. Clabbered milk is easy to digest since it is already partially digested. Its own natural acid assists protein digestion.

If milk is taken it should be raw, sweet milk or clabbered. Goat milk is the superior milk as it is so near the composition of human milk and is the easiest to digest. Raw milk tends to form a tough "cheese type curd" if taken in large quantities or if consumed rapidly. Sip it slowly and in small quantities for best results.

Pasteurized milk lacks the lactic bacteria for proper digestion and this is the reason for putrefying or decaying in the human system. Its pasteurized products should be avoided as well.

Dr. Charles Mayo has explained the difference between souring and putrefaction as follows; "Souring is a natural process in milk that comes with age, and to many is not objectionable. Souring prevents putrefaction. Preventing acid organisms which produce the souring makes the putrefaction process more rapid unless the milk is kept cold." He clearly pointed out that putrefaction is greater in pasteurized milk.

A Doctor Owes His Life to Milk

Dr. Estes, a Los Angeles physician, said he owes his life to milk. He was diagnosed as a terminal case and was given a short time to live. He defied the ultimatum and undertook simple and natural living habits. He made a complete and surprising recovery from the disease. Raw milk was a staple in his nutrition program. He said, "Milk is, in my opinion, the only medium through which perfect regenereation of the body can be obtained.

"I would advise those who are seeking health and wish to rebuild themselves, to become thoroughly conversant with the surpassing value of milk which carries all the elements necessary to build the body. Milk is the only thing which builds babies. If milk will build the body and health of a baby it will regenerate our bodies and lost vitality since, after all, we are only grown up babies.

"Malnutrition would not undermine our vitality and sap out our very lives if milk were substituted for the quantities of tea, coffee, alcoholic and soda fountain beverages which are annually consumed by the people."

Grapes and Longevity

When I traveled all over the world to find out the health secrets of the oldest people, I discovered that most of them lived where the grapes grow best. We find grapes that grow in the North all right, but they never become really ripe nor are they completely sweet. It was unusual to see that where these old men lived, the wooden crosses in the churches were decorated with carved clusters of grapes. The fences had grapes carved and molded into their structure. It seemed more than coincidental that the old men lived where the grapes grew so beautifully and sweet.

We find that in the Bible it says Noah's first work after the Flood was to start a vineyard. And the words grape and grapes can be found over forty times and the words vineyard or vineyards is found over seventy times. The Bible says:

"Eat ye every one of his vine, and every one of his fig tree, and drink ye every one the waters of his own cistern; until I come and take you away to a land like your own land, a land of...wine...and vineyards" (Isaiah 36:16-17).

It is interesting to find that so many ancient writings give the grape an important place, and giants are sometimes mentioned in connection with grapes.

Alvin F. Harlow refers to grapes as the superior fruit. He says:

"The grape is probably the oldest domestic fruit we have. The fruit and the wine made from it are frequently mentioned in writings, reaching back to the dawn of history. Apples are mentioned in the Old Testament, but there is no certainty that the word which King James experts translated as "apple" meant the apple as we know it.

"The grape has a very high value to the body both as food and medicine. It is mildly laxative, diuretic, and like all other fruits, is anti-scorbutic. It contains one of the four beneficient fruit-acids that are so useful to the body. These acids in the process of digestion release potassium, sodium, and magnesium, which are changed into carbonates and overcome by their alkalinity the acids in the blood.

"The average grape contains nearly 80 percent sugar; and scientists agree that grape sugar is one of the easiest of all fruit sugars to digest and assimilate.

"The grape also contains [organic or food] iron, which helps to build up the red corpuscles of the blood."

(— Correct Eating)

Dr. Holbrook praises the value of grapes when he says:

"The physiological effects of grapes are significant...They increase nutrition, promote secretion, improve the action of the liver, kidneys, and bowels, and add to the health.

"The sugar of the grape, which may often be as high as 30 percent, requires no digestion, but is taken almost at once into the blood, where it renders up its energy as required; so also of the water.

"The dextrin of the grape promotes the secretion of pepsin, and this favors digestion...The phosphoric acid, of which there is considerable, acts most favorably on all the bodily functions, and especially on the brain."

(— Eating for Strength)

We find the grape diet is easier on digestion, is quickly and easily absorbed and metabolized by the body with little vital energy needed. Grape juice is a lovely tonic drink, rich in minerals and organic nutrients which supply the blood with the nutrients the body needs. Its phosphoric acid is valuable to the brain.

Otto Carque has this to say about grapes:

"In Europe the so-called grape cure, during the harvest season, has become very popular. It is used in many health resorts in Southern Europe, where people live exclusively on the grapes for four to six weeks, increasing the quantity from three to six pounds daily, according to age and constitution.

"The grape-cure is especially helpful in diseases of the respiratory organs and kidneys, also in anemic conditions. The beneficial effect of this cure is chiefly due to the simplicity of the diet, which furnishes the protein and carbohydrates in the most assimilable form, while the larger proportion of the alkaline salts, such as potash [potassium], lime [calcium], magnesia, and iron, reduces the acidity of the blood."

(— Safe Way to Health)

The News Chronicle had this to say about grapes:

"Eminent doctors (of Italy) declared that grapes cured melancholy and spleen, obesity and indigestion, liver complaints and Bright's disease, gout and rheumatism, dyspepsia and biliousness, gastric and anemia, and almost every disease treated in hospitals and clinics — that it made old men young and improved the complexion of women."

"Ripley's Believe it or Not," November 6, 1930 said the Great Grapevine of Hampton Court Palace Gardens, England was planted in 1768 from a cutting from Valentines, Essex, England. He added that the parent vine was also quite large. The stem of the Great Grapevine is six

112

feet eight and one-half inches around; one of its branches is 114 feet long. And he tells us that the grapes are the black Hamburg variety. Each year the vine bears over 650 bunches weighing about two and a half pounds each. It was reported to have produced up to 2,000 bunches at times.

John Ott

We are becoming increasingly aware of the "hyperactive" child. It seems that there are more each year — they can't sit still and can't pay attention in classrooms. Parents don't know what to do with them. The well known scientist John Ott, a pioneer in the study of light, insists that artificial lights increase hyperactivity in children. These are found eveywhere — classrooms, parks, play areas and in the home.

Mr. Ott says, "Fluorescent light tubes are miniature cathode ray guns, operating on the same principle as X-ray machines and giving off trace amounts of radiation." They are not beneficial.

Research into light resulted in his move to persuade a Chicago light firm to make a full-spectrum fluorescent light fixture similar to natural sunlight. When these lights were installed in Florida schools the extremely hyperactive children immediately settled down, says Ott. Even some children with serious learning disabilities and who couldn't read improved markedly.

Several pieces of evidence disfavoring artificial light have been noted in Ott's experience. He grew geraniums under lights. "I noticed they grew better near the center of the fluorescent tubes than on the ends, where the cathodes are," he noted. In another instance a group of Sarasota youngsters with learning difficulties were studied. "We found that the televsion sets in their homes were giving off X-ray radiation. When the sets were taken away or repaired, all 12 of these children could be returned to regular classes within a matter of months," Ott said.

The problems don't stop with hyperactive children. "What starts this way in younger children is also responsible for campus unrest with older youths and it is a major contributing factor to our increasing crime and violence," Ott claims. Sodium vapor street lights are especially detrimental — usually pink or orange. "Some cities are completely flooded with them. People can't get away." They even kill trees along the streets.

This radiation attacks minerals and biochemicals in the body that we get through foods. "If artificial food coloring is removed from the diet, or peaks of energy are eliminated from our artificial light sources, then this interaction is broken," Ott explains.

His testimony before a House of Representatives subcommittee is responsible for legislation aimed at cutting X-ray exposure levels.

Gluten

We are inclined to think of wheat as one of the very starchy grains. Yet wheat alone of all the other cereals (except perhaps rye to a limited extent) contains enough of the protein, gluten, to supply the stickiness in a dough to make a raised bread. You simply cannot make a pure corn or oat bread. It takes the elastic nature of the gluten to enclose the bubbles of gas which make a bread light.

If you want to use the other valuable flours, such as whole barley, rice, millet, potato, cornmeal, flaxseed, etc., in your breads, add some gluten flour early in your mixing (e.g., to your yeast sponge), and this will carry the load of raising the bread with these inert flours. Replace 1/2 cup whole wheat flour with gluten flour for bread sponge, then proceed with your regular recipe.

Another outstanding benefit of the addition of gluten flour is the extra protein it supplies. Remember this especially in connection with those wishing to reduce starch intake—overweights and sedentary workers.

Gluten is made by washing the starch out of a high protein wheat. The gluten is then dried and ground into a flour. Naturally, it is quite expensive.

Gluten can also be used to make your own gluten steaks for a meat substitute or you can buy these ready prepared in cans at the health food store.

Chapter 11

Counseling the serious patient

Why Ill People Don't Take Action

It is very difficult to persuade sick people to take action where their health is concerned. Effort is painful: It calls for putting out energy, the very element sickness lacks. They have lost initiative and ambition. Problems like lack of motivation can be traced to a lack of calcium and other vital elements. Without calcium you can't fight the next problem that comes along. Without silicon all your energy and magnetism is gone. Such people want someone else to cure them (usually with pills from a bottle, with drugs or even surgery). Then they return to the same old habits that built these maladies in the first place.

I hate to tell you that sickness is sometimes a blessing. Sickness has moved more people into the health field than anything else. As soon as you get tired of being tired and sick of being sick, you will seek Nature's real health. It is not pleasant to go through sickness, but it is a necessary earthly experience.

A healthy person, on the other hand, is usually only too eager, enthusiastic, to add to the wealth of natural health he already knows. Most people don't know what it feels like to feel wonderful. The sick person, or one nearly sick, lacking vital energy, depressed, leans to despondency, hopelessness; he feels old and worn out. Good health has to be earned; it can't be bought. You have to work for it. It is a homework project where nobody can make the decisions for you. It takes a long time — at least a year. The secret is to put two summers together, because this is when you build reserves needed to get well. We need all the seasons and the foods that go with them to build health.

To just have a good body is nothing; to have a good mind is nothing. Without a heart any human being is dangerous. We find that a person who has a good body but doesn't know how to love can accomplish many harmful things. Mussolini, Hitler and Stalin were vegetarians. Think what they would have been like as meat-eaters!

Without a good mental attitude and a spiritual philosophy you can't get well. You have to start feeling good to start feeling good. Do you understand that? However, I still have to put good nutrition at the top of the list of the physical, mental and spiritual package for good health.

How Much "Health Stock" Do You Own??

A chemically balanced body brings joy for living, and that person is willing to take up the challenges of life. We find there is an abundance of what is commonly called "pep and energy." Mental work can be met with a feeling of being able to conquer and to overcome any obstacles. The strain of the average day's job of eight hours of work should not hurt anyone or produce any undue fatigue; we should be ready to carry on eight hours of recreation of whatever we would like to do after the work is done. We must make sure we have an evacuation of food residues and body wastes by moving the bowel more or less after every meal for the most perfect health.

Good health is usually brought on by a good inheritance, a vital inheritance. It was Dr. Oliver Wendell Holmes who said, "The greatest of all human felicities is to be well born." If we could have the constitution and have a vital stamina to begin with, our chances for a long life would be more assured. When a person lives in a good environment and on good foods, a good constitution is the one factor that will keep his body well organized and free from defects. His predisposition to disease can be kept at a minimum and his vital energy will allow him to do his daily tasks without any breakdown as he goes through life. Man is naturally long lived. He has a body that rebuilds, repairs, constantly. He is self-starting, self-rejuvenating, self-rebuilding and there is no reason from a scientific standpoint for the average person to die.

But through bad habits we break down under stress and strain and we are much lacking in proper education for the best part of our lives. In this day and age when there are so many problems produced through our environment, such as poor air, which can break down the breathing centers in the body, with the heavy carbohydrate foods breaking down the pancreas, with our intake of alcohol to break down the liver, kidneys and so forth, we find that the parents cannot give the children the constitution that they should have. It was an English physician who said, "Of this I am perfectly sure, that there is room for improvement to the extent of something like 100 percent in all our living conditions, that there is room for improvement of 100 percent in the average physical capacity for work, that there is room for improvement of 100 percent in happiness and usefulness in the average life in the community."

"If we would take this as a basic thought, we would find out that we are not living up to our capacity or to our potential. We find that our personal habits, environment and many other factors and our mental life, finance, marriage, and so forth, can easily counteract and overshadow the influence of a good inheritance, a good and strong body."

In this day and age most people know that cigarette smoking is bad, yet just breathing the air is probably as bad as smoking. We work in fume-filled factories and in apartment houses that are in need of clean, pure and fresh air. Of course, careless bowel habits are a great cause of disease and premature death. We find that constipation is almost universal among the people of civilized countries.

Great bodily strength is probably one of the most desirable qualities that we should perfect in our life, because without strength we cannot produce the proper blood circulation in our body. The average strength is adequate, however, to fit one for the ordinary activities of life. But if we have any endurance tests to perform requiring stamina and stress, we have to have that extra reserve built into our body in order to keep well under adverse condition. This is the emergency power we need to have stored in the muscles and in the nerve centers. When we are forced to call on extra power and energy to carry on, it has to come from the storage centers — the reserve force. This is one of the greatest reasons for keeping well and having a reserve power source, or extra batteries ready for any emergency that might come along.

Avoid the "Catarrh-Prone" Diet

I believe that the overabundant use of wheat in this country has brought in an overabundance of catarrhal discharges, bronchial trouble and so forth. While I do not feel it is the whole thing, I believe wheat is one of the things that adds to a heavy catarrhal condition when taken in heavy amounts. If 25 percent of our intake in the average American diet is wheat, this is too much. It is this overabundance that causes catarrhal elimination. Catarrh, in the Greek means "to follow down." When we have an excess amount of wheat, we need to get rid of it, and catarrh is the natural way of running it out of the body. Even in the elimination processes and healing crises we find that catarrh is developed as we liquefy and break down settlements that have accumulated in various parts of the body. This catarrh could be, of course, from other things such as an excess of milk or any food that we take in excess. [For more detailed information on catarrh and the healing crises refer to my book *The Doctor-Patient Handbook*.]

Allergies: Be Careful of Wheat & Milk

Allergies are the result of numerous causes, but I am convinced that the primary cause is poor food combinations and choices — especially overuse of wheat and milk products.

The affliction is a result of the acid and alkaline balance in the body being upset. With an over-acid con-

dition, catarrah is built up. Most allergies are related to inflammation of the mucous membranes. The purpose of these membranes is to throw off catarrh — an acid or phlegm accumulated in the body.

Research figures say the average person in the U.S. or Canada includes 25 percent wheat and 25 percent milk products in the daily diet. The other foods — vegetables, unrefined carbohydrates and proteins are sadly neglected. We don't get the variety we should on such a diet. (We recommend 6 vegetables, 2 fruits, 1 protein and 1 starch each day to help make up for the wrong balance in the past.)

Even though other starches such as brown rice, millet, rye, yellow cornmeal, buckwheat, barley and so forth are readily available, wheat seems to be the staple. In my practice, cutting out wheat and milk has done more good in controlling allergies than any alternative. Use the other grains and learn to make milk substitutes from ground nuts and seeds combined with liquids such as water. Use goat milk occasionally since it is not catarrh-forming like cow's milk. Soy milk powder makes a good substitute for milk.

Many people panic at the thought of giving up milk — insisting it is a perfect food — that it is a whole and complete protein food. As for today's pasteurized milk, stop to consider the pros and cons. During the heating process of pasteurization the one chemical element capable of preventing catarrh build-up — fluorine — is destroyed. Fluorine escapes as a gas when even low heat is applied. Due to its instability when exposed to heat, fluorine is the most easily lost element in foods. It is known as the "resistance element," wonderful for ridding the body of catarrh and acids.

You will find many recipes for the use of nut and seed milks, also soy milks in my book *365 Days of Menus and Recipes*. Seeds and sprouts are the survival foods of the future and for today. They are the most perfect foods because they contain everything necessary to foster a new life. They are "live" foods. The laboratory will never be able to duplicate their unique properties. That is a secret Nature refuses to give.

Many may say wheat is the staff of life and shouldn't be blamed for allergy troubles. Think of all the forms wheat comes in — pastry, wheat cereals, doughnuts, pancakes, pasta, noodles, bread, cakes, etc. The body is overloaded with these foods. In addition, the outside of the wheat and the germ, which contains the life force, is removed during milling to give the resulting white flour an eternal shelf-life. It becomes a dead food. Fluorine, we might point out, is removed with the outer portions of the wheat.

Allergies and Lymph Gland Congestion

In many allergy cases, lymph gland congestion is present. Exercise is the principle method of decongesting the lymph glands. Milk, we recognize, comes through the lymph tissue of the cow's udder. Liquid derived from the lymph system of this animal can add to allergy difficulties. For this reason we don't like to use cow's milk when the lymphatic system is in a weakened condition.

We find many ways of tackling the allergy problems. I prefer the elimination diet procedure. Juices or a short water fast is beneficial, followed by a healthy nutrition program.

Don't forget the ABC's of Allergy: Always Be Careful of wheat and milk.

Exercise Is the Best Stimulant

Many foods are used today to stimulate the human body. This is a mistake. Exercise is the only stimulation the body should get. Pure and natural nutrition is what we need to build a perfect body — not unnatural stimulants such as coffee, tea and other harsh condiments. Abnormal stimulation is opposed to healthful living, and in the long run, squanders our precious vital energy.

When food becomes a stimulant to the body, it behaves like all foreign substances — drugs, medications, intoxicants and other substances that create toxins or extreme reactions in the body. We know that stimualtion is always followed by depression — a let-down. If the vital energy needed for digestion of food is depleted, eventually we can no longer digest food properly and completely. Vital energy and vital body power must be preserved and guarded.

What You Digest, Not What You Eat, Counts

It is not what we eat that counts; what we digest really keeps the body fit. I am convinced many foods people eat today wear the body out attempting to digest it. Overeating can kill you faster than the worst foods in the world. Rest and pure foods, along with the proper exercise, are the three great curative powers that rebuild the human structure.

Through my practice the past 50 years, I have witnessed the wonders of nature cures possible through the return to natural, pure and whole foods. We have seen arthritis relieved, indigestion removed and ulcers disappear through proper feeding. In this day and age when pure air and water have all but disappeared, there are still those who insist that these things don't affect the health of the human body.

History tells us that in the golden days of the magnificent Roman Empire when that nation approached the final stage of decline, vomiting troughs were used at banquets as and aid for those gorging on rich foods. When Rome became a country of gluttonous gourmets, its downfall was assured.

How Important Is Hydrocholric Acid?

Increasing use of hydrochloric acid [HCL] for a number of ailments and diseases is seen. We know that without adequate stomach acid the body can't digest and assimilate calcium and proteins. Sodium is needed.

Arthritis: Many arthritics complain with gas and belching due to protein putrefaction. HCL is necessary to help keep calcium in solution rather than being deposited in the joints and tissues. Without sodium enough HCL can't be produced.

Epilepsy: It has been reported that the number of epileptic convulsions is lowered with the generous use of HCL. Glutamine and arginine availability is raised.

Anemia: Some believe that hard-to-correct anemia is partly due to a shortage of gastric HCL. We know that the older individual doesn't secrete as much HCL, and it may be a factor in pernicious anemia as well as in arthritis and in older persons.

Diabetes: HCL is said to bring about normal acidity to help restore natural secretion of insulin. Insulin can only function in an acid medium, so it aids the pH balance.

Cancer: A great many cancer clinics use HCL to help in detoxification and promote cell ionization.

Allergies: HCL is said to help break down protein complexes (allergens) that can cause congestion by getting into the blood stream through the liver.

Chronic Constipation: HCL helps establish the "friendly" bacteria in the intestinal tract by promoting correct digestion.

Mental Disturbances: It is believed that the brain cells of mentally ill persons are laden with toxic materials that upset the normal brain fuction. HCL aids better digestion to reduce toxin production and to help remove the toxins already produced.

What Causes Indigestion Distress?

Many people talk about indigestion. It really is a case of sub-acidity in the stomach when food doesn't digest well. There is usually a lack of hydrochloric acid in the stomach due to a shortage of sodium. Proteins need an acid medium for proper digestion. And meat requires more acid digestants than other proteins. Also, too many starches and sugars (refined carbohydrates) can produce indigestion symptoms. Overeating, unbalanced diets and wrong food combinations — such as heavy proteins with heavy starches — are common causes of annoying indigestion.

Confusing Hunger & Thirst Centers

We find that the brain contains hunger and thirst centers. The thirst center was intended to move us to drink water, not colas, coffee, tea, beer, other intoxicants and milk. Often we confuse these centers, eating when we are thirsty or drinking when we need a whole food. We develop abnormal cravings and short circuit the delicate communication system from the brain to the taste buds. For example, ten percent of the juice of almost any fruit is sugar. We can get far too much sugar by drinking juice, while we would be meeting our body's actual needs better by eating the whole fruit. Blood sugar levels aren't usually disturbed by eating the whole fruit.

When we discontinue sugar in the diet, beneficial things result. After a time the appetite and thirst centers of the brain begin to function normally once again. We automatically begin to make better, healthier choices of foods, especially natural foods.

Today when sugar-converting glands and organs are overworked, they get to the place where they are worn out and poorly functioning. We find they can no longer properly control the body functions, assimilation, conversion and elimination. When cells break down, disease is invited into the body. Glands become a party to the reduced functioning and inferior building material.

Good health is only possible with a good diet for optmum cell nutrition and building. We find that optimum cell nutrition goes along with properly working glands. A simple guide is to include everything the body needs and to eliminate everything harmful in the diet. When we use natural, pure and whole foods, we are increasing our vitamin and mineral intake. Our instincts for food selection are as good as any animal's if we give them the chance and don't pervert them with processed, sugared, spiced and artificially flavored foods. Have you ever seen an animal in the wilds dying of our civilized diseases such as cancer, diabetes, heart disease? No.

Only the Obese Die Young

We find that in the following table the death-rate is suprisingly lower in people called "skinny" and "too lean" by common weight standards. And they are 20 pounds below the average weight at that. The figures come from the research of insurance companies.

MORTALITY RATE

20 lbs. under average weight	89%
10 lbs. under average weight	90%
5 lbs. under average weight	91%
Average weight mortality	94%
5 lbs. over average weight	98%
10 lbs. over average weight	102%
20 lbs. over average weight	112%

Those who think they should weigh more should be careful. The death rate shows a corresponding lowering of health and vitality with added weight. So we find that the best average weight should be well below the national average — about 20 pounds below it!

Nature's Seven Best Doctors

How many of you stop to realize that perhaps the true doctor doesn't get the fee? Nature cures, and the doctor gets the fee. Doctors make a living on people who don't know how to live correctly. They have waiting rooms for you because they know you will get sick. New hospitals and new hospital wings go up daily.

We find that the seven best Nature Cure doctors are: 1. Sunshine; 2. Water; 3. Air; 4. Food; 5. Exercise; 6. Positive mental philosophy; 7. Spiritual mind. Stop and think about these a moment.

SUNSHINE: We find that all life depends on sunlight for its very existence. Without sunlight photosynthesis could not take place in plants and without plants we could not be here either. In many parts of the world sunbaths are a major form of therapy for many diseases.

WATER: We are told that over 90 percent of the nation's water supplies are polluted and unfit for human consumption. Pure water is an essential part of good health and all the old men I have visited drank mountain water. None of them knew about distilled water, though at times I believe it may be necessary to get rid of calcium and mineral salt deposits in the body. But, we don't drink water for the minerals it contains. Fluoride water softeners have caused much harm, and I believe water softeners are partly reponsible for some heart trouble symptoms. The inorganic sodium salts they add to it are harmful and can actually produce heart trouble. There is no actual evidence that fluoride [inorganic] added to water supplies or toothpastes prevents cavities. But we find that there is accumulating evidence pointing to the fact that inorganic fluoride is harmful to the body. When you perspire more, you need more water. My diet is 90 percent water, and this is necessary to get rid of toxic materials. The water content is so high because there are less proteins and starches, and it's half eliminating and half building. Several glasses of warm water are good taken upon arising in the morning. As for the question of how much water to drink, take enough so that the urine is very light in color.

AIR: Oxygen, the element we all need so much of, is part of the air. Most of the air near cities is polluted these days and detrimental to health. We must have pure, fresh air, and the best source for most people is higher altitudes. Deep breathing in the open air is wonderful for the bronchial system. Air baths are as important as sunbaths.

FOOD: Food can be our medicine. The basis of my work with foods is that it must be natual, pure and whole. If you don't pay for the best foods you will pay a doctor. One of the most important food laws is that it must be natural, pure and whole; it must be live food, not "dead" food that has an eternal shelf life. Any food that isn't capable of spoiling is not a good food. And we find that live food should be eaten soon after picking. Another food law is variety — a variety in kinds, colors and food elements. Vegetables are high in minerals, and fruits have more vitamins. Starches are for the left side of the body (the negative side) and proteins are for the right (or positive side of the body). If the left side of the body is broken down, you need starches and for the right, protein. Proteins build the body, and starches furnish it with energy for physical work; proteins are for mental work. We need animal foods such as goat milk and egg yolk for heat and the higher vibration they provide for the brain and nervous system. Lower vibration foods build the bones and tissues. We need a diet that is about 60 percent raw food for the enzymes and other nutrients as well as the roughage it provides. The diet should be 80 percent alkaline (fruits and vegetables) and only 20 percent acid-forming (starches and proteins). Proper combinations of foods are also important; it is best not to take starches and proteins together, or fruits and vegetables at the same meal. but perhaps one of the most important food laws is to eat in moderation. More graves are filled from people overeating than from what they ate. The long lived people of the world eat when they are hungry and not because they have an appetite. They are frugal eaters. Look to God's Garden for your nutritional needs.

EXERCISE: Good health also depends upon proper exercise. Without exercise the blood can't flow well and the body can't function efficiently. Exercise is every bit as important as rest, food and positive spiritual and mental attitudes. We must have exercise physically, mentally and spiritually. More physical exercise should be taken early in the day, because it is stimulating. Bernarr McFadden said that we die from the feet up. The blood can't get to the brain if we don't exercise. That's one of the reasons for using the slant board, Kneipp leg baths, grass and sand walking. Exercise encourages more oxygen to travel throughout the body, and all of us need more oxygen. We find that exercise is the only stimulation the body needs.

MENTAL PHILOSOPHY: We have to let go and let life flow through us. We can't depend on people and things for our happiness—it comes from within us. Seek knowledge, wisdom and guidance through life and follow your own path of evolvement. The good life comes from selecting the things that are best for us and traveling the higher road. My mother used to say, "What you are seeking, is also seeking you." Mind is the builder; we build a better body, a better life, a better outlook, a better philosophy through our thinking. If things aren't right, it's time for a change. The only permanent thing in life is change. We can build more acids in our thinking than all the alkaline broths can ever neutralize and we know acids are the grim reapers of death. Emotions of fear, hatred, miserly, self-pity and resentment are killers. Get rid of them. Diseases begin in the mind. Remember that the mind has power over all matter.

SPIRITUAL MIND: It is said in the Good Book that, "In my Father's House are many mansions." And it also says, "I have not given you a spirit of fear." The Good Book teaches that what you fear will come upon you. So, be afraid that good things will come to you. Know that the Garden of Eden is within, and your body is a temple of the Living God. Ennoble the Great Within we all have. "As a man thinketh in his heart, so is he." Beauty is a healer and it is truly within the eye of the beholder. The Chinese have a saying that what goes into the mouth produces indigestion and what comes out of it produces misfortune. We live on what we pour out, and if we give good we will receive good in return. To hate is to kill, so love your enemies for your own good.

Know that we were born to Love, born to Serve and born to Grow. It's not for us to hurt anyone. Don't step on toes; wear the other person's shoes. Under the law of compensation we reap what we sow. We get back what we give; we meet our actions again. I don't feel sorry for the man that dies, but for the man who never lives.

This brings to mind a story I heard one time:

A man went to Heaven but couldn't get in, and was told he would have to go down to Hell as he belonged there. Satan looked over his books and told him, "No, your name isn't here. You don't belong to us. Go back to St. Peter. St. Peter went through his books again and still couldn't find his name. Finally he said, "Say, here's your name in next year's book. You aren't supposed to be here for another 6 months. Who's your doctor?"

Yes, who is your doctor? Some of the best doctors in life are free. Nature's doctors: sunshine, water, air, food, exercise, mental philosophy and spiritual mind. Nature cures, but she needs an opportunity. She can build new cells, new tissues, new bones if you provide her with the best physical, mental and spiritual building material. Give the body, the mind, the spirit what it needs, and Nature will put those materials in the right places.

You Can Starve on a Full Stomach

There are many things we must consider in nutrition and the healthy way of living. We can starve on a full stomach; we can eat foods that are quite filling but empty of nutrients. We have many puffed foods today — foods that swell up in the intestines to give a full sensation. We look for foods that will not make us overweight, obese. So, we are settling for substitutes for real foods. Then, we find that in eating the "foodless foods" our bodies eventually become unbalanced and chemically deficient. We produce disease through the consumption of chemically unbalanced foods so common today. Then the diseases have to be treated. Abnormal cravings develop in an undernourished body — a chemically depleted body.

It is said that America is the best nourished country in the world. It may be true in terms of the amount of food we put into the stomach but it doesn't mean we have adequate nutrition for proper functioning in every organ of the body.

Alcohol is a toxin in the body. Heretofore, we have had all kinds of reasons for using intoxicating drinks. But, we have found recently that alcohol is an enemy of health. It can destroy the liver, keeping its cells from their job of normal detoxification of the blood. We find that a destruction of the cells of the brain is a result of the overuse of alcoholic drinks.

White sugar is one of the greatest alcohol producers we can put in the body. It helps set up an "alcoholic still" within the body. It has been said that William Jennings Bryan was a teetotaler, a man who was so against alcohol that he went about talking of the evils produced in the body by it, and yet he died of alcoholic poisoning. This man had some 13 hot cakes with sugar syrup on them the morning he died! They claimed that his death was due to an alcoholic stomach that was produced by these foods.

Dr. Roger J. Williams of the University of Texas says that there is a nutritional way of combatting disease. He believes this is probably the most important way of taking care of alcoholism and our other problems today.

Who Needs the Flu Vaccines?

Those who live a good life, a healthy life, those who live on good foods in a good climate in a rural district, up in the mountains, away from the average person, will not be susceptible to the "flus" (influenzas) as we have them in the city. We find that people live on a certain level of conciousness, and when flu takes hold in an epidemic form in the city, it's because everybody is living in the same level consciousness, and when flu takes an epidemic form if we're going to separate ourselves from other people, then we can in most cases avoid flu and other so-called contagious diseases and conditions. If you're bringing up your children to live correctly, most of the time they will not develop a chronic condition of disease expression. And flu is often a symptom of a chronic condition developed over a period of years from poor bronchial management. There are times when catarrhal discharges from the bronchial tubes can indicate the beginning of a chronic disease stage after we have suppressed symptoms for many years. (Flu comes from suppression in the past.) So if we can keep below that level where flu expresses itself, we will not have the catarrhal problems brought on by it.

Distilled Water and When to Use It

We find that in elderly people many of the arteries are hardened because of the type of foods they have eaten and the type of life they have lived. We are encountering Alzheimer's disease more often. Bones become brittle, and the body moves with difficulty. Elasticity is gone in the veins and the arteries and throughtout the body. No, of course, we use distilled water in these cases. Rainwater has been distilled by the heat of the sun, but we have to get rid of some of this mineral material from the earth. Filtering the water is not good enough. We need to use distilled water with no minerals in it; this will dissolve some of the excess minerals from the blood vessels, joints and tissues.

Distilled water is water that has been vaporized, cooled and condensed again, free of impurities. For mineral-hardened bodies, arthritis, rheumatism and premature "aging" due to encrustations that collect on the inside walls of the arteries (the same as our kettles), then distilled water is advised. It can be used as a great solvent. Of course, we must realize that fruit and vegetable juices are naturally distilled and carry the soluble biochemical salts and vitamins necessary for rebuilding and rejuvenating the body. We should not depend on the minerals in water to build a body. These materials must come from foods and natural juices.

An Unproportioned Body Is Unhealthy

It has been said that when the body is out of proportion, it is a sign that there are glands or parts of the body that aren't working properly. The pituitary gland affects the amount of water we have in the system; it affects our bone growth, and we have to exchange good nutrition for bad nutrition in order to take care of the *whole* body. We are today treating the disease; we are treating the end effect, the result, and we must make sure that we give the body all the materials it needs. To withhold any of these elements will not give us the whole body we must have. When the body chemistry is disproportionate, we find out that the body is also disproportionate.

Iridology Belongs to Nutrition

The only system we have today to see where we need to develop greater resistance to disease is found in the science of Iridology. In avoiding disease, we have to have the highest state of health and the proper chemical balance. This can be detemined in the analysis from the eye better than any other analysis or test that I know of today. Body chemistry is thrown off by all toxic conditions found in the body and by the lack of the proper biochemical elements. Without the latter, we get rid of these toxic accumulations in the body. Without considering the patient rather than the disease, we will never build up resistant factors that will prevent disease and maintaining good health.

Iridology shows which organs and tissue areas of the body are hyperactive or hypoactive, in need of biochemical nutrients. It reveals inflammation, congestion, anemia and toxic accumulations.

In looking at a patient I translate symptoms I find into a lack of certain chemical elements. I feed the patient the particular foods, tonics, herbs or special preparations that will help rebuild the areas of weaknesses found in their body.

Caring for a patient eventually always reverts to the chemical structure of the body. The chemistry of the food eaten becomes the internal chemistry that balances or unbalances the body. When the body becomes unbalanced — "dis-eased" — a revolution takes place. Disease is the symptom, rather than the cause of the pain and troubles. A strong constitution is vital for ease in recovery; it is not usually present in the patients I have handled. They have lacked the strength, the good inheritance, the power to carry on in the face of difficulties. So, they weren't able to survive on the fiery foods served in today's restaurants or to tolerate rich and heavy gourmet dining. The polluted foodstuffs and fancy additives, sugary and starchy desserts, French and Danish pastries, and so forth eventually weakened and sickened them. They could not remain healthy on such "civilized" diets. Manufactured foods, chemical additives, preservatives and highly refined and processed foods resulted in poor health and diseases.

A man once came to me with over 3,000 eye ulcers. He was allergic to the artificial fertilizer used in agriculture today. The condition left while he remained at Hidden Valley Health Ranch on a diet of produce from naturally composted soil. He learned a valuable lesson. He now lives where he can grow his own organic food.

Blood Stream: The "River of Life"

It is the blood that we depend on for the animate existence of man. It is in the condition of the blood that the condition of the body will show up. If this blood flows sluggishly or if it is foul, you will find the body cannot respond properly and the vital force cannot build healthy organs. A sound brain is not found in an unsound body. And you cannot build a sound body with a polluted blood stream. You have to supply that blood with the proper material in order to have that "river of life" nourish, repair and rebuild. We keep a stream of water clean by keeping the filthy substances out of it. This same law applies within our body. The body does the best it can with the blood that is coming to the cell structure and uses it to its best advantage. You can give the finest carpenter on the face of the earth rotten building materials and you'll find he cannot construct a good house. The house will be just as good as the materials he has to work with. Due to the unnatural bodies we have today, we have created a market for unusual invention including specially designed gadgets and beds, ear covers to sleep with, electric hot pads, perspiration eliminators and so forth.

This building material we have can go for days without water and weeks without food but only minutes without oxygen. The smoke-laden cities are not going to allow a person to get well or remain well or to have the body that we would like to have. A patient should find out how to purify his blood stream and how to keep it pure. To have health and strength, we have to have a pure and clean blood stream.

Your Blood Stream — Your Life Line

Note — that the blood stream has seven major functions in the body. Don't neglect this vital life line to health.

1. To transport nutrients (food and oxygen) to the cells.
2. To remove waste materials from the cells.
3. To provide the glands with material for the manufacture of various products.
4. To carry these products from the glands to the parts of the body where they are used by the cells.
5. To evenly heat the entire body and bring about the release of excess heat.
6. To guard and defend the body against the attack of poisonous substances, bacteria and viruses.
7. To heal the body when it is ill, injured or wounded.

Steps to the Healthy Way of Life

There is more to health than merely brushing our teeth and combing our hair — or caring for the outside of the body only. The body is a servant; it needs care and dressing up. You don't want a "Raggedy Ann" body accompanying you when you visit the king. Have a body that is in good working order, inside and out, the kind of body that can jump for joy when you want to show how good life feels.

There are other things to consider besides nutrition. Create your own recipe for a good day. Learn to think well of others. Don't look for the worst in people; see the good points. Don't allow life to disturb you peace of mind. The physical side of health is diet, exercise and rest. If you have a sedentary job, compensate for it by physical exercise. A tired body needs the slant board. Use forms of exercise different from exercise you get in your job. If one arm is used all day, do physical exercise to develop the rest of the body. If you are a mental worker, include physical exercise or work, to offset this. Keep in good company and take up hobbies you enjoy. Do the things you enjoy. Learn to find beauty in everything and appreciate the natural beauty around you. Get close to Nature. Choose good associations and aim for the noble and high goals in life. Remember: we were created for joy.

Of course, what we eat is very important — it will be walking and talking tomorrow. But, also remember that a positive mental outlook is as important as the care of the physical body. A healthy body is built of positive thoughts and actions.

What Is Disease?

The basis of disease is impaired function. In *Human Life, It's Philosophy and Laws*, Dr. H.M. Shelton says, "impaired health or disease is simply a lessened degree of action of the organs of the body taken as a whole, than is performed by the same organs in the highest state of health, together with such impairments of structures and secretions that flow naturally from such depressed action. The present health standard is a false one. Indeed it represents just the conditions of things described above. A true health standard would be the highest possible degree of healthy action in a perfect organism. Anything short of this is impaired health, disease. In this view the highest action in the most perfect organism which we know is the condition of disease. That is, mankind is sick and is far short of perfection. And those whom we call healthy, are just a little less sick than those whom we call sick. Or, to put it more naturally, those whom we call sick are only a little less healthy than those we call well."

Civilization, Domestication and Disease

Animals, when they are in their natural state, do not have disease. It seems that civilization and the domestication of animals is bringing on the sickness of both animals and man. We have the power and the vitality to build great resistance when we live in the correct manner. When we want to immunize our body we do it best by building our good health. And, of course, this is dependant upon sufficient rest, sleep, pure water, exercise, food, fresh air and so forth, and the mental attributes that keep us from getting sick. The best philosophy is that in order to avoid or to rid of disease, we have to build a healthy body.

The Worst Diseases Are in the Mind

If we don't start the day thinking properly, what we have in our mind can be far worse for us than disease. The mental and spiritual part of life can't be separated from the physical body. It was the late Senator Hubert H. Humphrey who put it quite nicely when he said, "I do feel good... I'm blessed with vitality."

In an interview on the "CBS Morning News," Senator Humphrey said, "One never knows about this crazy, strange, dread disease called cancer — what will happen to you, so I start out each day and say, 'Well here's another one. Let's go at it and let's enjoy it,' because if I spent any time worrying about myself, it would make me feel worse than the disease."

There Are No "Miracle" Cures

I am opposed to thinking for one moment that a carrot can "cure" certain conditions or that parsley is a "cure" or that any one food may "cure" any disease. However, I am one who believes that the chemical elements that are found in any of the foods are necessary at times to keep the proper chemical balance in the body. I believe that disease enters the body when our resistance is low in any organ because of a poor chemical balance. There are definite materials in each food that could be used to make that balance perfect in the body so that no disease would come. Rather than use any one food and call it a cure for a disease, I would rather say that we are balancing the body biochemically.

There are people who might say that certain foods may cure certain conditions. While we know that certain foods have an effect on certain organs in the body, that doesn't always mean they have a healthy effect. We find that some foods can act as diuretics and force the kidneys to work, but they do not necessarily provide all the chemical elements to bring them to normal. So we have to be careful.

For instance, with carrots, they claim that Vitamin A is high; but carrots have pro-vitamin A, an incomplete substance has to be converted by the liver into vitamin A, and many times producing conditions that look like jaundice if the liver isn't working right. The yellow pigment (carotene) is thrown out through the skin because it is an incomplete vitamin A, and the body can't handle too much at a time.

There are a lot of things that cause us trouble. We might consider that poor air is just as bad as poor food. Diet isn't everything in life. We find that a broth or a soup can be wonderful. But we find, too, that if we have too much of it or if it hasn't been made right — too much salt or too many spices — it can ruin all the good that might have come from it.

Laugh to Improve Your Health

One of the most beneficial health tonics is laughter, says a psychiatrist who has studied laughter and humor for 23 years. Dr. William F. Fry Jr. who has conducted tests at Stanford University with 65 subjects, says there are three good things that happen when we laugh, medically speaking.

There is an increase in adrenalin in the blood; this encourages more mental alertness. The heart rate is increased, like taking light exercise. Muscles relax. Surprisingly, there is not a decrease of oxygen in the blood, even though laughing has to do with exhaling. Dr. Fry also pointed out that laughter relieves tension and helps people come closer together. It wards off depression.

Die Laughing or Laugh and Live?

Norman Cousins, former editor of *Saturday Review* tells of his conquest of a terminal disease 13 years ago. Doctors gave him a 500-to-1 chance of surviving. In spite of severe pain and a rapidly worsening condition, he refused to give in. Che chose to cure himself with a positive attitude, large doses of vitamin C and *Candid Camera* reruns. He disregarded the medications doctors had recommended, as he did their prognosis.

Cousins checked into a hotel with movie films, a projector and his nurse. He began taking huge intravenous doses of vitamin C and watching *Candid Camera* classics. "I made the joyous discovery that 10 minutes of genuine belly laughter had an anesthetic effect and would give me at least 2 hours of pain-free sleep. When the pain-killing effect of the laughter wore off, we would switch on the motion picture projector again, and, not infrequently, it would lead to another pain-free sleep interval," Cousins was quoted in a recent issue of the *New England Journal of Medicine*.

After publication of the story, Counsins said he received 2,000 letters from physicians. "Many of them recounted similar stories in which they cited examples of where a positive approach to life—the desire to live—is so tremendously important," he said. He added that he is in hopes that his story can help save lives, but not raise false hopes in those with similar afflictions.

Your Choice of Food Determined by Taste

Our taste buds register four different sensations: sweet, salty, bitter and sour. The back of the tongue is more sensitive to bitter, the sides react more easily to sour and salty substances, while the tip perceives a sweet taste.

Among aquatic animals taste buds are distributed over the entire body. Fish also taste with their tailfins. The whale, which swallows unchewed or whole schools of small fish, has few or no taste buds.

Man is a moderate taster possessing 3000 buds. A pig gets more enjoyment from its food, with 5500 taste buds; cows have only 3500.

At least half the food we eat and think we taste is actually smelled. You cannot taste a rotten egg. You smell its rottenness. Greater pleasure is experienced from the smell of apples and oranges than from the tasting. A connoiosseur of fine wines will first smell the bouquet before drinking.

An interesting experiment is to place a clothes pin on your nose and then be blindfolded. Without your smelling sense, you will not be able to differentiate between a tomato and an orange or raspberry water and sweetened milk.

It is most important that our foods be prepared to bring out the most pleasant odors so our enjoyment and digestion will be of the best.

Chapter 12

How to stay well on $1.35 a day

How would you like to see a book on how to get well on 3¢ a day? Maybe you couldn't make it on 3¢ a day, but perhaps 35¢ or then make it $1.35 a day. Wouldn't it be nice to know a way you could get well the cheapest way possible?

Who Can Afford to be Sick?

First of all, sickness is quite expensive. We all know that. Sickness is a very expensive thing. The average cancer, for instance, brings in to the doctor $6,000; some of them may cost $12,000. That was five years ago, so it has probably been raised since then. A young lady in Hollywood, a movie actress, a short time ago had lung trouble, and this cost her $26,000 for her doctor bills alone for five days. Now if that actually had been done to me, I would think I would have died. I mean, if there was no other way, then have five days in the hospital with doctor bills of $26,000, why I would almost rather have died. The New Day doctor is going to be one who watches the fact that he has a whole person to deal with whenever he is treating a patient. Now, a patient is just as good as his reserves. He is as good as his reserve energy; he is as good as his supply of reserve chemical elements that he has in his body. If you have any type of sickness and you have to be treated, you will find that it is much easier to treat a body that has been taken well care of, than one that hasn't been treated well.

The Poor Get Well Faster!

So, this whole thing resolves itself down to one thing, and that is, what is the cheapest way of being well as possible? We find that the person who has the least money gets well quicker under the doctor's care. Both he or she and the doctor have more motivation, so to speak.

Medical expenses, like other commodities are priced according to what the traffic can bear. Did you ever hear that phrase used before? "Whatever the traffic can bear." If you drive in a Cadillac it is going to cost you more than if you come up in a Ford, and it might pay to come in a very cheap automobile when you see the doctor. I am, in a sense, joking; but there is something to it. Surgery is very costly; medicines are very costly. But are they necessary? Doctors are much less hesitant about

recommending expensive therapies, medications and operations when they know that a patient (or the patient's insurance company) can afford them.

How to Cut Doctor Bills

Well, they are necessary at times and we are all subject to them, and I am not saying that we don't need a doctor, but my topic is this, "How can we have the least amount of doctor bills; how can we get well and stay well on a few pennies a day?" The same thing that will prevent a disease will also cure a disease. So, this is something for you to think about. You must try to live in such a way that you avoid the disease, because disease is a very expensive thing. Few people realize that when they are sick they can do something for themselves, and I would like to suggest what you can do for yourself from a preventive standpoint.

Four Prerequisites for Getting Well

First of all, there are four things that you should take care of: 1. The nervous system. 2. The blood stream. 3. Exercise. 4. Rest. These four things should always be considered in getting well and staying well.

Care for the Nervous system

The first thing we should consider is how to save and conserve our nervous system. Now there are means of taking care of this nervous system, through the spine. We cannot maintain proper nerve supply with sedentary occupations or with occupations that are pulling on one side of the body, keeping it uneven, unbalanced. We have to have good posture. Every joint has to be mechanically exercised in a circular motion every day. This keeps the nerve supply active throughout the body. Without good posture, we interfere with the nerve supply. The nerves need silicon foods like sprouts and rice bran; they need nerve fats and phosphorus as found in eggs, cod fish roe and lean meat.

Healthy Blood and Tissues

The next thing is blood supply. You cannot have extreme prolapsus in the body; this interferes with the proper nerve and blood supply. If the transverse colon has dropped and is pressing against the pelvic organs, it presses against nerves and blood vessels and tissues that need blood.

Don't Neglect Exercise

Exercise helps take care of the nerves and blood circulation. We must have a good blood stream that takes care of the nerves, organs, glands and tissues, and that is accomplished through exercise and proper nutrition. We can use the bouncer exercises and slanting board to move the blood. We must take care of the stomach first in feeding our bodies, because if we don't take care of the stomach, we will not get enough good from our food to help the rest of the body. To take care of the stomach first, we make sure that we take plenty of the sodium foods such as whey, celery, greens, goat milk and cheese (table salt doesn't have the right kind of sodium). Don't think that just any one thing can get you well. Carrot juice never cured anybody. Carrot juice is not enough to cure a condition alone. We have to have other proper nutrients going along with it.

Sodium foods also help take care of the bowel. We find that most people have an underactive bowel, a toxic bowel, often with diverticula or bowel pockets. But, we can't have a clean bloodstream with a dirty bowel. So, we must clean up the bowel. The most thorough way I know of to clean up the bowel is through colemas, as described in my book *Tissue Cleansing through Bowel Management*. Colemas are like a cross between an enema and a colonic — more than an enema, not as extreme as colonics. We should all be having two or three bowel movements each day, and we do have them with a healthy bowel. Exercise helps tone the bowel. We should be taking two alfalfa tablets with each meal; alfalfa is one of the best supplements for the bowel. We need bulk — bran, fresh fruits and vegetables, whole grain foods, raw foods. Bulk keeps the bowel toned and healthy. A healthy stomach digests food well; a healthy bowel assimilates nutrients and gets rid of wastes rapidly; a healthy bloodstream carries a rich supply of nutrients; sufficient exercise moves the blood to all parts of the body, especially the brain which is most important.

Rest for Repair and Rebuilding

We cannot get well and stay well without sufficient rest so the cells can repair, rebuild and replenish themselves. The brain needs rest so the stresses of the day can be released. The nerves need rest. During sleep, the entire metabolism of the body goes down so cells can get the rest they need. I don't like to say everyone needs 8 hours of sleep. I know people who can get along on 6 hours and others who need 10 hours plus a mid-afternoon nap. If you know how much rest you need, develop the discipline to get it. If you don't know, find out. Sometimes we may have to fast or go on juices to get rid of a catarrhal condition, cold or flu; always have complete rest along with it.

Weighing the Costs of Food

The best foods are not always the least expensive foods. When we can buy foods or get them from a farm, we may be able to save by buying them in volume; then you can preserve them, can them, put them away. Talk to the produce man at your grocery store and find out when fresh fruit and vegetables come in, especially greens. Buy them fresh. Eat more raw fruits and vegetables in season. Leave the packaged and processed foods on the shelf. Find out where you can get raw goat milk and use it, not pasteurized cow's milk. Use whole grains for cereals in the morning. Above all, go by Nature's Law: "What is whole, pure and natural is best for us." And the second law is, "Get plenty of variety in your foods." Variety ensures that the bloodstream has the right nutrients for every cell in the body. Cut meat down to two or three times a week. That will save you a bundle, and you'll be healthier for it. Avoid sugar and white flour foods and products.

There are a few things you have to pay more for in order to get them right, because man is paid for his labor, and labor sometimes costs more than the material or food produced. We find that labor is more expensive than tomatoes today. There may be about 3¢ worth of tomatoes in a can of tomatoes, but what do you pay for it? You're paying for the cost of the can and for all the work that went into bringing that can to you. If you're buying fresh tomatoes, you're paying for planting, fertilizing, spraying, harvesting, washing, packing, shipping and store handling. When you can get to a farm, coop, farmer's market or direct sales outlet, and all of this labor isn't put on these foods, then you can beat some store prices.

There are farmer's markets, markets on corners that sell foods. If you know a place where you can get organic foods, shop there. Keep in mind that when you buy string beans directly from the farmer they are alkaline forming; four days after they are picked they are acid-forming. So, you can't even buy good string beans in any market unless they have been picked and shipped in less than 3 days. but as fresh as you can, however.

Natural, Pure and Whole Suggestions

Nutritious food has to be natural, whole and pure. People living on good wholesome foods will know the organic gardeners. Still further, we find if you're going to have two fruits a day, they should be completely ripe, a fruit fully ripened by the sun. The sun finishes fruit, brings it to complete ripeness. Otherwise, you are getting a green acid in all the fruits you eat. If you will go to the farmer and pick your own strawberries, raspberries and cherries, you can usually save money. And, it is good exercise for you. If you can pick your own foods you'll get by cheaper and stay healthier, but above all things when you come to a place where they sell fruit directly from the farm, you can depend upon the fruit being much riper. In other words, stores will put out green apricots to sell, but you can get a ripe apricot right from the tree.

I just gave you a couple of examples. There are 1000 more if you would get your food the cheapest way possible, directly from the farm. Find out where to get the freshest, cheapest foods. Seeking out these best foods is going to make better tissue, better health, a higher level of well-being.

Doctors are making a living on people who are not getting fresh foods as grown on the farm. Poor nutrition is undercutting our health and inviting disease. Well being may not come in a week, two weeks with better care — it could be a year or two but that is the same way with disease. We are either earning our way to better health or we are earning disease. Its our choice. You have to consider that for a few cents a day more, its well worth the money to have farm-fresh, ripe fruits and vegetables — not to mention fresh eggs, raw milk and perhaps other good foods. If you ever need a doctor, he is going to have the best possible body to take care of. You'll get well fast. But, aim for prevention.

I read a news item once that said in Boston no one had ever tasted a ripe blackberry. They have to be picked green for shipping into Boston. And I'm telling you if you have never tasted a ripe blackberry right from the vine, you've never had a "real" blackberry. You've never lived. And, a ripe apricot right off the tree has a flavor you'll never duplicate in the market. It is an impossibility.

These are some ways that will keep you well from a food standpoint. If you can keep well, you're going to spend the least amount of money for the doctor. If you spend more on good, fresh foods, you are going to save more on the doctor bills. This is what is eventually going to happen.

Exercise to Better Circulation

Now we come back to the third thing, which to me is very important. That is exercise, that's circulation. I don't know if you realize that good circulation must be developed in the body; circulation is automatic, but it's not adequate without exercise.

I think, personally, that the slanting board is probably the most necessary of all the exercise gadgets that I know. I feel it is one gadget you have to have. It doesn't have to be expensive. You can get a slant board from $20 to $50, or you can make one for yourself. You can adapt an old sign board, a door or an ironing board leaned on a chair to work out on. The idea is to lay head down on it, getting gravity to bring the transverse colon back into the proper position; to get some of the pressure off the abdominal and pelvic organs.

Secrets of the Slant Board

You find that you are also going to separate the vertebrae. It is these discs between the vertebrae that get flattened and compressed as we go through the years, interfering with the nerve supply that comes from the spinal column, the spinal nerves. As you grow older, you can get as much as 3 inches shorter than you were at age 20. It is the spinal discs that get shorter. We find out that we stand too long; we don't get enough rest and the first thing you know, we get compressed discs.

Lying head down on a slant board separates the vertebrae and discs, moves the transverse colon back up into place and moves blood into the brain where it is needed. Practically every patient that comes to see me is anemic in the head. They are troubled with brain anemia. You must feed it; you must take care of it. It is the most important organ you have. The average executive today, the secretary, court reporter — these people really need more blood in their brain. They don't exercise enough to move the blood there. We find that the upside-down slant board is one important way to get blood to the brain.

The "Jogger" for Internal Massage

There is another gadget that I think is absolutely wonderful, and this is what we call the jogger or bouncer, a small trampoline exercise gadget. And, now, I believe you can get a good one for from $35 to $100. Look for them on sale. Over a period of time, you will realize that this is one of the best investments you have made. It can be used indoors or outdoors, rain or shine. Because of the "give" from the springs, it will not jar the spine or bones.

I believe in the bouncer because you give yourself an internal massage everytime you exercise on it. The springs are forcing you up against gravity, and the internal organs which are all soft, bathed in liquids and fluids, will massage each other, and this is great for all of them.

Skin Brushing for Skin Breathing

The next gadget that I think is important is the skin brush. Buy a long-handled vegetable bristle brush. The brush, if you take care of it, will last a year. Use it to brush that skin, all over the body, every morning for 5 minutes. Twice a day is better. It is the best mechanical massage that I know, and it clears the dead skin scales away to allow the skin to breathe.

We have about 200 pores to the square inch in the skin, and if you take that brush and get right into those pores you will get rid of the top layer of skin. That skin is continually growing, as it grows the top layer dies. It is dead flaky material, and it has to be brushed off. You can help it, and you need to help it if you wear clothes. I consider the skin a third kidney because it is an elimination organ. We need to keep it clean and brushed.

I am convinced that wearing clothes contributes to the beginning of every disease. In using iridology, we find a black rim around the outside of most eyes and we call this the scurf rim. This shows that the pores of the skin are not eliminating properly. Toxins are being held under the skin. If you brush the skin you'll get right down to the next layer which is as clean as the blood can make it. If you have a clean blood stream and build a good clean skin, no bath will ever make your skin better than that new skin. Skin brushing is wonderful.

Nylon Clothes Encourage Health Problems

If you want to be well, beware of nylon clothes. We're sending all of our cotton things to China. The Chinese are going to be healthy in the future, and we're going to collapse from all of the unnatural nylon clothes we wear. Nylon cannot absorb the toxic material from your body. I've seen a lot of people, especially women, who have had leg troubles. We could get rid of most of them by getting rid of the nylon stockings they are wearing.

A Few Valuable Exercises

There are a few exercises I think are most important. One of the finest exercises for the abdomen is sitting on the edge of a straight-backed chair and leaning your head back so that your body is in about a straight line, a straight line from your legs right up to your head. Now, lift up the back and legs at the same time until you can feel the muscles of the abdomen really tight. Then, put your feet and head down, relax the abdomen for a second or two, and repeat — 10 times altogether (or less if it is hard for you). We call this the "Chest Leg Pull-up Exercise."

Another exercise I like is called the Alley Cat Exercise. If you don't know what the Alley Cat dances are, ask the young people, but it is also an exercise. When we do this exercise, we lift the right leg up high, bending the knee and swinging the leg to your left, while twisting the torso in the other direction. Then you've got a nice spinal exercise. Alternate five times with each leg for two or three repetitions.

Here's another one, and when you think about this exercise, think of a figure 8. First draw an imaginary figure 8 on the floor. Then, stand in the middle of that figure 8 and make the hips follow the outline of the eight. I have seen wonderful activity developed in the abdomen; I've seen congestions, cysts, and many things controlled and handled by this figure 8 exercise. We do the same thing with the lower extremities. Put your hands on your knees and move the knees in a figure 8. Notice how the ankles are doing a nice circular motion. Next, we are going to move the shoulders up on one side, down on the other, forming a figure 8.

For the neck, look straight ahead and move your head in a figure 8, first forward and back, then from side to side — figure 8's in two directions.

The last of the figure 8 exercises is Fred Astaire's exercise. One I learned from Fred Astaire. Now Fred uses a stretching dance movement to do this exercise, each hand grasping the forearm near the elbow, feet spread apart, leading with the elbow and shoulder first to one side then the other, in a figure 8. A spinal stretch, abdominal stretch, liver stretch—it's a lovely exercise. Repeat at least 10 times each direction, and do it to nice music.

Kneipp Bath and Better Circulation

If we cannot exercise, we have two other ways of getting blood to different parts of the body. We can go to the Kneipp bath to force blood to circulate and to come to the surface near the skin. Cold water on any part of the body drives the blood in, warm water brings it to the surface. So, we spray the legs with a hose, up to the knee, front and back, then walk briskly and let it dry in the air. Or, like the actual Kneipp baths, wade 30 feet in knee-deep cold water, then walk to air-dry the legs. Some people can't exercise, so then we use the water.

The average woman lives 8 years longer than a man in the United States. I seldom found really old women in my world travels, but I found lots of old men. Why old men and not old women? All of these men married 3 and 4 times because their wives died early. The secret was given to me by Dr. Paul Dudley White, who was President Eisenhower's heart physician. He said, "We die from our feet up...we die from our feet up."

All of these people who come to me sick and dying have cold feet and cold hands, and also a cold head. They don't have adequate circulation. The men were all working outside on uneven surfaces, wearing soft shoes. The wives worked out in the fields, too, but after a certain age, the women stayed in the house. She was walking on flat, even surfaces. She wasn't using her legs, and that's why she died sooner.

To get blood into your head, you're going to have to do it with your legs. One way is to walk on hillsides, another way is walking barefoot on sand or grass for 10 minutes every day.

A Case of Leg Surgery Prevented

A lady aged 75 was told by her doctors that they were going to have to amputate her legs at the knees. Her legs were covered with running ulcers, the circulation was so bad that they weren't healing — they were getting worse.

When she came to me, she said, "I'm 75 years old, and I don't want an operation at this age. Isn't there something you can do?" I persuaded her to walk down on the beach barefooted in the sand in about 5 inches of ocean water. She said, "I can't walk." I said, "You can walk 3 steps, can't you?" She said, "Yes." I said, "Do three steps the first day, six the next day, nine steps the next day and just keep walking."

Do you know that at the end of the month she was walking 3 miles? She went back to her doctor, and the doctor said, "You don't need the operation." I mean, if she could do this at the age of 75, you people who are only 40 or 50 have a good chance to build a good circulation. I'm exaggerating, but I am wondering if you see what we are talking about.

Older people often have trouble with varicose veins. In the iris of the eye I can see that the legs are essential to take care of. And, it has to be done through exercise. Don't ever think you can get well with food alone. Exercise is very important.

A Recap of Expenses so Far

All right, have you spent much money on the exercises so far? No, but I've given you some good ways to go. You may spend $1.50 on a skin brush, $20 on a slant board and $30 or so on a bouncer isn't that something? We have covered foods, too, but if you cut down on meats, eliminate processed foods and eat more fresh fruits and vegetables, you'll save on both your food bills and doctor bills.

Quiet is Necessary with Rest

I don't like to bring this out from a spiritual standpoint, but the Christ brought this out and said, "Come, all ye that are weary and heavy laden, and I will give you rest." Well, what do you suppose he did? Did he give them a pill, or send them to bed? No, he was talking about peace of mind, peace with God. All ye that are heavy laden, can you understand that? You need to be still. Be at peace. Did you ever hear, "He leadeth me beside the still waters."? Have you ever marveled over a mirror-like lake at dawn or sunset? It is very still, very, very still. You must take care of this outlook in your body. The attitude of stillness brings recuperation. You can't do it any other way. You see this has to do with your mental attitude, getting along with people, getting along with your finances, getting along with your marriage.

I heard of a lady the other day who couldn't get along with her husband, so she shot him. I've heard of a man next door to someone who played his TV so loud that the neighbor took a shotgun and blew that TV set to pieces. You must understand that people need peace and quiet. They can't stand excessive noise, or it gets to the place where, as the kids say, "They flip their lids." When you want to get well, you're going to have to "let go and let God." You're going to have to go this quiet way.

Super Salesman or Super Pressure?

We have been taught to skin the other fellow before he skins us. We have been taught to get there first with the mostest. This is the mental side of daily life, isn't it? Psychologically speaking, if you want anything, you've got to go and get it, and you've got to work hard to get it. They teach you how to do it.

Salesmanship is not easy. I've taken care of a man who received an award for selling more insurance than any other man in this country, and he was a wreck. He sold more insurance than anyone else, but I'm telling you he didn't do it quietly, he was out there every night. His wife said she saw him two Sunday evenings in the whole year. This man made a wreck of himself.

You Must Get Along with People

Getting along with people isn't easy. Public opinion is not easy, and because often we live on public opinion, we find when other people are unhappy we get unhappy too. I mean, we have so little harmony in this life, we have to get to the place where we can't look to anyone else for our happiness. We can't take the path of public opinion.

Learn What Love is Like

Often we don't know what it is to love, to love wholeheartedly. This is part of healing. If a person knows what it is to walk in obedience, as it is spoken of, and to walk in enlightenment, and to know humility, love, peace, harmony we find these are necessary to good health.

Now, I don't know how much it is going to cost you to have peace and harmony. Some of you may spend thousands of dollars with a psychiatrist without getting well. Did you know, the greatest suicide rate is among the psychologists and psychiatrists? More than any other profession? They're the men who know...they're the men who know, but the point is this, it isn't what you know but it is what you do with what you know.

Secrets that Are Priceless

We find that money is quite a valuable thing, but knowledge and wisdom are invaluable...priceless.

So, I am bringing this out for you to see that it isn't exactly money...it isn't exactly the doctor you are going to find, because you don't see him long enough for him to know you. In China, a doctor says he cannot do anything for you until he knows you six months. How many doctors will tell you to quit your job? How many doctors will tell you to straighten our your marriage or get a divorce? How many doctors will tell you that you better get your financial situation fixed up? How many doctors know you that well?

They take a thyroid test, and the thyroid is bad from all your emotional strain and stress. So, you take thyroid. It isn't a matter of going to the source of the problem and straightening things out. I am wondering if you realize that removing the potential cause of physical or mental breakdown is the cheapest way. Find out what is causing your troubles, get in there and remove it and you will find out that getting well requires, before anything else, that you stop breaking down.

That is the secret of the whole thing...stop breaking down. Now, there are doctors who are good; and we need doctors. I didn't bring this out to prove we should avoid doctors; but I say this, that first of all you should live correctly so that any doctor, when he works on you, is going to have an easier time to take care of you. If you have been living correctly, you're going to overcome a serious infection better than the person who has been living on coffee and doughnuts. A person who has an operation of any kind and who recuperates rapidly will be praised by his or her doctor. "I had a good patient to work on," they say. "You had a good blood count. We didn't have to give you any blood. You'll be out of here in two days."

Can you see the value of just doing the right thing? When you know that you're doing the right thing, you can expect the right things to happen to you. Right rights itself. The wise man takes care of his body as well as his mind. Life is not all spiritual. It is a matter of putting this all together.

Life Must Find a Balance

Balance is the most important thing you can have. Very few people go through life and think of balance. We have no value we place on health until we begin to lose it. Mother used to say, "Health isn't everything, but without health, everything else is nothing." That's how important it is. She used to say, "You can lose all your money and

you have lost a lot, and if you lose your health you've lost still more, but if you ever lose your peace of mind, you've lost everything." We need to see where the real values are in life. We haven't been taught to live. We need to learn to reach for the life more abundant. Can you understand that?

It isn't a matter of just working for good health. A person working for good health is a "health nut, an extremist." He has gone to the edges. But to realize that health interrelates with everything we do and feel and think, that's a start. I don't care if you only have 10¢, you've got to be happy with it. You cannot allow that to kill you. Doctors make a living on people who have lost money. Doctors make a living on people who don't get along with other people. Doctors make a living on your living. That's why I say there is life more abundant if you will put it all together and balance it out. Then you will find you're going to keep well.

When Do We Get Wisdom?

I feel sorry for the elderly more than anyone else. Often, we find that the elderly drag through life or they are drugged through life. They often have to seek rest homes the last part of their life. I think we should work as hard as we can at the age of 20 when we have no sense at all to keep good health so that we can have it at the end of our life. How do you teach this to young people? You don't. That is why I say the fool cannot see what is in the wise man's head, but the wise man can see what is in the fool's head, because he was once a fool himself. But, he doesn't know this until the end of his life. The wise man is not born, he is made.

So, when do we get wisdom? We get it at the end; we get it through terrific experiences, but the lessons in this book are only for those people wise enough to profit from more than hindsight. That is when you save money and peace of mind.

The Inexpensive Food Budget

When I said at the beginning of this chapter that you can help yourself for a matter of a few cents a day, there are meals that can be very inexpensive. Now, if you cook cereals in their natural forms, they are very inexpensive. But, if you want toasted puffed sugar-coated rice twinkle berries, you're going to pay $1.85 a box for it compared to 69¢ or 79¢ a pound for the cereal grain. Then, you'll pay again when you take your twinkleberry-caused arthritis to the doctor's office. We need to realize that we can have more simple foods; fried foods may taste better, but they lose much of the nourishment. When we get polished grains, we're losing vitamins and minerals. When we buy packaged, refined food, we're paying for a ticket to the hospital.

Get back to natural foods. There are ways of saving money. Buy a whole box of apricots when they come in. You can use 2, 3, 4 lb. Dry what you don't use for the winter. There is no dry fruit that is going to be better than what you can dry yourself. Did you ever think about getting a lug of cherries? Take 4-5 lb for your family, perhaps 6 lb. Dry them; there is no reason in the world why you shouldn't have a good high-iron food in the middle of winter, such as dried cherries. Use them for making juices and have black cherry juice in the middle of the winter. This is the highest iron fruit that you can get. In the winter time we don't have these things. There are economical ways, so many ways of saving money if you think about it and keep your eyes open.

Buy leaf lettuce instead of head lettuce. There is 100 times as much iron in leaf lettuce as in head lettuce. Learn to make some great salads — use raw grated carrots, beets, turnips, parsnips — add sunflower seeds, raisins — to be creative. Be creative with pure, whole natural foods, and you'll get by on less money.

A Thanksgiving Menu

Appetizer: Celery filled with happiness.

Soup: Cream of everything nice.

Roast Turkey: Stuffed with joy.

Salad: Chef's special, new ideas tossed with surprise.

Potatoes: Baked in smiles.

Peas: Rolling around in fun.

Dessert: Ice cream topped with love.

Drink: Overflowing with good cheer.

Bread: Buttered with patience and tolerance.

Blessings: We have much to be thankful for!

There is no sickness in spirit; no disease "within." To bring harmony to the body, get harmony within.

To get over being tired, stop wearing yourself out—either physically or often more important, with your thinking.

Health is an inside job? Whole health comes from whole living—physical, mental and spiritual.

The more truth you have the more alone you go.

What can we add to a carrot, an apricot—to make it better than the Creator did?

Olives, eggs, avocado oil and sunflower seed oil are high lecithin foods?

Kelp and dulse are both high in iodine, but dulse has manganese as well?

Authorities tell us that diabetes is increasing so fast that in 25 years there won't be anyone with it?

Chapter 13

Coping with intense stress

Stress Is A Major Health Attacker

Many experts believe stress to be the number one health enemy in the entire world. It can lead to such complications as ulcers, heart attacks, hypertension, migraine headaches and mental illness. It wasn't until about 50 years ago that stress was recognized as a major medical problem, and there is much to learn about the syndrome yet. Our modern fast-paced, got-to-get-ahead at any cost world is producing no little degree of stress.

Stress in the form of "flight or fight" feelings is familiar to everyone. Anger, fear, rapid heartbeat, clammy skin, exasperation, resentment, blood pounding in the ears are a few symptoms. Stress is not entirely a negative entity. It encourages action, the desire to succeed, but we can become addicted, caught up in the craving for the excitement of the stress syndrome so that we remain keyed up far longer than necessary. Nighttime is the time to unwind and relax, to sleep and let go of the daily stress patterns that are so engrained in our existence. Adrenalin, the stress hormone, can keep us tense, tight, unable to sleep or relax.

We find that adrenalin is still largely a mystery in the stress response, though it is under a great deal of study at the present time. High levels of adrenalin are linked to insomnia, high blood pressure and possibly to heart attack, stroke and other heart troubles in American men.

Some of the warning signs of stress are nervousness, irritability, lack of concentration and loss of muscle coordination. For instance, the desire to achieve doesn't cause as much stress as the obsession for power and control of people. Seeking inner perfection is better than the quest for power, it would seem. Adrenalin levels aren't raised as much in the loss of a loved one as in some other stress situations, for example those involving power struggles. Stress can be positive — joy, achievement, accomplishment and self expression. It does not have to be harmful.

To explain the "fight or flight" response a little better, during times of stress the body braces itself to either stand or run by releasing hormones into the bloodstream; this activates the autonomic nervous system that controls the involuntary muscles such as those that regulate digestion and blood pressure. The result will be an emotional response — rage, fear, alarm, resentment. Behavior changes are also noted. It has been found that those under chronic stress are more inclined to accidents. The chances of disease development are greatly increased. It is said that there is greater risk of rheumatoid arthritis, asthma, col-

itis, cancer, backache, pneumonia, neurodermatitis as well as the ailments mentioned above. Stress can also hasten old age symptoms.

The hormones released by stress signals are adrenalin from the outer layer of the adrenal glands and others from the thyroid and pancreas. These chemical messengers speed throughout the body at the direction of the pituitary gland and hypothalamus. The autonomic nervous system is responsible for the dispersal. The hypothalamus is the part of our brain that shapes and shades our feelings. The muscles of the body are made tense and ready for action through direction by the higher brain centers.

Of late there has been a dissatisfaction with the use of drugs and psychotherapy as methods of dealing with stress. Many are turning to Eastern philosophy, transcendental meditation, yoga, Zen and other self-administered relaxation techniques. Others are finding that simple rest is helpful; even short naps. Research suggests that meditation may be effective in relieving stress symptoms.

The home can be a place of stress if light, color, space and noises are not handled properly. Get rid of furnishings that clutter rooms and interrupt easy movement. A television set should not be in the bedroom — it is a place of rest and sleep only. Pay special attention to decorating colors. Soft tints such as green and blue are relaxing and quieting; add soft lighting to these color schemes. Have a comfortable family room large enough for the entire family to get together. If possible have a play room for small children to keep their toys and play on their own. Soft solid colors and small patterns in furnishings are better than large patterns and bright colors. Avoid a lot of red in the home because it is exciting and stimulating. It can produce stress. Subtle colors in general are restful and bright colors are exciting. Keep the noise of appliances and other noises down. They are the main cause of stress in the home.

Heavy drapes and plush carpeting cut down on noise. Upholstered furniture is better than hard furniture — wood, plastic, chrome. A shower curtain that is cloth with a plastic lining cuts down on noise. Buy the quietest household appliances you can get. Replace a loud telephone bell with a soft buzzer or even a flashing light. Soft music can cover outside noise to some extent.

Vacations can be stressful instead of relaxing. Avoid the popular crowded tourist areas. Do what you want and go where you want to go for vacation. You don't have to keep up with the Joneses, so to speak. Often shorter trips taken more often are more restful than an occasional long vacation. Get away for weekend outings often. Above all, do what you enjoy during vacations.

Meeting and Conquering Stress

Stress can lurk almost anywhere. We meet it every time we get behind the wheel of a car, especially during peak traffic hours. Learning to adjust to annoying traffic jams is important for handling stress and avoiding the greater chance of accidents. Learn to relax in traffic, listen to music and traffic reports on the radio. Always make frequent stops during long trips to avoid overtiring. Be alert for unexpected moves by other motorists at all times. Above all don't become angered to the point of losing your temper toward other drivers.

The way you stand, sit and sleep can produce stress. A straight spine is important in walking and standing or sitting. Sitting with the legs crossed at the knees is harmful because circulation is cut off, causing pressure to the nerves and blood vessels. A chair should be comfortable and the hips elevated slightly above the knees; it should support the lower back. Low, deep-cushioned chairs can cause the spine to curve and the back to slouch; they are not recommended.

When standing the feet should hold equal weight — spread apart enough to be a sturdy base. Shifting weight from one foot to the other is not good. Your legs should hold equal weight to keep the spine straight.

A firm mattress is important to keep the body well aligned — especially the spine. Sleeping on your back or side is better.

Many tend to use the same hand and arm for most tasks. This strains the head and neck and upsets body balance. Try using alternating hands.

Stand tall and proud — emotionally telling your body you feel good and are in control of all situations. This counteracts stress.

We find that TV viewing is not relaxing as we are led to believe. It is a perpetual stress situation — causing perspiration, rapid heartbeat, increased adrenalin flow and edgy nerves. Even the commercials are stressful because they are designed to pressure you into buying things you don't need and that are too expensive. We tend to identify with the characters on TV and react emotionally to their situations and predicaments. Emotional detachment prevents some of this stress. The news brings more stress, as we are faced with negative happenings daily — be it in our town or remote parts of the world. You should get up and leave the TV often to take your mind off what it is impressing upon your mind. Every hour or half hour, get up for a few minutes. Better yet, don't watch junky, stressful programs.

Noise is a prime stress offender. When privacy is invaded the stress is even more pronounced. Noise can lead to annoyance and even extreme anger, fatigue from loss of sleep, drug dependence, heart and digestion abnormalities. Try to keep from letting children get on your nerves with noise of play. Meditate if that is helpful.

The body must be biochemically balanced to handle stress. Certain vitamins and minerals are said to fight stress — Vitamins C, B-complex, E and minerals such as zinc, magnesium, calcium and potassium. A balanced diet is essential for preventing the damages of stress. The nervous system must be well nourished to handle pressure. A number of chronic diseases are directly related to stress.

Comfortable clothes reduce stress. Wear what makes you feel good — mentally and physically. Wear loose, casual clothes when possible. Go barefoot; loosen your tie and take off hot jackets when you can. Cotton clothing reduces stress by allowing the skin to breathe. Synthetics hold in acids that should be eliminated through the skin.

Follow an Anti-Stress Nutrition Program

A few simple guidelines can help reduce stress connected with the digestive tract, weight problems and inability to relax. Cut down on salt; it is a stress factor; so are animal fats, tea, coffee, cola drinks, chocolate, junk foods of all kinds. Include lots of unrefined foods in the diet and raw vegetables for bulk. Drink plenty of liquids, including spring water. Relax before meals and if not calm miss that meal. Get enough outdoor exercise. Include foods high in Vitamin C, B-complex, potassium, magnesium and calcium, as well as all essential nutrients.

Stress builds acids in the body that must be eliminated. Excess weight also adds to stress. Refined carbohydrates — especially sugar — create stress by the see-saw effect of low and high blood sugar.

Some specific foods that fight stress are low-fat meats, fowl and poultry, fish, low-fat cheeses, apples, apple juice, apricots (fresh and dried), bananas, green and wax beans, berries, broccoli, cabbage, brussels sprouts, cherries, corn, leaf lettuce, greens, melons, okra, parsley, peaches, fresh peas, potatoes (baked and eaten with skins), prunes, plums, tomatoes, watercress, brown rice, pineapple, yellow cornmeal, rye and millet, even goat milk.

To reduce stress, one psychiatrist recommends breaking your routine once in a while to do something special you like. Get off by yourself for 20 minutes each day and sit under a tree and read or watch the clouds. Married couples should take off at least one weekend a month to go somewhere, relax, unwind and enjoy themselves.

Stress Rating Scale

Rank	Life event	Stress Rating
1.	Death of spouse	100
2.	Divorce	73
3.	Marital separation	65
4.	Jail term	63
5.	Death of close family member	63
6.	Personal injury or illness	53
7.	Marriage	50
8.	Fired from job	47
9.	Marital reconciliation	45
10.	Retirement	45
11.	Change in health of family member	44
12.	Pregnancy	40
13.	Sex difficulties	39
14.	Gain of new family member	39
15.	Business readjustment	39
16.	Change in financial state	38
17.	Death of close friend	37
18.	Change to different line of work	36
19.	Change in number of arguments with spouse	35
20.	Mortgage over $10,000	31
21.	Foreclosure of mortgage or loan	30
22.	Change in responsibilities at work	29
23.	Son or daughter leaving home	29
24.	Trouble with in-laws	29
25.	Outstanding personal achievement	28
26.	Wife begins or stops work	26
27.	Begin or end school	26
28.	Change in living conditions	25
29.	Revision of personal habits	24
30.	Trouble with boss	23
31.	Change in work hours or conditions	20
32.	Change in residence	20
33.	Change in schools	20
34.	Change in recreation	19
35.	Change in church activities	19
36.	Change in social activities	18
37.	Mortgage or loan less than $10,000	17
38.	Change in sleeping habits	16
39.	Change in number of family get-togethers	15
40.	Change in eating habits	15
41.	Vacation	13
42.	Christmas	12
43.	Minor violations of the law	11

Stress, like life itself, is full of the predictable and the unexpected, as is demonstrated by this list ranking forty-three common experiences in terms of stress. (*J. Psychosomatic Res.*, 2:216, 1967.)

Excerpts from the Los Angeles Times:

California farmers are losing from $8 million to $10 million a year because of smog damage to crops, the Council of California Growers reports. The crops most susceptible to smog damage are tomatoes, lettuce, alfalfa, cotton, grapes and citrus fruits. Smog damage to crops isn't limited to the Los Angeles area. It's now moving into parts of the San Joaquin Valley, which produces more than $1 billion worth of farm products a year.

The San Francisco Bay area is recording increasing concentrations, too. And growers of lettuce, spinach and salad greens who have moved from the Los Angeles area to Monterey, Santa Barbara and Ventura Counties, now say smog has followed them there. Dr. John T. Middleton, head of the Air Pollution Research Center at the University of California at Riverside, says 26 counties in the state are more affected in varying degrees by smog. Farmers suffer from smog in three ways: (1) they must spend more money for irrigation because crops growing in contaminated air take longer to mature; (2) yields are reduced; and (3) quality is impaired.

Chapter 14

Hypoglycemia: the "in" disease

Sugar Coated Gourmet Foods

It is hard to believe that in all the ages of the past many of the discoveries that we have in foods and the culinary art have worked contrary to good health. We find that the rich, opulent and the gourmets have often departed from the natural foods and had special foods made for them. In more recent times, white flours, white breads and our white sugar products are creating mass havoc in the health of millions. As a consequence, entire societies have developed epidemic proportions of certain types of diseases. When commercial sugar was first made we find that only the right could afford it and they could only use it on special occasions. In our annals of history, Sir Walter Raleigh gave the market price of sugar at that time as 50 shillings — or about $12.00 a pound. But now it is cheap, everybody can use it and we are running well over 135 pounds a year per person in the United States.

Hypoglycemia, like heart disease, is very much a child of this century. Low blood sugar afflicts somewhere between 50 million people and half of the nation's population, according to experts.

HISTORY OF SUGAR

When sugar was first introduced to the European market it was more expensive than caviar and was used strictly for sweetening the palates of society's upper crust. In fact, it was so rare and valuable that, in 1736, sugar crystals were catalogued with precious stones among the wedding gifts given to Maria Theresa, the future queen of Hungary.

True Magazine 10-75

Those Harmful, Hidden Sugars

		Granulated sugar
cola drinks	6 oz.	3½ tsps
sweet cider	1 cup	6 tsps
choc. cake (plain)	4 oz.	6 tsps
choc. cake (iced)	4 oz.	10 tsps
brownies (unfrosted)	¾ oz.	3 tsps
donut (plain)	1	3 tsps
donut (glazed)	1	6 tsps
hard candy	4 oz.	20 tsps

av. choc. milk bar	1½ oz.	2½ tsps
ice cream	3½ oz.	3½ tsps
ice cream sundae	1	7 tsps
jelly	1 Tbsp.	4-6 tsps
strawberry jam	1 Tbsp.	4 tsps
gelatin (sweetened; flavored)	½ cup	4½ tsps
cream pie	1 slice	4 tsps
berry tart	½ cup	10 tsps
apple pie	1 slice	7 tsps
chocolate pudding	½ cup	4 tsps
plain pastry	4 oz. piece	3 tsps
sherbet	½ cup	9 tsps
pumpkin pie	1 slice	5 tsps
chocolate icing	1 oz.	5 tsps
white icing	1 oz.	5 tsps
maple syrup	1 Tbsp.	5 tsps
macaroons	1	6 tsps

Many hypoglycemic cases are not correctly diagnosed. Due to the strange array of mental symptoms, they are often considered as psychiatric cases, people in need of counsel and treatment. Many of the mental and nervous symptoms found in hypoglycemic cases can be changed by a high-protein, low carbohydrate diet. We find that there is more of a need for proteins for the brain, glands and nerves that are affected. The glandular system, particularly the adrenals, have been broken down and the insulin imbalance is one thing we note in many mental, nervous and behavioral troubles. Many times we need to add niacin and vitamin C to the diet to help stabilize the glandular functions in cases of hypoglycemia. These people must cut out all unsaturated fats. Vitamin B is very much indicated. Psychotherapy may be used as an adjunct when certain people suffer excessively from confusion and depression due to the "low sugar blues."

All sugars, baked foods, pies, cakes, pastries, are on the taboo list. We go for the high mineral content, especially of silicon. The pancreas is a silicon organ, so silicon is indicated for its repair. Silicon is probably the element that was lacking in their diet in years past, because silicon is found in peels, seeds, skins, and outer sections of nuts, cucumbers, potatoes, seeds, fruits and all kinds of vegetables. People develop a lack of silicon over a period of years and produce many of these problems that we find today.

The diet for hypoglycemia involves eating many small meals each day rather than two or three large ones. The slow trickle of protein-derived glucose in the bloodstream assures an adequate supply without the disruptions due to sudden sugar influx and just as sudden sugar "starvation" soon afterward. This diet must eliminate highly sugared foods and drinks, especially *all* refined white sugar foods. Even honey should be avoided. Severely limit the intake of natural sugars in dried fruits, and sweet fruits such as grapes, plums, cherries, dates. Dried fruits to be careful of include raisins, currants, figs, prunes, dried apricots, bananas, pears, etc. Take natural sugar foods only in very small quantities. Artificial sweeteners are *not* recommended either.

When carbohydrates are eaten, make them the unrefined kind such as whole cereal grains, vegetables and salads. Avoid all white flour carbohydrates. Coffee, tea and soft drinks are definitely not advised.

The high protein meals can be made up of meat, fish and eggs. Do not use pork or fatty meats. Milk usually doesn't do well with the hypoglycemic patient due to its lactose (milk sugar) content. Nut and seed milk drinks or soy milk would be better in place of cow's milk and dairy products. Cream and butter are high in fat; cheeses should be limited to a little cottage cheese or cream cheese because of the high fat content and lactose. Supplement the protein meals with low carbohydrate vegetables and fruits. Squashes are a good vegetable for the hypoglycemic patient. Limit potatoes and white rice due to their sugar conversion in the body.

Protein powders can be combined with vegetable juices; fish and tomato juice are good; have sliced tomato with protein. Use soy milk powder in drinks.

Some of the many symptoms of hypoglycemia (low blood sugar) are headache, leg cramps, nervousness, irritability, lack of concentraiton, drowsiness, insomnia, constant worry and anxiety, fainting, tremors, cold sweats, weakness, incoordination, staggering, convulsions, fatigue, muscular pains, vertigo, allergies, palpitation (pounding heart beat), arthritic pains, gouty arthritis, loss of libido, gastrointestinal symptoms, lightheadedness.

Patients suffering from hypoglycemia have often been treated for mental and emotional disturbances, even schizophrenia and alcoholism. Dr. Harry M. Salzer (M.D.) of Cincinnati, Ohio, defines relative hypoglycemia as, "...a clinical syndrome in which patients develop symptoms referrable to any system of the body as the result of a relative drop in blood sugar level in response to a high carbohydrate food intake and drinks containing caffeine."

Relative hypoglycemia hides behind a mask of numerous disorders, such as schizophrenia, chronic alcoholism, convulsive disorders, migraine, manic-depressive psychosis, hypertensive cardiovascular disease, depressive reactions, psychoneurotic depression and psychoneurotic anxiety, among others. According to Dr. Salzer, the symptoms may be classified as psychiatric, neurologic or somatic.

Psychiatric symptoms, according to Dr. Salzer, include depression, insomnia, anxiety, irritability, crying spells, phobias, lack of concentration, forgetfulness or confusion, unsocial or anti-social behavior, restlessness, previous psychosis, suicidal tendencies. Under somatic symptoms he places exhaustion or fatigue, sweating, tachycardia (fast heart beat), anorexia, chronic indigestion or bloating, cold hands or feet, joint pains, obesity, abnormal spasm. Neurologic symptoms are headache, dizziness, tremor (inward or external), muscle pains and backache, numbness, blurred vision, staggering, fainting or blackouts and convulsions.

Symptoms common to hypoglycemia and to many other ailments cause hypoglycemia to be often misdiagnosed or dismissed as something "all in your head." Some of these include fatigue, drowsiness, sharp hunger, trembling, sweating, rapid heartbeat, dizziness and headaches.

The Relationship of Hypoglycemia and Diabetes

Hypoglycemic symptoms may warn of approaching diabetes and lead to its early detection and treatment. In the pre-diabetic or early diabetic stage the patient may experience all the signs of functional hypoglycemia (different from organic malfunctions). The blood sugar level may rise abnormally high and then drop suddenly to normal. These severe variations touch off the symptoms. Sudden hunger and faintness are symptons of hypoglycemia, but frequent urination is a classic sign of diabetes, they may both be present.

A six-hour glucose tolerance test is suggested for these and other abnormal sugar metabolism symptoms. Often the doctor will give only the three-hour glucose tolerance test for diabetes; this is not sufficient for hypoglycemia testing. Family history of diabetes should be checked. The patient is also advised to lose weight if it is too high. If the glucose test results shoot up into the diabetic range and then drop back to the normal level, diabetes is suspected or the pre-diabetic phase. The patient is often placed on a high protein, low carbohydrate and fats diet, exercise and told to cut down on emotional stress causes; he may be warned that he is a potential diabetic.

We believe that diet and stress are key factors in controlling pre-diabetes and preventing diabetes; attention to these factors can also prevent further hypoglycemic symptoms. It is during the pre-diabetic stage that hypoglycemia warns of approaching diabetes.

The next stage is chemical diabetes. The glucose tolerance test will show a curve climbing abnormally toward the diabetes range and then dipping down into the hypoglycemic levels (low blood sugar). It can be months or years before the diabetes makes it definite appearance if the proper measures aren't taken.

Overt diabetes is the state that shows abnormally high

fasting blood levels of high blood sugar levels. The hypoglycemic dips disappear.

Hypoglycemic symptoms can be produced during diabetes if the blood sugar level is too rapidly lowered by too much insulin. There is hope, howerver, in diatetic and nutritional approaches to both diabetes and hypoglycemia. Hypoglycemia (low blood sugar) and hyperglycemia (diabetes — high blood sugar) can be overcome.

What Is Hypoglycemia?

A below normal level of sugar in the blood stream can be the cause of many symptoms related to hypoglycemia — low blood sugar. The millions of cells in the body must have a continuous supply of sugar through the blood to work properly. If hypoglycemia is present it is a sign that the body chemistry is out of balance. It can even lead to diabetes. Insulin and the adrenal cortex secretions control the blood sugar level. Such terms as hyperinsulinism, adrenal cortical insufficiency, and more commonly, "hypoglycemia" describe this condition.

What causes hypoglycemia? The pancreas and sometimes adrenals may atrophy from the heavy diets of refined carbohydrates and refined sugar. Protein must be added to the diet to allow the pancreas and adrenals to rebuild. How many times have you heard: "I'm too tired all the time." "I don't have any energy." "Why am I so nervous?" "I'm so depressed for no reason." And how many times is the doctor's answer the following: "It's in your mind." It's just nervous energy." Or, more seriously, some hypoglycemics are treated as mental and psychiatric cases. I believe it is one of the most misdiagnosed ailments we have today.

The causes of constant low blood sugar can be such things as periods of stress, over-excitement, poor diet or nervous system shocks. Some instances are infection, pain, overwork, burns, accidents, fractures, domestic troubles, drugs, pregnancy, lactation. Of course, a diet of refined carbohydrates and white sugar products are at the top of the list.

The pancreas and the adrenal cortex can be broken down so that proper control of the blood sugar level is no longer possible. The liver also enters the picture because it must maintain the right glucose levels. Many things can overwork and damage it: excessive alcohol, smog, toxins in the body, tobacco and coffee or tea and toxic chemicals found in foods.

Adrenal and pancreatic weaknesses are often passed on to the infant if the parents have the problem. The same may be true of the adrenal glands. These children often start out with problems such as colic, chronic diaper rash, respiratory disorders, allergies to formulas, etc. from adrenal weakness.

Some experts believe that a deficiency of B-complex vitamins can contribute to hypoglycemia. These vitamins may be short in the diet or poorly assimilated. Proper carbohydrate metabolism is related to these vitamins, and thus they have to do with control of the blood sugar level.

Blood sugar control is held to a narrow margin for best health since the body metabolism reacts to too much or too little glucose. If the controls are called on too often they are broken down or become less efficient. Thus, we can become less tolerant to sharp changes in blood sugar levels. We find that glucose can be made from fats and proteins besides carbohydrates. The advantage to proteins and limited fats is that glucose from their conversion is absorbed into the blood stream slowly enough that the balance of the regulating organs is protected. If, however, we decide to have a coke, for example, an overload of glucose is rapidly "dumped" into the blood and the glands must overwork to balance the blood sugar level at the proper concentration. Eventually the adrenal glands can be exhausted trying to *raise* the blood sugar back to the correct level. The pancreas reacts so fast to the excess glucose concentration, secreting extra insulin, that this *reduces* the blood sugar level suddenly and too far. But we find that weak adrenal glands can't raise the blood sugar back to normal easily, and this causes hypoglycemia symptoms.

Protein drinks and snacks are valuable in keeping the blood sugar near normal. Soy, seed and nut milks are well to use along with vegetable juices, tomatoes, squash, limited cottage cheese, egg yolk. A good source of B-complex and silicon is needed. Eliminate all stimulants. Rebuild the glands with protein.

A Sample Hypoglycemia Diet

Upon Arising:
Three glasses of warm water to cleanse the stomach. Follow with 4 oz. fresh juice.

BREAKFAST:
Fruit (other than sweet or dried fruit); or 4 oz. fresh fruit juice; 1 egg or cottage cheese or yogurt, if desired. (Soft boiled egg.)

2 Hours After Breakfast
4 oz. fresh juice (vegetable is preferred)

LUNCH:
Soup; generous raw salad (vegetable) with a little health mayonnaise or other dressing; steamed vegetables; whole grain cereal or unrefined vegetable starch; health beverage.

3 Hours After Lunch:
8 oz. nut or seed milk or protein powder drink, and/or vegetable juice.

1 Hour Before Dinner:
4 oz. fresh vegetable juice.

DINNER:
Raw vegetable salad; steamed vegetables; one protein: meat, fish, fowl or vegetable protein; Health beverage.

2 to 3 Hours After Dinner:
8 oz. nut or seed milk; or protein powder drink, with vegetable juice.

Every Two Hours Until Bed:
4 oz. of nut or seed milk or vegetable juice or protein powder drink.

ALLOWED VEGETABLES:
Asparagus, avocado (protein), beets, broccoli, brussel sprouts, cabbage, cauliflower, carrots, celery, corn (starch), cucumbers, eggplant, lima beans (protein), onions, peas, radishes, sauerkraut, squash (large winter squashes are starches), parsnips, turnips, tomatoes, string beans, leaf lettuce, watercress, parsley.

ALLOWED FRUITS:
Apples, apricots, peaches, pears, berries, melons, pineapple, oranges, lemons, tangerines, grapefruit.

ALLOWED BEVERAGES:
Herbal teas, whey, vegetable juices, limited fruit juices, nut and seed milks, soy milk, protein powder drinks. (*Not* sweetened with honey or dried fruits.) Avoid grape and other sweet juices.

ALLOWED DESSERTS:
Unsweetened gelatin and fruits occasionally.

ALLOWED PROTEINS:
Eggs, fish, fowl, meat, cottage cheese and yogurt, avocado, nuts, protein powders, legumes, seeds.

ALLOWED STARCHES:
Corn, baked potatoes and sweet potatoes occasionally, whole grain cereals: rice, millet, buckwheat, rye, yellow cornmeal. Breads and bakery goods are to be avoided.

TABOO FOODS AND BEVERAGES:
Avoid entirely alcoholic beverages, colas and soda pop, carbonated drinks, liquors, wine, beer, cocktails.

Avoid candy, chocolate, sugar and other sweets such as cake, pie, pastries, puddings, etc.

Avoid dried fruit and sweet fruits such as dates, figs, raisins, prunes, grapes, persimmons, bananas; and their juices.

Avoid all refined starches and carbohydrates such as spaghetti, noodles, macaroni, doughnuts, jams, jellies, marmalades, honey, etc. (Only Tupelu Honey is allowed occasionally.)

Prevent Future Diabetes Today

As with all diseases, prevention is the real cure. Diabetes is no exception. About two million Americans have diabetes and don't know it, according to some experts. It ranks fifth among the nation's killers, says the American Diabetes Association. Millions have a genetic tendency toward the disease.

Diabetes mellitus is a complicated malfunction where the ability to properly metabolize sugar has been lost. There are many types, affecting many age groups. Diet, exercise and weight loss have been successful in controlling many cases. One type comes in childhood or early adulthood, while another is likely to be noted in middle age or later life.

British nutrition researcher Dr. John Yudkin, M.D., reports experiments in which rats that were fed sugar developed a decreased glucose tolerance similar to human diabetes. The average sugar intake in the U.S. has recently been placed at 1 teaspoon per half-hour, 24-hours, every day of the year! Dr. Yudkin further states that, ''In human subjects, a high-sugar diet maintained for several weeks has been shown to reduce sugar tolerance, and a low-sugar diet for several weeks has been shown to improve it.''

Classic signs of diabetes are: (1) Fatigue and frequent urination; (2) Increased appetite accompanied by weight loss; (3) Heavy thirst; (4) Toe or finger cramps or pain or vision changes; (5) Cuts or bruises take longer to heal; (6) Women may note a genital itch. Any diagnosing should be left to a physician.

Alcoholism and Hypoglycemia

Alcoholism is a disease which makes the afflicted unable to quit drinking by choice. The more they try to quit the more difficult it becomes. They can leave alcohol for short periods, but they return to the vicious cycle. If the alcoholic stops, he experiences acute cravings, physical and mental tensions, anxiety, thirst and irritability. These and other symptoms are temporarily alleviated by more alcohol. The three stages of alcoholism are excessive drinking, addiction to alcohol and finally chronic alcoholism. A common characteristic among all alcoholics is the craving syndrome that starts with the first drink.

Some of the theories of the causes of alcoholism include abnormal sugar metabolism, especially hypoglycemia. Also, some believe it has to do with hormone deficiency of the thyroid, adrenal glands, pituitary or glandular imbalances of various types. Dietary shortages of minerals, vitamins, enzymes or amino acids are another possible cause. Liver dysfunction and allergy are other candidates. These factors are summed up as allergy, abnormal carbohydrate metabolism, dietary deficiencies, glandular imbalance, liver dysfunction, and brain disorders.

Research has shown that some 20% of the U.S. populace is susceptible to addictive qualities of alcohol; for the other 80% it acts as a tranquilizer. Also, if the person smokes, the need for the sedative qualities of alcohol is much greater. Further studies reveal that an enzyme dysfunction can be genetically inbred and transmitted to descendants, which makes for difficulty for an inability to successfully handle intoxicants. (The American Indian, for example.)

The now famous "alcoholic rat" studies at Loma Linda University in California revealed some surprising facts about diet and biochemical imbalances. Ninety-six rats began the study; they all had a choice of drinking water or a 10 percent ethanol alcohol solution in water. Thirty rats became moderate ethanol patrons in five weeks on a high carbohydrate diet. Researchers divided the 30 into three groups for a 16-week study. One group was fed the high carbohydrate diet already begun; one group received the same diet with mineral and vitamin supplements; the third group were given a balanced human diet.

Rats on the high carbohydrate diet alone drank about 49.5 ml. of ethanol per week (the equivalent of over one quart of 100 proof alcohol for a human). Rats on the supplemented carbohydrate diet drank about 16.8 ml. ethanol a week. The rats on the balanced diet drank only about 7.0 ml. of ethanol on the average.

It was noted that ⅕ of the rats didn't acquire a taste for alcohol in the first five weeks study. *But* the addition of sugar to the ethanol mixture made these rats the heaviest of all drinkers! How much did they consume? Up to 70 ml. per week! When one half of these rats received a balanced diet, their alcohol consumption immediately dropped.

The six-hour glucose tolerance test for sugar supports the theory that 70 to 90 percent of alcoholics have underlying hypoglycemia. A general diet program of high protein, moderate fat intake (balanced between saturated and unsaturated), and extremely low in simple or quickly and easily assimilated carbohydrates (sugar and starch) is the best means of curing the addition. Refined carbohydrates (white sugar and flour products) should be totally eliminated from the diet. Only moderate unrefined carbohydrates and low carbohydrate vegetables and fruits should be emphasized. This is the basic hypoglycemia-based diet. Niacin supplements and B-vitamin complex along with 4 grams of vitamin C per day are also recommended.

Dr. Roger J. Williams, University of Texas biochemist, says that at least 50 percent of the alcoholics would be helped by a hypoglycemia-base diet and vitamin-mineral supplements. He states:

"I know of scores of individuals who have made at least partial trials with tremendous success.

In some cases every testimony is that abolishment of appetite [for intoxicants] has been complete and lasting, something little short of miraculous....I have not the slightest hesitation in recommending to alcoholics and to those who may have the beginnings of an alcohol problem, that they try the nutritional approach."

The Mt. Sinai School of Medicine, The Bronx Veterans' Hospital and New York Medical College conducted research in which volunteers took a pint of 86 proof whiskey daily for four weeks. We find that the conclusions were that continued drinking of alcoholic beverages reduces sexuality to the point where some men become impotent. The scientific reasoning is that the alcohol stimulates the liver to drastically raise its destruction of the male sex hormone — testosterone — by producing up to five times the amount of the liver enzyme that breaks down this sex hormone.

Dr. Emanuel Rubin of Mt. Sinai said, "The findings go a long way in explaining the sexual problems of alcoholics. This effect is produced by alcohol in ANY form — whiskey, wine or beer. The total amount of alcohol is the only thing that counts."

Diet Is Linked to Alcohol and Drug Abuse

What is the most serious drug abuse problem in America? Alcoholism and problem drinking. We have some 10 million alcoholics and more than 26 million problem drinkers.

There are millions of tobacco addicts besides. The World Conference on Smoking and Health found that the drug effect of nicotine caused more deaths yearly than heroin.

Coffee, tea and cola drinks are universally "enjoyed" because they contain caffeine, known to stimulate the central nervous system. People who use them often are actually drug users.

Drugs are all mind-altering substances, many of them addictive narcotics. Their effect is in the influence over the central nervous system — the brain and spinal cord. This is the master control system of the entire body.

Many doctors and nutritionists associate highly seasoned, rich foods and meats, among other stimulating foods with the "need" or desire for stimulants and drugs. Many researchers say the problem drinker loves spicy and highly seasoned foods and meat. They further state that correct diet can change these cravings. Among the taboo foods are spices, hot sauces, pepper, mustard, vinegar, coffee, tea, meat and all highly seasoned foods.

Chapter 15

Expectancy, infancy and childhood

"A child should be educated 25 years before it is born."

Anticipating the New Baby

Often the news of expectancy is a surprise and unfortunately not always welcome. The mother must consider diet, personal habits, exercise, mental activity and spiritual philosophy. She should give considerable attention to mental, physical and spiritual health of the baby from the moment of conception. If she fails to properly prepare for the new arrival with positive and loving efforts, the infant will be poorly equipped for meeting the harsh outside world as a separate entity. The mother provides the foundation for the child's venture into life. At the time of birth she relinquishes forever her ability to shape many faculties of the new family member. Thus all care should be taken to ensure the best start in life before birth on the part of both parents and all family members.

A harmonious environment, free from any antagonisms or unhappiness is vital. Mental harmony in the home life is conducive to a healthy and happy mother and baby — before and after delivery. The child is marked through the senses the mother develops and keeps active before and after conception and birth. The senses we want highly developed in the infant can become dormant if the mother does not concentrate on them during pregnancy. The mother can transfer her philosophy and beliefs to her new offspring — be they positive or negative...So convey the higher principles in life to the child..the higher and lovelier aspects.

Mozart's mother took up music before conception. Napolean's mother followed her husband in the battlefield before he was born. In a similar manner genetic strains are developed and cultivated in animals. The equestrian species is a good example. The cutting horse or the race horse is bred for its respective career and often sold before foaling. The owners have confidence that they will become the champions they were bred to be. Dr. David Smith found in his research that more of the chronic alcoholic mothers he surveyed had normal babies. Most were stunted in growth with nervous disorders and lowered IQs. Pregnant mothers should avoid drugs, even aspirin, according to the FDA due to potential harm to the unborn babies and to the mother during delivery. Again, the baby can be affected by virtually everything the mother does.

While visiting New Zealand we watched a girl perform who was capable of making 35 turns standing on her head on bicycle bars. When we questioned her about the talent, she explained that both parents had been circus performers before her.

Inherent weaknesses can be diminished the moment we start to live correctly. They can be controlled and overcome. Even back "unto the fourth generation" it is said that we inherit the weaknesses of our mothers and fathers and other ancestors. Now is the time to start reversing the trend toward inbred weaknesses — genetic weaknesses. Start with your own body. Make the next generation better for our being here.

The Natural Childbirth Movement

There is a trend toward having children at home through natural methods once again. It is to our best interests to make an extensive study of the rediscovered technique. In 1975 over 3,000 children were born at home in California alone. In many cases the delivery under anesthetics, drugs, fast deliveries, forced labor, are destructive to the child physically and mentally. It is encouraging to see an increasing number of doctors enthusiastic about working with natural childbirth methods.

The modern "convenience" of medical science in helping children come into the world under such artificial and abnormal conditions is often detrimental to both mother and infant. At times, however, and for some individuals and their lifestyle, natural childbirth is not indicated or recommended. While natural childbirth is on the increase, births by Caesarian section also increased in the late 1970s, possible because of deteriorating physical condition on the part of many women. However, even with the best of health care women's bodies differ widely, and we cannot say how a women should give birth. Expectant mothers must decide for themselves. Yoga classes, yoga exercises and training, natural childbirth classes for the expectant parents are available and worth looking into. The child will mean more to the family and the family more to the new addition if the birth and preparation for it is a joint adventure.

To bring a new baby into the harsh world of bright lights, cold air, spanking, rough impersonal hands and harsh voices of strangers can be damaging during the first few moments of stark reality. Under proper and soothing conditions, warm colors, dim lights and soft music the infant's introduction to the world can be cushioned and inviting to its senses. The new parents who consider these things are nurturing a better soul relationship with their child.

Special Health Care During Pregnancy

The mother-to-be should get plenty of fresh, clean air, sunshine, exercise and mental stimulation during pregnancy, along with a good nutrition program. Exercise is very necessary during this time such as hiking, walking and swimming. Avoid strenuous exercise, however.

A few other things should be considered. From the time of conception the mother should avoid tight-fitting garments. Breathing exercises to increase lung capacity are essential. Do these in the fresh air and in sunshine often. It is critical that the expectant mother not be bored and idle. She must stay busy and happy, doing good things for the rest of the family and others. She should cultivate a beautiful spiritual philosophy for the health of herself and the new family member.

We recognize that the smoking is detrimental at any time—but especially so during pregnancy. The same goes for alcohol consumption. The smoking habit destroys Vitamin C and alcohol is an enemy of B-complex and other nutrients.

Sunbaths are important for the making of Vitamin D. Lack of it is known to cause rickets in babies and small children. The body of the expectant mother must have all necessary chemical reserves to give the child all it needs to begin life. The child is forced to rob from the mother's body if the elements are not supplied as needed. The mineral building blocks are crucial for the proper use of vitamins in the body. When sufficient calcium is not readily available to the growing fetus, calcium is drawn from the bones and teeth of the mother. There is an old saying: "A tooth for every child." This is not necessary if the reserves are there.

The expectant mother must use extra care in her nutritional program to assure the greatest amount of health for herself and the new baby. She needs special foods to take care of herself and prepare best for the new arrival. Begin the day with a natural fruit juice blended with an egg yolk. Include more raw vegetables and fruits in the diet. Make juices of these; have them in salads and blended drinks. For extra protein add more sunflower seeds, sesame seeds and almonds in the form of butters and drinks for easiest assimilation.

Have additional sodium, calcium, silicon and iron foods during pregnancy. The calcium level in the body should be especially high at this time to guard against calcium depletion in the mother. More greens are essential to the mother and child before birth for iron, calcium and other mineral elements. Add parsley, beet greens, turnip greens, spinach, kale, chard and comfrey leaves. Steam lightly, blend in drinks and add raw to salads.

Some of the cravings, if not abnormal, should be indulged moderately. Heavy starch foods should be quite limited; select only the unrefined starches and carbohydrates. (Of course refined carbohydrate products are taboo.) Meats should be limited to fish and occasional fowl. Some of the best proteins are eggs, unpasteurized cheeses (aged), raw milk and cultured milk products. Goat milk is preferred. Use nuts and seeds and a few dried legumes, though legumes are high in starch. The best starches are yellow cornmeal, brown rice, rye and millet. Baked potatoes and winter squashes are acceptable in moderation.

Raspberry leaves may be steeped and the tea used as a base for vegetable drinks for aiding in an easier birth. Raspberry leaves also contain many valuable vitamins that will help supply the body with nutrients for this all important period. A pint of raspberry tea can be included in the daily food regimen. To prepare the tea, cover a handful of leaves with boiling water; place a lid over this and allow to steep one hour or longer. Strain and use the tea alone or as a drink base.

Tender Loving Care of the New Arrival

New babies need exercise; roll them after the bath and take them out into the fresh air and sunshine (not during the noon period when rays are harshest). Give them gentle body massages after the daily bath until the skin turns pink. Handle them as little as possible at other times. Keep babies warm and comfortable, but not over-clothed and smothered.

Use a soft, natural bristle skin brush before the daily bath. This encourages good skin activity and healthy skin. A gentle stomach massage, using a kneading movement, can help in case of bowel congestion for better elimination. Massage the skin all over with a coarse towel following the daily bath. The skin is the third kidney and must eliminate many wastes daily. Use a pure vegetable soap or castile soap on the baby's skin; avoid oils and powders because they clog the skin and interfere with skin elimination.

If the infant's diet is suitable, there should be no difficulties with proper elimination. If there are occasional flare-ups of constipation or diarrhea, use an enema.

The Natural Food for Your Baby

Mother's milk contains the colostrum necessary to begin the infant's bowel movements by establishing a high ratio of "friendly bacteria" in the intestinal tract. Nature intended mothers to breast feed their young ones. If, however, there is not enough milk for the needs of the baby, the mother should add a generous amount of greens such as vegetable tops (beet and turnip greens), spinach, parsley and chlorophyll to her diet. The results will be a well adjusted and healthy growing child. A new baby needs the feel of closeness to the mother during feeding time. Never force the baby to eat if it is not hungry.

The mother's diet must be adequate in vitamin and mineral content for her milk to contain all the baby needs. Many are not stored in the body. Begin early to supplement vitamin C by fruit and vegetable juices so the milk will be nutritious; add a calcium supplement to the diet to be safe. Get a lot of sunshine for vitamin D in the body.

Mother's Milk and Chemical Residues

Needless worry to nursing mothers has been brought on by the DDT scare and the chemical fertilizer and pesticide controversies. The solution is to continue breast feeding, since no ill effects have been linked to breastfed babies. All commercial milk and milk formulas are possibly polluted. There are no findings that prove a baby is safer and healthier on formulas. Rather, the reverse may be the case. Doctors and scientists agree that mothers' milk is still the best food for new arrivals. A mother should avoid the use of hair tints and permanents, personal and household aerosols and sprays containing chemicals and chlorinated hydrocarbons. I believe that exposure to chemicals and even commercial formulas may be responsible for later diseases and poor health.

Why Is Breast Feeding Best?

Tiny babies must be fed often because their digestive system is undeveloped and small. Breast milk is the perfect temperature and quickly and readily available. The little one up to 12 or even 15 months of age should have all liquids at blood temperature — never lower or higher. Formulas are made from processed milk that has been altered by heat; it is no longer a perfectly whole and natural food for baby. Mother's milk is always raw, natural, pure, whole and fresh. Vitamins and minerals can't be duplicated as Nature made them as formulas and artificial additives. Mother's milk digests rapidly and much easier than formulas.

Infants who nurse don't get constipated as often as formula babies. Digestive upsets are less likely in the nursing child. Skin disorders are uncommon in the breastfed offspring. Respiratory infections such a pneumonia, colds and bronchial troubles are not likely in the nursed little people. It has been found that the sucking exercise of nursing helps develop stronger and wider jaws, more room for permanent teeth later. Nothing can duplicate the closeness and aura of love that binds the mother and baby through nursing. This encourages a happier and well-adjusted baby — physically and mentally — and helps the child grow up with a good mental outlook on life in general.

Studies have shown nursing mothers less likely to get breast cancer later in life. Spacing pregnancies is much easier for nursing mothers, according to a large study.

Mother's milk is three times higher in vitamin C than cow's milk. Studies show that the infant nursed for at least six months is healthier than the solid food or formula baby. Cow's milk is known to cause iron deficiency anemia since it is so low in iron. Many babies have allergic skin reactions and other allergy symptoms to cow's milk. Mother's milk is many times richer in milk sugar and galactose than cow's milk. Proper completion of the myelin nerve sheaths depends in part on galactose. An article in *Environment* magazine said that canned milk has a very high level of cadmium, tin and lead. Lead has been found to be a contributing cause to hyperactivity in children and cadmium is linked to high blood pressure and other disorders. The tin was not mentioned as harmful.

A Texas A & M University research scientist says that breast feeding may protect against heart disease in later life. Tests indicate that mother's milk — with its high cholesterol content — actually builds immunity to cholesterol deposits in veins and arteries.

A study of 383 grade school children found that those who had nursed walked and talked sooner than formula reared children.

According to V.G. Rocine, "Milk drinks require an alkaline stomach or they produce more trouble. Milk is acid-forming except as it comes warm, directly from the animal (or mother). By the Divine Law it should be sucked from the udder."

The Truth About Commercial Baby Foods

Babies thrived on food directly from the family table and made in the kitchen at home long before baby food became a multi-million dollar business. Adulteration is common in processed baby foods. They use a lot of water, refined sugar and salt, not to mention additives and preservatives such as MSG and sodium nitrate. Sugar is used liberally for the purpose of making the taste pleasing to adults. This early sugar exposure often leads to a sweet tooth, obesity, tooth decay and other sugar related disorders. Some $200 million worth of commercial baby food is sold each year. The advertising campaigns are elaborate and hard-hitting. It is in the baby foods and sugared formulas that the child is introduced to dangerous sugar addiction. Sugar upsets the calcium metabolism in the body and often leads to glandular imbalances. There is no reason to give babies either sugar or salt. Research has shown that infants can't taste salt until the age of three.

How Long Should the Child Nurse?

This depends a great deal on the health of the mother as well as the infant. If the mother's body becomes depleted of calcium and silicon, the condition can be irrepairable. Many a mother hasn't taken care of herself sufficiently to avoid serious depletion of biochemical reserves with each child. The child takes the best from the mother, for her own sake as well as the child's the mother must eat wisely and well. Generally, I believe a child whose mother is healthy can nurse 9-12 months.

Weaning With Goat Milk

Goat milk is the ideal food for weaning the child, being nearest to mother's milk in composition and properties. It is easy to digest and is weight building. Its fat globules are five times smaller than those found in cow's milk — making it much easier to digest. If cow's milk is used, it is necessary to remove some of the cream; goat milk is naturally homogenized.

WEANING OR SUPPLEMENTAL FORMULA

1 oz goat milk or certified raw milk
3 oz distilled water
1/2 oz pure cream
1 tsp sugar of milk

MENU SCHEDULE FOR WEANING

6 o'clock—Milk formula (above)
8 o'clock—Fruit or fruit juice
10 o'clock—Cereal and milk formula (above)
2 o'clock—Milk and steamed vegetables or pureed vegetables
4 o'clock—Broth or celery and parsley soup
6 o'clock—Cereal and milk formula (above)
8 o'clock—Fruit or fruit juice
10 o'clock—Milk or milk formula (above)

Distilled water may be used for the infant first and gradually begin to use less. Vary as weaning advances. After a couple of weeks, depending on the child and the reactions, use straight goat milk or raw milk (or milk substitutes). If goat milk can't be tolerated, try cow's milk (raw). Begin introducing other foods at this time. Include foods high in silicon, calcium, fluorine and iron, among others. Emphasize these minerals most. As we have said, it is best not to give the youngster meat until about age 7.

Supplemental Diet at Weaning Time

1. Orange juice (tree ripened only), with some pulp, diluted with distilled water.

2. Fresh tomato juice, grape, papaya, pineapple and apple juice.
3. Figs and prunes, raisins and dates — soaked for about 12 hours (revived) and then pureed or mashed. Also their juices.
4. Any fresh, uncooked fruit, pureed, mashed or cut into tiny pieces to introduce the child to the new taste and texture.
5. Any whole grain cereal, including brown rice, millet and yellow cornmeal that has been steamed in a double boiler over very low heat several hours or thermos cooked overnight. Cream whole grain cereals. Other good cereals are oatmeal, cream of rye and creamed whole barley.
6. Any fresh vegetables in season — steamed, mashed or cut into tiny pieces or pureed in a blender. It is best not to have more than two varieties at a sitting. Use very small quantities at first. Add broths made of carrots, parsley, etc.
7. Replace part of mother's milk with goat milk gradually to assure a natural and healthful break.
8. Do not flavor baby's food. The natural flavor of foods is adequate and healthier. If the child displays a dislike for a cereal, flavor with a little fruit juice concentrate, unheated honey or dried fruit. DO NOT USE SALT OR CONDIMENTS.

Further Suggestions for Weaning Time

At or near weaning time, the amount of goat or certified raw milk may be reduced by substituting soy milk powder mixed with water to for a consistency similar to milk. This may be used in weaning the baby. Try avocado and zapote in the milk or part coconut milk.

When the infant is well on the way to being weaned add rice water, barley gruel, soaked milk and berry juices (without seeds). Mash young tender carrots with goat milk, especially when the youngster is older and starts teething. Add fresh figs and soups made of carrots, parsley and celery. Add some juice of sweet fruits — fig and prune. Introduce raw vegetable juices, soft boiled eggs, tender omelets and souffles, spinach toast (stale bread), fish bone broth for bone development and teeth building, if not vegetarian.

After the First Birthday

Special care should be taken to start the one-year-old out right with sound nutrition to guard against future abnormal cravings and peverted tastes of unbalanced diets. Any food in the toddler's diet should be easily digested and dissolved, especially when they are learning to chew solid foods. Ripe and soft fruits, eggs, milk, some whole grain steamed cereals, baked apples, and bananas, cottage cheese, avocados, etc. are good first "adult" foods. Serve a variety of steamed vegetables and baked white and sweet potatoes. Mash vegetables well or puree in a blender at first. Use cream soups. Don't give them foods with tough cellulose fibers.

Serve the youngster simple meals with only a few kinds of food per meal. Avoid meat entirely until about age seven. They should be allowed NO refined starches and carbohydrates — especially white flour and white sugar. Breads made of baking powder and soda are not good for children (or adults for that matter). Serve stale whole grain toast occasionally for older children. Don't allow refined sweets. A few natural sweets such as dried fruits and honey can be allowed once in a while. No condiments — salt, pepper, vinegar, pickles, mustard and harsh spices or seasonings should be given to children.

Youngsters are extremely active and therfore must get plenty of rest. An afternoon nap is good for all children, and they should be in bed by sundown. Late hours and excessive T.V. viewing are as detrimental as "junk foods."

Raising Children Without Dental Braces

Cracker-like foods can be introduced at teething time to develop the jaws. The teeth need proper exercise. Many children have narrow jaws. The teeth need proper exercise. Many children have narrow jaws today and v-shaped dental arches. This is partly due to a lack of calcium in the mother's body. She didn't have sufficient calcium to properly finish the baby's body. Many times this is indicated in the "crooked" little finger and in other fingers not growing straight.

Wire tightening devices (braces) and straightening-out bands are necessary to straighten crooked teeth to try to compensate for the lack of jaw development. By chewing properly and adequately, the jaw structure can be developed fully.

In the case of my own ten-year old son, we gave him a carrot to chew and spit out before meals to try to prevent braces by straightening the teeth as they came in. (The carrot didn't spoil the appetite for regualr meals because he spit it out.) Over a period of months, the jaw developed and the teeth straightened. We didn't need to put braces on his teeth after all.

Children should not be allowed to select their own foods. A survey has shown that preschool children have a great deal of influence over what their mothers buy in the supermarket. On the average, children attempt to put something in the shopping cart every two minutes, and we find they are successful 45% of the time. The mother must select proper foods. The child may be allowed to choose, occasionally, from what she offers.

It would be interesting to know to what extent T.V. influences a child's recognition of and selection of particular products in a supermarket. Incidentally, 15 mothers particapated in a T.V. experiment, cutting their children's T.V.-viewing time to one hour per day for four weeks. Most children become calmer, more outgoing and performed better in school, quickly and painlessly adjusting to the T.V. "rationing."

Teaching Children To Eat the Right Foods

If the mother's attitude is positive and cheerful, the child responds favorably. This is particularly important at feeding times. Set good examples for children in all things. The old addage "Do as I say, not as I do" is not the way to manage children successfully.

Do not go to extremes with sweet foods, even fruits, when bringing up a child to eat right. They must be taught to eat the foods that are best for them. Their natural inclinations can't be trusted. The real diet trouble is with parents who don't start the child on the right foods. A mother complains that her children will not eat vegetables or certain "health" foods. That is only because they have never been allowed to get hungry enough to eat what is placed in front of them. Foods have often been used as bribery tactics; they were probably forced on the youngsters. If the child didn't eat what was on his or her plate, dessert was withheld. If the child is not taught to eat the right foods for the right reasons at a young age, parents will be raising a doctor bill! Start the child out right.

The memories of weaning and early food regimens have lasting effects into adulthood. Most of those who overeat have childhood memories associated with foods, possibly bribery to get them to eat certain foods. They were rewarded for eating certain foods "good for them" with desserts and sweets or candy. "Sympathy foods" is the term I prefer to use. When the grownup hasn't been treated well or things go wrong they turn to sympathy foods from childhood experiences to soften a wound or substitute for happy times.

It is the responsibility of the parents to know what foods are best for growing children. Start the child out right on natural foods from the vegetable kingdom and some fruits and their juices. Youngsters are naturally opposed to salty foods. It is generally the parents who salt their children's food and set the example by salting their own food excessively. Most Americans use 8 to 10 times more salt than their bodies need, and too much salt has been shown to lead to hypertension. The harm in sugar, not to mention cost in doctor bills, should be obvious.

Children seem to know when they should eat. Don't be afraid of fasting them for health reasons. Don't force food on a child if he or she does not feel up to eating. They should not be allowed excessive fruit in place of vegetables.

The habit of snacking between meals is harmful and should not be allowed unless the snacks are occasional and limited to fruits, fruit juices, vegetables or vegetable juices.

Greens, chlorophyll, blackberries and grapes (Concord) are high in iron. Fluorine is found highest in raw goat milk — it is destroyed in pasteurized milk. Calcium foods are milk, grains and seeds. Silicon is high in brown rice, whole grains (unpolished) and oat straw tea; also in rice polishings. Vegetables, especially greens, should be in the daily diet of the child since they are higher in minerals or cell salts. Fruits have more vitamins.

Mealtime should be a happy and relaxed time when the family gets together. Serve children foods similar to what the adults eat. Don't make a fuss about their eating. Avoid making threats, praises and giving them excessive attention. Don't try to hurry them, and assume the food will be eaten quietly, without a big production. Be an example to the child. Serve a variety of foods.

Natural Remedies for Diarrhea

Scraped apple is effective in cases of infant or toddler diarrhea. Scrape a fresh, peeled apple and give in small quantities.

V.G. Rocine suggested several aids for child diarrhea. "Homemade" rye meal bread, dipped in boiling water until soft or dipped in goat milk helps in some diarrhea conditions. Roast dry rice in oven until brown; then cook in boiling water until kernels crack. Pour off liquid and give two to three times a day for severe diarrhea.

Including Vegetables in School Lunches

My son, while in grade school, said the other children at school made fun of him because he took vegetables to school and had them in sandwiches. I explained that vegetables were important for carrying water in the intestinal tract since bread dries out alone. He went back to school and told his friends who had called him a rabbit at least he wasn't a constipated rabbit!

Expanding Your Baby's Diet Program

Milk is the most important food for the first few months of a new baby's life. Gradually introduce the following, in addition to mother's milk or goat milk. As weaning time advances, these foods and beverages can take the place of some of the milk. We find that certain cases make vegetable drinks useful and necessary at an earlier age. If an infant suffers from diarrhea or cannot tolerate his formula or shows other digestive upsets, the following vegetable "bottles" can be invaluable.

Use the blender often. It is especially good for baby and toddler food preparation.

CARROT BOTTLE
4 tsps. cooked (steamed) carrot
¼ cup juice from steamed carrots
¾ cup soy milk
2 Tbsps. steamed millet, ground fine

Liquefy for 2 minutes in blender; strain. Fill baby's bottle and heat to blood warm in top of double boiler.

SPINACH BOTTLE
3-4 spinach leaves
2 slices steamed carrot
¼ tsp. honey or yellow D sugar
1 cup soy milk

Dip spinach leaves in boiling water to wilt. Liquefy all ingredients for 2 minutes; strain. Fill bottle; warm.

TOMATO BOTTLE
1 small ripe tomato
1 cup goat milk or raw milk
2 Tbsps. steamed cereal
*   (millet, oatmeal or arrowroot, ground fine)*

Blend in liquefier 2 minutes. Strain; fill bottle. Warm.

CARROT MILK
1-½ cups goat or raw milk or milk substitue
¾ cup carrot juice (or less)
1 Tbsp. honey

Mix well; warm slightly.

APPLE BOTTLE
¼ apple, cut up and peeled
2 half-inch slices banana
½ tsp. honey or fruit concentrate
¾ cup goat or raw milk
2 Tbsps. coconut powder

Blend 2 minutes; strain; fill bottle; warm slightly.

Baby's Introductory Solids

BANANA SOUP
½ cup milk (goat or raw)
½ cup grape juice
½ banana
a little honey or fruit concentrate

Puree well in blender. Warm slightly if desired.

AVOCADO SOUP

½ cup milk (goat or coconut)
½ cup pineapple juice
½ avocado
a little honey or apple concentrate

Puree well in blender. Warm slightly if desired.

CARROT SOUP

¼ cup carrots chopped
¼ cup water
1 tsp. arrowroot
1 tsp. butter
½ cup warm milk

Steam carrots in water until tender. Thicken with arrowroot; remove from heat. Add remaining ingredients and puree in blender.

HOMEMADE TEETHING BISCUITS

1 egg, beaten
2 Tbsps. Yellow D or date sugar
2 Tbsps. blackstrap molasses
2 Tbsps. oil or water
1 tsp. vanilla
¾ cup oat flour (or rice flour)
1 Tbsp. soy flour
1 Tbsp. flaxseed meal
1-½ tbsps. whey powder

Blend egg, sugar, molasses, oil and vanilla; mix dry ingredients and add to liquid mixture. Roll out very thin on lightly floured board (⅛" to ¼"). Cut in baby-sized crackers or triangles. Bake at 350 deg F. on unoiled cookie sheet about 15 minutes or until crisp and golden. Remove and cool; store in tight-lidded container or in refrigerator.

Bananas Are Baby Pleasers

The banana is high in vitamins and minerals. It contains generous amounts of Vitamin A, some B-1 (thiamine), B-2 (riboflavin), B-6 (pyridoxine), vitamin C, potassium, phosphorus, calcium, iron and some niacin. A single banana has about 85 calories. It contains no saturated fatty acids; the small amount of fat it contains is unsturated. Bananas are easy to digest and assimilate. For the higher nutritional value use very ripe bananas, even dead ripe. Mix them with other fruits. Following are some suggestions. Berry juices or fruit concentrates, dates, figs, raisins, persimmons, pears, cherries, peaches, papayas, mangos, nectarines, avocados and plums. Use bananas in the toddler and older child's diet often.

Avocados Are Food For Baby

The avocado is an excellent fruit and a source of easily digested protein, though the protein is low. It has 11 essential vitamins and 17 minerals. Vitamin A is high (carotene); it contains iron, vitamin E, abundant potassium. It has a good supply of riboflavin, pyridoxine, thiamine, folic acid, pantothenic acid, niacin, choline and vitamin C. Half an avocado has a average of 132 calories; 19 calories per tablespoon. (And it has no cholesterol.) Other minerals found in the avocado are manganese, magnesium, sodium, calcium, phosphorus and copper, among others. Try the following ideas for baby for introductory solids. Mash and sweeten with a dab of honey or fruit concentrate. Mix with such fruits as bananas, apricot, scraped apples, prunes, dates, figs, pears, peaches, nectarines, applesauce, berries and raisins. (Revive dried fruit by soaking in boiling hot water, except dates).

Best Baby Vegetables

Use steamed vegetables such as asparagus, carrots, squash (summer and winter), zucchini, peas, green beans, cauliflower, greens, spinach, yams, baked white potatoes, beets, parsnips, turnips and broccoli.

Best Baby Fruits

Acceptable fruits are apricots, apples, peaches, nectarines, avocados, bananas (starch), tomatoes, pineapple, persimmons, grapes, berries (without seeds). Use some dried fruits, revived first except dates, such as figs, prunes, currants, raisins. Give berries to the older children and make sure seeds are strained off.

Best Baby Juices

Some of the good juices are tomato, vegetable juices, apple, grape, pineapple, raspberry and apricot or peach. Use juice concentrates also; and the juices of some dried fruits moderately.

Best Baby Sweeteners

Sweeteners should be kept to a minimum; use ony natural (no refined) sweeteners. Raw honey, blackstrap molasses, date and Yellow D sugars, maple sugar and syrup and fruit concentrates can be used occasionally. Use sweet and dried fruits as sweeteners at times. No white sugar or chocolate should be allowed — ever. For an occasional treat use carob flavoring in place of chocolate and cocoa.

Best Baby Grains and Cereals

Try a variety of grains (steamed or vacuum cooked) such as yellow cornmeal, rye, rice, oatmeal, millet, barley, buckwheat and soy. Cream these for younger folks.

Best Desserts for Bigger Babies

Don't make the mistake of launching the child on a sweet tooth habit early in life. It will be difficult to control from that time on. Make sure to start the baby on vegetables even before fruits. Use fresh fruits as desserts moderately. Puddings, custards and yogurt are all right once in awhile.

Best Baby Proteins

Use cheese (aged raw), cottage cheese, eggs, some nut and seed butters for older children. Leave out meat until about age seven.

Overview of Baby Diet

Be careful of food additives, chemicals and preservatives in most commercial baby foods. Read labels and learn to make most baby food in your own kitchen — from natural, pure and whole ingredients. Avoid prepared, processed, refined and sugared or salted foods.

Recipes For Little People

MASHED CARROTS
½ cup steamed carrot
1 Tbsp. goat milk or soy milk

Place in blender and puree until smooth. Serve slightly warm.

FRUIT FLAVORED YOGURT
¼ cup plain yogurt or thick clabbered milk
1 Tbsp. coconut or soy powder
¼ cup fresh fruit of choice

Place in blender and puree until smooth. Use such fruits as banana, avocado, peach, nectarine, pear, apricot, persimmon.

NUT MILK
½ cup goat or soy milk
1 Tbsp. raw nut butter
1 tsp. honey or molasses or maple syrup

Place in blender; liquefy at low speed a few seconds.

PUREED VEGETABLES

Place about ½ cup liquid in blender (water, milk, milk substitute, tomato juice, vegetable broth or stock or vegetable juice). Add steamed vegetables gradually through hole in lid with motor running at low speed.

PUREED FRUIT

Place sliced fruit in blender; whirl until smooth; add honey or fruit juice concentrate to sweeten (only if necessary) and a small amount of liquid if thinner consistency is desired.

FRESH APPLESAUCE
1 large sweet apple, cored and peeled
¼ cup apple or pineapple juice (unsweetened)
½ tsp. apple concentrate (optional)

Cut an apple. Place juice and concentrate in blender; add half the apple pieces; blend. Add remaining apple chunks and blend until smooth.

OATMEAL PORRIDGE
1/2 cup water
1/6 cup rolled oats
dash sea salt

Combine ingredients in saucepan with tight fitting lid or in top of double boiler over water; bring to simmer and continue to cook over very low heat until tender. Remove from heat and allow to stand covered for 5 minutes. Serve with a little fruit concentrate of pureed sweet fruit if necessary.

COTTAGE CHEESE PUREE

Blend ½ cup cottage cheese (raw preferred) with fruit such as pineapple, pear, peach, apricot, strawberries, blackberries, banana or avocado. (For younger children strain off seeds first.)
Blend ½ cup cottage cheese with pureed steamed vegetables such as carrots, peas, spinach, other greens, parsnips, broccoli, cabbage, asparagus, cauliflower, beets or squashes.

MILK SHAKES

1. Place 1 cup goat milk and 1 Tbsp. molasses in blender. Mix.
2. Place 1 cup goat milk and 1 Tbsp. carob powder in blender. Mix.
3. Place 1 cup raw milk and ½ cup revived dried fruit in blender. Puree.
4. Place 1 cup soy milk, ½ tsp. vanilla, 1 egg yolk and 1 tsp. fruit concentrate in blender; mix.

5. Place 1 cup coconut milk and ¼ cup avocado in blender; mix. Add honey if necessary.
6. Place 1 cup nut or seed milk and ½ cup steamed carrots in blender. Add date sugar or maple syrup for a treat. Mix.

FRUIT GELATIN
1 Tbsp. plain gelatin
¼ cup boiling water
1-¼ to 1-½ cup fruit juice or fruit puree

Dissolve gelatin in boiling water. Add fruit juice or fruit puree. Chill until set.

CREAM OF TOMATO SOUP

Place 1 part tomato puree in stainless steel saucepan; add ½ to 1 part milk. Warm only. Add dash of lemon juice or broth powder if baby is older.

POACHED EGG

Gently drop 1 egg into simmering water or milk or tomato juice. Cook just until white is set. Spoon water or milk over egg while cooking.

FRUIT-NUT BUTTER

Mix revived dried fruit or other fruit with raw nut or seed butter (unsalted) other than peanut butter. Use enough butter to flavor as desired.

RAW, WHOLE MILK: Certified raw milk is acceptable if goat milk is not available. Give them cottage cheese occasionally.

EGGS: Eggs should be in the daily diet. Poach, soft boil or coddle slightly.

MEAT: It is not necessary in the child diet. For protein use raw milk, eggs and some nuts and seeds (ground or butters). Meat may be added to the diet at age seven.

VEGETABLES: Steam or bake — never boil or use high heat or open utensils for preparing, give them plenty of raw salads and vegetables.

CEREALS: Serve as a starch once a day. Prepare by steaming in a double boiler or by thermos cooking; always use very low heat. Cereals may be creamed or pureed for smaller children. Use sweetening of cut-up sweet (revived) dried fruits occasionally. Use only the natural, unrefined cereals found in natural food stores.

SUGAR & SWEETENERS: Refined sugar should *never* be given to children. It leaches calcium, so important to growing bones and body tissues. Dental decay is attributed largely to refined and artificial sweets and white flour products. Use fruits and fruit concentrates or (revived) dried fruits for occasional treats. Allow honey, maple syrup and Yellow D sugar in very limited amounts.

BROTHS & SOUPS: Make them as natural as possible and avoid heavy, cream or thickened soups using milk, cream or starch thickeners. Vital broth is good for children and barley and green kale soup — for growing bodies.

BREAD: Stale bread and dry toast are best (if bread is allowed occasionally). Encourage children to learn to chew well and thoroughly by giving them hard foods. Most bread does not encourage proper chewing.

RICH DESSERTS: Never allow children to have rich and heavy dessert. For occasional desserts allow natural sweet fruits or (revived) dried fruits.

VEGETABLE & FRUIT JUICES: For occasional snacks between meals these may be given.

APPETITE CONTROL: The appetite of children comes naturally. Never bribe, coax, force, punish or threaten to make them eat.

HERBAL TEAS: Oat straw tea is excellent for children since it is high in silicon. Use other herb teas as health drinks for children.

SALADS: Try adding raisins, chopped dates and ground nuts or seeds to salads to make them more appetizing and appealing. Serve a salad as the first course and wait for it to be eaten before bringing additional foods. Make gelatin salads with fresh fruit and fruit juices. Combine salads with flavorings of carob, fruit concentrates and a little honey. Make cottage cheese salads with nut butters, fruit concentrates, shredded vegetables or cut up fruits.

OTHER FOODS: The growing child needs a generous amount of calcium, calcium control (Vitamin D), iodine, iron and silicon, as well as other minerals and vitamins. For meal suggestions V.G. Rocine mentioned the following: Chicken bone broth with whole (brown) rice, parsley and steamed cabbage is a good meal for the growing child. Halibut bone broth and goat buttermilk are also good foods. Try pineapple gelatin with goat cream, whole rice muffins, creamed carrots with Russian rye bread, creamed cabbage with whole wheat bred, goat milk with whole grain cereals (creamed for younger children), whole rice pudding with fruit sauces, steamed spinach on soy bread, rye bread with a glass of goat milk, goat cottage cheese with corn meal muffins or ripe olives and fruit salad make good combinations.

Chapter 16

Renewed youth for the geriatric

"A long life lived is not always good enough; but a good life lived is always long enough."

We find it frequently said that life expectancy is longer today on the average than ever before in history. However, the advocates of this popular misconception don't see a need for nutritional reforms and don't consider the state of world health standards. Health in the civilized countries is declining in ratio to the increased use of refined and chemical laden foods. Present statistics are deceiving because life spans have increased largely due to reduced infant mortality, reduction in epidemics and infectious diseases and scientific medical advances in surgery.

The Social Security Administration in a recent year announced that 8,300 Americans were over 100 years of age, receiving Social Security benefits. Doubtless, there are more, living on their own means. Women in the US live an average of 75.3 years and men 67.6 years, an increase of 27 years for women and 21 years for men since 1900. Women have more illness, take more medications and have more operations, but they live longer than men because they are more likely to take action than men when they get sick, the experts say. We find that infant mortality rates per 100,000 births have dropped from 728 in the early part of this century to 15 in recent years. Medical advances can keep more people alive for more years, but the quality of health and the level of chronic disease has become almost a scandal.

In short, more grow older but life expectancies for the individual is little changed. The 50-year-old person in the mid-1800s could expect to live 20 years more and in the mid-1900s only 22.5 years longer. The real point we want to bring out is that we have gotten to the place where we live slightly longer, but life is often miserable, filled with suffering, degenerative diseases, inactivity and lack of productivity. This is no way to exist. So many of the elderly are so broken down and pained that they would rather not survive at all.

It is said that one million two hundred thousand elderly people are in rest homes and half of them suffer from senility. They make up one fourth of the suicides and fill one third of the hospital beds. In 1976 they made up 10 percent of the U.S. population and they are expected to make up 17 percent by 2015. Two-thirds of the Federal Health funds have to go to their care. The National Institute on Aging was formed in 1974 to study the problems of aging. But very little attention is paid to the research involving nutrition and better health for the aging, let alone increasing their life span. Studies on vitamin E, C, calcium, sodium, silicon, selenium and RNA effects on aging are mostly ignored.

Senility and Alzheimer's disease have both been associated with high serum cholesterol, high triglycerides, clogging of the fine blood vessels of the brain and the extremities and poor circulation. The high cholesterol levels are said to be related to deficiencies in vitamin B-6, magnesium and lecithin as well as to excessive intake of hydrogenated fats and foods fried in hot fat. RNA, considered an anti-aging factor by some experts, is highest in sardines — 2 times higher than other fish, 100 times higher than tuna, 10 times higher than lamb or beef. High RNA foods include asparagus, mushrooms, lentils, pinto beans, nuts, wheat germ, bran, chicken liver, beef liver and the dark meat in poultry. An 8 oz. can of sardines has 5 times as much niacin as a bran muffin, more calcium than a pint of milk and as much iron as an 8 oz. serving of spinach.

Although we use a great deal of animal proteins in the U.S., the kind of preparation, the amount eaten and the condition of what is eaten leave much to be desired. In the U.S. 40% of the diet is protein; in Africa 11%, Near East 9% and Far East 5%. Different types of deficiencies and imbalances plague each part of the world. When we eat cheese, considered an excellent protein, we don't realize it is not a whole food because the whey has been removed. Whey is rich in biochemical sodium, vitamins, lactose and amino acids while low in fat. We can eat whey with cheese to get more of the food value from it. Senility, I believe, is related very closely to poor eating habits over many years.

Aging, to a great extent, is still a mystery to science. Most of the cells of the body are replaced in time. Why aren't they replaced perfectly, year after year? Part of the answer lies in nutrition. Dr. Alexis Carrel kept a chicken heart alive for over 20 years by feeding it fresh egg yolk. The tissue of the heart, to all appearances, renewed itself perfectly, but finally died when students forgot to feed it for two days. It has been claimed that the key to aging lies in the DNA and RNA of the cells. ATP (adenosine triphosphate) can be interfered with, disrupting the energy-production cycle which gives life to cells.

Raw Milk Drinking and Longevity

One of the strongest arguments in favor of milk (raw of course) is in the fact that centenarians and people famous for long lives have lived largely on it. We find that goat milk is a part of the daily food plan for many of the old people of the world — often in the form of clabbered milk and whey from cheese-making. Due in part the development among adults of lactose intolerance and the prevalant use of pasteurized milk, it is, in general, in disfavor with many dietitians. Lactose intolerance comes with prolonged disuse of milk in favor of the stimulating and toxic beverages so common today — colas, soda pop, coffee, tea and alcoholic drinks. Renin, that causes milk to curdle, stops flowing in the stomach. Milk guards health and youthful joints — especially goat milk that is high in the youth element (sodium). Milk should be taken raw and goat milk is the top choice.

We find the following records of milk and longevity: Margaret Patton, of London, England, lived to be 137 and enjoyed good health to within a few days of her passing away. For many years, the records vouch, she depended on milk.

Thomas Parr, an Englishman, lived to 152 years of age, and used milk and its products profusely in his diet. As the story goes, he died within one week after being summoned to the King's court where he was wined and dined to death — ironically, in honor of his unusual and dignified age.

Jonathan Hartop, also English, of Yorkshire, lived to be 138. It is said that at 136 he walked nine miles to a Christmas party; he ate very little and his only beverage was raw milk. Peter Czartin lived to 184 in Austria. He is said to have fasted regularly as a religious observance and his diet was milk and Hungarian dark bread.

Raw milk, especially goat milk, and specifically in the form of clabbered milk, has been in the diet of many of the oldest people I have visited around the world, in search of the secrets of longevity.

Many Factors Affect Life Spans

The average life span for Americans is 72.5 years, according to the latest research figures. Women outlive men up to about seven years. We find many factors influencing the general life expectancy in the U.S. Our fast-paced and highly stressful lives take their toll as do the physical abuses of the body. Our minds can cause severe aging symptoms if they are not controlled and well-adjusted to our lifestyles and adapted to the pressures we face daily. We have listed the most important influences on the number of years you may expect to survive.

INHERITANCE: If your family is known for living past age 70 you have a good chance of living longer too. For each five years your parents lived beyond 70 add a single year to your life expectancy.

GEOGRAPHIC AREA: We know that pollution and stress in cities is extremely high. Studies show that city people die four years sooner than those in small towns or in the country.

AFFLUENCE: The middle class seems little affected by money matters. But we find that the very poor and the wealthy lose three years from their life on the average.

EXERCISE: Three years may be added if you take moderate exercise, on a regular basis. For vigorous fitness programs five years may be added.

WEIGHT: For the over 40 age group, subtract a year for each five pounds above the normal weight. Measure waist and chest and take off two years for each inch your waist measures larger than your chest.

INTOXICANTS: If you are a heavy drinker, knock off 10 years!

SMOKING: Those who smoke a pack-a-day lose three years. For a pack and a half subtract five years. Over a pack and a half a day costs you 10 years! Pipe and cigar smokers shorten their life two years.

MARRIAGE: Married people outlive singles by five years. Take off a year for each ten years of single adult life.

MENTAL ATTITUDES: The calm, easy-going person adds five years. But the nervous, high-strung, emotional person has to give up one to five years.

REGULAR HEALTH CHECKUPS: Research has found that they extend your life three years.

Sound Nutrition for the Geriatric

Old age is so often accompanied by senility, loss of memory, failure to recognize people, arthritis, asthma, osteoporosis. . . The list goes on and on. What we find with this list is malnutrition and often a neglected program of exercise.

Osteoporosis is loss of calcium from the bones, or rarification. It is due to lack of calcium in the blood stream and in the diet. Calcium becomes more difficult to assimilate with age — especially because the flow of hydrochloric acid (HCL) is greatly reduced in many cases. Many substances are also known enemies of calcium in the body. White sugar, cola drinks, white flour and refined cereal products are the main antagonists. The less the flow of HCL, the harder it is to digest and assimilate calcium. Much of it passes out of the body.

Many older people try to save on the food bill without knowing the value of sound nutrition. This is unfortunate because many are laid up in hospitals and in rest homes with broken unhealthy bones that take many months to mend, while arthritis, blindness and senility are blamed on just "old age" when poor nutrition is the basis of much suffering and diseases. It would seem that the addition of supplements such as calcium, sodium, phosphorus, vitamin D (that works so closely with calcium), vitamins C, A, B-Complex, lecithin and a good diet could prevent some of the premature aging and heart-breaking suffering of the "aged." Many of the ailments can be linked to a calcium deficiency or calcium out of solution due to a shortage of sodium in the body. A few supplements — vitamins or minerals — can't be the magic answer, however. We must look to Nature and natural living. Wholistic health is a vast subject with no magic formulas.

The crusading nutrition authority, Dr. Roger J. Williams, Professor of biochemistry at the University of Texas, believes that the illnesses and diseases of old age and aging could be slowed down greatly and in many cases completely avoided by proper nutrition. We agree. Dr. Williams expressed his views in an article in *Geriatric Focus* magazine as follows:

"Enumerating various changes characteristic of aging [impaired vision, hearing, memory, strength and endurance; insomnia; loss of libido and appetite for food; aches and pains; increased tendency toward constipation, arthritis, diabetes, arteriosclerosis, osteoporosis, senility, etc.], he said: "I want to call attention to the idea that every one of the cells and tissues somewhere in the body have to perform their functions properly; and also that every one of these failures is related to cell and tissue nutrition...

"Without concerning ourselves with the problem of whether there is an irreversible aging process in all cells that cannot be overcome, we can state with assurance that the longer cells are furnished with the necessities of life, including good nutrition, the longer they will continue to remain in good working order."

Zinc and Rheumatoid Arthritis

Recent research suggests that zinc is deficient in the blood of rheumatoid-arthritis sufferers. Dr. Peter S. Simkin ran a test in which he gave 24 patients zinc sulfate, 220 milligrams three times a day or a placebo, a look-alike capsule with no value. It was noted that the patients receiving the zinc sulfate had improvements in symptoms of joint swelling, walking time and morning stiffness.

Over 60 Diets Often Lack Zinc

At Purdue University many Americans over 60 have been found to lack zinc in their diets. The study showed 59 percent of the test group of people to be taking less than the recommended daily allowance of zinc. Symptoms of a shortage of zinc included a diminishing sense of taste and wounds healing poorly and slowly, according to Dr. Janet L. Gregor, Assistant Professor of Foods and Nutrition who conducted the study.

Charlie Smith, Sardines and Crackers

Several years ago I went down to see the oldest man in America, Charlie Smith, in Barstow, Florida who passed away a couple of years ago. He was 134 and has lived mostly on sardines and soda crackers for about the last thirty or forty years! I couldn't believe the man could live so long on that diet. But, as I thought more about it, I realized that that's probably a more healthy diet than many of us are on. Sardines could be called a *whole* food. He was getting the bones, the scales, the fins; he was getting everything that could build every part of the body. And there's a possibility that he was getting nutrients he could digest easier at his age. It's possible that he had something that we have yet to find out.

Dr. Benjamin S. Frank discovered the RNA factor in sardines that retards the aging process. Yeast is considered a good RNA source. But we find sardines [small ones] have about ten times the RNA of yeast.

Charlie Smith attributed his long life to "enjoying your income while you live because you can't take it with you when you die." And he said his favorite hobby was talking. He was born in Liberia, Africa in 1842, kidnapped by slave traders at the age of 12 and then sold at a slave auction in New Orleans to a Texas rancher.

"The cell is immortal. It is merely the fluid in which it floats which degenerates. Renew this fluid at intervals, give the cell something upon which to feed and as far as we know, the pulsation of life may go on forever."
—*Alexis Carrel*

149

Los Angeles Herald-Examiner,
Thurs., May 13, 1976

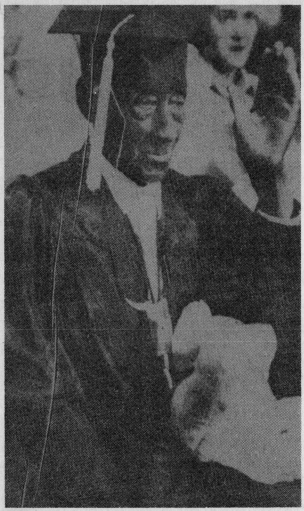

With his Winnie the Pooh bear in tow, Charlie Smith waits to receive diploma in Florida.

133 Years Old
Former Slave Receives Diploma

BARSTOW, Fla. (AP) — Charlie Smith, a former slave who signs his name with an X, received an honorary high school diploma Wednesday for a storehouse of knowledge no one can match.

The honor was bestowed for his years of experience — all 133 of them. Smith, considered by Social Security Administration to be the oldest person living in the United States, also received a telegram from President Ford.

Smith carried his Winnie the Pooh bear, a black purse and his attache case to ceremonies at the Polk County School Board.

"It takes a lot of coaxing to get him to put those things down, even in his room." explained a nurse from the convalescent center where Smith now lives.

"My warmest congratulations to you as you receive this honorary high school diploma from the Polk County school system." Ford's telegram said. "This recognition reflects the affection and respect in which you are held by your fellow Floridians and it symbolizes this nation's continuing dedication and concern for its older citizens. I hope that this will be an especially happy occasion for you."

Smith, in traditional cap and gown with beige hush puppies visible beneath the robe, sat proudly in the front row of the auditorium.

"This won't get you into college." school superintendent Homer Addair quipped as he presented the diploma, which read:

"This certifies that Charlie Smith, through the experience gained in his 133 years, has acquired a vast store of knowledge which qualifies him for his honorary high school diploma."

Born in Liberia, Africa in 1842, Smith was kidnaped by slave traders when he was 12 and sold at auction in New Orleans to a Texas rancher who gave him his name and a birthday of July 4.

He says his favorite hobby is talking, and his secret for a long and happy life: "Enjoy your income when you live because you can't take it with you when you die."

Memories of a Century Plus a Decade

In the Las Vegas Indian Colony home lives a woman 110 years young. She was born in January, 1867 when there was no water, air or food pollution, no jets, Am-Trak trains, nor modern technology complete with nuclear energy and atomic bombs. Stella Smith was married and never bore children but took care of the children of many others. During her school days she learned basket weaving and how to read and write. She recalls fond memories of a life filled with laughter, many friends and enjoyable though hard work. She retains her faculties and a good memory of bygone days and people who shared her past. But she says they have all passed away and everything has passed away. She is alone with her three dogs now.

Stella has gotten to the place where she walks less, but enjoys the hot sunshine and still has youthful joints that allow her to cook and weave baskets. She notes that Indians are hard workers. She has two boarders she cooks for; the meals are simple: beans, hot bread, tortillas, potatoes, gravy. She still uses her own remedies though she won't tell their ingredients, and she says she has never been very sick. But she doesn't dwell on death either. Her days begin at sun-up with cleaning her small house, making beads and baskets or sewing.

The simple, dignified and proud lady doesn't really know why she has lived so long. But she gives a few hints. She doesn't drink alcoholic beverages and has never smoked. She has always liked people and gotten along well with them—talked to them and made them laugh. She values her freedom and shrewdly judges people though she loves them.

Is Shangri-La in Ecuador??

Writer Grace Halsell put out a book called *Los Viejos* about the unbelievable villagers of isolated Vilcabamba, Ecuador. Los viejos means oldsters in Spanish. Nine members of the villiage of 1,000 are over 100 years of age. In other statistics of this quaint village it is said that in 1972 the population was 819 with seven men and two women over 100. This is remarkable compared to the U.S. with fewer than 9,000 centenarians in over 200 million people!

Vilcabamba is in what is called the sacred valley and is located about 260 miles below the Equator. It is peacefully untouched by the pressures and technology of civilization. They never heard of pollution. The air, water and food supply are clean and pure. The climate is mild, even and warm — allowing them to spend much time in the open outdoors working close to the land. They keep active though their lives are serene and peaceful like the quiet valley. They accept what life brings them day by day and keep a positive outlook — giving and receiving love generously. They love life and yet have no fears of death. Life there is always calm.

Teams of researchers, doctors and scientists have gone to study this remarkable "lost world." They have found the people free from arteriosclerosis and circulation problems, with no heart disease in present or past generations. The "Los Viejos" don't need doctors, dentists and hospitals. They treat their own ailments with herbs and fasting. Broken bones are a rarity. This calcium-type people have strong, heavy bones. They are as strong and unyielding as the ground they till.

Natural foods are a key to their longevity and wonderful health. They have no refined cereals, flour, grains or white sugar products. Their food consists of only natural, pure and whole foods — corn, wheat, barley and oats for cereals. Fresh vegetables include leaf lettuce, carrots and other root vegetables such as turnips, potatoes, yucca and sweet potatoes; beans are a staple. Other foods they depend on are eggs (a few), cottage cheese, clabbered milk, some yogurt, bland white cheese (aged), nuts and seeds. They make a soup from animal bones that is high in calcium and sodium. Sweets consist of papayas, mangos, bananas, figs, pineapple, watermelons and oranges. For sweetening agents they have occasional treats with a brown sugar called panela and molasses — both containing iron and zinc. They eat very little meat.

They don't have grocery stores or refrigerators and almost never use canned foods, refined foods or processed products.

These earthy people are thin because they work vigorously and avoid overeating. The average American diet is 3,300 calories a day, while the Los Viejos consume about 1,200 daily. Their diet is low in protein and fats; carbohydrates are strictly the complex unrefined kind. They walk everywhere and get much exercise in the fields.

The sparkling river running through the valley gives a feeling of rejuvenation with one bathing. Whatever the secret of their fountain of youth, we could take a few lessons from their way of life free from stress and degenerative diseases.

Survival Tips from Around the World

Thirty-four keys to longevity are presented in my book *World Keys to Health and Long Life*. I traveled the globe in search of keys to keeping well, happy, productive, active and long lived. Definite laws of Nature must be observed for long and healthy lives full of meaning and reward. I found that three principles — knowledge, wisdom and guidance — were a vital part of man's existence.

The Tapestry of Success.
Accomplishments are not everything in life, and most of the long-lived people had little or no schooling. What they accomplished was in the realm of Nature — according to her laws. Their greatest education came from Nature through natural food, pure air and water, sunshine and tranquility.

Soil Is the Giver of Life
There were no old men living on brown soil, dust bowls or where trees and vegetation were sparse. All the old people lived on the rich, black soil with the elements for man's proper nutrition. It is said that 85 years ago the topsoil in the U.S. was some 80 inches deep. Today it is about 8 inches or less. Yet life depends on rich and abundant topsoil.

Civilization's Major Disease
Doctors deal with people daily who lack minerals — chemical elements and cell salts — and vitamins. These people suffer from a man-made malnutrition — a deficiency dis-ease. Dr. D.W. Cavanaugh of Cornell University has said, "There is only one major disease, and that is MALNUTRITION. All ailments and afflictions to which we may fall heir are directly traceable to this major disease." Body tissues break down through everyday use

and must be replaced and rebuilt. The body reaches out for the elements it needs — that must come from the "dust of the earth." If that dust is deficient then the bodies built from the food that grown in it will be malnourished and deficient. An unbalanced soil can't produce healthy and balanced plants, animals or humans.

Temperance: The Greatest Key

One of the greatest long life keys is that the old people ate very little. They had small meals and many had only a single meal each day. Many drank liquids at one time of day and had solid food at another. The older the people became, the less they ate. These wise people didn't overtax their digestive systems. We found they rarely smoked, used almost no alcoholic beverages and had very little meat in their diets. Most had been married and enjoyed their families.

Calcium Builds Strong Bodies

The families of the old people had lived in the same regioins for centuries. Their bodies had molded to the climate and conditions where they resided. The body contains more calcium than any other element, and strong inheritances are built with calcium. They had excellent genetic backgrounds and calcium helps promote these.

A Natural Foods Foundation

All the oldest people of the world lived on natural foods — berries, seeds, sprouts, greens from the field. They build good health on natural, pure and whole foods. These unbelievable people lived where grapes grow. Cabbage is used often as a sulphur food for body heat during cold winters. Their diets were high in sodium, the youth element, found highest in whey, the by-product of cheese making. Goat or sheep milk was used in place of cow's milk; it is much higher in fluorine for strong hard bones and teeth and for resisting infections. Herbs of the fields such as comfrey, garlic, rose hips and chammomile prevented or relieved most of their small ailments. Few vegetarians were among the oldest men of the world. But we found that those who ate meat had it only two to three times a week. Protein sources were generally apricot kernals, walnuts, almonds, sunflower and sesame seeds and clabbered milk.

Exercise for Good Circulation

The old people were active — bending, stretching, reachings, lifting, pulling, pushing — to promote good circulation. Too many of us lead a sedentary life — sitting and working in stuffy offices with artificial light or driving automobiles. The blood must be active for a long life. The men lived the longest lives, probably because they continued working in the fields in the sunshine and fresh air long after the women began to stay at home, sitting more and exercising less.

The Old People Were Lean

We found that the centenarians weigh about the same as at age 20. Obesity is recognized as the number one killer in America — surpassing deaths attributed to cancer, heart diseases, diabetes and alcoholism. Science is finding that it is a disease in itself.

A Golden Rule for Longevity

The last old man I visited in my worldwide search was in Baku, Russia. He traveled down from the highlands on horseback. I inquired if he had ever been sick. He had never taken a pill or a drink of alcohol. He was mystified as to what a diet was. To my question of what rules he followed to reach the age of 153 he replied, "I didn't know I was going to live so long, so I don't have any rules."

We can all take a lesson from these words of wisdom. We should know what the natural life is and live it. We are under rules today; we are numbers; we must walk on the right side of all the traffic. We live in rooms of artificial sunlight. We engage in many other activities of a destructive nature. The goal is to return to Nature — where good health reigns. Her rules are actually less binding and strict than the doctrines of civilized society.

Man Cannot Live by Bread Alone

Dr. Stephen Smith (1823-1922), born in Onondaga County, New York, was a sickly child, unable to retain his food and was placed on an exclusive diet of bread and milk. For the first 70 years of his life he took no other food. When he passed his three-score and ten, he allowed himself a little wine with this diet. He was a surgeon in Bellevue Hospital, New York, for a full 60 years and was long the oldest and most distinguished doctor in the country. He contributed a great deal to the establishment of a board of health in the city, state and nation. He lived to the age of 99-1/2 years.

Chapter 17

Are we conquering degenerative diseases?

"60% of the cancer in women and 40% in men is attributed to diet."

The Focus of Vested Medical Interests

The vested interest of the medical profession is in disease, not health and preventive medicine. Less than 3% of the doctors in the U.S. practice preventive medicine. The principal studies of medical researchers and scientists are concentrated on disease. It was stated recently: "Cancer is the most profitable disease members of the American Medical Association have." In a recent year, statistics showed 14,000 deaths from stomach cancer and 81,000 from lung cancer. It is calculated that the average cancer case is worth about $7,800. This is a reflection of our amazingly short-sighted concept of paying people to cure, rather than to prevent sickness and diseases — especially the chronic and degenerative afflictions.

Doctors must make a living, too. Under the present health system, doctors forced to prevent disease and keep people healthy would go bankrupt in most instances. They would put themselves out of business. It is said that 56% of America's M.D.'s make $50,000 a year or more; 18% make at least $80,000 annually. Are they making it from your diseases??

The World Health Organization (WHO) reports that most countries' health services are not in keeping with the population growth in quality or quantity. They warn that a major crisis is near. There are over 1,000 institutions that train doctors. "Most of the world's medical schools prepare doctors, not to care for the health of the people, but instead for medical practice that is blind to anything but disease and the technology for dealing with it; a technology involving astronomical and ever increasing prices; they prepare doctors for cure rather than for care...(doctors are) trained predominantly to look at episodes of diseases, paying little or no heed to the whole man, and to his interaction with society."

A famous surgeon of London, Sir Arbuthnut Lane, had this to say in an address to the American College of Surgery in Chicago: "Our hospitals are crowded with sufferers from tuberculosis, rheumatism, arthritis, and gastro-intestinal diseases, due to wrong feeding, impure food and air, and lack of hygienic knowledge. There is convincing evidence that if men will eat natural foods, adopt right habits and take sufficient exercise, the diseases of civilization will be kept at bay."

For example, the Addiction Research Foundation of Canada predicted a rise of 72% in alcohol consumption over the period 1972 to 1984, indicating that cirrhosis of the liver may become the fastest rising disease in Western Civilization and perhaps the third leading cause of death among men 25 to 64 years of age. On the hopeful side, a recent study of 3,000 men by Dr. Kenneth H. Cooper of the Institute for Aerobic Research in Dallas, Texas, showed that the risk of heart attack was significantly lowered by regular exercise over a 3-year period. After regular exercise they had lower cholesterol, triglycerides, glucose, uric acid, blood pressure and body weight — the six major risk factors in heart disease. The men had taken up swimming, jogging, biking and other exercises.

Senate Approves Millions for Conquest of Cancer

WASHINGTON (UPI) — The Senate Wednesday approved President Nixon's call to make the final conquest of cancer a prime national goal, beginning with $332.2 million this year to search for its causes and cures.

Sent to the House on a 79-1 vote was legislation to create a semi-autonomous Conquest of Cancer Agency within the National Institutes of Health (NIH) responsible for seeking an end to the dread diseases.

Backers predicted the new assault could lead to the "final breakthrough" against cancer — but warned it will take some time.

"It is extremely important that the bill not create unrealistic expectations of quick success," said Sen. Peter H. Dominick, R-Colo., the measure's floor manager.

"Cancer is in reality many complex diseases, none of which is yet well understood. There have been several important breakthroughs recently, but more are necessary, and they cannot be forced. There is simply no basis for predicting with any certainty when they will come."

But Dominick and others stressed that the new emphasis on conquering cancer and sharply increased funding should provide researchers the impetus needed to make the final breakthrough possible.

The bill was a compromise between Nixon's proposal to establish a cancer-cure program within NIH and others to create a completely independent cancer agency.

As approved by the Senate, the Cancer Conquest agency will be independent within NIH, with its director reporting directly to the President and seeking its budget separately from other health units.

Sens. Gaylord Nelson, D.-Wis., and Alan Cranston, D-Calif., strenuously opposed this organizational structure on the grounds it would erode other NIH efforts and prompt those searching for cures to other diseases — such as heart ailments and arthritis — to seek similar independent status.

But Sens. Edward M. Kennedy, D.-Mass., and Jacob K. Javits, R-N.Y., sponsors of the alternative approach for a completely independent agency, enthusiastically endorsed the compromise.

The current National Cancer Institute would become the nucleus of the new Cancer Conquest agency and the current National Cancer Advisory Council would be replaced with a 19-member board of scientists and laymen to advise it.

Including the $100 million extra for cancer research approved by Congress earlier this year, the agency would have $333.2 million to begin operations, with appropriations increasing yearly.

Perhpas we are looking into the wrong places for the answer to the dread disease of cancer. Dr. Frank Rauscher, Jr., director of the National Cancer Institute had the following to say in a Washington report. "...The vast majority of cancer cases are caused by the way Americans live... 60 to 80 percent of cancers are caused by something we eat, we drink, we smoke — the way we live." If more of the dollars were spent in teaching people how to live to avoid cancer and other degenerative diseases the U.S. could be a much healthier nation as a whole and much less money could be spent on building institutions to match our health — hospitals, clinics and mental institutions. Why can't we live so that we don't have so much disease and suffering?

60% Cancer in Women Linked to Diet

Cancer researchers informed a recent Senate House Sub-Committee that 60% of all cancers in women and 40% in men are linked to diet. This included cancer of the breast, liver, prostate, kidney, stomach, colon and rectum. According to the testimonies, U.S. citizens eat too much — especially fats, salts, sugar and cholesterol. At the hearing doctors claimed that *too much* attention has been paid to cancer from chemicals, food additives and smoking and *too little* attention to dietary factors. Experts gave the advice that Americans should eat less, have meals with variety, including more fresh fruits and vegetables and whole grain cereals. Such diets would help *prevent* cancer, they said.

Possible Dietary Causes of Cancer

It was Lucile Steel in *Food Science — Nature's Supreme Healing Art* who gave the following common causes of cancer through wrong diets.

1. Pastries, sweets and excess starches.
2. Pickles, vinegar, spices and condiments.
3. Eating foods too hot or iced cold.
4. Eating too much and too often.
5. Laxative dosing, irritation therefrom.
6. Eating a preponderance of dead or devitalized foods.
7. Polluting the blood stream with vaccines and serums, which are degenerated animal infection.

Disease Doesn't Suddenly Strike

With more independent studies and reports linking cancer and other degenerative diseases to faulty diets, why isn't the public enlightened? No one has come forward to give any relief to the cancer victim on valuable insights into its prevention for the future. We wait until we have the condition diagnosed and then wonder what hit us so suddenly. We build these maladies over a period of 18, 20, 25, 30 years. It takes many years to build any chronic, degenerative disease. It came from what we began to eat, sometimes when still children.

Are We Winning the Cancer War??

Cancer takes the lives of 350,000 each year in the U.S. alone. Dr. Dean Burk testified for the NCI (National Cancer Institute) that 90 to 95% of the time in extending the life of cancer victims by even 5 years, conventional cancer therapies are failing. He gave these statements before the U.S. Superior Court. He termed government drug agencies and the American Cancer Society "self-perpetuating bureaucracies" which refused to admit that their vast knowledge in the treatment of cancer might be wrong or could be improved upon. Dr. Burk is head of the cyto-chemistry division of the NCI and has 46 years of cancer research experience. He further alleged that the federal and state drug regulatory agencies and the American Cancer Society are "intentionally misleading" the general public about the malady... They make highly misleading statements in an effort to befuddle the public," he said.

After the Saccharine Scare, What Next??

When we consider carcinogenic substances we can't forget saccharin and the findings of Canadian scientists that linked it to cancer. This reminds me of the joke about the man who wasn't using sugar anymore. He was using an artificial sugar substitute and finally developed artificial diabetes.

While saccharin can take the place of sugar as a sweetener we find this is simply substituting one health hazard for another. Neither sugar nor saccharin is a true food, but saccharin is a substitute for sugar just the same The irony is that sugar, a contributing cause to diabetes, has been replaced by a synthetic substance linked to cancer.

Those whose health is endangered by sugar should realize that the answer is not to take another dangerous substance. We find saccharin is a coal-tar product, and all coal-tar products are carcinogenic in their activity. The big problem today is not so much in taking care of disease, but in refusing to give up foods and activities that we know are strongly linked to disease.

We don't want to bring in any scare tactics here about cancer. But if there is anything that is producing cancer or is cancer-forming, we should see how far we can stay away from it. If we live in a pure environment, on natural, pure and whole foods we are insuring ourselves against disease.

This reminds me of the story of three men who went to apply for the job of driving the king's carriage over mountain roads. The first man bragged, "I can safely drive that carriage as much as 12 inches from the cliff edge." The second man said, "I'll bet I can go within six inches, the king will be safe as in his own castle!" But the third man got the job because he said, "If I'm driving the king in that carriage, I'm going to stay as far away from that edge as I *possibly* can!"

Obesity Is Linked to Diabetes

Obesity is one of our most serious "diseases" and points to the fact that the body's chemical balance is greatly disturbed. The door to further disease is wide open. Diabetes is strongly associated with obesity, and it is said that every 20% in excess weight doubles the chances of diabetes in the future. Women are 50% more susceptible to diabetes than men. Diabetics are also 25 times more likely to go blind, 27 more times likely to get kidney disease, 5 times more prone to suffer from gangrene and twice as likely to have heart disease. We know that one type of hypoglycemia is the beginning stage of diabetes and some authorities say up to 5% of the U.S. populace has hypoglycemia. Our refined diets of sugar and white flour products — especially combined — are greatly responsible for the prevalence of these diseases.

The American Diabetes Association tells us that over 80% of adult diabetics were overweight before they developed the affliction. Most are 5% or more too heavy at the time diabetes is diagnosed. The association adds that fat alone doesn't cause the condition, but it raises the risk of diabetes in those predisposed to the malady.

An Insulin Shortage to Come??

Diabetes is the third ranking killer in the United States — behind heart disease and cancer. The National Commission on Diabetes says the number of diabetics will double every 15 years at the present rate. There are some 10 million diabetics today and it is found three times as commonly in poor people and 20% more often in non-whites. The potential of diabetes doubles with each decade a person's age increases.

Each ounce of insulin produced requires 1,500 pancreas glands from cattle. At the present rate of doubling diabetes every 15 years, there may soon be a shortage of insulin. This is something for us to think about.

Alternate methods of handling diabetes and more so in preventing it must be found. New ways of dealing with diabetics include the use of hydrochloric acid and digestive enzymes to normalize the digestion. Intense research is needed to provide viable alternatives.

In *Food Science,* Lucile Steele observes, "It has been stated that every over-weight person is a potential diabetic. Fleshiness indicates over-eating and over-working the pancreas as a result. Our ancestors didn't eat the huge quantity of cereal grain foods and starches we consume today. These foods weren't refined and devitalized of their nutrients. In addition, 100 years ago the annual consumption of white sugar was about 11 pounds per capita; today that figure is over 105 pounds."

Heart Disease: The Number One Killer

A National Institute of Health Advisory Committee has warned Americans that death and disease from arteriosclerosis in the country has reached epidemic proportions. The group stated that 36 million are stricken each year; deaths are in excess of one million yearly and rising fast. This accounts for more than 70 percent of all deaths.

Jeremiah Stamler, M.D., a heart researcher, says there are basic risk factors in the cause of heart disease. They are:

1. High cholesterol levels of the blood.
2. High blood pressure.
3. Any current cigarette usage.
4. Overweight by 25 percent or more.

Two other factors are heart irregularity and high levels of blood sugar, (also possible indications of diabetes).

John Yudkin, M.D., Ph.D., professor of nutrition at Queen Elizabeth College of the University of London says, "We have yet to find an exception to the parallel that exists between high sugar intake and heightened incidence of atherosclerosis, as manifested by coronary heart disease." He goes on to say that the mass cultivation of sugar cane about 1900 skyrocketed the sugar intake in civilized countries to over 100 pounds a year.

Studies of Increasing Cancer Vulnerability

Though cancer is the second leading cause of death in the U.S. it strikes terror in the hearts of all. How can we cut the danger out of cancer, as well as other degenerative diseases? Nutrition has much to do with all degenerative and chronic diseases, as we have stated, but so do other factors.

A study of 1,500 children who underwent radiation therapy shows that one-third had cancer 32 years later.

In 1976 the wire services carried the following: "The government was urged to curb X-ray treatments which are now suspected of causing up to 6,000 cancer deaths each year...nearly 17 a day. HEW estimates that 95% of the radiation Americans are exposed to comes from X-ray machines. Every year more than 130 million people are X-rayed."

Following the bombing of Hiroshima, the increase of cancers among the survivors were estimated at tenfold.

Cancer of the colon is found largely in societies in which the members are heavy beef eaters. Vegetarian societies are usually immune.

Studies that compared the cancer rate among Japanese in their native land and Japanese in California show a much higher incidence of colon cancer in Japanese Californians.

Krebs and the Nitriloside Theory

Some researchers are convinced that natural food substances having an anti-cancer effect are found in the seeds of fruits and grains. These nitrilosides are said to retard the growth of cancer cells or to "arrest" the invasion of the disease. Another theory suggests that the underdeveloped societies have rare cancer occurrences where the diet is high in nitrilosides. Civilized nations that consume refined foods with little or not nitrilosides are said to have high cancer rates.

According to Dr. Ernest T. Krebs, a biochemist, "Nitrilosides are non-toxic, water-soluble, sugary-looking accessory food factors, found in the seeds of almost all fruits and in over 1,200 plants." He names several rich sources; wild crabapple, hawthorne apple, wild grasses, quinces, peaches, plums, apricots, cherries and apples. The seeds of these foods must also be eaten. Blackberries, huckleberries and gooseberries are also said to be excellent sources of nitrilosides, according to Dr. Krebs.

Legumes he includes are lentils, mung beans, lima beans, garbanzos, shell beans and some garden peas. Whole grains rich in nitrilosides are millet, buckwheat and flaxseed.

Many researchers and scientists give credibility to the theory. Studies point to the fact that primitive peoples have a natural cancer protection through their unrefined diets. Civilized countries like the U.S. have increasingly depended on refined foods, processed and packaged foods, "dead" foods with "eternal shelf life."

Physical and Mental Health Parallels Crime

Crime, insanity, immorality and physical disorders have increased so markedly in the last few decades that we wonder where they come from. I am convinced that the foods we eat can produce wars and crimes and immoral acts. Insanity, schizophrenia and a lot of our mental disorders are being controlled through megavitamin therapy, showing that there are alternative ways of doing things. We need to research this further.

From a wholistic health perspective, when we have a criminally sick person, he is also physically sick. It is only in the last couple of years that they have considered alcohol a toxic element in the body, defining alcoholism as a disease. It may be that bizarre sexual behavior and violent tendencies are linked more to diet than most people realize.

"The new method now much used of cooking foods in closed vessels without adding water preserves the minerals and most of the vitamins."
—*Dr. Herman H. Bundeson*
Former Chairman, Chicago Board of Health

Chapter 18

Staying afloat on the chemical flood

Staying Afloat on the Chemical Flood

In America, amazingly, we are told we are the best fed nation in the world. And yet we are saturated with additives, soda pop, tobacco, alcoholic beverages and other "privileges" of a wealthy, well fed nation. Advertising campaigns tell us these products will do us no harm.

Ignorance combined with gluttony and vanity have brought civilizations to ruin in other times. The rich Romans ate and drank from vessels coated with lead, kept wine in lead containers and used lead-based cosmetics. Their life expectancy, historians have estimated, was from 22 to 25 years, and the deterioration in the health and mentality of the ruling class due to lead poisoning may have contributed to the fall of the Roman Empire.

What about our civilization? The marvels of modern chemistry have given us DDT, polyvinyl chloride, food additives, asbestos, fluorides, saccharine, and various other substances that make our country an increasingly dangerous place to live. A study by Mt. Sinai School of Medicine found that millions of office workers could be exposed to asbestos levels far above levels established for cancer risk. Tall office buildings erected from 1958 to 1970 may be contaminated. Recently Britain has banned butylated hydroxytoluene and butylated hydroxyanisole, common additives to many foods in this country, due to cancer risk. Chlordane, a long lasting chemical spray, has been linked to cancer of the nervous system and leukemia, and the government allows its sale without a warning label. The FDA ignored warnings by scientists that red dye #40 was a carcinogenic, as shown by tests on mice, and said it should be left on the market two more years while more testing is done. In the U.S. we consume over a billion pounds of food additives a year, not to mention the chemical fed to beef cattle and chickens that our bodies take in through what we buy in the market. Diethylstilbestrol, fed to cattle to fatten them fast on 11% less feed, is a possible carcinogen in humans.

Despite the 1970 Occupational Health and Safety Act, millions of Americans are still endangered by the chemicals in food, water, air, work spaces and industrial processes. When will we learn?

Present-day man hasn't developed a true health standard to live by. However, the standards of natural living and natural health were set up long ago. If we followed the right standard of how to live and proper nutrition, we would not have advanced to the chronic disease, epidemics we see everywhere today — especially emphysema, heart disease, diabetes, arthritis and cancer.

Several reasons make progress in health difficult. First, people are reluctant to change habits and customs; we all have set likes and dislikes, patterns of living handed down to us from our parents. Secondly, the vested interests in the food and drug industries are powerful — but they are only meeting the supply and demand balance. The commercial food industry is huge, growing by leaps and bounds. Someone is buying their processed foods by the millions of tons. With so many sick and degenerative diseases on the rise, maybe we should reassess where our interests really lie. To whom do we really owe loyalty and allegiance?

Food Defined Medically

Dorland's Medical Dicitonary defines food: "anything which when taken into the body, serves to nourish or build up the tissues or to supply body heat."

It says nothing about "foodless", "junk" and "empty calorie" foods, does it? What about the chemicals, additives, colorings, flavorings, preservatives, texturizers and other additives said to "improve" the food we eat? Do we live to eat rather than eat to live?

Authorities in the field of nutritional science believe that sugar is a contributor to the increasing diabetes and hypoglycemia (low blood sugar) in the U.S. Sugar, they tell us, adds nothing of value to food.

Additives actually add nothing to nutritional value; often they are included to mask the inferior quality of foods. Many additives and artificial ingredients are questionable at best.

Monosodium glutamate (MSG) is an additive that has been under consideration for years as health hazard. Biochemists at Washington University found in 1969 that big doses damaged brain cells in young mice. As a result of these findings some manufacturers withdrew the additive MSG from their products, especially baby foods. MSG is used heavily in flavor restoration for canned, packaged, frozen and precooked foods [convenience foods]. Chinese cooking uses MSG commonly. One fourth teaspoon of MSG can produce side-effects, according to reports, such as allergies and digestion distress.

Research findings point to the fact that the taking of a minute dosage of a carcinogen over a period of years can be far more detrimental than larger occasional doses [such as used on test animals]. In addition you will find that a substance that is not cancer-producing alone may react fatally with a true carcinogen to enhance its power [acting as a catalyst]. It is well known that the combination of two or more chemically reactive substances in the body can multiply the damaging potential. (The term for this action is synergism.)

The American Food and Drug Administration discovered that *one-tenth* of the lethal or fatal dose of two specific chemicals, ingested at the same time, can kill both rats and dogs. This example shows how unrealistic is the faith of the scientific experts in the "safe levels" of certain food additives.

Biochemists are just getting into the study of human cells and gene reproduction. Studies so far are to the place where they recognize the decline in cellular health and tissue integrity. These adverse changes take many years and possibly many generations. But isn't this the way cancer works? It takes 10 to 20 years or longer to appear and then those afflicted wonder what suddenly "hit" them. (In 1970 some 117,085 deaths were attributed to cancer; the 1900 figure was only 26,721.)

Processing and chemical additives in today's foods are no laughing matter, but then most of what is made light of isn't either. The following appeared in the Washington Post: "H. Herbert Fox tells me that the other night he ate some delicious citric acid mixed with propylene glycol, assorted glycerides, butylated hydroxyanisole, butylated hydroxytoluene and propyl gallate. Until he read the full list of ingredients on the package, Herb had been under the impression that he had just been munching on some tasty corn chips."

Nitrates, salts used to process bacon and some meats has been used for many centuries, but researchers are considering them as possible carcinogens in combination with amines in the form of nitrosamine compounds.

Saccharine, a synthetic sweetener, finally came to the attention of the FDA in recent years. The *Times* stated the the FDA may ban saccharine as a cancer hazard; rats fed large doses of the sweetener were found to have tumors in the blood stream. At that time "safe levels" were established, pending further study. (Even minute amounts leach Vitamin B-1 from the body.)

Agricultural and Industrial Health Hazards

DDT, the pesticide spray now banned in this country, observes no boundary lines either on land or sea. It has been found even in the Antarctic among the seals and penguins, and we find it is especially toxic to sea animals. Levels in food have gotten so high that DDT banning began a few years ago in many other countries along with various organochlorine pesticides. Sweden completely banned DDT in 1970 for two years. England banned its use in garden and homes. But, other nations still allow its

use. We know the effects of pesticides and other chemicals linger in the soil for up to ten years, longer in some cases, and they often end up in our food, accumulating in our bodies as highly toxic settlements.

MERCURY has also been in the news for several years as found in fish — both in lakes and the seas. According to many sources the levels are still rapidly increasing around the world. Areas severely contaminated may be unsafe for centuries! In 1970 almost a million cans of tuna were recalled from the U.S. supermarket shelves because they contained high mercury levels. The larger the fish, the more mercury it is apt to have. When mercury combines with water it is changed to a lethal methyl mercury. The tiny sea-life organisms take it up and pass it up the food chain to concentrate in larger fish and finally to man and animals that eat them. By that time it is much more concentrated. In 1972, the World Health Organization (WHO) issued a warning that the "insidious poison" mercury was threatening fish eaters. Japan was noted for high levels of mercury in humans at that time, as that country depends almost entirely on the sea.

LEAD is a considerably more serious threat to health than many of us realize. The main sources are from car exhausts, factory wastes, also paint, canned foods, toothpaste, glazed pottery and other commercial products. It is suggested by research that the interference with blood enzymes by lead can take place at well below the level of noted metabolic effects. We find that canned meats are likely to contain lead from the sealing of the cans, along with canned milk. Aluminum foil also contains lead, and it can be found in drinking water in polluted area. Professor Epstein of Harvard University stated that he believed 80 percent of human disease is due to environmental origin, and he specifies industrial pollutants and technology as causes. More doctors are relating the patient to the total environment.

DES, the synthetic carcinogenic female hormone (diethylstilbestrol), has been used in force feeding and [U.S. Department of Agriculture] has publicly admitted that new methods of testing revealed in a random sampling of 10 cattle and sheep that they had DES residues "in excess of amounts found to have produced cancer in laboratory animals." DES residues are serious indeed. The Massachusetts General Hospital found a rare form of cancer in more than 100 young women whose mothers had been given DES 15 to 20 years before to guard against miscarriages. France, Sweden, Holland, Switzerland and 17 other countries are reported to have banned the use of DES, "because the benefits are believed to be outweighed by the risks — especially in view of the latency period of ten to twenty years in which cancer cannot be detected." Argentina and Australia, along with the US have banned the use of DES—the three largest beef-producing countries. Eight U.S. specialists in cancer-causation have said that the theory of "toxicologically insignificant" levels is scientifically unsupportable, as the present knowledge of carcinogens is not large enough to allow the setting of any "safe level for man."

PENICILLIN & OTHER ANITBIOTICS are widely used in livestock and poultry feed to assist in quick weight gains and disease suppression. We find the use of such antibiotics as penicillin and chloramphenicol in livestock raising is being seriously questioned by medical authorities. It has been found that transferable drug resistance is possible. This means that some varieties of disease-producing bacteria have recently become resistant to many common anitbiotics. According to British researchers this resistance can also be transferred from one bacterial strain to another *and* to non-harmful bacteria in the human intestinal tract when treated meat and poultry is eaten.

The Disasters of White Bread Diets

The work of Dr. P.C. Elwood showed that iron in the form used in bread — ferrum radactum — was almost unassimilable by the body. An editorial in the British journal, *Lancet*, raised serious doubts about iron-fortified bread . It said, "A considerable sum of money is spent in Britain each year in adding to flour a form of iron which has been shown to be almost completely unavailable to man." American bread also contains inorganic iron that can't be assimilated.

Biochemical research is finding that the amount of a nutrient in food is not nearly as vital as its quantity ratio to other elements. In an article in *Health Today*, "Our Most Neglected Science," Hugh Sinclair pointed out that in white flour there is twice the amount of potassium in ratio to magnesium as compared to whole wheat flour. The ratio of cadmium to zinc is one to twenty in white bread and one to one hundred twenty in whole wheat flour. An excess of cadmium displaces zinc, the trace element that helps in healing wounds and promoting normal growth. Too much cadmium is thought to encourage high blood pressure and more of it is found in the tissues of smokers than non-smokers.

It might be interestng to note that the inferior quality of white flour products makes extra quantities necessary to satisfy the need for nutrients. And we find that the lack of fiber also causes overeating of these products as well as constipation. This is probably a factor in so much obesity today, in addition to many other illnessess, such as diabetes, hay fever, colon cancer, etc.

These products are all classed as "dead" foods that can't support good health. People must have live foods for good health. Professor E. V. McCollum of Johns Hopkins University says, "Eat only those foods which spoil, rot or decay, but eat them before they do."

The compulsory "enrichment" ingredients include synthetic niacin, thiamine, inorganic iron and inorganic calcium.

A Few Consequences of White Flour Additives

POLYOXETHYLENE MONOSTEARATE is an emulsifier that makes flour absorb more water, up to six times its weight. Tests in feeding hamsters food containing it cause many symptoms such as ulceration, severe diarrhea and bleeding from the genito-urinary tract. And they all died within a few weeks. The greatest danger to humans is that it makes body cells too absorptive and so poisins such as pesticide residues are absorbed more readily. Also, we find that it upsets fat absorption. Dr. Hueper, a U.S. cancer authority, found that this emulsifier caused cancer in experimental rats.

AMMONIUM CHLORIDE is used to ferment the dough. And we find it is also an ingredient in antifreeze for cars and in soap powders.

POTASSIUM BROMATE makes more air stay in bread while it is baked to keep it light and puffy. Britain and other countries permit this chemical. The same additive is used in home permanents with a warning not to drink it.

PROPIONIC ACID (sodium or calcium propionate) slows the growth of mold and makes the bread stay fresher longer. We find that it is naturally occurring in cheese, but the synthetic form used in flour processing is derived from ethylene, carbon monoxide and steam. This additive interferes with the enzyme that makes calcium assimilation possible [nearly everyone lacks calcium]. But it is also used in powders and ointments for treating athlete's foot!

Therefore we can think of at least five good reasons for avoiding white bread and white flour products. First, because most of the vitamins and minerals are removed during milling of the flour, and the balance is distorted in the remainder. Second, bran is removed. Third, the germ of the wheat is taken out. Fourth, chemical additives and chemical treatment further deplete the flour and threaten health by accumulating in the body as toxins. And fifth, it is constipating without roughage.

Beatrice Trum Hunter has a lovely description of the purpose of manufacturing chemical-laden white bread in her book *Consumer Beware*: To create the biggest loaf, with the greatest speed, the least work, the longest shelf-life and with the greatest economy.

Why You Should Avoid Processed Foods

Processed meats such as luncheon meats, corned beef, and ham generally contain monosodium glutamate, sodium nitrate, sodium nitrite and other preservatives. The USDA and FDA have found residues of cancer-forming substances (nitrosamines), believed to be brought out by high temperatures, on well-cooked, crisp bacon. Eppley Institute researchers suggest that Vitamin C helps counteract the formation of such carcinogens.

Many other processed foods are known to contain antiocidants to prevent rancidity; these are made from petroleum and thus are possible cancer-producers according to some authorities. The two most common are BHT and BHA — Butylated hydroxytoluene and butylated hydroxyanisole. These few primary additives show you the dangers and what to look out for in food shopping. Look for labels that state "no preservatives," "free from additives," or "contains no chemical dyes," etc. Learn to be a detective shopper to guard your health and the health of your loved ones. Processed food may be cheap, but doctor and dental bills aren't! If you don't buy the natural, pure and whole foods you will buy lots of doctor and hospital and dental services.

Soft Drink Contents

Besides the high sugar content, many soft drinks and soda pop contain emulsifiers, anti-foaming agents, artificial flavorings, artificial colorings and preservatives. They have *no* nutritional value. Cola drinks have a high phosphoric acid content that damages teeth greatly. Dr. Clive McCay of Cornell University found that human teeth placed in a cola drink began dissolving within two days. Just as with alcohol, soft drinks can lead to cirrhosis of the liver and reduce the desire for healthy foods such as proteins. The phosphoric acid in colas can also prevent assimilation of iron. Some 90 million colas a day are consumed in about 138 countries.

Soft Drinks Vs. Fruit Juice

NUTRIENTS	(12 oz.) TOMATO JUICE	(8 oz.) COLA DRINKS
Protein (gm.)	3.6	0
fat (gm.)	0.7	0
carbohydrates(gm.)	15.0	19
calories	75.0	78
calcium (mg.)	25.0	0
phosphorus (mg.)	54.0	0
iron (mg.)	1.5	0
vitamin A (I.U.)	3800.0	0
thiamine (mg.)	0.2	0
nicotinic acid (mg.)	2.7	0
ascorbic acid (mg.)	60.0	0
riboflavin (mg.)	0.1	0

The Possible Hazards of Food Additives

The average American consumer has faith in the policing of the commercial food industry by the FDA. But we find that a recent estimate of the number of chemicals in our food is 7,000! Why do we have so many? We have gotten to the place where convenience, speedy preparation, attractive appearance, shelf life and prestige living are the rule. The advertising campaigns of major food firms are impressive and seductive. But we pay for all this in terms of lower health and more disease, while the profits of the food industry are tremendous.

Senator Abraham Ribicoff has said that, "...we each consume every year more than four pounds of chemical preservatives, stabilizers, coloring, flavoring and other additives." This was brought out at a hearing on "Chemicals and the Future of Man." This is something to think about.

How thorough are the tests that "insure" chemicals safe for human consumption? Tested food additives have been checked for the dosage needed to cause almost immediate health. What about the untested additive labeled "Generally Recognized as Safe" (GRAS)? When an additive is put on the GRAS list, the FDA has to prove beyond a doubt that it is harmful. And we find out that the substances that are tested on laboratory animals such as rats, mice, rabbits, and so forth must prove lethal within 24 hours to two weeks of the dosage. They decide what dosage is needed to kill 50 percent of the animals during this time. But we find out that this lethal dose for 50 percent (LD/50) doesn't take into consideration the long range effects on users or the mixing with many other additives that can accumulate in the body. The industry also considers the "benefits" as compared to the possible dangers to the consumer. If it is profitable and lets the consumer save a few cents — for instance, in DES and other hormones to stimulate beef growth — often it is deemed safe.

We believe foods should be guaranteed safe, not just "Generally Recognized as Safe." The only way we can assure this is to grow our own organic food or secure an organic supply — food that is natural, pure and whole — the way Nature gives it to us. If any substance is remotely connected with a possible cancer risk, why not see how far we can stay away from it? The lab testing and red tape are much too slow for those who value their health. Every day we have new chemicals added to the list already in foods. How often is one removed?

We have gotten to the place where we can't blame it all on the food industry. If that food wasn't selling, it wouldn't be there. They would replace it with something new. Somebody is buying billions of dollars worth a year. Maybe they are buying my share and your share, too. The best voice we have is in our food dollars. Learn to be a discriminating shopper. Read labels and be suspicious of chemical names and ingredient abbreviations. Find out what goes into your foods and where they come from. Get acquainted with farmers and fruit growers who don't use chemical agriculture methods. Nature and her foods have been around thousands of years longer than the Jet Age supermarkets. She has a clean record.

If consumers refuse to buy the refined, adulterated, chemical-saturated foods and chemically-treated white sugar and white flour products, the food concerns will get the message. They keep monthly research checks on what the consumer buys. If we demand reform we can get it. We already know how money talks for the manufacturer. Why don't we let them hear from our dollars? The industry produces what sells.

Mass Mercury Poisoning in Iraq

Iraq, the land known for the first cultivation of soil, is mostly barren today. In 1969 and 1970 it suffered extreme droughts resulting in crop failures. Its ten million people were left short of seed for planting the next year so their government decided that the peasants would be provided with the best imported wheat berry seeds available. They ordered 73 tons of Mexipak, a hybrid developed by the Rockefeller Foundation wheat-improvement station in Mexico. Cargill, an American grain concern, took 63 tons of the order.

Iraq government officials requested that the grain be treated with a methyl-mercury fungicide to ward off wheat blight. (The USA and Canada, among other countries, have banned its use due to damage to the environment and destroying of fish and wildlife.)

In mid-September of 1971 sixteen thousand tons docked at Basrah in southern Iraq. The grain had been sprayed with a pink dye to warn that it contained a deadly poison and was intended for planting only. However, we find that the warning was printed in Spanish. And within a few weeks it was being used to feed farm animals and even to bake bread. The government failed to issue strong and well-publicized warnings; many peasants were unaware of the danger and others thought it was government deception. Due to over-buying, the treated wheat was doled out free of charge with repayment expected from next year's crops. The farmers hearing of the free grain sold their stock so they could get more, still unaware of the danger in having to depend on the poison grain through the winter. It is ironic that the Iraqi peasants had suffered from poison grain tragedies in both 1956 and 1960, on a smaller scale.

By mid-January the hospitals were filling with poison victims, and the government started a "hush-hush" attempt to reclaim the poison wheat. They had no desire to have the news spread to the outside world. By February the officials discovered that mercury-poisoned meat was in the retail markets. A two month ban was issued on meat until fresh herds could be imported. The country was encountering the worst mass poisoning in history.

The Iraq government released figures of 6,530 poison cases and 459 hospital deaths, but the poison grain probably reached nearly every village in the country. Experts privately estimated the death toll at some 6,000! Many never got out of their village and were buried in unrecorded graves. Up to one hundred thousand were said to be permanently injured. There is no cure for mercury poisoning, and traces three times as high in the new-born infant as in the mother have been found.

Mercury poisoning is slow, without an immediate warning, so many of the people thought they were safe. For weeks or even months the mercury is undetected in the system until the level is high enough to damage the brain and nervous system. As the brain faculties are attacked, one by one, balance, sense of touch and feeling, sight and hearing are deadened. An unknown number suffered crippling, deafness, blindness, brain and nerve damage. Almost no village was left untouched, and some whole families were wiped out.

A moral to this story might be to communicate to people in a language they can understand. Sprays, poisons, pesticides are in everything today — the soil, water, air, food supply. Such poisons should not be used; we should not have to beware of them, whether in food or seeds for planting, and so forth. The residues can be found everywhere. If we used only natural, pure and whole foods we would be safe from environmental poisons. Organically grown food is safe.

The Rise of Health Foods and Stores

Many people insist that they can't afford "health foods" because they cost so much more than supermarket brands. Granted, a few of the staples cost more, but when you consider the cost of processing, packaging of manufactured unnecessary foods, they are nearly the same. It will be found that natural foods go farther because they taste more satisfying due to more roughage and more vitamins and minerals. If you are interested in health, give up packaged cereals, canned and process meats, biscuit, bread and cake mixes, soft drinks and sweets. Be willing to give up the pre-cooked, ready-to-eat, "instant," refined, processed and chemically treated foods if you seek good health. There is no compromise. Invest in the initial cost of setting up a healthy kitchen and see what the lovely results are. You won't regret the change. Move up to natural, pure and whole food or wholistic health.

Who are the "health food" store customers? Since the national press is taking note of so-called food "faddists" and "cranks," this "cult" must be gaining momentum and popularity. At look at the customers in the average natural foodstore takes in retired and Social Security pensioners, teenagers, dentists, doctors and their wives, young housewives, mothers and many movie, television and stage personalities. Within the last few years in the US, the growth of these stores has been over 250% and in some cities as much as 1500%. Britain reports nearly one thousand as compared to about one hundred a decade ago. Countless other countries of the world are taking up the idea of organically grown foods.

The fact that there is a giant difference between organic food and artificially grown produce was brought out by an article in *Organic Gardening and Farming* by Nancy Butler called "What Makes a food Organic?" It said that there is scientific evidence for a decline in the trace mineral content of artificially grown grain and that generally the organic produce is better for human health. We are aware also that there is a reduction in the quantity of protein in artificially grown foods.

Natural foods have become sufficiently popular to find their way onto supermarket shelves. Even some airlines have dietetic and additive-free meals available if called for 24 or 48 hours in advance. Check for them yourself.

4,000 Approved and GRAS Additives

Since 1958 the FDA has issued formal regulations that allow the approved use of some 3,000 food additives. Another 1,000 are on the GRAS list (Generally Regarded As Safe). $15 billion worth of chemical food additives are used by the processed food industry. They are largely unidentified chemicals used in artificial flavors and colors as well as for waxes, bleaches, extenders, clarifying agents, emulsifiers, softners, thickeners, hydrogenators, curers, buffers, sprout inhibitors, deodorizers, fungicides, sweeteners, conditioners, anti-oxidants, fortifiers, dryers, alkalizers, anti-foaming agents, firming agents, stabilizers and buffers. They embalm foods to make them appear fresh and most don't need refrigeration as a result. The counterfeit "freshness" is eternal, but the food is dead.

Typical GRAS additives are butylated hydroxyanisole and butylated hydroxytoluene, commonly known as BHA and BHT. They are anti-oxidants made from petroleum that give foods a long shelf life without the cost of refrigeration and the chance of rancidity. Read a few labels and you will find them in dry cereals, candy, gelatin desserts, shortening, ice cream, dairy foods, processed meats, peanut butter, margarine, chewing gum, salad oil, dried fruits, potato chips, meats, fish, dressings, roasted nut snacks, etc. Several health crusaders have pointed out for many years that these additives cause allergic reactions and are harmful to nerves. Many countries, Britain included, have banned the use of these additives. But in the U.S. the "eternal shelf life" and corporate profits are more important than health it would seem.

MSG (monosodium glutamate) is widely used in the food industry — almost fifty million pounds are sold each year. It serves as a flavor enhancer in over 10,000 processed foodstuffs. Foods from fruits to sea foods, canned to frozen), soups, snacks and "convenience" foods, TV dinners, dressings, processed meats, tenderizers, candy, poultry, baked products, "meat extenders" and animal feeds. Industry officials report that MSG is the most widely used chemical flavoring agent.

Since MSG is a derivative of sea weed, soybeans, wheat and corn gluten or sugar beet by-products it is considered safe by the FDA. It has been used since 1907, but more recently a study found it to produce permanent brain damage in laboratory test animals.

I have decided to write another book, and we will be working on this very shortly. It is going to have a very touching title, BE SMART, ANY JACKASS CAN GET SICK. The idea for this book came to me one night in a restaurant after I had given a long evening lecture. It was late, and as I sat awaiting the arrival of my food, I noticed a very large man with long ears sitting in another booth across the way from me. This man was eating "thunder bread," baked beans and pickles, topped off with a huge cup of Norwegian Gasoline (coffee to you). He did skip the dessert, but the final touch came as he passed the counter on his way out and drank a "fizzler" to alkalize his acid combination! It was at that moment, my friends, I knew I must write a book on just what real jackasses we can become in our eating habits.

Chapter 19

Are you a poor health statistic?

"Thousands upon thousands have studied disease; almost no one has studied health."

—*Adelle Davis*

Diet: Its Effect on Physical and Emotional Health

We find that medical science today is preoccupied with labeling diseases and placing patients in neat categories. If they don't fit they are told their problems are "in their head" or just need a tranquilizer. Those suffering from stress, depression, anxiety, hypoglycemia, and nerve symptoms often get Valium or Librium. Yet, biochemistry has linked diet to emotional health in many cases, and more doctors are hearing about megaional vitamin therapy of late, especially in cases of alcoholism, schizophrenia and hypoglycemia.

A look at statistics will show us that some 800,000 people a year are hospitalized with mental disturbances and illnesses. In a recent decade, the number of psychiatrists increased by 40%. All other diseases would have to be combined to equal total mental illnesses, with the exception of dental troubles. During the past two decades, the suicide rate among the 15 to 24 age group has more than doubled. We find that in the 17 to 24 age group almost 40 percent have developed chronic ailments. Over 25 million in this country take the leading tranquilizer (Valium). Along with this decline in mental and physical health our nutrition has dropped rapidly, too. Our national health is so bad that present health standards are based on *unhealthy* people. I have never found a well person even in my world travels. We don't know what optimal health is. So we can't accept the current so-called health standard.

The U.S. Department of Agriculture made a survey recently that found only half of 7500 families surveyed had a diet that reached the Recommended Dietary Allowances of protein, calcium, iron, vitamin A, thiamine (B-1), riboflavin (B-2) and ascorbic acid (vitamin C). In the uppermiddle class income group 37% of the diets were lacking these elements. Other surveys have shown serious lacks of such nutrients as vitamins D and E.

It should be brought out that the recommended daily allowances of vitamins and minerals are minimum and not adequate in many things. The National Research Council set the requirements purposely low and many elements aren't even considered as necessary to human nutrition. In others the Minimum Daily Requirements haven't been established. The requirements of individuals differ too greatly to establish R.D.A. levels.

What is the solution for health? Rely only on natural, pure and whole foods — organically grown; have a lot of raw foods. Get rid of white sugar and white flour products in the diet. Leave behind processed, packaged, additive saturated and chemically preserved "foodless" foods. Get fresh, clean air and lots of sunshine. Depend on a few supplements — always from natural sources — when necessary. Now is the time to turn to Nature.

Statistics on Our Deteriorating National Health

A report on Human Nutrition by the U.S. Department of Agriculture and the State Universities and Land Grant Colleges, plus other surveys and research figures give us the following information.

Heart and vasculatory diseases caused over one million deaths in 1967. The fact that vegetarians have one-sixth the heart attack rate of the national average shows that improved diet could reduce that figure by at least 25%.

About 49.1% of the U.S. populace has one or more chronic health problems representing 102 million people. Better nutrition could reduce this by 10 million.

5.2 million persons are severely or totally disabled. 25 million show this affliction. Improved nutrition could reduce this by 10%.

200,000 babies are born each year with birth defects, of which 20% are estimated to come from environmental causes, according to the March of Dimes.

20 million suffer from arthritis, including 200,000 children. Fifteen million workdays are lost each year due to arthritis amounting to 3 billion dollars in lost wages. Eight million could be freed of pain through nutrition.

As for dental health one half of all those over 55 have no teeth. 1967 saw $6.5 billion spent for dental services. By the age of 2 nearly half of U.S. children have cavities. By age 15 the average figure is 11 missing, decayed or filled teeth. 40% of the population receives dental care, and 98% need it. 60% of the people either don't have the money or the desire to see a dentist. Cavities are commonly a sign of calcium deficiency due to an upset of the glandular balance by excess sugar consumption. In a recent year, Americans bought 28.6 million gallons of mouthwash to combat bad breath — again a sign of bad nutrition. 50% could be reduced in expenditures and occurrences of poor dental health.

Diabetes and carbohydrate diseases, (including hypoglycemia), caused an estimated 3.9 diabetic deaths in

1967. 79% over 55 show impaired glucose tolerance. 50% of these cases could be avoided through proper nutrition.

Obesity is seen in 30 to 40% of adults; in those over 40 years of age, 70% are obese. One in 3 food dollars is spent eating out, while the average American consumes 1,500 pounds of food per year. Again, the average amount of excess weight for half of all Americans is 10 pounds. We average 187 pounds of beef, 290 eggs and 18 pounds of ice cream, and our fat and oil intake averages 52 pounds per person per year. Sugar intake is up to 135 pounds per person annually. Proper diet could reduce the number of overweight persons by 75%.

Eyesight is also poor; 48.1% or 86 million persons over three years of age wore corrective lenses in 1966. 90% of those over 45 wear glasses. The number could be reduced by 20% through better diet.

Allergies affect 22 million (9%); 16 million have hay fever and asthma; 7-15 million people are allergic to cow's milk. U.S. consumers spend over $500 million a year for allergy remedies and treatment and lose 25 million working days. Sound nutrition could reduce the irritation of allergies by 20%; 90% could change the dietary program to avoid milk.

Digestive disorders are common; about 20 million cases of acute conditions occur annually; 4,000 new cases appear daily; 14 million have duodenal ulcers. This could be reduced by 25% in acute cases and $1 billion saved.

Cancer was found in 600,000 people in 1968 and 320,000 died of the terrible disease that year. The use of chloroform in cough syrups, linaments and toothpastes has been banned by the FDA because it causes liver cancer in mice. How many additives will eventually be linked to cancer? The list could be very long. Better nutrition could account for a 20% reduction in incidence and deaths.

The 5 million estimated alcoholics at the time the government report on human nutrition was issued (1971) has since doubled. These people lack sufficient protein, Vitamin B-complex — especially B-1 and B-6 — Vitamin C and magnesium. an estimated 33% of these could be helped by better nutrition.

The number of graduates from U.S. medical colleges has risen by 168% since 1930, while the population has risen only 72%. Who is supporting all these new doctors? Apparently, those with poor food habits and unhealthy lifestyles. About 20 million operations are performed in this country yearly. Employed persons lose an average of seven and a half workdays a year due to illness, while experts say school children average 6 colds per year.

In 1975 the average daily cost of hospitalization was $131.20, which has more than doubled in the 1980s. This doesn't include doctor bills, surgery or medications. In 1976 Americans averaged $102 for doctor's expenses and $215 for hospital expenses. Many who need hospital care but who cannot afford it simply live with whatever problems they have. Bad nutrition guarantees a ticket to the hospital or a life of misery with chronic problems.

Here are extracts of Table 1:
Magnitude of Benefits From Nutritional Research

Health Problem	Magnitude	Potential savings from improved diet
Heart and Vasculatory	Over 1,000,000 deaths in 1967	25% reduction
Respiratory and Infectious	141 million workdays lost in 1965-66; 166 million school days lost.	15-20% fewer lost days
Mental Health	5.2 million people are severely or totally disabled; 25 million have manifest disability.	10% fewer disabilities.
Early Aging	About 49.1% or population have one or more chronic impairments: 102 million people.	10 million people without impairments.
Reproduction	15 million with congenital birth defects.	3 million fewer children with birth defects.
Arthritis	16 million afflicted	8 million people without afflicitons.
Dental Health	½ of all people over 55 have no teeth; $6.5 billion public and private expenditures on dentists' services in 1967.	50% reduction in incidence, severity and expenditures
Diabetes and Carbohydrate Disorders	3.9 million overt diabetic deaths in 1967; 79% of people over 55 with impaired glucose tolerance.	50% of cases avoided or improved.
Osteoporosis	4 million severe cases; 25% of women over 40.	75% reduction
Obesity	30 to 40% of adults; 60 to 70% over 49 years.	75% reduction

Alcoholism	5 million alcoholics; ½ are addicted; an- billion from absentee- ism, lowered produc- eism, lowered produc- tion and accidents.	33%
Eyesight	48.1% or 86 million people over 3 years wore corrective lenses in 1966; 81,000 became blind every year; 103 million in welfare.	20% fewer people blind or with cor- rective lenses.
Allergies	22 million people (9%) are allergic; 16 million with hayfever/ asthma; 7-15 million people allergic to milk.	20% of peo- ple relieved; 90% of those allergic to milk.
Digestive	About 20 million in- cidents of acute con- dition annually; 4,000 new cases each day; 14 million with duodenal ulcers.	25% fewer acute condi- tions; over $1 billion in costs.
Kidney and Urinary	55,000 deaths from renal failure; 200,000 with kidney stones.	20% reduc- tion in in- cidence and deaths.
Muscular Disorders	200,000 cases	10% reduc- tion in cases
Cancer	600,000 persons developed cancer in 1968; 320,000 persons died of cancer in 1968.	20% reduc- tion in in- cidence and deaths.
Improved Growth and Development	324.5 million work days lost; 51.8 million people needing medical attention and/or restricted activity.	25% fewer work days lost.
Improved Learning Ability	Over 6.5 million men- tally retarded with I.Q. below 70; 12% of school age children need special education.	Raised I.Q. by 10 points for persons with I.Q. 70-80.

The U.S. Isn't Alone in Disease Increases

The world faces faster and more widespread sickness and diseases in the near future. Britain admits that its national health is rapidly deteriorating and gives the following reasons and statistics. We find that they men- tion chemicals and additives in food processing, agriculture, animal husbandry practices and industry as some of the causes.

Cardiovascular diseases are now the cause of over half the deaths, striking younger and younger age groups. Scotland lists coronary heart disease as the commonest cause of death under 35 and in the United Kingdom it is the most common overall death cause. They attribute chronic bronchitis to the reason for over 30,000 victims each year. They add that migraine headaches attack 5 million. Their cancer deaths in 1970 totalled 117,085. (The figures were only 26,271 in 1900.) Cancer of the large intestine (colon) is the second leading cause of death after bronchial carcilnoma (cancer). Mental illness is another of their prime maladies. During the 10- year period from 1957-1967 it increased 6 times. Almost half of their hospital beds are filled with the mentally ill (46.6%) and the largest group are the schizophrenicsk (divided personalities). Suicide rates are also rapidly rising.

Another affliction is diverticular disease which affects 30% of the people over 50. Their studies indicate it is due to the diets lacking fiber — especially refined sugar and white flour products. Diabetes is on the rise, linked to sugar consumption, especially, along with refined starches. They also list peptic ulcers, varicose veins, con- stipation and obesity — also linked to lack of fiber as one cause. Nearly half of Britain's populace is fat, and 20 per- cent are children.

Britain's Dr. H.M. Sinclaire has maintained for many years that animal tests with feeding show that over- fed, overweight children who mature earlier may also die at an earlier age. He has added that being fourteen pounds overweight is more dangerous to health than to smoke 25 cigarettes a day. (Lecture to the Royal Institute of Public Health and Hygiene) We recognize that obesity is a sign of a body imbalance and/or malnutrition and possible future disease.

One of the most tragic findings is the rise in young children of degenerative diseases, such as cancer. Cancer is considered the second most common cause of disease in children today, not only in Britain but the U.S. as well. America reports that in children between 4 and 14 leukemia is "the deadliest disease...claiming 1400 victims a year," it was stated in *Time* Magazine, "and that after accidents, it is the third leading cause of death in this age- group."

What are the implications of these statistics and findings? Diseases that were uncommon a century ago are rising and new ones appearing along with the "civilized" diet and living standards, and side effects of modern drugs. The present ratio of 10 hospital beds to every 1000 persons is inadequate in Britain, and hospital building programs aren't keeping up with the illness and disease rise. Their recent health surveys have uncovered surprising and extensive nutritional deficiencies blaming much of it on refined sugar and white flour. Sir Robert McCarrison observed years ago "...that it is the less obvoius manifestations of such deficiencies that are of importance in Western countries." He added that to recognize this fact was necessary for the prevention and cure of many of man's common sicknesses.

It was Professor Max Rosenheim who wrote in *Lancet*, "It must increasingly be the purpose of the medical profession, and of all who work with it, to aim at prevention rather than cure..." *Lancet* carried the following by J.N. Morris: "To improve health, lift the burdens of chronic disease, and reduce the death-rate, the main hope surely lies in prevention." Prevention, he said, must include "patiently trying to teach individuals and families healthier living."

Some Alarming Facts and Figures

Dr. U.D. Register, Chairman of the Department of Nutrition at Loma Linda University says that a diet rich in legumes reduces cholesterol levels even with large quantities of butter fat eaten. Vegetarians suffer less from heart attacks as shown by these and other of their experiments. A study was made of Seventh Day Adventist Church members. A group of its men who ate no flesh meat were found to suffer only 60% as much heart disease as other American men. If heart trouble developed, it was much later in life.

A vegetarian diet usually lowers weight and guards against heart trouble by lowering cholesterol. The main danger in this regime is the B-12 deficiency often noted in vegetarians; this can lead to anemia or neurologic damage. If animal products such as eggs and raw milk (goat milk preferred) and its products are added, the danger is mostly avoided.

Some 475,000 U.S. citizens have gallstone surgery each year, and 16 to 20 million suffer occasioal attacks. Cholesterol is usually the cause, according to the Mayo Clinic. We find that most Americans don't get enough lecithin to balance their high fat diets. Salt is another culprit in diet. According to Dr. Lot Page of Tufts University, "Salt is the single greatest cause of high blood pressure, and people should eat less than ¼ teaspoon per day." 15% to 20% of Americans have hypertension, the main cause of heart disease and strokes.

Americans now consume nearly 5 pounds of meat and fowl a week. This is twice the amount of Sweden, 50% more than Britain, and 5 times the amount of Japan. The U.S. total is about 254 pounds per year per capita.

U.S. consumption of staple foods is rapidly declin-

ing. New "convenience" and processed foods are taking their place. The use of dairy products had been lowered 21%, vegetables 23% and fruit 25%. Soft drink consumption had risen 80%, pastry 70% and the other snack foods 85%. An over-view shows a decline in the average diet at the same time. In 1955, 60% of a survey group, according to the USDA, had an adequate diet; in 1965 the figure had dropped to 50%.

Many researchers maintain that the decline is directly related to the increase of many diseases and illnesses. These include heart disease, diabetes, hypoglycemia, some cancer forms, hypertension, obesity and tooth decay among others. some nutritionists estimate these cost Americans $30 billion a year.

A chief bandit is refined sugar. We average two pounds a week. Children eat as much as 140 to 150 pounds a year, almost three pounds a week.

A 1971 National Nutrition Survey ordered by Congress found great deficiencies in the U.S. diet. Anemia, vitamin A deficiency, calcium deficiency and dental caries incidence were alarming.

At least 25% of our population is dangerously overweight.

Packaging is on the increase. Packaging materials went from 412 pounds to 591 pounds (43%) per person between 1958 and 1971. Fresh produce consumption dropped 11.3% from 90.2 pounds in 1958 to 80 pounds per person in 1970.

Americans eat 30 pounds of frozen French fries a year; this is a rise of 460% since 1960. During the same period fresh vegetable consumption dropped by 7%.

In 1971 "snack" food sales totaled $3.4 billion by themselves. The yearly increase is estimated at 6%.

In 1974 there were 104,000 dentists in the U.S..

About 325 million acres are farmed in the United States. Since 1950 that figure hasn't changed much, but the number of people living and working on farms has decreased 50%.

American agriculture produces far less energy than it uses. It depends almost entirely on petroleum and natural gas for fuel, fertilizers, herbicided, pesticides and chemicals and drugs used in raising livestock and poultry.

Organophosphates have replaced the DDT farmers used to rely on. These are appearing an increasing levels in foods. Their effects aren't as long range as DDT, but they are an even deadlier poison. Methyl parathion, one of the organophosphates, is one of the deadliest.

Wholistic Health is Crucial

The emphasis on wholistic health is vital, Dr. Alexis Carrel, who pioneered organ transplanting says in his work *Man, the Unknown.* "Man thinks, invents, loves, suffers, admires and prays with his brain and all his organs." He continues, "In illness the body preserves the same unity as in health. It is sick as a whole. No disturbance remains strictly confined to a single organ." Human organs can withstand tremendous punishment, but there is a breaking point. The heart pumps blood through 60,000 miles of blood vessels in the body and is the body's strongest muscle. Obesity, lack of exercise, high salt intake, drugs, alcohol, coffee and smoking can harm any heart.

Every single cigarette affects the lungs and blood by polluting; coffee harms the kidneys, nerves and heart; alcohol hurts the stomach and the liver. All drugs are potential time bombs—their effect is cumulative in the body and lowers vitality with continued use. Medical science lists about 203 causes for the headache, and all headache suppressants and remedies contain harmful ingredients of coal tar derivatives or caffeine. They can promote kidney troubles later.

Disease "Suppression" Is Rising

Tonsil removal operations are the most common single surgery in the U.S., followed by hysterectomies, many of which are not necessary. A report in the *New York Times* states: "Increasing numbers of surgeons are rushing their patients to the operating tables, more out of considerations of monetary gain than of sound medicine." Antibiotics are used which are capable of causing damage and complications themselves. Iatrogenic disease, those resulting from medicine or medical methods or medical men, are on the rise. There are some 20,000 varieties of drugs designed to suppress disease and illness. The list grows annually by several hundred. Most of the people of the world would prefer to escape from pain rather than getting to the cause and slowly overcoming it through Nature. Only Nature can restore balance and health within.

Tooth Decay Is a World Epidemic

Cavities reach 98 percent of the U.S. population at some time during their lives. The first 35 years are the most cavity prone. Over 100,000 dentists are kept busy and are unable to keep up with the cavities and other dental work.

A government survey made in the early 1960's showed an adult to have an average of 18 decayed, missing or filled teeth in the assumed total of 32. A study of the military draft indicated that the average draftee required one extraction and about six restorations in addition to other dental work.

Americans spent $4.7 billion dollars in 1971 for dental work. No more than 40% of the public saw a dentist. An estimated $2billion was laid out for dental caries. Tooth decay occurs faster than dentists can restore teeth and fill cavities.

During the food rationing of World War II, Norway cut back on sugar and other refined carbohydrates and raised the intake of potatoes, vegetables, milk and bread. Statistics showed a steady decrease in caries from 1942 to 1946. In 1947 they were rising in keeping with the return of sweets and other refined carbohydrates.

In 1821 the U.S. used about 10 pounds of sugar per capita. By 1931 the consumption was at almost 108 pounds. It has continued to rise over the past decades. In 1963 industry used 8 billion pounds of sugar; 12 billion pounds were used by 1967. The increase for only four years was 33%! The average per capita consumption now is over 135 pounds per year.

Tooth decay is often a sign of chemical imbalance in the body due to using too much sugar. The resulting calcium deficiency weakens many bodily functions and opens the door to other chronic periodic problems.

Glasses Indicate Poor Nutrition

It is alarming to find that 88% of the people of the US, aged 45, wear eyeglasses. A large portion of younger people also wear them. It is becoming more common to see very small children, even preschool ages, in glasses. Why are American eyes so bad? Drugs, surgery and corrective lenses are becoming more and more prevalent.

There must be a correlation between poor eyesight and the large quantities of "foodless foods" consumed so freely; add the oceans of soft drinks known for carbonic acid. Dr. Hunter H. Turner wrote in the 1944 *Pennsylvania Medical Journal* that he believed carbonic acid found in soda pop taken in such large quantities was responsible for the great increase in myopia (near sightedness).

Maybe we should pay more attention to what our eyes see. They are the body's most complex organ.

What Is the Real Price of "Miracle" Drugs?

It has been reported that no antibiotic yet devised is completely free from possible harmful side effects. In 1965 Montreal General Hospital disclosed that 25% of the deaths reported by the public medical service were the results of adverse drug effects. Drugs are generally of two classes — first antitoxins and toxins, secondly the class of "anesthetics" which affect the nerves. Aspirin, a coal-tar product related to carbolic acid, is in the latter class. 19 billion aspirins are sold each year. Quoted as a "cure-all" for many symptoms, it is know to have 20 possible adverse side effects. Dr. William Beaver says that medical claims of the four leading pain relievers advertised on T.V. are "misleading or deliberately deceptive." Dr. Robert Mendelsohn, assistant director of Chicago's Michael Rees Hospital, states that 30 million patients are hospitalized in the U.S., and one million are there due to adverse drug reactions. Dr. Joe C. Nichols, M.D., author of *Please Doctor Do Something* says, "One of seven babies born in America today comes into the world with a birth defect." What are the causes?

Dr. Nichols also said, "America is one of the sickest and worst fed nations on earth."

Antibiotics and Their Reactions

While penicillin, streptomycin, chloromycetin and other wonder drugs can do much good they have been misused and abused. Since the invention of penicillin in 1941 millions of lives have been saved. But through overuse and misuse, much harm has also been done.

Reactions and side-effects reported from antibiotics are: headache, mild to severe skin reactions, nausea, hypertension, drug fever, vomiting, anemia, asthma, colitis, severe bleeding, nerve damage, shock, limb numbness, secondary infections, blood cell destruction, blurred vision, liver damage, jaundice, insomnia and toxic reaction of the spleen.

It is also reported that 25% to 50% of the antibiotic doses have been unnecessary.

Amphetamines: The "Pep" Pills

"Pep pills" such as benzedrine, dexedrine and so on excite and stimulate the nervous system and body functions. This often gives the false impression of well-being and increased energy. Other uses include appetite curbing and to keep alert and awake when sleep is indicated.

Some of the side-effects are: insomnia, diarrhea, fainting, drowsiness, dry mouth, head ache, agitation, nervousness, rapid heart beat, skin rash, blurred vision, disrupted liver function, habit-forming tendency and reduction of white blood cells. With these "uppers" usually "downers" or sleeping pills are required.

Tranquilizers — Peace for a Price

A study by the Drug Enforcement Agency has shown that a leading tranquilizer causes the greatest number of drug-related illneses in the U.S., followed by alcohol, heroin, marijuana and aspirin. The figures were drawn from a study of 200,000 cases of drug misuse. A common tranquilizer taken by 1 million men interferes with sexual function. About 60% of the men surveyed reported trouble in sexual performance. Reports have linked many deaths from a lethal combination of alcoholic beverages and sleeping pills. Marijuana, according to Dr. Milos Novotny of the University of Indiana, contains a higher concentration of cancer-causing hydrocarbons than cigarettes.

"Senile" Elderly Often Suffer from Drug Misuse

It is estimated that a million Americans diagnosed as senile really suffer from a misuse of prescribed drugs — doses too large and harmful drug combinations. So says the National Institute for Drug Abuse. Experts give their reasoning for the problem: 1. Older people are given new drugs with little knowledge of the side effects; 2. the dosages are much too high; 3. combinations of drugs come from different doctore; together they can produce symptoms diagnosed as senility.

Dr. K. Warner Schaie, a psychologist and director of the University of Southern California's Gerontology Research Institute says, "One out of every four elderly persons presumed senile, who aren't in institutions, are actually simply disoriented by misused drugs. On a national basis, this means 600,000 to 700,000 people over age 65. Among the long-term nursing home population, the figures are even more dramatic. Out of 626,000 so-called senile residents, perhaps 300,000 — or one out of two — are actually suffering drug-induced disorientation that could be easily reversed."

Dr. Paul Lofholm, consultant to the National Institute for Drug Abuse says, "First, everyone knows that children need different dosages of drugs than adults. But it's only now being recognized that the adult dosages of most drugs should usually be cut in half for an old person because he absorbs and excretes the drug at a much slower rate." He adds that specialists often treat various diseases not knowing what other doctors have prescribed. The medications can have adverse reactions when combined.

"The average housewife peels her vegetables, thus throwing away the part directly underneath the skins containing the most plentiful amount of mineral salts; then the remaining portion is boiled and the water, which has dissolved out more minerals, is thrown away."

—Dr. Charles H. Mayo

Chapter 20

Are you chasing the bran wagon?

"We should have been getting enough roughage in the first place."

Protection Against Colon or Rectal Cancer

More intestinal cancer is found in the last part of the bowel, the sigmoid colon, than any other section. Cancer of the colon or rectum ranks second to lung cancer — leading cause of cancer deaths. Some 49,000 die each year of cancer of the colon or rectum (colorectal cancer) and 99,000 cases are diagnosed annually. Most of the colostomies are performed because of trouble in the last part of the bowel. After all, we hold more waste material in this area. Holding it three or four days makes it concentrated in drugs and toxic by-products, and the constant absorption by the body can be degenerative in its results.

We have to consider roughage necessary, and the diet we recommend has plenty of roughage to carry the excrement and the intestinal waste to a quick elimination from the body. Bowel tone is developed by working against this roughage. The six vegetables, two fruits, one starch and one protein program is high in roughage. By experience we have found that the average person having only one bowel movement a day has quickened peristaltic action to the place where they have two bowel movements each day. People who have been under our care have reported only one bowel movement in three days or four days, but they soon increase to the point where they were having one or two bowel movements a day.

Diverticulosis is the single most common condition of the colon. About 30% of those over 40 have it, and up to 70% over age 70 have this condition of bowel pockets that harbor toxic material. About 40% of the American people are said to carry diverticula. We have found that taking care of the bowel improves many of the symptoms diverticulosis; and many symptoms of indigestion, bloating, acid and gas problems disappear. Whenever there is distension or bloating, it is possible that this bowel pocket condition is causing pressure symptoms and toxic conditions. Appendicitis can result.

It is said that our bodies do not absorb water from the intestinal tract, but I know the fecal material becomes hard and dry in the large colon, so water must be absorbed. We also absorb toxins from this fecal material — through the bowel wall into the blood stream. With balloon conditions in the bowel, there can be much absorption, and this can become the seat of a low-grade in-fection. It is only through making sure that we have the proper movement and elimination of toxic bowel material that it can be improved. Exercise of the bowel from the outside of the body is not always enough. We have to start from the inside and work out — work on the inside as on the outside.

The average doctor believes that diverticulosis is incurable and pays very little attention to the condition. I know we should pay more attention to it than anything else in the body, because from this point every organ is affected if a low-grade infection of the colon develops. The one thing we should make sure of is a proper bowel movement every day. We must answer Nature's call. We must keep these bowel pockets or diverticula clean, as cleanliness is the beginning of our routine in keeping well. Cleanliness is not only proper for the outside of the body but also for the inside.

Do You Get Enugh Roughage?

I feel we are using too little roughage in the average American diet today. Salads are taboo with most children. We aren't taught to eat the roughage we should have early in life. We take orange juice instead of eating the whole sections of the orange. We have apple juice instead of eating the apple for the roughage it contains. It is no wonder that the Ralston Club was established some years ago to encourage members to add bran to their diets in order to get the roughage they lacked. Many members of this club attributed their good health to the fact that they had taken extra bran in the diet. Well, they should have had this bran or roughage in their diet in the first place! They shouldn't have continued eating such soft foods, such mushy foods, that they had to add bran for good bowel movements.

Caring for the Sensitive Digestive System

The basis of our teaching is that if you live in the right way in the first place, you won't have to worry about roughage, diverticulosis or bowel disturbances through life. If we leave the bowel long enough without exercising it properly, in time, it loses tone and loss of tone in any part of the bowel is a good invitation for gas pockets to form. The bowel is a very insensitive organ and doesn't warn of disturbances until they are far advanced in many cases. (This is another reason for the prevalence of colorectal cancer.)

However, I believe there are some people who cannot take the extreme form of roughage, and we should be very careful because diverticulosis can eventually get into an extreme, irritable state. In this condition we find that the ulcerous, sensitive, acid-bearing tissue cannot take extreme roughage in the form of bran, strings, seeds and so forth. It is at this time that we have to work for healing. Working for healing is making sure that we have enough raw foods that can eventually get into the blood stream to go back and heal the bowel wall and take away that acid, sensitive condition that has built up. You do not correct this condition by taking bran. We start with natural foods, possibly in juice form, until the body has become properly balanced biochemically. It's the chemically well-balanced body that will eventually heal the bowel wall tissue. Of course, we do have to get into the roughage foods eventually. We build bowel tone by adding a little bit of rough foods at a time to the diet.

Success Records of Natural Roughage

Experiments in England have proven that by adding bran many of the patient's symptoms have disappeared. One of the great doctors in London, Sir Arbuthnot Lane, surgeon to the King of England, changed his procedures entirely. He found that by taking care of patients through nutrition he could help them tremendously. By taking care of the intestinal tract and using the proper natural foods, he was able to overcome cases of arthritis, rheumatism, goiter and growths in the body without operating as in the past. His work is a classic example for the Nature Cure advocate seeking the proper knowledge of how to get well through the correct dietary procedures.

Arnie Werlin, one of the great teachers in the past, advocated roughage in the diet for healing. He just added more natural foods. In his work in Europe he was able to produce many unbelievable changes in a person's health through just changing their diets.

Dr. Kristine Nolfi, of Denmark has produced tremendous changes in people with natural foods. It was using the skins, peelings and seeds of fruit and vegetables that quickened the bowel movements and produced less toxic materials in the bowel. I am convinced that the whole body responded because less toxic waste was produced and bowel contents were expelled faster and more regularly.

Otto Cargue, one of the champions of good health in this country using natural foods, went back to the Nature Cure methods. When we stop and think about the average person's diet and compare it with what God gave us in seeds, grains, nuts, you will find that we have become a nation of milk and bread eaters. The bread is lacking in roughage because it is made from refined white flour. When you look at the roughage the average person has in his diet, you wonder how his bowel works at all. He does not have enough material for his bowel to work against to develop and keep good bowel tone. You develop a muscle by using it. This is why it is necessary to have roughage within the bowel. No one can really be well living on less than 60% raw food daily. This is a law; if you can't take any raw food at all at this time, healing is necessary. If you use raw food, use raw food with roughage — plenty of raw vegetables and hard raw fruits. If raw food is not easily tolerated, use other roughage food.

I have never heard of a doctor who helped a patient through Nature Cure methods unless that patient had natural foods with natural roughage and the biochemical elements the body must have — the dust of the earth.

Juices Don't Give You Roughage

There are many foods we can take in juice form, but I still feel it would be better if we return to the natural way of life and eat the fruit or vegetable. Those who are short, however, in the biochemical elements should possibly take the greater concentration of elements they can get from fresh juice. When it comes to grapes, for instance, the grape has a wonderful peeling on it. As we chew that grape peeling it becomes very bitter. This is potassium that grapes are high in. There's also a good deal of silicon in grape skins. This is something we don't find within the grape. We can use grape skins in liquefied form and whenever we need roughage to tone the bowel.

Properly Prepared Grains Add Fiber

Grains can be either constipating or laxative, according to the way they are prepared and the form they take. Whole grains are good for intestinal activity, but flours made from them are constipating. Wheat bran is well known as a remedy because it adds bulk to the system. One or more tablespoons per day are often recommended for cases of constipation, but the individual tolerance must be carefully considered. Yellow cornmeal, you will recall, is an excellent laxative cereal to serve once or twice a week. Quick cooked cereals and processed cereals are not approved. It is best to slowly steam whole grain cereals over low heat or use vacuum bottle cooking in a heated thermos.

Sprouts Are Excellent Roughage

One of the best roughage foods for the bowel is sprouts. It is one of the finest fiber foods, not too irritating or harsh and scratchy, but one most people can tolerate. It gives the colon a good work out against the cellulose bulk of the sprout.

Alfalfa Tablets: Bulk Magicians

One of my most effective remedies in taking care of diverticulosis is alfalfa tablets. They are made from the fiber of the alfalfa leaves. After being swallowed, the tablets swell as they absorb liquid and digestive juice, then break into particles of fibrous leaf bulky enough for the bowel walls to work against. The chlorophyll found in alfalfa tablets helps clean the bowel and to sweeten the putrefactive bowel pockets in diverticulosis.

Potential Damage By Harsh Laxitives

I do not believe in laxatives — of any kind — even natural products. There are times when they are necessary; but get off them as soon as possible. Developing natural bowel tone is the goal we should work for. One of the worst problems in this country is our snack habit of coffee and doughnuts — made with fine white flour — or sandwiches — made with peanut butter and white bread. I don't believe in bread or any white flour products. No bread should be eaten without having plenty of raw vegetables, even sprouts, along with it. Vegetable fiber carries the liquid to hold bread particles in suspension and move waste material along rapidly.

Our Disastrous Coffee Breaks

Coffee breaks, I think, are one of the poorest ideas we have in America. First, it's degenerating in its bowel effects; it is stimulating with no compensation. The energy boost we get from drinking coffee leaves the body depleted. Coffee is one of the greatest destroyers of the "friendly bacteria" in the large intestine. Another objection is that it has no roughage; elimination must be taken care of through the kidneys and liver — which overworks them over a period of years, and eventually can break them down entirely.

Good Teeth — Good Digestion

We found that those natural people who lived on rough and raw foods had the best teeth, and this is important to all good digestion. Those people who have lived on soft foods developed tooth decay and gum disorders. Dr. Price, studying the primitive peoples of the world, found that they were almost invariably free from carries.

In examining children in the Philippine Islands in years past, it was noted that almost ⅔ of them had perfect teeth. The defects in the remainder were so slight as to be almost undectable. It was found that the highlanders of Scotland had wonderful teeth because they lived on coarse and rough foods. Soft foods are usually poor in calcium (lime) and the vitamins and minerals the body must have. Hard, dry foods require vigorous use of jaw muscles and promote the flow of saliva. A liberal saliva flow and strong jaw muscles are both necessary for good teeth development. Greens, coarse vegetables, bran and acid fruits that stimulate the flow of saliva are all important means of promoting healthy teeth and gums. Our white sugar, fine flour breads and the hot and iced foods and drinks are most objectionable from the point of dental health and hygiene.

Benefits of Quickened Elimination

According to John Harvey Kellogg, Battle Creek Sanitarium, the person whose bowels move once a day usually has a motility period of 50 hours or more. When the bowels move thoroughly three times a day, the motility period is reduced to 16-24 hours. So foods that have a lot of fermentation, putrefaction, have the greatest chance of being absorbed by the body as toxins. Dr. Kellogg said that the breakfast residue is discharged some time between supper and bedtime; the dinner residue between breakfast the next morning and not later than soon after breakfast; the supper residue after breakfast or not later than soon after dinner the following day. When this normal motility rate is maintained, the time that the food residues remain in the body for breakfast will be from 13 to 15 hours, for dinner 17 to 20 hours, for supper 15 to 20 hours. This is the reason we should eat breakfast like a prince; lunch like a king and supper like a pauper.

When the solid body wastes are dismissed in a prompt regular manner, there is not time for putrefaction to take place. Germ life, waste material, abnormal and toxic bacteria, will not have the opportunity to develop. Harmful bacteria develop in the colon when there is a dormancy or reduced motility of the intestinal wall. When the bowel is clogged or choked up we hold three or four meals in the bowel and are in arrears to eliminate waste that has been breaking down in the bowel. The waste product of half a dozen or more meals packed into the colon undergo putrefaction and can poison the rest of the body by absorption through the intestinal walls into the bloodstream.

We have to encourage motility in the bowel when there is not enough roughage to carry waste materials along. It is well to guard against excessive and heavy carbohydrates and proteins where motility is concerned. Include a greater amount of nonputrefactive foods such as fruits and vegetables along with meals.

The bile represents the alkaline body elimination while the urine is the acid waste material. Like the colon waste, the kidney material must be kept moving along well. In order to keep a healthy body urea, uric acid and other waste by-products must be speedily and efficiently eliminated. Ammonia, indol, indican and other putrefactive products are eliminated through the kidneys.

Chapter 21

Refried carbohydrates: health menace

Sugar Intake

Professor John Yudkin said in *Lancet* that: "...there is reason to believe that some of the diseases of civilization—obesity, dental decay, myocardial infarction (heart disease) and diabetes—are at least in part caused by the fact that our diet...shows a persistently high intake of carbohydrates, much of which comes from sugar."

per year for the average 12- to 20-year-old, perhaps more. The per person average across the country is now up to 135 pounds per year, as compared with 4 pounds per year in the 1700s. Sugar is a calcium leach, upsetting the calcium-phosphorus balance in the body, destroying B vitamins and fostering disease-producing bacteria and fermentation in the colon. People here spend over $800 million on chewing gum each year, about 200 sticks per person; a stick of gum has a teaspoon of sugar in it, while sugarless gum contains sweeteners known to have toxic effects, possibly linked to cancer.

Raw sugar is little better. Kleen-raw is a trade name for refined sugar sprayed with molasses to color it brown. Cane and beet sugar must be heated for sugar formation. Yellow-D is highest in vitamins and minerals, Golden-C is second; both are low. Americans eat only one pound of honey per year on the average.

Carbohydrate Fermentation: Health Attacker

Henry C. Sherman, Ph.D., Professor of Food Chemistry at Columbia University, gives an important summary of food values: "Fruits, vegetables and milk are now seen to have higher food values than were hitherto known, because they serve (as meats, sweets and most fats do not) to make good the mineral and vitamin deficiencies of the bread-stuffs and other grain products."

To Professor Sherman's classification of valuable foods, add the lighter meats, lamb, fowl, and fresh fish; also, cheese, goat milk, and egg yolks. The latter foods replenish the nervous system, and healthy nerves are required for all bodily activity, including digestion.

Research has shown that a diet high in refined carbohydrates stunts growth in young males but not females, due to the decrease of growth hormone production in males.

If excess starch is eaten, even of whole-grain products, fermentation is likely; it is certain with refined starches. Few foods have been so robbed of nutrients in the refining procedures as white flour and sugar.

The average family uses sugar and starch to excess, partly because they are cheaper, but mainly because a craving or abnormal appetite is developed for these foods. Chemically they affect the body like alcohol — the more indulged in, the more craving is set up. Sugar and starch are a lethal combination because sugar hastens decay or fermentation and the whole meal is more or less decayed. We find these combinations in pies, cakes, cookies, puddings — taste-pleasing but unhealthy dishes. Add candy, soda pop and ice cream and a "still" or "vinegar works" is established in the human stomach. Acid is rapidly produced.

Refining Removes Vital Nutrients

Four-fifths of the vital elements in white flour have been removed by milling, leaving the carbon end.

Polished rice is not widely used in the Orient. However, here great quantities are consumed. In removing the little brown coat from unrefined rice, it is robbed of vitamins and minerals. It becomes a "dead" food and has been the cause of many beriberi outbreaks in such countries as the East Indies, Japan and the Philippines. According to reports, Filipino babies were fed an extract of rice polishings to counteract nerve disorders, and they recovered quickly.

In Labrador, beriberi afflicts the people who live almost exclusively on white bread and its products. Fruits and vegetables are rare in such a snowy, cold country.

Food budgeting has always been greatly stressed in the American kitchen. That should be a thing of the past when you learn that you pay the doctor in the long run if the proper foods aren't obtained.

According to Walter H. Eddy, Professor of Physiological Chemistry, Columbia University, prisoners in Java were experimented on with the rice diet. Out of 150,266 prisoners fed on white rice (polished), 4,201 developed beriberi, while from the 96,530 fed unpolished brown rice, only 9 were afflicted with the disease.

Most commercial cereals compare to polished rice

from the standpoint of nutrition. They simply serve as sugar carriers and cream bases. Some processed cereals are as much as 50% sugar, more than some candy bars. Sugar should not be used on any cereal because of fermentation.

Starchy foods are commonly eaten with fats or sweets — cream, butter, jam — giving the body a double dose of carbons. Most people have taken to this diet three times a day, or more often. One starch serving daily is adequate for the body's needs. It is as much as can be efficiently digested and burned as fuel. (Fewer times per week serve ill people better.)

It is much safer for the individual to eat a fruit breakfast, due to the lowered body vitality following the long night's fast. It is incapable of digesting heavy foods in most cases. Fruit may be eaten with honey and raw cream, or supplemented with cheese, raw milk (goat is best) or egg — raw yolk or soft boiled.

Any feeding regimen should recognize the laws of food combining and food compatibility. To digest starches the body requires an alkaline medium; with protein meals an acid medium is called for. The four most important considerations are:

1. Starch does not combine well with meat, cheese or egg yolk. (Egg whites are difficult to digest and should be used aerated only occasionally.)

2. Starch does not combine well with acid vegetables or acid fruit.

3. Starch doesn't combine well with cooked fruit or sugar.

4. Starch combines with dried fruit.

How Many Carbohydrates Do We Need?

What percentage of the normal diet should consist of heavy carbohydrates (starches and sugars)? Roughly 10 to 20 percent. One meal of starch in 24 hours will furnish enough heat for the average person in winter; in summer one every 36 to 48 hours will do. This estimates the average digestive capacity for carbon foods and the body's need for them.

Otto Carque, one of the noted food chemists of the world, had the following to say in *Vital Facts About Foods*. "We should always remember that we cannot extract vitamins and present them in separate form as body-building material, any more than we can dissolve an apple into its various elements and try to live on them. Vitamins, can only be active when they exist in combination with other elements in natural food."

He said in warning the public against artificial vitamin forms: "Consequently, all artificial preparations are more or less unbalanced simply because the fundamental knowledge necessary for their manufacture is entirely lacking. Only living plants can give us all the factors necessary for the maintenance of health."

Formidable Enemies: White Sugar & Flour

White flour and sugar are made into pastries and sweets, and the average child receives a huge quantity of them. This is why acidosis is so common among them. infect the tonsils. If the child is oxygen starved, adenoids infect the tonsils. If the child is oxygen starved adenoids may also develop. Inflammation will continue in the guise of intestinal "flu", colds, childhood diseases and tonsilitis. Intestinal inflammation is a result of fermented food. What the child needs is a change of diet, eliminating all stimulants, rich and foodless foods.

The "False" Sugar Prophets

The extensive advertising campaign labeling refined white sugar and its products favorably is seen in the following quotation from one of their supporters. This doctor stated: "Treat candy and other forms of sweets as food. Remember that they have a place in a well balanced diet just as all other varieties of food have. Pure candy is a safe and requisite food for children as well as for adults. It has one advantage over plain sugar in the diet in that it contains not only the sugar by variable amounts of other needed food elements, depending upon the type of candy selected. For instance, candies which contain nuts , milk, cream, cocoanut and chocolate or molasses afford a supply of mineral salts. All the vitamins are found in candy, which contains milk, raw fruits, butter and eggs."

We do not agree at all with such statements showing nutritional ignorance. Another paragraph by the same man continues: "Finally, I should like to set at rest any apprehension that may exist regarding the harmful effect of candy upon the teeth. There is no scientific basis for any such belief. Candy may collect around the teeth as other foodstuffs will, and this may be a factor in decay of the teeth. But the remedy in such a case is to keep the teeth clean rather than go without food. Sugar has nothing to do with the formation or preservation of the teeth."

Had you realized any physician anywhere in the world would hold such a view? White refined sugar is the greatest stimulant outside of drugs and alcohol. It depletes calcium from the body. It is the deadest of the "dead foods," so to speak. It floods the body with glucose, and promotes acid, "the grim reaper of death" in the body.

Sugar's Affinity for Calcium

Sugar has great affinity for lime (calcium) as stated by Dr. A.D. Birchard in *Philosophy of Health* Magazine. He explains that a thousand parts of water can dissolve one part of lime, but if sugar is added, the water can dissolve 35 times as much calcium. This accounts for the calcium starvation of the present civilized generations in heavy sugar consuming countries, especially America. Dr. Birchard says, "The human body, unless otherwise fortified by an abundance of unrefined food such as milk and whole grains, must be prepared when indulging in refined sugars and starches, to surrender calcium from its own tissues, depriving the growing bone structure of its building material, eating into teeth and handicapping all the normal functions of metabolism and natural immunity against disease."

Children & Calcium Deficiency

Dr. Philpots, of Melbourne, Australia, after 15 years working in the Children's Hospital says: "I have seen children at the age of 18 months to two years, with their teeth decayed down to the gums and badly abscessed, caused by incorrect diet. A complete lack of vitamin foods, extended over a period of years, produces sickly children with bad teeth.

Frailty indicates ill health and disease in children. Look for the cause in the diet. If it is there, remove it. Leg aches and other "growing pains" are often a sign of a calcium deficiency.

Candies, puddings, cakes, pies, fried foods, other pastries, gravies, pickles, jellies, preserves, sweetened fruit and drinks, devitalized and sweetened cereals and white flour products are among the taboo foods for raising healthy children. Such foods promote frailty and sickness.

Food which should be fed to growing children are:

1. Clean (raw) unpasteurized milk — generously fed. (Goat milk is the champion.)
2. All vegetables except dry beans and dry peas, which are difficult to digest.
3. Fresh fruits other than bananas (that have to be ripe and mellow).
4. Cooked fruits sweetened with honey, dried fruit or pure maple syrup.
5. Cottage cheese, buttermilk and clabbered milk..
6. Chicken, lamb and occasionally other meats except pork. (This does not apply to the vegetarian regimen.) (Children under seven are best without meat.)
7. Whole-grain bread with raw butter.
8. Whole-grain muffins or biscuits.
9. Whole-grain cereals to be eaten dry with honey and maple syrup. Revived dried fruit may be added.
10. Whole-grain cakes and cookies made with molasses, maple syrup and raw sugar. Serve only occasionally.

Is Bread the "Broken" Staff of Life?

It is tragically ironic that as the "affluent" nations grow richer their national health grows poorer. The so-called "primitive" peoples enjoy superior health in many countries. Infectious diseases used to be the principle causes of shorter life expectancies. They have been overcome but epidemics of chronic disease have taken their place. Today the life expectancy statistics are little improved. We face agonizing and torturing degenerative diseases at increasingly younger ages. Even some doctors are speaking of the 20 to 25 years of health abuse before the results begin to catch up. The Westernized nations have the most advanced medical science and the most disease.

In the U.S. diabetes is rising rapidly along with arthritis, ulcers, heart disease, sterility and cancer. One of the reasons is poor diet. When healthy rural people adopt the "civilized" diet of refined foods, they, too, start attracting the "civilized" diseases. The obvious junk foods are recognized, but what about the staples in our diets — pasteurized milk and its products, white sugar, white flour; the man-handled foods? What about the absence of natural, pure and whole foods? Bread, the staff of life, is a case to illustrate. The pale, fluffy, white cake-like bread so many Americans eat is a far cry from the heavy, wholesome, chewy whole grain breads that were once the staple for older societies.

From Whole Grains to Refining

A look back into history shows bread to have a special place in Egypt, Greece and Rome. But we find that this was made of whole grain crudely ground between millstones, retaining all the components. The bread resulting from this process had considerable roughage left in. It was symbolic of the simple rural life. The wealthier class during the Middle Ages preferred whiter flour made by sifting the coarse flour through simple sieves. Thus brown flour became known as the symbol of the lower classes.

Then came the Industrial Revolution and machine milling. By the beginning of the 19th century, white flour products were becoming common, even to the poor. Mass advertising campaigns praise the "purity" and "superiority" of white flour products as the Western standard of living rose.

The first part of the grain to be discarded was the bran, and some white flour authorities insisted it was an irritant to the digestive system. The next parts of the grain to go were the testa, aleurone and finally the germ . The aleurone is rich in protein, minerals and fatty substances, and the germ contains high protein, natural sugars and wheat berry. However, they contain nearly all the valuable nutrients. The part that remains (endosperm) is almost pure starch, high in gluten.

Is Refining an Improvement?

With the ushering in of the Industrial Age and growing populations, more wheat was urgently needed. The steel plow that turned up the virgin soil in America was invented in 1840 and, unfortunately, the soil was heavily used but not replenished and restored due to the call for increased wheat crops. Then came the refining mills, so grain shipping could be replaced by more economical flour shipping. The wheat germ and its oil was removed largely because it was likely to go rancid in long jouneys. And the opening up of the fertile U.S. prairies made world trade quite profitable. So, the germ was removed for commercial purposes.

The bran, or outer covering, was also removed to make the flour more white and "pure." Now these processes make for different kinds of bread. There is the white bread from white flour, brown bread from brown flour and bran (without the germ) and wholemeal bread from the brown flour, bran and germ. And Hindhede's bread in Denmark was wholemeal with extra bran for more roughage.

What Is Really Missing?

The germ is the living part of the grain that is intended to start the new plant and to make it grow. This oily part of the grain is for the sexual system of the animal or man who eats it. It strengthens the whole organism through revitalizing the reproductive system.

The bran covers the wheat berry to protect it as skin protects any living thing. It has more than a mechanical function, because the organism can regrow this "skin' when injured and store substances beneath it that are necessary and strengthening.

The remaining part of the grain is chiefly starch for feeding the infant plant. When this is finely ground into white powder it does not go rancid because it has become a "dead" food.

Chemically Treating White Flour

Before milling, the grains are treated with methyl bromide to prevent rancidity and spoiling in the bins. This chemical is retained to some extent by the grain, according to studies, along with the pesticide residues before harvesting. It is uncertain whether or not the methyl bromide contaminates milled flour. (*Cereal Chemistry*, Jan. 1971, p. 34 suggests that the chemical is retained in part by the grain.)

Aging must follow the grinding of the grain. Artificial aging is brought about by several chemicals. Chlorine dioxide, a bleaching and aging agent, is widely used today because it combines the two steps.

Is it ready for bread-making yet? No. After it is bleached, aged and sterilized it must be conditioned for use in sophisticated machinery. For this, calcium stearyl-2-lactylate and sodium stearyl fumarate are commonly used. For softening and emulsifiying to maintain freshness (or mask staleness) lecithin, polyoxyethylene monostearate, stearyl tartrate or partial glycerol esters are added.

But we find the bread could still beome stale over a long shelf period, so chemical staleness-inhibitors are needed. These include mono- and diglycerides, diacetytaric acid and esters to make the bread "look" fresh. They don't really keep it from spoiling; but they give that illusion. The poor quality of grain in the bread may be partly responsible for the staleness. (The crops are artificially stimulated to grow on depleted soils.)

The scientific journal *Die Starke*, Vol. 21, 1969, pp. 305-315 said that bread becomes stale because there has been a decrease in the amount of protein. A higher quality whole grain flour would not become so stale so readily.

Now For The Baking

The bread is still not ready for baking. Commercial bread doughs have the additions of mold and "rope" inhibitors and preservatives to keep black mold from appearing if the bread is not fresh. Main ingredients are calcium propionate and sodium propionate. Other additives that have been used are sodium diaceteate, bromates, persulphates, acid calcium phosphate, ammonium chloride, fungal amylases, bacterial proteases and others.

But we find out that more important than these chemical additives are the natural elements removed in the commercial milling process.

What Does "Enrichment" Mean?

"Enriching" white bread was introduced on a voluntary basis in 1941. From 1943 to 1946 it was made compulsory. Financially speaking it is beneficial to restore vitamins B-1, B-2, B-3 and iron. The iron is usually the inorganic ferric form the body can't assimilate, and the vitamins are synthetic.

The term "enrichment" is misleading. Milling robs 40% of the chromium, 30% of the choline, 50% of the pantothenic acid, 86% manganese, 16% selenium, 78% sodium, 60% calcium, 77% potassium, 85% magnesium, 71% phosphorus, 78% zinc, 76% iron, 89% cobalt, 77% vitamin B-1, 67% folic acid, most of the vitamin A, 80%

vitamin B-2, 81% vitamin B-3, 72% vitamin B-6, most vitamin D and 86% vitamin E. Much of the food value is in these substances. If a thief stole your car and left you a bicycle, would you consider yourself enriched?

How Does the Deficient Flour Effect You?

Many biochemical elements are necessary for proper human nutrition. It has been found that most heart attack patients lack chromium. Chickens and other research animals became sterile when manganese was taken from their diets. Rats and chickens without selenium showed liver deterioration. Zinc helps wounds heal faster and benefits the reproductive system. Cobalt has been used in anemia. Calcium is the "knitter" for bones, teeth and general body repair. Joints lose their youthfulness without sodium and when calcium is taken out of solution to deposit in joints. Joints and stomach become acid. Magnesium is the body relaxer and promotes good elimination. Phosphorus is required with calcium for the brain.

DNA and RNA manufacture and function depend on B-1, B-12 and folic acid in particular. Pantothenic acid is used to produce body hormones. Vitamin A is vital for good vision and clear skin. B-2 is important to good digestion and to the mucous membranes along with the nervous system. B-3 is needed for good digestion and calm nerves, too. It fights pellagra. B-6 aids in metabolizing and strengthens bones. Vitamin E is the heart and circulatory vitamin and the reproductive and anti-aging vitamin.

Whole grains contain the proper balance of these and other elements. This is why we approve of whole grain cereals. They have everything needed for reproducing life. They are the seeds of life.

We might mention that white rice is polished and white sugar is refined to the "pure" state, removing all vitamins and minerals. The dark molasses left from sugar refining, full of vitamins and minerals, is fed to livestock or used to make rum.

Are there any other reasons to avoid "pure" refined white foods?

Typical enriched white bread from the U.S. is made from 70% extracted flour — 30% of the wheat has been removed by milling. The part missing is the bran and germ — the parts containing the richest vitamins and mineral. A measured amount of three B Vitamins (B complex) are added to the flour in the form of synthetic vitamins, and some iron is added in the same manner. The foregoing was stated in an article from the *Journal of the American Dietetic Association*.

Following is a comparison of the mineral content of 100 grams of whole wheat flour and refined white flour. Note what is lost in the manufacturing process. There is a difference in natural and man-handled foods. Man has broken down and re-organized chemical balances.

	Whole Wheat Flour	White Flour
Potassium	453 milligrams	151 milligrams
Phosphorus	380 milligrams	127 milligrams
Magnesium	157 milligrams	30 milligrams
Calcium	51 milligrams	20 milligrams
Iron	5.1 milligrams	1.4 milligrams
Manganese	4.0 milligrams	.8 milligrams
Zinc	4.4 milligrams	1.9 milligrams
Copper	.4 milligrams	.2 milligrams

Whole wheat contains up to 1100 micrograms of pantothenic acid, a B-complex vitamin, while white flour has only 300. Wheat germ has up to 1,750 micrograms of pyridoxine. One hundred grams of white flour contains 1.7 milligrams of vitamin E. Following bleaching it may have as little as .9 milligrams. Whole grain flour contains up to 3.4 milligrams of Vitamin E.

Some minerals listed are considered "trace" minerals, but their importance is demonstrated elsewhere in this volume. They have proven their necessity in the human diet.

Essential amino acids, forms of proteins which must come from food, since the body can't manufacture them, are largely contained in the wheat germ. The amino acid lysine, one of the essential amino acids, is especially deficient in white flour. The *Journal* article states further that "serious consideration should be given to the advisability and feasibility of including such nutrients as lysine, vitamin B-6 (pyridoxine), vitamin B-12 and essential fatty acids in the enrichment formula." Still there is no mention of vitamin E. We all know its importance in the daily diet. It is vital to health.

Refined Vs. Unrefined Carbohydrates

The average American diet is grossly overloaded with refined carbohydrates; namely, refined white sugar and flour products. Fruits, sugars, white flour products such as pies, cakes, bread, rolls, donuts, refined cereals and grains are high in carbohydrates. Vegetables grown underground are unrefined starches (carbohydrates); such as potatoes (sweet and white), parsnips, beets, carrots, turnips; corn, large squashes, pumpkins and rice are others. Depend on unrefined carbohydrates and beware of all refined foods.

Chemically, a carbohydrate is made up of carbon hydrogen and oxygen atoms, and easily absorbed through the intestinal walls. The body utilizes starches for heat and energy along with sugars and fats. Excesses are stored as fat for future use. The digestion process breaks down carbohydrates into simple sugars absorbed directly into the blood stream. The digestion begins in the mouth to convert starch to usable sugars; saliva contains a digestive enzyme to start the process.

Cut down as much as possible on refined carbohydrates, known as "empty calorie" foods. Stay away from white sugar, candy, soft drinks. Use the natural unrefined starches from whole grains, fruits, vegetables, raw milk (goat milk preferred) and its products. Refined foods encourage unwanted pounds and inches. Many experts estimate the average daily calorie intake in the U.S. is 3,000 calories or more. This is way too high for most occupations. Research proves that the slim individual outlives his obese counterpart. If the diet consists of 10-15 percent protein calories and 25% fats the rest is carbohydrates or starches. If these are refined foods there is great potential for damage to health.

Many an infant is launched on the "sweet tooth" road by sugar in baby formulas and foods. It is known that a fat baby is not healthier than the lean infant.

One starch per day is a good idea—but make it an unrefined starch. Stay with steamed cereals such as cornmeal, brown rice, millet, rye, barley,, buckwheat, all whole (unrefined) grains, of course. Other good starches are baked potatoes, both white and sweet, winter squash (banana, hubbard, etc.), corn-on-the-cob, and the starchy vegetables. Use bread sparingly if you must eat it, and make your own whole grain breads for best results. Bake them well but slowly. Always chew starches thoroughly.

Did You Know That...?

According to the *Guinness Book of World Records* the Irish public consumes the largest total calories per day; the figure was 3,450 in 1968. (Compare it to the 1,200 of Los Viejos of Ecuador.)

American people drink more carbonated soft drinks than any other population. In 1972 the average was 30.3 gallons per capita. Cold juices, not in the total, came to only 5 gallons per person. Coffee consumption was at 35.6 gallons each and tea was 7.2 gallons per person. Coffee decreased that year and tea increased.

Iceland dwellers eat the largest total of refined sugar, averaging 5.29 ounces a day per person. (Present U.S. figures are probably rivaling that figure.)

The largest candy consumers are the British. Britain ate 7.8 ounces a week per person in 1971. Scotland's total was over 9 ounces alone in 1968.

What's in a *Soft* Drink?

Soda pop consumption almost doubled during the 1960s. Do you know what you're drinking? Most people don't. In 1973 the U.S. drank some 34.8 gallons per capita. According to researchers soft drinks are loaded with sugar, caffeine, phosphoric acid and many other chemical additives. What is its claim to fame? Its principal ingredient is water and that is what the human body needs most. A suggestion is to stay with "natural" water — not carbonated drinks with carbonic acid.

Those Hidden and Harmful Sugars

Where else does sugar hide? It is high in most canned fruits, soft drinks, many fruit juices, bread, ice cream, cereals and many foods you may not suspect. Look at the labels. Watch for dextrose, sucrose, corn syrup, etc. (Alcohol is made of empty carbohydrates, also.)

Canned fruit (1 serving)............ 3 teaspoons
Chocolate candy (2 oz.)............. 8 teaspoons
Chocolate cake (6 oz.)...............15 teaspoons
Fruit pie (1 slice)...................10 teaspoons
Gum (1 stick)...................... ½ teaspoon
Ice cream (2 scoops)............... 8 teaspoons
Jam, Jelly (1 Tablespoon)........... 3 teaspoons
Soft drinks (12 oz.)................. 8 teaspoons

Read labels and spot more hidden sugars such as dextrose, sucrose, maltose, etc.

Sugar: The Subtle Enemy Number One

Refined sugar is an invention of civilization and could be its ruin ultimately. It is now linked to hypoglycemia, diabetes, heart disease, arthritis, gout, hardening of the arteries, heart attacks, ulcers, tooth decay and general conditions of poor health, according to many researchers. It is the body's greatest calcium leach. It is the grim reaper of death due to its acid production and carbonic acid residue. It is a boon to the food manufacturing industry for its huge profits. It goes hand in hand with industrialized agriculture.

Why Is Sugar a Deadly Enemy?

Sugar as a continuous staple in the diet over a period of years causes a perpetual over-acid condition. Refined sugar is nothing but empty calories and in addition leaches minerals and vitamins from the body — notably calcium. In an effort to protect the blood from this acid condition, calcium is drawn from the bones and teeth causing decay and crumbling. Too much sugar eventually harms every organ and part of the body. It is first stored in the liver in the form of glycogen and later in the form of fatty acids in the least exercised parts of the body, such as the stomach, hips, buttocks, thighs. From there, where it is relatively harmless, it attacks the vital organs such as heart and kidneys. The nervous system, lymphatic and circulatory systems are invaded as well as the entire body tissue system. The brain, the body's most vital center is damaged eventually. Resistance to germs and bacteria and general impaired functioning are noted along with a loss of the valuable B-complex vitamins.

Research has proven that refined sugar consumption

leads to dental caries, obesity and major diseases such as heart ailments, diabetes and cancer. Sugar is only one of the causes, but a major one. Add refined white flour products and the other dead and devitalized foods making up the majority of American diets, and we are confronted with a life or death choice in nutrition. Which will it be?

Thirst and Hunger

Among the various metabolic centers in the brain there is also a hunger and thirst center. If the water content of the blood gets too low, the thirst center sends an impulse to the pharynx which contracts. It is this contraction of the pharnyx that we feel as a "dry throat" or as thirst. The hunger center is a brake mechanism. It brakes the activities of the stomach and intestine as long as the blood contains sufficient food. If the blood becomes deficient in nutritive materials, the inhibitory effect is relaxed and the intestines become active (one can hear rumbling in an empty stomach).

A feeling of hunger informs us that the blood lacks nutritive materials. Hunger is not particular; the body cries for any kind of fuel. Our appetite sees to it that we choose a mixed diet as required by the metabolism of the body. If a heap of barley is placed before a chicken, it eats with a great deal of appetite, and then stops. Is the chicken satisfied? No. It has only been satisfied with again begins to eat with appetite.

The digestive apparatus has two tasks. Its first task is to break down the large food molecules so they can be transported through the body. Large molecules cannot pass through the cell and tissue walls. Starch must be broken down to sugar, oil to soaps and protein to amino acids before they can pass through the cell walls. The second task of the digestive apparatus is to transform the foreign molecules of food into specifically human molecules.

The first phase of digestion takes place in the mouth. First of all, the food we eat must be thoroughly chewed. For total digestion and absorption, the particles must be small enough so that the chemicals and enzymes liberated in the intestinal tract can do their job properly. In the course of mechanical treatment of food, it is saturated with secretions of the salivary glands. The digestive glands do not wait until food has entered the body to begin functioning, but produce their secretions as soon as the brain is stimulated by sensory impressions (the odor or sight of food). The ferment (enzyme) contained in saliva is known as amylose, because it digests starch (amylum). It splits the large starch molecules into dextrins and these again into malt sugar. The food is then swallowed and passes through the esophagus into the stomach.

178

Chapter 22

Avoiding the "foodless food" traps

"We are what we eat; but we are also what we don't eat."

If man handles every morsel of food which goes into his mouth he will not be as complete as he should be and he will suffer accordingly. Our main purpose is to outline a better diet course. God never meant us to have to mend this human body so often or so drastically. He gave us the proper foods from his garden to live on. There can't be a godly thought left in a French fry, in white sugar or white flour. Some of us must be brave — stand up and be counted. Whose side are we on if we build bodies which have to be vaccinated? Bodies susceptible to disease? Why not live so that we are immune to disease? Where does health come from? Does it come from jogging? Does it come from Christian Science? Does it come from mental awareness? Does it come from meditation alone? Where it really comes from is nutrition.

At the dawning of a new day — a new age — someone should be forthcoming with new nutrition knowledge. Nutrition has more to do with health than any other single factor. Many try to disallow this philosophy. They say it doesn't matter that carcinogenic substances are entering the body. This is a cancer day. Who is attempting to prevent its ravages? I have no quarrels with manufacturers. I like Danish pastry, donuts, pasteurized cheeses — I like everything I shouldn't from a health standpoint. But I became sick of being sick many years ago. I had to leave it behind.

This work is not for the person who doesn't care — who doesn't want to build good health — who wants to buy his way through life, who wants to "put on the dog." This text isn't for the person who wants to show off, who wants to cover acne and other skin ailments with salves and ointments, who wants to treat constipation with laxatives. It isn't for the person who wants to go through life with a medicine chest full of drugs, who can't enjoy a meal because an alkalizer must follow. Many people buy insurance to take care of them when they become sick and disabled — most of them know they will be sick. They do nothing to prevent it.

The worst nutrition robbers are white flour and refined sugar. A U.S. Department of Agriculture survey disclosed that the annual per capita consumption of "empty calorie" foods totals 164 pounds: 102 lb. of table sugar, 88 lb. of white flour, 53 lb. refined fats and oils, 14 lb. corn sugar and 7 lb. white rice. In a news release, the National Macaroni Institute claimed that Americans eat 2 billion pounds of pasta a year, 40% spaghetti, 30%

macaroni, 20% egg noodles and 10% miscellaneous. (That's a lot of white flour.) The trend has been away from a few natural sweets, to refined sugar products in huge amounts; and from whole grain flours to bleached white flour. Sugar and white flour are the most common and detrimental products on the market. Their use has gained great prominence in a short century and a half. The human body makes changes and adaptations much slower in general. To enact such extreme dietary changes in such a short span of time is to invite the disaster and lowered vitality so many in our society now face. The human body is not capable of changing so fast even if it was beneficial. It takes many generations for the body to adapt to a radically new diet, yet we find that 10,000 new products entered the market in a recent year.

The popularity of refined white flour is due mainly to excellent advertising and top salesmanship. Whole grain flour doesn't have a very long shelf life; bugs and rodents get to it if at all possible. White flour, easy to transport and to store, became a status symbol from its first appearance for its purity and whiteness. People don't realize that it has been robbed of nutrients. Nature produced the proper food for man to start out with and to keep him in good health for a lifetime. Why should we interfere with the superior nutrition of Nature?

What Happens to Commercial Granola?

We find that cracking grains to roll or shred them destroys the life force of the seed (whole grain). The outer sheath is removed in processing and the inner nucleus is exposed to the air for oxidation. This destroys the life force, and the oils are dried out. As the oils are oxidized they become rancid. (Rancidity is actually the oxidation of oils.) Refrigerate the product to prolong the life force as much as possible. In the heating and toasting of granola the enzymes are destroyed and the rest of the oils dried out — the Vitamin E and lecithin are lost.

It is even popular now to puff granola! Muesli, a raw cereal, is far superior to toasted, roasted, crackled granolas, especially the commercially processed varieties. Granola is what we consider a "compromise" food — a step in the right direction, if it isn't puffed!

Alternatives to the Refined Starch Diet

Try to get away from using too many white flour products (wheat) in your diet. Cut down on starch by using artichoke and spinach noodles occasionally. Cut down on the number of starches — one good starch per day is enough — and make that unrefined.

If you insist on bread once in awhile — though I don't approve of it — have pumpernickel and rye bread that have been baked the slow way. Serve corn bread occasionally.

Yale University researchers found that artichokes make the food eaten after them tast better and sweeter. And the Jerusalem artichoke contains a quality carbohydrate called inuin. Serve them raw in salads or as a steamed vegetable starch. It is one of the best starches you can serve.

I believe in the whole grain steamed or vacuum cooked cereals most. The four best, of course, are rye, rice, millet and yellow cornmeal. You find they don't have to be served at breakfast. They should be steamed over very low heat to preserve the lecithin, vitamin E and other oils they contain. One reason I don't approve of bread is that most of it is baked quickly in high heat that destroys all the oils and makes it a bowel-binding food because it doesn't carry water or oils.

Serve other whole grain cereals, but remember that wheat and oats are high in gluten and fattening. But you could try others such as buckwheat, barley and wild rice.

And we find that some of the other starches to include are baked potatoes (white and sweet). Eat the skin and serve them with a mealy texture. Use the large squashes such as hubbard, acorn, banana and try pumpkin once in awhile. One of the most important food laws is to be sure you have a variety — and those in season.

We don't approve of "hotcakes," so to speak, but once in a while you could serve them made from buckwheat or cornmeal (yellow) and buttermilk. While I don't condone many baked goods, if you insist on having them occasionally have corn bread, rye muffins, date bread, banana bread, bran rolls etc. (The bran is extremely important to the intestinal tract.) Waffles are a little better than hotcakes because they are dextrinized. Dextrinization is the heating of the flour and changing it into an easier to digest starch. Starches have to be transformed from starch to sugar, and all the stages in between that we can put these foods through will help to make them easier to digest. However, most of the commercial products add to these foods — as in frying doughnuts. They can be dextrinized, but the grease (heated oil) that goes with them makes them highly indigestible. Toast is dextrinized. By the time it is burned, however, it becomes a carbon which is detrimental to the body; however; carbon can absorb gas and if this is a problem with intestinal disorders, non-gas producing foods are to the advantage. Use brown rice flour and rice polishings in baking since they are rich in vitamin B and silicon. Baking powder should be avoided, but when it is used make it a natural product. Yeast is a better leavening agent. (Try a variety of different flours to get away from too much wheat flour.)

Sprouted grains and seeds are one of the finest alternatives to the refined and high starch diet. Serve them daily in salads and other recipes. Eat them as snacks.

Preparing Starches for Best Digestion

We find out that starch digestion begins in the mouth with the enzyme ptyalin secreted in the saliva. It is important to chew starches to the liquid state. There's an art to properly preparing starch foods; if the individual has a weak digestive system for starches they should be slow cooked or steamed thoroughly, always extremely low heat. The way we prepare cereals (whole grain) they could be planted in the ground after cooking and they would still sprout. Slow cooked cereals are usually tolerated by most digestive systems. Sprouting is another excellent way of taking grains and seeds. (They provide extra bulk for the intestinal tract and silicon from the shaft.)

Refined white flour that has also been bleached has nothing much left but pure starch. Avoid it and its products and stay with the whole grains and their products. Include bran in bread recipes, for bulk. An easier to digest bread can be made from ⅓ unbleached flour and ⅔ whole grain flour; add bran and soy flour, if you wish, along with rice polishings. It should be slow baked.

Rice is a good starch (unpolished brown rice) and one of the finest foods for reducing. I don't go to the extreme with diet, however and I don't approve of the macrobiotic diet unless it is professionally supervised. The rice diet is the most common of this type. Rice can also bring down high blood pressure better than anything. They used to use rice back in the Carolinas for high blood pressure, hypertension and for that the rice diet is wonderful. The Chinese don't have high blood pressure with rice as the staple part of their diet. To prepare rice properly it should be steamed over very low heat in a tightly covered stainless steel vessel or vaccum cooked in a wide-mouthed thermos bottle.

I lived with people in Guatemala, Central America where you see these people working with yellow corn meal. Ninety percent of these peasants' diet is yellow corn. They don't have any trouble with bowel elimination! Yellow corn meal is the highest thing in magnesium that helps in constipation. Serve it once or twice a week, steamed as you would other cereals.

If you have a good bread once in a while it is not so bad for you. But bread today is rapidly baked and the Vitamin E and other oils are destroyed. When you take out the oils you take out the lubrication that it needs to go through the bowel and constipation results. Cereals do not cause this problem. The bread doesn't hold water so it dries up in the intestinal tract. So I believe in cereals as a starch. Once in awhile you can have bread. As we say, "It's not what you do once in a while that counts; it's what you do most of the time."

Never eat bread unless you have vegetables with it. Vegetables carry water; bread does not. I taught my children not to eat bread unless they also ate celery, green peppers or carrot sticks with it.

Vitamin A and carotene (pro-vitamin A) are both damaged by heating, only in the presence of oxygen. But we find out that most foods are cooked in the presence of oxygen. Foods should not be cooked in open vessels, stirred much during cooking nor pureed or mashed when hot. Steaming is the best way to cook since the steam largely replaces air. Add seasoning at the time of serving. DO NOT FRY FOODS.

Ascorbic acid is injured by heat when an alkali is present, such as by addition of soda when cooking. We find that soda also is detrimental to several B-complex vitamins; thus it should be avoided in cooking and baking when possible. Baking powder is not much better. Only the natural kind should be used, and only occasionally. Replace soda and baking powder in recipes with bakers' yeast.

Stimulants and Condiments

The average American guzzled nearly 27 gallons of soft drinks in a recent year, according to the National Soft Drink Association. Another report claimed Americans drank 400 bottles (or cans) of soda pop. According to nutrition experts Dr. Emery Thurston and Dr. U.D. Register, cola drinks are the worst of the "junk foods" because of the high sugar content and the caffeine, which is in a far more potent form than in coffee or tea.

Coffee, Tea and Cocoa

Americans average two cups of coffee a day, and coffee contains a stimulant named caffeine. It is a known poison capable of producing stimulation to the reflexes, extreme cramps, staggering walk and convulsions of a tetanic nature, if taken in large quantities. Two grains of caffeine can violently excite the blood and nervous system and also cause heart palpitation along with it. One cup of coffee has between 100 and 150 mg. of caffeine, about the same as a medical dose. Nondairy creamers, often used by diet-conscious coffee drinkers, are saturated fats which raise cholesterol levels in the blood.

Dr. H.H. Rusby, chemist and Dean of the College of the City of New York, says:

"Caffeine is a genuine poison both acute and chronic. . . If its use is persisted in, it results in per-

manent disorders of the heart function, and of the brain circulation. The 'coffee heart', like the 'tobacco heart', has become a familiar term with life insurance examiners, who know well the damaging effect of this heart poison. The effects of caffeine on blood pressure are well known. . . It is not unusual to see a blood pressure drop 20 to 40 points in cases of high blood pressure after the disuse of coffee."

Theobromine, closely related to caffeine, also has a similar harmful effect upon the body.

When tea was first introduced to England, about 1665, it was mistakenly eaten from bowls as if it were spinach. For many years after that disastrous experiment, it was considered a deadly drug; those selling it were thought disreputable. In England and Ireland and other countries where it is used so liberally, it is admitted to be a common cause of insanity.

Coffee was not known to the Romans and Greeks and we find it first with the people of Arabia at about the 15th century. Holland was introduced to it in the 17th century and it soon traveled to the West Indies.

J. Wood, M.D., had this to say about some 100 coffee and tea cases:

"Of these 100 cases, 20% complained of persistent dizziness; 19% of indigestion; 45% of headache; 20% of despondency; 19% of palpitation of the heart, and 15% of insomnia."

Caffeine, theobromine, theine and tannin are foreign substances to the body, so the body cannot use them as it would food. These toxins are picked up by the bloodstream and are carried to the heart, liver, kidneys, brain, pancreas, spleen and various glands and cells where it does damage to the entire body. A South Africa study showed that tea reduces assimilation of iron from vegetables like corn and rice.

Other Irritants

In one experiment a rabbit was fed a gram (7.5 grains) of pepper daily; in 27 days the test animal died. The liver was found to be hardened and the cells of it were degenerated. The kidneys were highly congested. Dr. A.D. Birchard says this of condiments:

"Man is the only animal that deliberately commits suicide by (slow) self poisoning. He is the only animal that spoils his food before he eats it. The average individual suffers constantly from chronic poisoning of some kind, due to the food he eats, either in wrong combination or in excessive amounts, or by adding to it injurious substances for the purpose of stimulating a jaded appetite.

"Instead of going without food until he has an appetite for the simplest of foods, he tries to whip up an appetite by the use of irritating and injurious condiments; or he doses himself with poisons of various sorts. He begins the day perhaps with a poison dose, in the form of coffee, to wake him up, or maybe a drink of whisky or bitters to get an appetite. Probably he finds an afternoon cup of tea necessary to cure after-dinner stupor and at night he needs a narcotic to put him to sleep, and in the morining a cathartic to move his bowels.

"With all his other poisonings, he deliberately spoils his food by putting into it toxic substances, which by the means of acid, biting, and burning flavors, which belong to the poison class and are unfit to be eaten. These substances used for their flavoring properties and having no food value, are known as condiments."

—Philosophy of Health

Salt, peper, mustard, vinegar, spices and other condiments cause stimulation, congestion and irritation of the stomach and bowels. Add tobacco and whiskey to the list of stimulants and condiments and don't stop there, by any means.

Dr. Hal Bieler, M.D., has this to say about salt: "In the days of our forefathers, salt solution was used as an embalming fluid. The ancient Egyptians used oils, spices, and salt in their mummy wrappings. Today we mummify the living with salad dressings made of mineral oils, spices, and salts. You can see any number of these mummies walking the streets. The dry skin, shrunken bodies and white hair bespeaks the hardened livers and sclerotic kidneys. I often wonder why it is necessary to embalm such bodies after they are dead."

"They are already 'pickled to the gills.'"
—Philosophy of Health

50 Billion "Cholesterol" Burgers a Year

We find that a study released in the late 1970s says Americans consume some fifty billion burgers each year, and the figures are rising rapidly. One leading burger chain plans to open a new outlet each day for the next ten years. The hamburger has become the symbol of the U.S. diet, it would seem. It is like the tortilla of Mexico and Italian spaghetti. It may be more American than apple pie.

The tremendous growth of fast food chains shows the popularity of the practice of eating out. Major fast-food chain franchises in the USA had a total advertising budget of $262,350,000 in a recent year, most of which went to TV ads. Typically, music, special effects, exaggerated excitement and parent approval are used as TV ad gimmicks to attract children to products. Consumer Reports magazine says that Americans eat a high percentage of meals out. The sales figures of the fast food chains in 1976 was a whopping $13 billion! The price of hamburger has been fairly stable, but we find that the flooding of the market with the over-produced beef has to come to an end. When this happens the fast food chains will fight for the hamburger supply. It has been estimated that the number of fast food outlets will rise from 28,000 to 43,000 by the time there is less beef on the market.

Almost half of the $25 billion a year Americans spend for beef goes for ground beef. How much beef do we eat? In 1935, each person consumed about 117 pounds per year. By 1970, we find that figure was 180 pounds per capita. That is quite an increase in just 40 years. The eating of fresh produce has dropped sharply during this time. Potato consumption, for example, has been reduced from 198 pounds a year each in 1910 to 91 pounds in 1970. That's quite a drop. Choice "steak" beef is fed corn, whole lower quality beef cattle are fattened on other grains because corn is more expensive. We are seeing more "grass fed" beef on the market.

Billions Spent on Junk Food

Americans spent over $130 billion on junk food in a recent year, up from $110 billion five years before. Snack foods alone, such as potato and corn chips, pretzels, crackers, etc. brought in $20 billion. Pickles came to over $123 million. In a typical year, Americans eat 20 billion hot dogs. This junk food leads to the $200 billion Americans spend annually on health care.

Top nutrition experts from the Institute of Nutritional Research, the Department of Nutrition at Loma Linda University, and other institutions rated the 10 worst junk foods as follows:

1. Cola and other "soft" drinks — because of the harm done by caffeine, sugar and acids in the body.

2. White flour products — because vital nutrients are removed and because chlorine dioxide, a potential toxin, is used to bleach flour.

3. Sweet rolls and pastry — because not only the white flour is bad, but sugar and fats are added, loading these items with calories.

4. Chocolate bars and candy — because of the high sugar content, fat, and frequent impurities and foreign material.

5. Fruit drinks — because they are 90% water, sugar and chemicals and only 10% fruit juice.

6. Heavily salted snack foods — because high salt increases water retention, leads to high blood pressure and contributes to obesity.

7. Hydrogenated fats (such as margarine and solid shortenings) — because they are high in calories, low in nutrition.

8. Potato chips — because of the lack of nutrients and salt.

9. Frozen desserts and ice cream — because most are

chemical concoctions lacking any nutritional value.

10. Imitation foods (dairy substitutes, instant breakfasts, etc.) — because they are fragmented foods, too incomplete to be of use to the body.

Have you stopped to think what these figures and trends mean to our health standard? We get to the place where this fried food is very high in fat and cholesterol-producing. It isn't a matter of the fat that's in meat, but that the high heat in frying will produce a cholesterol-forming deposit in the body. Heated oils have produced more cholesterol in this country than anything else.

Senate Committee Goals on U.S. Diet

We find that Congress is finally taking note of the fact that the U.S. average diet is detrimental to our health. It was Senator George McGovern (D-S.D.), who said, "The public is confused about what to eat to maximize health," in a report called "Dietary Goals for the United States." The report says the average diet since the turn of the century "may be as profoundly damaging to the nation's health as the widespread contagious diseases of the early part of this century."

The committee suggested a great increase in the complex carbohydrates — fruit, vegetables and grain products. They said that today's diet is at least 60 percent fat and sugar, rather than the fruit, vegetables and grains used at the turn of the century.

The blame for the "junk food" diet was partly laid on television advertising campaigns. This is not so pronounced in raw staples because product and brand name gimmicks aren't possible. Commercials and other ads don't say anything about the lack of nutritional value in their processed and convenience foods.

The committee set some general dietary goals for the American public: (we agree with some of them).

Unrefined carbohydrates should account for 55 to 60 percent of the diet rather than 46 percent now. (To this we would add that up to about 65 percent should be carbohydrate, but only fruits, vegetables and one unrefined starch per day; have about six vegetables and two fruits to make the balance. Leave all white flour products alone.)

Reduce sugar consumption that makes up 24 percent of the average diet to 15 percent. (We realize that there is enough sugar in fresh fruits, and carbohydrates and proteins are converted to sugar as needed by the body. Have no refined white sugar or foods that contain it. Limit sweeteners to Yellow-D sugar, honey, dried fruit, molasses, date sugar, maple sugar and other fruits.)

Reduce salt consumption, (currently 5 times the average per capita use in the rest of the world). Common table salt is heated excessively in processing and becomes inorganic and harmful to the body; cut down on salt and make that only evaporated sea salt; try vegetable broth powders to replace both salt and pepper.

Reduce cholesterol consumption by half, down to about 300 milligrams a day. (We believe the greatest cholesterol producer is in frying foods and heated oils in cooking generally. Don't heat oils and don't use oils that have been heated in processing; stay with cold-pressed oils and use moderately.)

Reduce fat intake from the average 42 percent to 30 percent. Saturated fat, the report said, is 16 percent of the diet and should drop to 10 percent. Polyunsaturated and monounsaturated fats that make up about 26 percent of the diet should be down to 20 percent. (We realize that there is enough fat in the balanced diet of one protein a day if you vary these and have nuts and nut butters, raw milk and dairy products, avocados, ripe olives and so forth. Oil and lemon dressings and others dressings with oil should be used only occasionally and those oils cold-pressed; if you use butter, add it after cooking and use it sparingly; avoid hydrogenated margarine.)

The report also suggested that we eat less meat and more poultry and fish. (We think meat, if you aren't vegetarian, should be held down to three or four times a week and one or two of those fish — white fish with fins and scales. Protein and starches are both over-sold in advertising. This is why we recommend only one protein and one starch a day. Most people have neglected raw foods and especially raw vegetable salads for most of their lives. Cooked food is robbed of much of its nutritional value. Make over 60 percent of your diet raw.) The report also said to substitute nonfat milk for whole milk. (We believe you should avoid pasteurized milk and its products entirely. Use raw milk and for the best health make that from goats. We agree that butterfat should be cut down, (but we don't approve of margarine). They attack the egg as cholesterol producing and we want that qualified. The frying of eggs and any food makes them cholesterol producing; if the egg yolk is taken raw or soft cooked, the lecithin, vitamin E and other brain and nerve elements are preserved; the white is best left alone except for having it aerated once in awhile.) They said to stay away from high sugar and salt foods. (We agree and we find that this should go for foods with white flour, chemical additives, preservatives, artificial coloring and flavoring; and of course all refined white sugar is out.)

The report also takes into consideration the fact that Congress should finance a "public education program" on television, in the schools and school cafeterias and the U.S. Department of Agriculture Extension Service. We support this suggestion.

Can Grocers Pass a Nutrition Quiz?

It is unfortunate that we must patronize health food stores for the most natural, pure and whole foods and nutritional guidance. Are grocery stores and supermarkets disease food stores? The lack of nutritional knowledge among grocers is quite pronounced. Yet, why shouldn't they be nutritionally aware enough to help consumers make better food choices?

Dr. Hazel Fox, Professor of Food and Nutrition at the University of Nebraska made a study of Nebraska grocers to see how educated they were in food and nutrition. Her coworker in the survey was a dietitian of the Veterans Administration Hospital in Grand Island, Polly Stansfield. Both independent grocers and managers of large supermarket chains were included.

Some of the following questions were in the questionaires. The answers are true or false. See how your own nutritional knowledge measures up.

1. One slice of bread has more calories than a 2-ounce portion of roast beef.

2. Gelatin desserts are good quality proteins.

3. Strawberries, cantaloupe and green peppers are good Vitamin C sources.

4. Milk and dairy products are among the best sources of calcium.

5. Corn oil margarine contains more polyunsaturated fatty acids than those of primarily hydrogenated vegetable oils.

6. Peanut and olive oils are not polyunsaturated oils and, thus, do not lower cholesterol.

7. Nondairy cream replacements are high in polyunsaturated fats.

8. The handling and storage of food in the grocery store influences the nutritional content.

9. Healthy, active children benefit by eating concentrated sweets, candy for example, for energy.

Compare your answers and score to those of the grocers.

1. FALSE. Only one of our four grocers answered it correctly.

2. FALSE. Almost none answered this question right.

3. TRUE. One third knew that these were good Vitamin C foods.

4. TRUE. Nearly all gave the correct answer.

5. TRUE. Fewer than half knew which margarines had the highest polyunsaturated fat levels.

6. TRUE. Not even one third said peanut and olive oils are not sources of polyunsaturates.

7. FALSE. Not even one out of four recognized that non-dairy creamers are not high in polyunsaturates.

8. TRUE. Over two-thirds knew this answer.

9. FALSE. Just one in three gave the correct answer.

The combined scores averaged out to the equivalent of a D on nutritional awareness. When asked where their dietary knowledge came from many said they had had some formal nutritional education — in high school or short courses. These took in seminars and conventions to "keep up to date." The majority felt that they had no responsibility in educating the public about nutrition. Nearly two-thirds mentioned that they had discussed nutrition with store patrons.

What do these findings mean to consumers? Their job is to sell food, though many grocers said they would rather sell nutritious foods. At least this positive observation is good. What would the answers of the food industry be? (Their largest profits are in the "convenience," packaged, highly processed and "junk foods.") America has become the land of the dollar foods — for profit, not nutrition.

The grocery market and the school cafeteria should be prepared to educate the public about good nutrition for optimal health. Some supermarket chains have expressed interest in giving more nutritional information on products with their brand names. At least this is a small step in the right direction.

"Weeds" and Flowers as Foods

It is interesting that many weeds and flowers are some of the best foods we have. They often grow wild and require no cultivation. For instance, the daylily has been a part of Chinese herbal remedy lore for many centuries. In one book called *Materia Medica,* we find a description of getting juice out of the root after pounding it to a mush and using the tender shoots boiled as a tea. The flower of the daylily is used even today as food. The flower is picked as it is opening and considered a gourmet delight. A biochemical analysis show it is made up of protein (a good percentage), minerals, low in fat, fiber roughage and is high in Vitamins A and B. The fresh buds might be higher still in these elements. The tender shoots can be steamed as you would any greens. Use the flowers, dried or fresh, in soups, salads, omelets and other dishes. Use them as you would sprouts.

This is just one example of the free food in Nature. There is a possibility that we are cheating ourselves out of a lot of very lovely things in life because we don't know all the things that are good to eat. We have never had to "scratch" for food like people in the past did. They had to "scratch" the earth and cultivate and hunt for themselves. Food wasn't available at the corner supermarket. They were tough and independent and resourceful people. They had to be. But we may turn again one of these days to the weeds and edible flowers. You might be surprised at how much they have to offer nutritionally. (And, they are organically grown.)

Truth never fears investigation.

Chapter 23

The answer to food faddism

Will The Real Faddist Please Stand Up

Science is dictating our lifestyles — our mental, physical and, in many cases, spiritual lives. If a person takes it upon himself to care for his own body, for his family's health, for his own well-being physically, he is considered an "oddball" or a "nut" who refuses to conform. In this way he is often left on his own, isolated from the mainstream of society and left to survive on his own "fringe benefits." More individuals every day are realizing that there is a better way to insure their family's nutritional needs. By spending extra time studying health and paying extra for the natural, pure and whole foods, insisting on the best for themselves and those they care about, the rewards in better health are realized. These people are, nevertheless, considered "food faddists," "quacks" and "health nuts." In the long run this unconventional minority will be the healthy group and have the last laugh.

Stamp Out Food Faddism

"Food faddism is indeed a serious problem, But we have to recognize that the guru of food faddism is not Adelle Davis, but "Betty Blocker." The true food faddists are not those who eat raw broccoli, wheat germ, and yogurt, but those who start the day on "Sugar Blinkies," gulp down bottle after bottle of soda pop, and snack on candy.

"Food faddism is promoted from birth. Sugar is a major ingredient in baby food desserts. Then come the artificially flavored and colored breakfast cereals loaded with sugar, followed by soda pop and hot dogs. Meat marbled with fat and alcoholic beverages dominate the diets of many middle-aged people. And, of course, white bread is standard fare throughout life.

"This diet — high in fat, sugar, cholesterol, and refined grains — is the prescription for illness; it can contribute to obesity, tooth decay, heart disease, intestinal cancer, and diabetes. And these diseases are, in fact, America's major health problems. So if any diet should be considered faddism, it is the standard one. Our far-out diet — almost 20 percent refined sugar and 45 percent fat — is new to human experience and foreign to all other animal life...

"It is incredible that people who eat a junk food diet constitute the norm, while individuals whose diets resemble those of our great-grandparents are labeled deviants..."

—(Editorial, Nutrition Action, Mar.-Apr., Science, May 16, 1975).

To quote a food industry pamphlet on foods and additives, "Protein is not the body's only nutritional requirement. But even adding the proper amounts of fat, carbohydrate and water to the diet is not enough. The vitamins and minerals, so often listed on food packages, are absolutely essential, not merely to health and growth, but to life itself. A well-balanced diet should contain all of the essential vitamins and minerals the body needs, but they are not always present in adequate amounts in everyone's diet. Food additives, in the form of vitamins and minerals, help insure that the body's needs for those substances are met."

To answer the claim, for example, one breakfast food was shown to be equal to five bowls of the natural cereal when the "proper" vitamins and minerals were added to their regular cereal. But they didn't tell you what those vitamins and minerals and other additives were made of. This is where the detriment comes to the body. The carcinogenic agents are found in the synthetic additives that are used today. Convenience foods are laboratory made foods with laboratory made chemicals added to them.

A newspaper columnist spoofed the dry breakfast cereal industry by suggesting that the box often has more nutritional value than what is inside it.

We recognize that the addition of iodine to the diet and to the water has helped many a person, especially in the Great Lakes area and the Pacific Northwest, where the soil lacked sufficient iodine. But in many cases we find they use this for criterion for all the other minerals that come out of a laboratory, and we also are finding today that these laboratory additives have a carcinogenic effect in the body. We have to be careful when we speak about the additives when we speak of what we place in the human laboratory (body).

We realize that foods containing a deleterious substance are to be considered unsafe even if the substance is required. But that is not the whole story. We find out they use such substances if they are necessary in good manufacturing practice and a "safe level" has been established. But I'm wondering if we are encountering a synthetic material that has side effects, cumulative effects, time bomb effects over a period of years. Manufacturers have used synthetic colors which should be certified as to their purity according to the Federal Food and Drug Administration (FDA). Yet, a "pure" substance can be "pure" poison. Those things marked pure aren't necessarily pure **foods.** The body is not meant to take anything into its realm but **pure food.** When they say all color additives are subject to constant scrutiny and retesting by both industry and the FDA, we find this is changing constantly. They are changing these colors after they have used them for years because they have found out the colors have caused many deleterious effects. To have a substance that is said to be safe by scientists does not mean it is safe by Nature.

The FDA and food companies are calling these foods safe, but that's speculation based on short-term testing. As the body changes, the acids in the body change; vitality goes down and we may develop a predisposition toward some disease simply as a result of the accumulated amount over a period of time. A better way to look at this is that if we could do without these substances, these additives, it would be to our advantage health-wise. Furthermore, we have to consider that these additives may have no effect whatsoever in many generations of mice and rats, which still does not prove they are harmless. Scientists are getting into gene testing today. And it's going to be sometime before we will recognize eventual consequences to health due to using these carcinogens, colors, flavors and so forth so promiscuously today. Many times they test a single additive to find the effects that it has on the test animal, not realizing that in actual life, countless additives mingle and accumulate in various combinations with the body chemistry. We have some 3,000 food additives on the market. If they added up all the effects of all these synthetic materials, it wouldn't take many years of our lives to accumulate conditions that would be "hazardous to our health."

For example, the oil of calimas is listed as a flavoring additive. The researchers say that to get an amount comparable to that which caused effects in rats, a person would have to drink 250 quarts of vermouth a day for life. But they never considered other additives such as flouride in the drinking water that can add to this to create detrimental effects.

Sixteen synthetic additives have been placed in white bread. After many years of holding these materials in our body as fatty acids, the liver eventually breaks down and/or the kidneys and other organs break down under the toxic load.

I'm in agreement with Nobel Prize winning geneticist, Professor Joshua Lederberg, when he says, "There is no way to insure that the risk of any substance or process is really zero. The reasonable question to ask is whether the benefits of a particular additive are commensurate with its possibly insidious risk to health." We can't afford to take any chance if in the end result that 250 bottles a day in 10 years would cause a cancer. This is a cancer day and we should begin to remove every single substance that has any possibility of producing cancer or any of our other diseases today or tomorrow.

"Dear General Foods,
What happens when I eat a preservative?"

In response to the question of the danger of preservatives in foods, (General Foods) states that "...an orange is a mixture of some 225 chemical compounds. And among these is — of all things — a preservative. It's called Citric Acid, and it's put there not by men but by nature." They go on to say, "The body can't use Food; it uses chemicals." What happens now is a process of picking and choosing. The chemicals that the body can use, it uses. Those it can't use, it eliminates." They explain that citric acid is subject to this choosing and is useful in the body's metabolism. "But the key point is: the body doesn't choose between chemicals based upon whether they have chemical-sounding or natural-sounding names...The digestive system does care about two things: what the chemical is, and how much of it is there."

They also say, "Salt is a chemical (sodium chloride). It's not only useful in diets, but both the sodium and chloride are essential to good nutrition. Too much salt, like too much of anything, can be harmful...." The organization that governs the use of preservatives and other food additives is the U.S. Food and Drug Administration. Its policy, as published in one of its own periodicals, is:

"FDA allows food additives to be used only if there is a practical certainty that no harm will result from their normal, allowed use over a lifetime. The permitted amounts of additives vary depending on the kind of food, the safety limits of the additive, and the least amount needed to accomplish the desired result."

"The FDA arrives at this amount as follows. It determines the maximum 'no-effect' level of an additive in test animals, and then prescribes an appropriate fraction of that amount (usually 1/100th) as the maximum allowed in a food for human use."

They conclude, "In short, our preservatives meet both government standards and General Foods standards. And those are very exacting standards indeed."

Under a 'Back to nature' heading they have this to day: "Sodium propionate, for example, is a chemical produced naturally in Swiss cheese during its making. It's used in baked goods such as cakes and breads to retard the growth of mold.

"We use sodium benzoate in Log Cabin (R) syrup to retard growth of molds and yeast. It's a compound formed from sodium and benzoic acid, both of which are found naturally in foods.

"Citric acid is an antioxidant — that is, it prevents browning of fresh food. You'll find it in citrus fruits such as lemons and oranges — and as a preservative in many foods, ours and others.

"But not all naturally occuring preservatives do the job, or else food would never go bad or spoil. So we use a variety of other preservatives, among them the antioxidant BHA which you'll find on the labels of many food products, ours and others. This preservative and all others we use, falls well within FDA regulations."

As a concluding thought in the article they say, "Our reasons for telling you all this are a mixture of helpfullness and pride in our products. The more you understand about food, the better off you'll be. And the more you understand about our foods, the better off we'll be."

Answering the "Today's Food land Additives" Booklet

Their statements:

"Scientists have learned that everything from our memories to our emotions has a chemical base. By changing the chemistry of the brain, they can manipulate the memories and emotions it stores. Similarly, by altering the chemistry of food, scientists can add to its nutritive value, extend its storage life, enhance its taste or otherwise change it from its original state."

Answer: No one has proved that chemical interference with the brain, usually via drugs, is either natural or harmless. Toxic substances can cause temporary euphoria, great pleasure, while destroying brain and nerve tissue. The fact that pleasure is produced means little in terms of health. Some additives have been proven harmful, and doubtless more will be in the future. The fact is, our nation faces a real health crisis, and we must consider the evidence against additives.

"If your morning platter of scrambled eggs carried a list of its chemical make-up, it would take you a good part of the morning to finish reading it. Consider the following partial catalogue: ovalbumin, conalbumin, ovomucoid, mucin, globulins, amino acids, lipovitellin, livetin, cholesterol, lecithin, lipids, butyric acid, acetic acid, lutein, zeaxanthine, phosphates..."

Answer: Yes, these are wonderful. But, they were put together by Nature's God, the Creator, not by men who don't know whether the future will show one or more of these ingredients to be toxic and disease producing. Man makes mistakes, regardless of intentions.

"There is no scientific reason to believe that naturally-occuring substances in foods are more or less safe than man-made substances," said Timothy Larkin, special assistant to the Commissioner of the U.S. Food & Drug Administration. Some chemicals in the "natural" foods we eat not only have no known nutritional benefits but are in fact highly toxic." For instance the potato contains a poison — solanine, (in the eyes and green peel).

Answer: Of course, Nature produces toxins, and we avoid those we know about. Similarly, we must make every effort to identify and avoid man-made foods and food additives which we have reason to believe have toxic effects in the body.

"A trace of cyanide lurks in apricot jam and a hint of arsenic in shrimp. Tiny amounts of known cancer-causing agents exist in kale, cabbage and charcoal-broiled steak."

Answer: There is no way to justify adding potentially carcinogenic substances to foods, no matter what we find in Nature or in natural foods. We find that a healthy body can process and eliminate many foreign substances, but there is a limit at which the body defences begin to breakdown and toxic substances are retained. Wisdom dictates that we avoid all possible harmful chemicals in foods when we have a choice.

"Why don't get sick from the 'poisons' we eat every day? Primarily because the levels we ingest are so low, they have no harmful effect. As the Renaissance physician Paracelsus put it, *Sola dosis facit venenum.* Only the dose makes a poison. In addition, the body has a number of its own chemical weapons to break down or otherwise render toxic substances harmless."

Answer: Illness and disease may take a long time to manifest after tissue irritation, toxic settlements and low grade infections begin. These go on at what doctors call the subclinical level — unidentifiable, invisible. Many additives will not likely cause problems for 10, 15, 20 years or so. Yes, the body, if it is healthy, will rid itself of many toxic or waste substances—but many Americans are not healthy.

"In the last 30 years the American life-style has changed radically. There are vastly more working women today...Tasty, nutritious meals are still planned, prepared and served by women — and men as well — who have spent the day working not in the kitchen, but in an office or factory. Those meals would be impossible without the additives that make convenience foods a reality."

Answer: Salads with one starch or one protein are just as easy to prepare and are for safer than packaged food with eternal shelf life.

"Additives, along with improved processing, packaging, and distribution, have made seasonal foods a year-round affair.

"What is perhaps most important is that foods keep far longer than they did in our parents' time.

"Additives are also used to provide essential vitamins and minerals to the diet, to add flavor to foods, to make foods easier to cook and to perform a host of other functions we now take for granted."

Answer:....It is not always wise to eat foods out of season. Over the thousands of years of man's history, seasonal foods were the only foods available until canning was developed, and man's body is adapted to seasonal foods. As for added vitamins and minerals, they are useless unless they are in a form the body can use.

Definition of Additives

"The 1958 Food Additives Amendment to the Food, Drug and Cosmetics Act defines food additives as 'any substance the intended use of which results or may reasonably be expected to result directly or indirectly in its becoming a component or otherwise affecting the characteristics of any food.'"

"Translated from the 'legalese', that means that food additives are components of food. That includes everything from sugar and salt to preservatives such as sodium propionate to vitamins such as ascorbic acid (Vitamin C) and to colorings such as carotene."

The FDA further divides additives into two categories — intentional or direct and indirect. "Intentional or direct additives...substances purposely or directly added to food. Indirect...not added directly to food, but which have migrated into it as a result of growing, processing or packaging."

Answer: We are not interested in technical definitions as much as safety and good nutrition. The fact is, when people avoid processed food and eat mostly natural fresh, whole and pure foods, the sick get well and the well feel better.

"A list of additives arranged in order of amounts consumed is headed by ones most familiar to us — sugar (sucrose), salt (sodium chloride) and corn sweeteners (corn syrup, dextrose and fructose). These three chemical compounds account for 93 percent by weight of all the food additives used in America. The next 5.5 percent is accounted for by 30 more additives. These include such common substances as yeast, citric acid (a natural component of lemons and oranges), baking soda, vegetable colors (such as the red from beets), mustard, pepper and the carbonated gas that gives soda its pop. The 1900 other direct and indirect additives on the list make up the balance of 1.5 percent.

"How much of those additives do we actually eat in a year? According to the President's Science Advisory Committee the amount of various food additives normally eaten in a year ranges from a high of 102 pounds per person of table sugar, to 15 pounds of salt and 13 pounds of dextrose, and 9.3 pounds for all the remaining additives together. The average use per person of each one of those remaining 1900 additives in a year is 0.08 of an ounce. And even this figure exaggerates the use of most additives. In fact, the use of fully half of those 1900 additives totals less than .000016 pound per year."

Answer: Just as trace elements and tiny amounts of vitamins can have a profound effect on the body, so can small amounts of additives when they interact with other additives and chemicals of the body itself. As for sugar, it should be classed as a drug, not a food. Sugar depletes the body of calcium and vitamins and contributes to endocrine imbalance. Salt contributes to hypertension, the predecessor of cardiovascular disease.

Additives for Nutritive Value

"These replace or add to foods the essential vitamins and minerals that are either partially lost through processing or may be lacking in the diet. They began to find their way into the U.S. food supply after World War I, when studies showed that some nutritional deficiencies existed in the country despite our abundant food supply."

Answer: It seems to me those deficiencies and others still exist, only worse. The disease statistics — especially chronic disease statistics — have increased as use of processed foods has increased. Of course, there are other causes — pollution, stress, drug abuse, alcohol, smoking, overworking, sexual depletion — but foods have the most effect on health.

"The term 'coal tar' derives from the early research in the dye-stuff industry which focussed on coal by-products to get coloring agents. Today the materials for food coloring are directly synthesized in such a pure form that their original source could not be identified. Synthetic dyes require certification, which means chemical testing and approving by the FDA."

Answer: "Pure" means nothing unless it goes with "whole and natural."

"And, by the year 2000, the U.S. Census Bureau says we must be prepared to feed at least 300 million people in America alone. Synthetic foods — particularly the 'analogs' which stand in for scarce animal proteins— will help in this monumental task. Additives will ensure that these new foods are as nutritious as their counterparts in nature and that they satisfy consumers' tastes."

Answer: My understanding of additives is different. I understand they are used to increase shelf life and profits by making the product more attractive to the potential consumer — visually and to the taste. I doubt if we will have enough doctors or hospitals to take care of those whose health breaks down if present rates of illness and disease continue to increase, and unless we have some miraculous breakthroughs in nutrition. The latter are more likely to come from edible algae, yeast and natural substances than laboratory concocted foods.

"Scientists have pointed out the upheaval which would result if food additives were removed from the American scene. Much of the food supply would literally halt within a few weeks.

"With only 5 percent of the U.S. population growing food for the remaining 95 prcent, much of the food would spoil before reaching the dinner table, if it weren't for additives."

Answer: That may be true, but we should be working toward the goal of supplying fresh, whole, natural, pure food just the same. If we had applied the same ingenuity to marketing fresh natural food as we have to developing and marketing processed foods, we would have a much healthier country.

"Today authorities estimate that enriched cereal products (other than breakfast cereals) provide 13 percent of the iron, 20 percent of the thiamine and 9 percent of the riboflavin in U.S. diets."

Answer:...The results are evident in the current health statistics published by government agencies and in the dropping achievement statistics of school children. We are losing the battle for health, and unless we turn back to Nature's ways we cannot expect improvement.

The "Philosophy of the Minimum"

"...the FDA uses what it calls the philosophy of the minimum. They sum it up as follows:

"A tolerance or limitation will not exceed the smallest amount needed, even though a higher tolerance may be safe.

"After determining the maximum amount that will not produce any undesirable effect on the most sensitive test animals use, 1/100 of that amount is normally the maximum allowed for use in foods by man."

"It is quite human to think of desired safety — in anything — in the realm of 100 percent only. Such 'perfection' is literally impossible."

"With absolute safety impossible, relative safety, consonant with the benefits and risks, is thus the goal... The final regulation for approval usually specifies the foods in which the compound may be used and the maximum quantities permitted.

"When consumers hear that a chemical is suspected of being toxic or hazardous, they really have no way of knowing whether the effect represents a true problem, or is the result of inadequate record-keeping, inappropriate test procedure or some other unknown variable."

Answer: There is more to this problem than meets the eye. An additive tested as "safe" on laboratory animals may react very differently in a human body in which dozens of other additives are circulating. Tests, to be valid, should simulate actual life conditions as closely as possible.

"And here is the paradox of poison. Even such a toxic substance as arsenic cannot be classed categorically as a poison, for in small quantities it has been and is being used as a therapeutic agent. Curare, the deadly poison of South American Indians, has found a role in medicine. And digitalis, the heart stimulant, has surely saved thousands more lives than it has ever threatened in its natural form as the poisonous plant we know as foxglove."

Answer: The fact that some toxic substances have some beneficial uses does not adequately address the problem of toxins and potential toxins in foods, nor does it justify adding unnatural substances to foods.

"The question is then, when does a substance become a poison? The answers...lie in what toxicologists call the Dose/Response Relationship. It states that every chemical — even those with the most toxic potentials — has a safe dosage level. This is called the 'no effect level.' A level of exposure at this dosage produces no effects because the body can isolate, excrete or change the chemical into a nontoxic form. Only when the level of exposure exceeds the body's capacity for defense will the effects begin to occur."

Answer: We must take into account long-term effects, "time-bomb" effects, and chemical interactions among the various additives. The basic problem is that substances are being introduced into bodies not equipped by Nature to handle them.

"In Japan and Iceland stomach cancer is the major killer. In America stomach cancer has dramatically decreased in recent years. But we hold the record for lung cancer and cancer of the large bowel or colon.

"Food has something to do with this universal human misery, as does virtually everything in our environment, but it is tragically unclear as to just what the relationships are.

"There is some evidence that nitrosamines (formed in the body) are capable of causing cancer in laboratory animals when given in large enough doses.

"The problem is that nitrosamines are not necessarily formed from the small amounts of nitrates ingested by eating cured meats. In addition, nitrosamines are not known to be responsible for cancer in humans.

"In eating natural foods like spinach, beets, radishes, eggplant, celery, lettuce, collards and turnip greens, we take in more nitrates than we get from cured meats and fish.

"The conflict then is between the very remote risk of cancer, against the very real and measurable risk of botulism, which can be prevented by the use of nitrates.

"It seems that most carcinogens must be activated by the host's metabolism. Accordingly some groups in the population have been identified as being more susceptible than others to exposure to carcinogens."

Answer: This simply evades the main issue, which is the responsibility food suppliers have to do everything in their power to provide clean, healthy food without adding preservatives or other materials which may be toxic to humans.

"...any substance the intended use of which results or may reasonably be expected to result directly or indirectly in its becoming a component or otherwise affecting the characteristics of any food." This makes it law to test substances that may be added to food, under the 1958 Food Additives Amendment to the Food, Drug and Cosmetic Act. Substances were classified as "Generally Recognized As Safe" or GRAS.

The Delaney Clause of 1958 specifies: "No additive shall be deemed to be safe if it is found, after tests which are appropriate for the evaluation of the safety of food additives, to induce cancer in man or animal."

Food industry officials charge that it goes far beyond the necessary safety standards. "...virtually any food could be banned under the provisions of the Delaney Clause. Even some common food and additives, including sugar and salt have been used at one time or another to stimulate cancers in laboratory animals. Moreover, as some scientists have pointed out, since every animal probably contains in its body at least a few molecules of every stable chemical in the environment, including carcinogens, nature herself could not obey the Delaney Clause."

Answer: I believe our country would benefit tremendously if sugar and salt were banned under the Delaney Clause, which is understandably inconvenient to the food industry. I approve the GRAS classification provisions as a step in the right direction.

The following problems are outlined by the FDA's chief counsel:

1) The scientific data available are seldom adequate to make a possible black-and-white judgment on the safety of any food or drug.

2) Even when a substantial collection of safety data does exist, the scientists seldom agree on its meaning and significance.

3) Even assuming there is adequate scientific data and agreement on its meaning, there appears to be no consensus on the degree of risk that would be acceptable with respect to the marketing of any food or drug.

4) Whatever the latest safety issue may be, there is enormous and continuing public pressure for the FDA to resolve it promptly and decisively.

5) Regardless of the decision, those who disagree with it will continue to vocally and emotionally pursue the matter through all available channels, while those who agree will remain silent."

I agree that the FDA is in an unenviable position in its role as watchdog over the food and drugs the American people ingest. Education and experience are the only long term solutions to resolving the controversies that arise over particular foods, additives, drugs, etc. Perhaps it takes a breakdown in national health to alert the people and the government to the fact that something must be seriously amiss in the lifestyle of the people. The whole point is that our survival as a people depends on learning from our mistakes, not repeating them endlessly.

What Is A Fear Of Food?

The moment a person lives on correct food as God made us to live, we find out that fears are all taken away. The only time I see health conscious people fearing foods is among those who want to combine their foods perfectly. These people have fears in their life. I think that we have to take out this fear, because fear is bad for digestion and everything else. Let us put it this way: Nature doesn't put food in perfect combinations, either. And I feel that I have to put food combinations at the bottom of the list. Now there are some people who should try to take care of their combinations. And, of course, I do believe that starches and proteins shouldn't be combined — especially the really heavy ones. We can't emphasize

too often that the crux of the philosophy is to live on NATURAL, PURE and WHOLE foods. The other basic "laws" should follow — and they are easy to follow.

60% raw food daily (or more)

80% alkaline and 20% acid foods

Proportion: 6 vegetables, 2 fruits, 1 starch, 1 protein daily

Variety: various foods and colors of foods

Avoid eating more than you need

Combinations: Separate proteins and starches

If we live on the natural foods and follow the foods as given in the Good Book such as white fish with fins and scales, we don't have to worry. For instance, when we talk about the shellfish we find that most of the ptomaine poisoning cases recorded in California come from shellfish. Invariably you find that when people go into different things they get into trouble. So, wipe out these fears about foods. We don't advocate extremes, but rather the middle path to accommodate the average person living in society.

People Who Fear Food

Picture yourself this morning in a coffee shop about to order breakfast. As you scan the menu, bacon and eggs with toast and coffee sure sounds good. But wait.

Eggs carry cholesterol, and isn't bacon loaded with preservatives? Better have a natural fiber cereal with nonfat milk instead. And make it whole wheat toast with margarine. Decaffeinated coffee too.

Sound familiar? It's an acute case of what researcher Ruth Gay calls "fear of food."

Gay, who recently devoted a year to the study of the history of diet, observes that supermarket shelves, "the great barometer of what America eats," are covered with the earthy broiwn and green colors of natural food.

Why this obsession with appearance and purity in our diets?

One reason, Gay suggests, is the rising concern over pollutants and chemical preservatives in what we eat. But Gay goes a little deeper. The science of nutrition is barely 50 years old, and many attitudes about food are still well seasoned with the "helpless analogies and dramatic conclusions" of 19th century medicine.

According to Gay, "with food and drink, we are still vulnerable to the claims of superstition." Good fads come dressed in pseudoscientific reasoning and peppered with medical terminology. But in essence, they appeal to the residue of magical thinking mixed with food. Thus, sour milk is thought to have healing properties, yogurt gives a long life, cornmeal and cheese help ward off decline.

White bread is shunned for the maore natural-colored wheat. Ironically, for most of European history, the rarer white bread was considered a sign of wealth and freedom. The peasant, munching on his black bread (which may have been more nutritious) case envious eyes on the nobleman's classy white loaf.

The modern pursuit of whole wheat and coarse pumpernickel has turned one of Europe's oldest food ideals upside down.

Gastronomical fears are overcome with one all-purpose incantation: "Whatever is natural or colored brown is good for us."

Gay does not suggest that contemporary concern with the quality of food is groundless, only that it is magnified and mystified by superstition and social custom.

Since 1956, per capita consumption of milk has not kept pace with the population growth. In 1962, the per capita consumption was 124 quarts in the nation (119 in California).

Milk consumption is influenced by income and number of children in the family. Milk consumption increases as education increases in low and middle income families. Households with higher total incomes and highest food expenses use the largest average quantity of milk.

Families with children consume greater quantities of milk. After the age of 6, more males than females drink milk. Amount used declines in young adulthood. Non-white families drink more evaporated milk, chocolate milk and buttermilk, but less fluid milk than whites. On the whole, more milk is used in summer than winter. Where vending machines are accessible, milk consumption goes up.

—Facts from "California Agriculture"

How to Substitute for White Sugar in Recipes

As honey should not be heated, it is better to use a good raw sugar, such as Yellow D or old-fashioned brown sugar instead of white sugar in quick breads, yeast breads, cookies, pies, cakes and other cooked desserts. Upon occasions, honey and molasses may also be used. When they are used instead of sugar, it is usually necessary to reduce the liquid called for in the recipe also. There is no exact rule that can be followed every time in substituting, but the following can be used as a guide. Some honey is thick, some thin; this alters the amount of liquid required. When mixing a cake, combine the honey with the liquid called for and adjusted in the recipe.

1/4 cup of honey for each cup of sugar. Reduce the liquid 1/4 to 1/2 cup less.

1/2 cup molasses for each cup of sugar. Reduce the liquid 1/4 cup less. Add 1/4 teaspoon baking soda per 1/2 cup of molasses.

Molasses is rich in vitamin B and also has very good protein value, is rich in iron. Honey is about 2-1/2 times sweeter than sugar, so in substituting this must be remembered. Also when using honey, it is well to try several kinds for taste and preference, since there are as many flavors of honey as there are flowers in the field.

Chapter 24

Fasting and elimination diets

Remedial Effects Of The Fast

Fasting can be a dangerous procedure unless it is under proper professional supervision. We recognize that animals in fasting have a sense of knowing when to eat again. But man has built such abnormal cravings from living on the culture of his parents and his ancestors and his upbringing, that the result is warped mental attitudes as to how he should go without food. So it is best to have proper supervision and guidance while fasting. During the fast, waste and morbid materials can be stirred up and eliminated so suddenly that this is alarming to many people. While I don't believe that correct fasting is harmful and I know it is the quickest way of getting well, it should not be taken to the extremes. It is a wonderful remedy, in full harmony with the philosophy of the cause of disease when properly used. It rids the body of harmful toxic materials that can lead to disease. Fasting is comparable to a sponge being squeezed, and during the fast a person may develop a fetid breath and a coated tongue. These reflect the foul condition of the digestive organs. The putrefying materials removed in fasting are the most important aspect. However, we must realize that fasting does not build a good body. It is through introducing the biochemical elements through the right foods that we rebuild and regenerate the body.

I don't advocate prolonged fasting in diabetes, in hypoglycemia and in tuberculosis. In fasting, many times the tubercular patient can break down the calcification that surrounds the seat of the old tubercular lesions in the lung structure. To break this open at a time when the patient may not be as young, strong and vital as needed to handle the crisis — is often not advisable. The diabetic can experience symptoms of convulsions and even coma can result. The hypoglycemia patient can run into serious mental disturbances with dangerous consequences even during a glucose tolerance test.

Proper fasting is probably one of the most potent and, incidentally, one of the cheapest of all the natural remedies. There is an erroneous idea that by going without food we lose our vitality and our energy, but the opposite is actually the effect usually experienced in fasting. It takes vital energy to get rid of toxic settlements and morbid waste materials through the body's elimination channels, but we save this necessary vital energy through refraining from digesting food, activity, exercise or even talking and walking.

Historical Notes On Fasting Practices

Mayor W.C. Gotshall, of the New York Athletic Club, in the official publication of that organization made some interesting historical observations about the art of fasting through the ages. He wrote an article called "Fasting for Efficiency" in which we find the following quotes.

"There is nothing new about fasting. Among the ancients it was recognized as a sovereign method of attaining and maintaining marked mental and physical efficiency. Socrates and Plato, two of the greatest Greek philosophers and teachers, fasted regularly for a period of ten days at a time. Pythagoras, another of the Greek philosophers, was also a regular faster, and before he took an examination at the University of Alexandria, fasted for forty days. He required his pupils to fast for forty days before they could enter his class . . . .

"Fasting at times mostly involuntary, was a regular practice of the ancient Jews. Moses fasted for forty days and forty nights. The vitality of this race is also well known as well as the longevity of the members. Many of the great Hebrew Prophets, such as Abraham, Isaac, Moses, Amos, Hosea, Rehoboam, Job, etc., lived to be over 120 years of age.

"Among the early Christians, fasting was among the rites of purification. Saul of Tarsus, St. Paul, fasted regularly. The remarkable spiritual, mental and physical ascendencies of St. Paul are familiar to all Christians. All of the Apostles fasted regularly. Today the Catholic Church still has its fast days."

Mark Twain's Account Of Fasting

The writer Mark Twain tells the story of the ship "Hornet" that burned at sea in 1866. The crew and single passenger survived by taking to a small open boat in mid-ocean. The passenger, Peter, had taken the voyage at the insistence of his doctor since he suffered from tuberculosis.

"The third mate told me in Honolulu that the 'portyghee' had lain in his hammock for months, raising his family of abscesses and feeding like a cannibal. We have seen that in spite of dreadful weather, deprivation of sleep, scorching, drenching and all manner of miseries, thirteen days of starvation 'wonderfully recovered' him. There were four sailors down sick when the ship was burned. Twenty-five days of pitiless starvation have followed and now we have this curious record: 'All the men are hearty and strong; even the ones that were down sick are well except poor Peter.'"

Peter, of course, was the tubercular consumptive passenger and the account says that he was improved. We see that the forced abstinence from food and juices can accomplish much healing in the body.

Fasting Hens For Health And Profit

A former patient of mine owns thousands of chickens in San Marcos, California. After learning fasting and proper dieting here at Hidden Valley Health Ranch, he applied what he learned in reverse of usual scientific test procedure. Doctors, chemists and scientists usually experiment first on animals, then try what they have learned on humans. This man found the good in fasting that could be used for human beings and went home and applied it to his chickens. Now he finds that in fasting his chickens when they molt, the molting season isn't as long. They give better egg production over the year when they are fasted occasionally. They are also in better health due to an occasional fast. Is this Nature working in reverse?

Many people would want to know how long he fasts them. It depends on the condition, season, time of year and so forth. Farmers are interested in getting the largest egg production they possibly can.

Dr. George Weger, of Redlands, California was quite successful in fasting his patients. He said, "The fast permits the body to free itself of the over-load of poisons previously stored in the tissues, and encourages the re-establishment of normal secretions, as well as nervous energy, to stimulate normal peristalsis."

He further states, "Real vital resistance is very rarely lowered by fasting. Temporary muscular weakness should not be classed as lowered vitality."

Doctors Who Know The Value Of Fasting

Dr. Arthur Vos was convinced that fasting was of great value. "In fasting all parts of the body, from the largest organ and the largest bone to the smallest fiber and the tiniest cell, give up their accumulations of debris which are then cast out of the body! No waste matter, no decay, no poison is omitted. All must go! In fact, so necessary is the method of fasting for the health of the body, so needful for the sanity of the mind and for the purity of the moral life, and so reluctant have people in general been to practice it that every religion on earth from the very

beginning of time has inculcated the practice of fasting in its ritualistic teachings."

Dr. Styles points out that the brain and nerves remain intact almost until the last in fasting. The blood holds near normal also. He gives a table to explain what takes place when one fasts.

Tissues Affected By Fasting

Fat	97%
Muscle	30%
Liver	56%
Spleen	63%
Blood	17%
Nerve centers	0%

Here we find that fasting is far different than starvation. We can starve on a full stomach if the food elements we need are not in that food.

Benefits Of Fasting One Day A Week

A one day a week vacation from food would be greatly beneficial to everyone. Of course, many people are against the idea, believing that they would starve. For those who fear going without food, it is not suggested, but anyone would improve his body by going on water or even juices a day a week. Water gives the body a total rest.

If fasting on juices, have them every three hours; make the day a restful experience, without work, especially heavy work. Don't travel, run around or engage in strenuous activity; avoid heavy mental and emotional strain also. Do something quiet that you enjoy most and do it calmly and leisurely.

Sunday is a good day of rest from foods. Why not try going on vegetable or fruit juices, better still water, a day each week? Give the chef a day off and the stomach a much needed holiday. The gesture will be appreciated and rewarding healthwise.

The Mechanics of Proper Fasting

The purpose of fasting is to allow the body a chance for complete rest — mentally, physically, psychologically, psychically. The state of rest allows greater energy, and vital forces are able to throw off toxic material and body poisons that accumulate over a period of time. Often the debris has built up over many years of wrong diets and incorrect living habits.

Many would ask how much water to drink during the water fast. The individual must be considered. Some are hydro types — they hold water — and must be careful not to add more water. Often in this case a half glass of water every two hours through the day is sufficient. Others need more water and can easily handle a glass every hour to flush the toxic wastes from the body. Distilled water may be used to pull toxins from the body, but it is not crucial.

Don't take water in large gulps; sip it slowly. Drink cool water but not ice cold. Take extra water if fasting during the hot summer due to extra water loss through perspiration.

Enemas should be taken for the first few days; then reduce these to every other day or every third or fourth day, depending on the duration of the fast.

Get maximum rest, along with mild exercise. Walk or hike on level ground. Avoid over-exerting the body, as this is a major consideration of the fast program.

Discontinue the use of ALL supplements during the fast.

Grape juice is good in catarrhal conditions, as a blood purifier and also acts as a laxative.

Correctly Breaking The Water Fast

The best way to break the water fast is to follow five, six or seven days on water with one to two days on juices — vegetable (preferred) or fruit. An eight-ounce glass every three hours is recommended. The enema should have been discontinued one or two days previously.

It is well to consider that some persons can't tolerate citrus pulp or juices well. These are not necessary in breaking the fast. The vegetable kingdom is as effective and perhaps easier on the digestive system. They can be diluted with water.

Following the juice phase, shredded steamed carrots the following morning is one of the finest bulk cleansers for the bowel and can be easily tolerated for breaking the fast. Steam or wilt the carrots for one to one-and-a-half minutes. This moves toxins along. Repeat the carrots for the noon meal. For dinner a small salad can be added.

Take juices at 10:00 a.m. and at 3:00 p.m. during this time.

Second Day: The morning meal may be juice (fruit) and fresh fruit. Have juice at 10:00 a.m. Vegetable juice and a small salad can be the noon meal. Take juice at 3:00 p.m. The evening meal can consist of one cooked (steamed) vegetable, juice (vegetable) and a salad.

Third Day: Proceed the same as for the day before, except for adding a second vegetable (steamed) at noon and also with the evening meal, if desired. Depending on personal choice, the breakfast can be a soft boiled (3-minute) egg or a tablespoon of nut or seed butter. Add this to the fresh fruit and juice for protein.

Fourth Day: Begin Dr. Jensen's Health and Harmony Diet (Ch. 38) without the starches.

Fifth Day: Add starches (one per day suggested).

Correctly Breaking The Juice Fast

After three to five days on juices — vegetable or fruit — the first meal (breakfast) should consist of shredded, wilted carrots. The second meal (lunch) can include fresh fruit and juices (fruit); make the third meal of the day salad and one steamed vegetable. Begin Dr. Jensen's Health and Harmony Diet the next day.

Break the seven-day juice fast in the same manner.

Notes On Longer Fast Periods

Consider taking juices for three days if the water fast is extended to 14 days. However, depending on the individual, this is not essential. The 21 day water fast should end with juices at least three days before any solid food (steamed carrots).

Discontinue enemas three to four days prior to eating solid food. Resuming natural bowel movements is very important.

Take NO supplements during the fasting period.

Other Menus For Breaking A Fast

Breakfast: Eight-ounces of any one of the following (warm or cool):

No. 1 — Diluted canned or fresh tomato juice.
No. 2 — Diluted orange juice (fresh) or grapefruit juice.
No. 3 — Raw skim milk or goat milk (preferred).
No. 4 — Cambric tea (half milk/half water).
No. 5 — Pineapple juice, lemon juice and water; equal parts.

Lunch: Same.
Dinner: Same.

The following menu may be taken for a few days, or even a week if the stomach has difficulty adjusting to the normal diet after a fast, or use the above menus. In cases of illness where fasting is not advised, or in chronic gastritis and hyperacidity with general enervation and stomach trouble or poor food digestion, it is useful. Also it can be used when there is trouble handling roughage and healing is needed.

Breakfast: 1 pint (or less) warm skimmed milk or goat milk, either raw.

Lunch: 1 pint warm skimmed milk or goat milk. (raw milk).

Dinner: 1 pint warm skimmed milk or goat milk. (raw) 3 oz. each pineapple juice and water (warm or cool).

Balance Elimination And Body Building

Elimination diets are numerous and many are good. Realize that diets must be supervised; harmonious living and balanced eating must be the aftermath of fasting and elimination. If you stayed on elimination diets all the time you would eventually be eliminated entirely. My diet is half building and half eliminating. You shouldn't need to fast so often when you are on my Health and Harmony Regimen.

Many times elimination diets call for enemas in the transition period and in entering into a new way of living. Often the effects of past diets call for enemas. Flaxseed tea is considered the best enema to use during these times.

Elimination and transition diets are important, but don't forget the building side of health; it must follow all transitions to a better way of health.

Three Day Transition Diet Procedure

First Day: Vegetable or fruit juice (not citrus) — one glass every two hours.

Second Day: Breakfast — steamed dried fruit (or revived), or fresh in season. 10:00 a.m. — glass of vegetable juice. Lunch — finely shredded carrots, steamed for three minutes. 3:00 — glass of vegetable juice. Dinner — finely shredded carrots, steamed three minutes, and one other cooked (steamed) vegetable.

Third Day: Breakfast — steamed dried fruit (or revived), or fresh fruit in season. 10:00 a.m. — glass of juice. Lunch — one cooked (steamed) vegetable, fruit or vegetable salad. 3:00 — glass of juice. Dinner — fruit or vegetable salad, one cooked (steamed) vegetable and cottage cheese (raw preferred).

Seven-Day Transition Diet

First Day: One glass of juice every three hours — one half pineapple juice, one half water. (If diabetic, take one half grapefruit juice, one half water.)

Second Day: Glass of all-carrot juice every two hours.

Third Day: Breakfast — steamed dried fruit (or revived), or fresh fruit in season. 10:00 a.m. — glass of vegetable juice. Lunch — finely shredded carrots, steamed three minutes. Raw fruit. 3:00 — glass of vegetable juice. Dinner — finely shredded carrots, steamed three minutes. Raw fruit.

Fourth Day: Breakfast — diced orange (or other fruit) and/or steamed dried apricots. 10:00 a.m. — juice of any kind, vegetable preferred. Lunch — one cooked vegetable, a fruit salad. 3:00 — juice of any kind, vegetable preferred. Dinner — vegetable salad, with sour cream or yogurt dressing, one cooked vegetable, a baked potato.

Fifth Day: Breakfast — diced orange (or other fruit) and/or steamed dried apricots (or revived). 10:00 a.m. — juice of any kind, vegetable preferred. Lunch — fruit salad, one cooked vegetable, yogurt. 3:00 — juice of any kind, vegetable preferred. Dinner — raw vegetable salad, cooked vegetable, cottage cheese (raw preferred).

Sixth Day: Same as fifth day, except add an egg yolk to breakfast menu (soft cooked).

Seventh Day: Health and Harmony diet.

We cannot nourish the soul or develop our gifts by negative thinking.

Eleven-Day Elimination Procedure

There are a great number of elimination procedures and many are excellent. Basically, the same results are obtained by most of them. The key is in allowing less food, having simpler foods and food combinations, more watery foods (water carriers) to make a transition in the cells of the body.

Persons in good health and those who have the average physical disorders can safely use the Eleven-Day Elimination Regime. However, patients who are feeble should not attempt the program without complete professional supervision. Tuberculosis sufferers should be especially careful and have the best supervision and assistance.

Modify the general outline to suit the individual, the time available and the medical history of the patient. Examples are: fruits, vegetables and broths for one day; fruit alone for one day; or one, two or three days of vegetables only.

Vegetable broths, lightly steamed vegetables and salads are a suggested routine for the average person new to this type of program. Citrus fruits are extremely harsh for most people.

A hot bath is beneficial each night during this routine. Enemas are recommended for the first four to five days; then discontinue for natural bowel movements. For the first three days, take only juices and water; distilled water is preferred. Grapefruit juice is also acceptable. Drink one eight-ounce glass of juice every four hours during the day. For the next two days, take fruit only — such as grapes, melons, tomatoes, peaches, pears, plums; use dried fruits such as figs, prunes, peaches, soaked overnight (revived) and baked apple.

Follow this procedure with six days of a citrus fruit breakfast. Any kind of fruit or fruit juice is allowed between meals. Lunch should consist of a salad made of three to six different vegetables and two cups of vital broth. Two or three steamed vegetables and two more cups of vital broth is suggested for the evening meal. If hungry, take fruit juice before retiring.

Serious and faithful obedience to the dietary outline is essential for anyone genuinely interested in better health. Eat enough but don't overeat.

Vital Broth

2 cups carrot tops
2 cups potato peelings (½-inch thick)
2 cups beet tops
2 cups celery tops
3 cups celery stalks
2 quarts distilled water
1/2 tsp vegetable seasoning
1 carrot and 1 onion for flavor (optional) grated or chopped

Finely chop all ingredients. Bring to a slow simmer and continue to simmer about 20 minutes. Strain the liquid and discard the solid residue.

When the above regime is completed, take up my Health and Harmony Regimen, (Ch. 38).

When To Use The Elimination Diet

The Eleven-Day Elimination Regime is valuable for the transition from the old way of living — "coffee and doughnuts," so to speak—to a healthy way of living. It is also an aid in the following conditions of the body:
    General body cleansing two or three times yearly;
    During a crisis period;
    For weight reduction;
    For stiff joints;
    For over-large hips;
    For constipation troubles.

Turnip Diet For Catarrhal Conditions

In cases of asthma, bronchitis trouble and any catarrhal or mucus conditions the turnip diet may be beneficial. Turnips are higher in vitamin A than carrots and have wonderful powers of cleansing and breaking up effects when used in an elimination diet for catarrh. Use the white turnip.

In this diet turnips may be prepared several ways — juice, greens, raw shredded, steamed or in a soup form. Turnip combinations add variety and may be used alone or with the regular balanced daily eating regimen. The turnip juice may be mixed with pineapple or apple juice to make it more palatable. Add raw turnips, shredded or diced, to salads with cut up dates or revived raisins.

Follow the turnip diet for periods from three days up to two months—depending on the circumstances of the ailment. A doctor should supervise the program.**

1. Three days on turnips alone is a good diet to begin with.
2. Three days a week for one month on nothing but turnips.
3. One month of nothing but turnip combinations.
4. Have just turnip juice mixed with other juices (alone).

It has been noted that during the time of Nazi concentration camps, the people who had to survive on nothing but turnips, had no asthma or other bronchial troubles. Those who had asthma when the ordeal began, had gotten over it by the time they were released.

SPECIAL NOTE

For those interested in one of the most effective cleansing regimens yet developed, my book, *Tissue Cleansing Through Bowel Management*, provides the details of lthe colema treatment program. This describes possibly the best way of removing the old mucus lining of the colon and cleaning out bowel pockets (diverticula).

Breaking A Fast

3 days of water. Follow that up with one day of juice, one glass every three hours. Regular diet next day—no starches in the day following regular diet.

5 to 7 days of water: two days of juices, one glass every three hours. First meal: sliced oranges, fresh soft fruit and juices. Second meal: shredded, slightly wilted, steamed carrots and juices. Third meal: salad and one cooked vegetable; juices at 10:00 and 3:00. Next day: regular diet; no starches. Next day: regular diet.

10 to 114 days of water: Two or three days: juices every three hours. Use variety; first juice should be one patient desires most. First meal: sliced oranges or soft, fresh fruit and juices. Second meal: shredded, slightly wilted carrots and juices. Third meal: shredded carrots again and one cooked vegetable. Next day: same. Add salad at noon; juices at 10:00 and 3:00. Third day: regular diet; no starches. Nut butters or seed butters added for lunch. Nut milk drink added to supper meal. Fourth day: regular diet; no starches. Fifty day: regular diet.

3 to 5 days of juices: First meal: sliced oranges or shredded, wilted carrots. Second meal: fresh fruit and juices. Third meal: salad and one cooked vegetable. Next day: regular diet.

7 days of juices: Same as above.

"The individual can affect his tooth substance by his diet, even after he has reached adult life."

—Dr. Percy E. Howe

Chapter 25

Normal weight for a healthy body

Normal Weight For A Healthy Body

In gaining and losing weight, remember it is more important to have a healthy body then to be a few pounds over or under the standard weight chart. No one knows what each individual's ideal weight should be. Weight charts are based on average weights of heavy and thin people of the same ages. But few are average. Heredity plays a decisive role in physical builds.

The correct way to determine if your body proportion is symmetrical is to study your body curves before a full length mirror. When they are smooth and well rounded, your weight is probably normal. However, when bulges protrude around hips or flabby tissue hangs from arms, health and weight are not good.

Work to normalize functions of every organ in the body and weight accordingly normalizes. The same applies to gaining weight. Begin a healthy living program assisting Nature in adjustments.

Losing Weight Correctly

Low-calorie foods are for reducing, leaving out the sweet flavorings and using grapefruit juice as a base, along with the pulp. The pulp neutralizes citric acid in the grapefruit, preventing the stirring up of body acids. Persons plagued with stomach disturbances should know this. Fresh fruits can safely be used in a reducing diet— peaches, pears and apples — particularly apples. Try liquefied fresh apples. Sectioned orange with pulp, a cut apple and a small amount of pineapple juice for a base is a tasty weight-reducing beverage.

Successful Weight Gaining

Combinations of dried fruit, banana and pineapple juice are excellent weight builders and as in-between-meal snacks. For intensified weight-building add flaxseed tea to the diet. Add it to liquefied fruit drinks such as bananas, dried peaches, prunes or raisins, along with a little soybean milk or a tablespoon of nut butter to disguise the flaxseed flavor. Use sweet bases such as apple juice concentrate, as opposed to citrus juices, for weight fortifying.

What Causes Obesity?

1. Lack of exercise.
2. Over-eating of all foods.
3. Over-eating of the high calorie foods.
4. Too much liquid, especially sugared and alcoholic stimulants.
5. Too much salt in the diet. Salt holds approximately 70 times its weight in body fluids.
6. Lack of vital minerals and vitamins necessary for proper glandular function.
7. Poor elimination.

Fattening Foods: Helpful & Harmful

Good fattening foods are nuts, avocados, dried fruits, honey, yellow corn, whole grains, (thermos cooked), cream. Detrimental fattening foods are: heavy denatured, refined starches such as white bread, white rice, pearled barley, white sugar, chocolate, concentrated oils, fatty meats.

Thinning Foods: Beneficial and Harmful

Beneficial reducing foods include citrus fruits (grapefruit and lemon best), pineapple, tropical fruits, berries, melons, vegetable juices, tomatoes, leafy vegetables, non-starchy vegetables, skim milk, whey, health teas such as strawberry, pine needle. Harmful thinning foods are spices, stimulating foods, mineral waters, coffee, tea, fried foods, pepper, prepared and embalmed foods, vinegar, patent medicines.

The Rounds Of Reducing

Follow the Eleven-Day Elimination Regimen. Weight loss from five to ten pounds is usually noted. Use rye crackers in place of bread, following the Balanced Daily Eating Regimen after the Elimination Regimen. If bread can't be omitted, eat only one slice per day. Drink no milk and dilute cream with water. Eat only fruit for breakfast and work for the healing crisis, or purification process. Leave the table a little hungry. Exercise daily and eat plenty of fruit and vegetable salads. At times glandular foods are beneficial in weight loss. Keep calories low.

The Angles Of Gaining

Go through a cleansing process by following the Eleven-Day Elimination Regimen. Follow with the Daily Food Regimen. Exercise at least one hour per day, in the open air. Cares and troubles must be dropped. Get plenty of sleep, especially by retiring before nine o'clock each night. Reduce mental strain and eyestrain. Use deep breathing exercises to calm nervous tendencies.

Weight-building meals are baked potatoes with butter, spinach and cooked vegetables, omelet, baked carrots, custard and salads. Drink half goat's milk and half water. Base the daily diet on the Balanced Daily Eating Regimen. Have cream on fruits in the morning. A combination of celery, apples and cottage cheese or goat's cheese is weight inducing; or celery, nuts and dried fruits such as raisins, dates, figs. In some cases, glandular foods should supplement regular meals.

Stomach And Bowel Inflammation

Flaxseed tea is a wonderful aid for stomach and bowel disturbances and inflammations. Mix it with raw vegetable juices or flavor with a little lemon. Prepare by boiling one pint of water to which 1 tablespoon flaxseed has been added for 6-7 minutes; strain off seeds. Discard the seeds. Flaxseed tea can also be used as an enema for excessive gas, colitis and bowel inflammation.

Plain water enemas are best for emptying the lower bowel. If inflammation is present, use enemas of flaxseed tea; use 1-½ pints to an enema. If the mixture is very thick, dilute with water. The knee-chest position is best in the average case. Often a change to a new diet will cause temporary disturbances, especially the addition of raw food and salads.

Rice water is mucilaginous as a drink, and pleasing to a weak or inflamed stomach.

Wheat Bran Tonic For Deficienies

Bran is one of the highest silicon foods. It has the elements needed for body tone and power most people lack. The 16 chemical elements are in a satisfactory proportion in bran water. Wheat is called the "staff of life," but we have broken that staff by the refining of the wheat grain. Bran was brought to my attention by Dr. McFerrin of Florida. Since that time I have had many marvelous successes with bran packs on various leg ailments such as eczema, pimples, boils and others. Great results have been attained by using it as a blood building tonic because of the high silicon content.

To get the best results, make a bran tonic according to the following directions: Bring one cup sifted bran in three cups cool water to boil. Don't allow to boil even a few seconds. Remove from heat and cool. Strain off the liquid into a quart canning jar and refrigerate overnight. The starch will settle to the bottom. Pour off very carefully without disturbing the starch; stop pouring the instant the starch begins to come up. Drink three or four cups liquid daily, half an hour prior to meals. Follow this program for two or three months for best results. A pinch of celery salt, garlic salt or vegetable broth powder may be added. Take either warm (not hot) or cool. Children will accept this drink if fruit juice concentrates are added to enhance the taste. The addition of liquid chlorophyll makes a nutritional drink. It is one of the outstanding bloodstream tonics.

The Method Of Measuring Calories

A calorie is the unit of measure determined by the heat it provides in food form. Do you know how they are measured? A device called the Bomb Calorimeter is used, It is made of two chambers, one inner and the other an outer chamber. The inner chamber is full of sugar (4 oz.) and the outer contains water. The sugar is set aflame and burned. The heat from the burning sugar is measured by degrees in the water. When 1 pound of water is raised 4 degrees Fahrenheit that is a unit of heat or a calorie. The degree of heat and amount of energy produced in the Calorimeter is about the same as that oxidized (burned) in the human body. For example, one ounce of protein is equal to 120 calories in the Calorimeter and 113 in the body.

What Are Your Calorie Requirements?

An adult needs about 1 calorie each hour for every 2.2 pounds of body weight; this decreases in advanced age. In the first year of life the largest number of calories is necessary for the body weight. It drops until puberty and rises at that time. Women require fewer calories than men, but the same nutrients, for the body metabolism. This may be because women have more "padding" or fatty tissue. During adult life calorie requirements are near constant, until old age. The infant below one year old needs more calories per body weight because the body processes are running at a higher speed than at any other time in life.

Cold climates call for more calories to maintain a uniform body temperature. When sufficient heat is not generated by the body, more is produced by the act of shivering; this converts energy to heat. Protein food digestion requires more calories. Calories from starch foods tend to collect in the body's inactive areas if not physically exercised off. It is stored to later be converted to energy as needed. The number of calories burned depends on the use of large muscles. Using smaller muscles does not utilize as much caloric energy. For example, fast typing does not use as many muscles, and as large muscles, as walking slowly.

Individual calorie requirements differ, especially according to the type of work done. Obese individuals don't need very many calories; physical laborers need more than mental workers. (Mental workers need more protein calories and physical workers require more starches.) A rule of thumb is to allow 16 calories a day for each pound of ideal body weight.

Calories Burned Per Hour For Various Activities

Activity	Per Pound Ideal Weight
Awake, Reclining	0.50
Bicycling	1.10
Bookbinding	1.10
Carpentry	1.56
Dancing	1.95
Dishwashing	0.93
Dressing & Undressing	0.81
Driving Car	0.88
Eating	0.65
Exercise, Light	1.10
Moderate	1.88
Strenous	2.90
Very Strenous	3.90
Ironing	0.93
Knitting	0.73
Laundering	1.05
Painting	1.56
Peeling Potatoes	0.75
Playing a Cello	0.98
a Piano	0.84
a Violin	0.77
Ping Pong	2.50
Reading Aloud	0.69
Running (5.7 m.p.h.)	3.70
Sawing Wood	3.12
Sewing by Hand	0.72
by Machine	0.74
Singing	0.79
Sitting Relaxed	0.65
Skating	2.10
Sleeping	0.43
Standing at Attention	0.74
Relaxed	0.69
Stone Working	2.60
Sweeping	1.09
Swimming	3.25
Tailoring	0.88
Typing Rapidly	0.91
Walking Downstairs	2.36
Slowly	1.30
Moderately Fast	1.95
Very Fast	4.22
Walking Upstairs	7.18
Writing	0.69
Vacuum Cleaning	1.78

How Much Should You Weigh Ideally?

Insurance figures show that the person ten to twenty pounds under the national average weight is much healthier. We believe that you should weigh the same as you did at about age 20 if you were in good health and the weight was normal. One method of reducing goes as follows: subtract your weight at age 20 from your weight at the present time. This is the amount you want to lose.

We find that to lose weight, the calorie count and amount of food has to be reduced. For each pound lost you have to burn up 3,500 calories. For instance, cut down 500 calories a day for each week and you can loose a pound a week. That would be 52 pounds a year.

Multiply your weight by 20 and subtract one percent for each year over age 20 to get the number of calories needed to stay at your present weight. The formula is: Calories to keep present weight = 20 x present weight minus one percent for each year after age 20.
Mathematics:

If you are 45 years old, weigh 146 pounds and you want to reduce to the 120 pounds you weighed at age 20, here's how to figure it.
Calories to maintain present weight:

45 yrs.	146 lb.	2920 cal.	2920 cal.
-20 yrs.	20	x25%	-730 cal.
25 yrs.	2920 cal./day	730 cal.	2190 cal.

1% x 25 yrs. = 25%

Your desired weight loss is 146 pounds minus 120 pounds or 26 pounds.

Decreasing your present calorie intake by 500 calories per day will net you a pound a week weight loss. To lose 26 pounds, then, will take 26 weeks if you eat 2190 calories less 500 calories or 1690 calories a day.

Calories to maintain weight at 120 pounds:

45 yrs.	120 lb.	2400 cal./day	2400 cal.
-20 yrs.	20	x25%	-600 cal.
25 yrs.	2400 cal./day	600 cal.	1800 cal.

1% x 25 yrs. = 25%

So, to maintain your weight at 120 pounds, you should stick to a diet of 1800 calories per day. If you wanted to reduce a little more slowly, you could simply use the 1800 calories per day guideline until you reached 120 pounds. That would take about 34 weeks instead of 26.

Scientific Basis Of Food Combining

It is well known that undigested or partly digested food in the intestinal tract can produce toxins and poisons for the tissues and cells of the body organs to take care of as best they can. They do this under great strain, especially to the organs of elimination. Such unpleasant symptoms as gas, indigestion, intestinal pain and disturbances may be the result. And we find that over a period of time organs can be damaged or diseased. We don't approve of the use of condiments, vinegar, alcohol, tobacco, carbonated beverages, common tea, coffee and very hot or very cold foods or drinks. These also retard the digestive functions in the body. Proper food combining ensures the most efficient digestion of foods and their best assimilation. Why use vital energy to try to digest improperly combined foods? Keep meals simple and properly combined for the best use of vital energy, and the most efficient metabolism. Be kind to your digestive organs and don't overwork them; help keep the bloodstream pure and waste products easily eliminated.

The Role Of Enzymes In Digestion

Digestion is made possible by the presence of enzymes, the body's catalysts that make biochemical processes take place. There are many different kinds of enzymes, and each has functions with certain kinds of foods. Without them we couldn't digest and assimilate foods. For instance, the first enzyme is ptyalin found in the saliva when starches are being chewed. However, if an acid food is eaten with it, the flow of ptyalin is stopped. This is why we don't recommend the combination of starches and acid fruits or subacid foods. Ptyalin converts starches into maltose for further digestion by the enzyme, Amylase, produced by the pancreas. This enzyme splits maltose into polysacharides (multiple sugars), and still more intestinal enzymes change these to simple sugars (mono- and di-saccharides) that are absorbed through the walls of the small intestine. The liver stores sugars for later use in the form of glycogen.

We find out that limited starch digestion takes place in the stomach until HCL (hydrochloric acid) secreted through the stomach walls stop it by saturation with an acid medium. (Starch digestion takes place in an alkaline medium). When the food mass passes into the duodenum it is again in an alkaline medium because it is neutralized by the secretion of bile from the liver along with more enzymes and cell salts and pancreas alkaline secretions. It is here that the food mass is converted to the materials in useable form the body can assimilate and metabolize.

Separate Proteins and Starches

Why aren't concentrated proteins and starches combined? They must have completely different digestive juices to prepare them for body assimilation, and this is why we suggest you don't take them at the same meal. While starch digestion begins in the mouth, protein digestion doesn't start until the food reaches the stomach. A generous flow of HCL is required for protein digestion because it must have an acid medium and this is where we find the protein-splitting enzyme pepsin. This enzyme partially digests the proteins by splitting them down into peptones. When the food mass reaches the small intestine it is met by the enzyme trypsin from the pancreas. This and other enzymes break down the peptones into polypeptides and amino acids that can be absorbed by the bloodstream through the villi in the intestinal wall. We know that amino acids are considered the building blocks of the body and eight of them are called "essential" because they can't be produced by the body; they must come from protein foods. Until they are needed as proteins the amino acids are stored in the liver.

Starches and other carbohydrates don't need the generous flow of HCL like proteins, just enough to emulsify the food mass. If starches and proteins are taken together the starches absorb much of the pepsin that should be used for protein digestion. So the proteins can't be properly broken down into peptones, and this results in putrefaction (proteins) and fermentation of starches. And we find out that gas is caused by this fermentation. Over a period of time ulcers can develop from this continuous indigestion; these in turn could lead to malignancies.

It is found, too, that sugars taken with proteins interfere with protein digestion; and only one protein should be taken at a meal to help avoid overeating.

To illustrate these correct and incorrect combinations, don't have meat (protein) and potatoes (starch) at the same meal. And we find, also, that double proteins such as both eggs and cheese should not be taken at the same meal. Meat and bread or eggs and potatoes are other incorrect combinations.

Using Concentrated Carbohydrates Alone

Examples of concentrated carbohydrates are grain foods, bananas, dates, raisins, figs and other dried fruits; potatoes, corn, some dried beans and peas, tubers and coconut. It is well to take only a single concentrated carbohydrate per meal to help prevent overeating. For instance, sweet potatoes and corn shouldn't be taken at the same meal. (We already mentioned that double or more proteins is not good at the same meal for the same reason.)

Limit Fats and Oils

Little stomach activity is necessary for the digestion of fats and oils, so the HCL flow is limited. They are noted for taking longer to digest than other foods. If they are combined with other foods, such as with proteins, the protein digestion is greatly slowed down and this can cause stomach discomfort. We don't advocate the use of very many fats and oils in the diet for these and other reasons.

Do's and Don'ts for Fruit Combining

We find that melons and berries should be taken alone, not combined with other fruits, for best digestion. And acid fruits don't combine well with sweet fruits (i.e., pineapple and dates). Fruits and vegetables should not be taken at the same meal. When sugars are taken alone they pass quickly through the stomach and digest in the small intestine, but if they are taken with proteins they are held up in the stomach and this encourages fermentation. Starches and sugars don't mix well because the saliva doesn't contain the ptyalin needed to begin starch digestion if sugar is present. In the warm, dark and moist stomach, the sugars can ferment if held too long, especially when they are eaten with starches. (For example, cereals sweetened with sugar or honey.)

Further Combining Notes

Juices and all juicy foods should be taken at the first of the meal, or juices at least 30 minutes before the meal. These foods leave the stomach quickly, unlike the concentrated foods. Liquids in the form of soups and juices or teas, and so forth tend to dilute the digestive juices and this slows down digestion. The small intestine is where the absorption of the food takes place, but if the food isn't properly combined in preparation for the stomach and intestine, trouble can result.

Remember to chew foods, to the liquid state, and salivate or chew even liquids. (For best results it is better to drink half an hour before meals or not to take liquids until about three hours after a meal.) And, too large a variety at a meal overworks the digestive system and can enervate the digestive organs eventually. Simple meals are best.

A Simple Guide To Carbohydrates

Carbohydrates are composed of sugars, starches and cellulose. The union of carbon with oxygen in the blood stream of the body produces heat through the process of oxidation.

The conversion of starches into sugars is initiated by the chewing process which mixes saliva with the starches. Without this process grain and cereal starches could not be assimilated. (This is the underlying reason for not recommending starches for babies before they have teeth for the chewing process.) Starch digestion is finalized in the intestinal tract.

For digestion ease, foods which contain the least percentage of carbohydrates are the easiest to assimilate. They also build a better and more chemically balanced body. The more delicate the health condition, the fewer carbohydrates we should eat.

Following is a percentage chart as a handy guide to the use of carbohydrates. Some of the foods listed are necessary to sustain life. Those in the 5% column are acceptable. In severe problem cases, select only carbohydrates from the 5% column. Heavy starches from the 20% column must be balanced at the same meal by 5% constituents.

Carbohydrate Chart

5 Percent
Artichokes
Asparagus
Broccoli
Beet Greens
Brussels Sprouts
Cabbage
Cauliflower
Celery
Cucumber
Dandelion
Eggplant
Endive
Leeks
Lettuce
Mushrooms
Okra
Radishes
Rhubarb
Sauerkraut
Sorrel
Sea Kelp
Spinach
String Beans (canned)
Swiss Chard
Tomatoes
Vegetable Marrow
Watercress

Fruit
Ripe Olives (20% Fat)
Grapefruit

Nuts
Butternuts
Pignolias

10 Percent
Beets
Carrots
Kohlrabi
Onions
Pumpkin
Squash
String Beans
Turnips

Fruit
Blackberries
Gooseberries
Lemons
Oranges
Peaches
Pineapple
Strawberries
Watermelon

Nuts
Black Walnuts
Brazil Nuts
Filberts
Hickory
Pecans

15 Percent
Green Peas
Lima Beans
Parsnips

Fruit
Apples
Apricots
Blueberries
Cherries
Currants
Huckleberries
Pears
Raspberries

Nuts
Almonds
Beechnuts
Walnuts (English)

20 Percent
Baked Beans

Bread
Brown Rice
Green Corn
Potatoes
Shell Beans
Lentils
Lima Beans
Navy Beans
Soybeans
Shredded Wheat
Whole Rye

Nuts
Chestnuts (40%)
Peanuts

Fruit
Bananas
Plums
Prunes

Acid-Alkaline Food Chart

Alkaline Fruits:

Apples and Cider	Loquats
Apricots	Mangoes
Avocados	Melons, all
Bananas, (speckled only)	Nectarines
Berries, (all)	Olives, sundried
Breadfruit	Oranges
Cactus	Papayas
Cantaloupe	Passion Fruit
Carob, pod only	Peaches
Cherimoyas	Pears
Cranberries**	Persimmons
Cherries	Pineapple, fresh if ripe
Citron	Plums**
Currants	Pomegranates
Dates	Pomelos
Figs	Prunes and Juice**
Grapes	Quince
Grapefruit	Raisins
Guavas	Sapotes
Kumquats	Tamarind
Lemons, ripe	Tangerines
Limes	Tomatoes

Applying The Acid/Alkaline Food Theory

Food chemistry is based on this chart philosophy. The dietary ratio should be 80 percent alkaline foods and 20 percent acid-forming foods. The acid-binding (alkaline) elements are calcium, potassium, sodium, magnesium and iron. Acid-forming elements are phosphorus, chlorine, sulfur, silicon, iodine (and also bromine).

Biochemistry divides foods, like the above/biochemical elements, into alkaline-forming (most fruits and vegetables) and acid-forming (most starches and proteins). We find that alkaline blood and an alkaline body promotes a good health and vigor. The acid state is associated with toxic and enervated body. Acids are the grim reapers of death. Body organs and glands depend on secretions that are alkaline for optimal health.

A good regimen to follow is to have two fruits a day, preferably at breakfast, six vegetables (or more with salads), a good protein and a good starch to maintain the 80/20 ratio. A raw salad with both the noon and evening meal is suggested. Have the starch at noon and the protein in the evening, or reverse them if you want.

We build acids mentally during the day when the sun is up, and the night is when the alkalinizing moon rises and we should rest. Negative thoughts and attitudes such as fear, hate, gossip, unhappiness, anger, selfishness, jealousy, lack of love build acids as do overwork and late hours and polluted areas. Rest, sleep, fresh air, sunshine, laughter, good companions, love, happiness, joy, satisfaction and a positive philosophy encourage alkalinity.

Acid Fruits

All preserved or jellied, canned, sugared, (dried) sulphured, glazed fruits; raw with sugar; bananas, if green tip; cranberries; olives: pickled, green.

(** denotes slightly acid)

Alkaline Vegetables
Artichokes
Asparagus, ripe
Bamboo shoots
Beans, green, lima, string, sprouts
Beets and tops
Broccoli
Cabbage, red and white
Carrots
Celery, entire
Cauliflower
Chard
Chayotes
Chickory
Chives
Collards
Cowslip
Cucumber
Dandelion greens
Dill
Dock, green

Dulse (sea lettuce)
Eggplant
Endive
Escarole
Garlic
Horseradish, fresh
Jerusalem Artichoke
Kale
Kohlrabi
Leek
Legumes, except peanuts & lentils
Lettuce and romaine
Mushrooms** (most varieties)
Okra
Onions
Oyster plant
Parsley
Parsnips
Peppers, green or red
Potatoes, (all varieties)
Pumpkin
Radish
Rhubarb (oxalic acid)
Rutabaga (swede)
Salsify
Sauerkraut (lemon only)
Sorrel
Soybeans**
Soybean extract
Spinach
Squash
Taro, baked
Turnips and tops
Water chestnut
Watercress

Acid Vegetables:
Artichokes
Asparagus tips, white
Beans, all dried
Brussel sprouts
Garbanzos
Lentils
Rhubarb

Alkaline Dairy Products:
Acidophilus culture
Buttermilk
Koumiss
Milk, raw (freshly drawn) (human), (goat, cow)
Whey
Yogurt
Clabbered Milk
Kefir

Acid Dairy Products:
Butter
Cheese, all
Cottage cheese
Cream
Ice Cream, ices
Sherbert
Custards
Milk: boiled, cooked or pasteurized, malted, dried, canned

Alkaline Flesh Foods:
None (bone and blood only are alkaline-forming)

Acid Flesh Foods:
All meat: red meat, fowl, fish
Beef tea
Shellfish
Gelatin
Gravies

Alkaline Cereal Grains:
Corn, green (1st 24 hours)

Acid Cereal Grains:
All flour products
Buckwheat
Barley
Breads, all varieties
Cakes
Corn, cornmeal, corn flakes, starch and hominy
Crackers, all
Doughnuts
Dumplings
Grapenuts
Macaroni and spaghetti
Noodles
Oatmeal
Pies and pastry
Rice
Rye crackers

Alkaline Miscellaneous:
Agar
Alfalfa products
Coffee substitutes
Ginger, dried, unsweetened
Honey
Kelp (edible)
Teas, unsweetened
Yeast cakes
Rest and sleep
Positive thoughts (joy, etc.)

Acid Miscellaneous:
All alcoholic beverages

Candy and confectionery
Cocoa and chocolate
Soda Pop
Coffee
Condiments as: Curry, Pepper, Salt, Spices, etc.
Dressings and thick sauces
Drugs and aspirin
Eggs, especially whites
Ginger, preserved
Jams and Jellies
Flavorings
Marmalades
Mayonnaise
Preservatives as:
  Benzoate
  Sulphur
  Vinegar
  Salt, brine
  Smoke
Sago (starch)
Sodawater
Tapioca (starch)
Tobacco, Juice, snuff, smoke
Vinegar
Lack of sleep
Overwork
Worry
Negative thoughts: fear, hate, misery
Late hours

Alkaline Nuts:
Almonds
Chestnuts, roasted
Coconut, fresh

Acid Nuts:
All nuts, especially roasted
Dried coconut
Peanuts

Neutral Foods:
Sugar, refined
Oils: olive, corn
  cotton seed, peanut,
  soy, sesame, etc.
Fats, and other greases

Easily Digested Foods

Vegetables
Artichokes
Asparagus
Beans, Tender String
Beet Greens
Beets, Tender
Broccoli

Butter Beans, Green
Cabbage, Chinese
Cabbage, Curly
Cabbage, Red
Cabbage, Savoy
Carrots, Tender
Cauliflower, Tender
Celery
Chard, Swiss
Chayote
Corn-on-the-Cob, Tender
Dandelion
Dwarf Nettles
Leek Leaves
Okra
Onions, Green

Peas, Tender Young
Rhubarb
Romaine
Spinach, Tender Garden
Spinach, New Zealand
Squash
Tomatoes, Ripe

Miscellaneous
Alfalfa Bud Salads
Almond Oil
Clover Blossom
Cod Liver Oil
Coconut Oil
Honey

Meat, Fish, Cheese & Eggs
Cheese, Roquefort
Clam Broth
Duck, Broiled Wild
Eggs, Omelet, cooked slightly
Fowl, Young Wild
Game, Young
Gizzard Broth
Goose
Lamb
Liver — from young animals
Oysters
Oyster Broth
Quail
Roe
Squab, Broiled
Shad
Tuna, Broiled
Whiting

Dairy Products
Goat Butter
Goat Buttermilk
Whey

Fruits And Vegetables
Apples, Custard
Apples, Baked
Apples, Mellow
Apples, Sun Dried
Apricots, Sweet Ripe
Avocado
Blueberries
Blueberry Juice
Brambleberries
Cherries, Black, Ripe
Cloudberries
Currants, Ripe Black

Currants, Zante
Elderberries
Figs, Fresh
Figs, Sun Dried
Fruit Pudding
Grapes
Lemon
Nectarines
Olives
Peaches, Ripe
Pears
Persimmons

Pineapple
Plums, Blue Damsons
Plums, Fresh
Prunes, Stewed Sweet
Prunes, Sun Dried

Pumpkin
Strawberries
Strawberries, Wild
Tangarines

Daily Requirements

We find that everyone needs the required amounts of liquids, enzymes, minerals, vitamins, proteins, carbohydrates and fats. Make sure you get the balanced requirements.

1. Several eight-ounce glasses of liquids including water, fruit and vegetable juices; raw milk and cultured milk products are liquids and also foods.

2. Supplements of wheat germ, dulse, rice polishings, flaxseed, sesame and sunflower meal. (A teaspoon per serving; ¼ tsp. dulse).

3. Two servings of fruit (best served at breakfast).

4. Six servings of vegetables; (include some in raw salads at noon and with the evening meal). Use many green leafy vegetables and tops. Serve one root vegetable and a top vegetable together.

5. One serving of a good starch such as steamed millet, rice, rye, yellow cornmeal; baked potatoes, baked winter squashes, etc.

6. One serving of a good protein such as cheese, eggs, fish, meat (if not vegetarian); soy beans, nut or seed butters, lentils, garbanzos, tofu, vegetable protein.

7. Raw salads count in the vegetable total, but more vegetables than the suggested six are a good practice. Have a raw salad with the noon and evening meals.

Minerals

Calcium: Milk, Greens, Cereals, Cheese, Egg yolk, Broccoli.

Sodium: Whey, Celery, Romaine, Watermelon, Asparagus, Goat Milk, Okra, Dates.

Magnesium: Nuts, Green Vegetables, Celery, Figs, Apples, Lemons, Yellow Cornmeal.

Copper: Almonds, Beans, Peas, Green Vegetables, Prunes, Raisins, Liver, Grains.

Iodine: Kelp, Green Vegetables, Garlic, Pineapple, Dulse, Pears, Seafoods.

Phosphorus: Milk, Cheese, Meat, Fish, Fowl, Nuts, Egg Yolk, Grains.

Potassium: Dried Fruits, Legumes, Dried Beans, Nuts, Lean Meats, Cereals, Vegetables, Dried Olives.

Sulfur: Cauliflower, Cabbage, Spinach, Brussels, Sprouts, Onions, Peas, Egg Yolk, Barley, Carrots, Dried Figs, Eggs, Legumes, Oats. Dates, Beans.

Chlorine: Goat Milk, Watercress, Avocado, Cabbage, Coconuts, Tomatoes, Celery, Fish, Dates.

Iron: Apricots, Peaches, Bananas, Blackstrap Molasses, Prunes, Raisins, Beets, Greens, Egg Yolks, Figs.

Manganese: Green Vegetables, Beets, Citrus, Bran, Peas, Kelp, Dulse, Egg Yolks.

Cobalt: Liver, Green Leafy Vegetables, Almonds.

Zinc: Wheat Bran, Germ, Seeds, Milk, Eggs, Onions, Oysters, Green Vegetables, Nuts.

Fluorine: Milk, Cheese, Carrots, Garlic, Green Vegetables, Almonds, Beet tops.

Silicon: Barley, Apples, Grapes, Dates, Rice Polishings, Parsnips, Nuts, Seeds.

Vitamins

A: Milk, Eggs, Yellow Fruits, Green and Yellow Vegetables, Tomatoes, Butter

B_1: Brewer's Yeast, Wheat Germ, Liver, Heart, Kidneys, Legumes, Whole Wheat.

B_2: Milk, Cheese, Brewer's Yeast, Organ Meats, Lean Meats, Green, Leafy Vegetables.

B_3: Whole Grains, Meats, Fish, Fowl, B. Yeast, Potatoes, Legumes, Peanuts.

B_6: Whole Wheat, Brewer's Yeast, Blackstrap Molasses, Whole Bran/Germ.

Pantothenic Acid: Brewer's Yeast, Liver,

Folic Acid: Chicken, Beef/Lamb Liver, Legumes, Spinach, Asparagus.

B_{12}: Beef Liver, Kidney, Leg of Lamb, Ham, Bananas, Peanuts, Kelp.

Choline: Egg Yolk, Liver, Beef Brains, Kidney, Wheat Germ.

Biotin: Peanuts, Beef, Liver, Eggs, Dried Peas, Beans, Cauliflower

Inositol: Brewer's Yeast, Wheat Germ, Dried Peas, Beef Heart, Oranges, Peanuts.

C: Citrus, Berries, Cabbage Family, Asparagus, Chili Peppers, Melons.

D: Fish Liver Oils, Egg Yolk, Milk, Butter, Sprouted Seeds, Sunflower Seeds.

E: Cold-pressed Vegetable Oils, Sprouted Seeds, Green, Leafy Vegetables, Eggs, Nuts, Grains.

K: Green, Leafy Vegetables, Tomatoes, Cauliflower, Egg Yolks, Soybean Oil, Liver.

Proteins

Meat
Poultry
Fish
Seafood
Gelatin
Seeds
Legumes
Soybeans
Eggs
Yogurt
Cultured Milks
Cheese
Butter
Cottage Cheese
Goat Milk
Nuts

*Carl C. Pfeiffer, MD, calls sulphur "the forgotten essential element"
because of its general neglect by nutritionists and the average person,
despite the fact that we need about 850 mg of this element per day.*

Onion Pack

*Slice 1 large onion in small frying pan and cover tightly; use no fat or water.
Cook until onion is hot. It will simmer in its own juice.*

*Place hot onion slices in muslin bag or cloth and fold to cover area doctor
recommends. Make another pan of onions and have ready to replace first pack
when it becomes cool (in about 5 minutes). Put first onion slices in pan and
reheat. Change packs as soon as they become cool. Continue for 1/2 hour a day
or as directed by doctor.*

HEALTH HINTS

*There are various remedies besides diet
which can be used, such as exercise, breathing,
water treatments, etc. Here are a few unusual
ones that may be of interest.*

*Many times we can relieve pain by using a
comb in the palm of our hand, with the teeth of
the comb held firmly against the tips of the
fingers.*

*A golf ball, because of its curve, is a fine
thing to be used for exercising the metatarsal
arch, working the foot back and forth on it.*

*Many times, for lower back pains, learn to
walk with the soles of the feet turned in for
relief.*

*For car sickness, manipulating the web of
the hand with the thumb and forefinger for 4 or
5 minutes will sometimes give relief,
alternating with each hand.*

*There are various techniques for driving
blood into different parts of the body. This
may be accomplished through breathing in the
full breath and applying pressure to a specific
organ or area, relaxing while exhaling.
Inhaling the full breath and holding drives
blood into the liver area. Quick inhalations
and slow exhalations are good for the body.*

*Many times, a joint problem may be
relieved by wrapping the area in a towel wrung
out of cold water, then wrapping with a dry
towel to hold in the moisture. This will help
relieve stiffness and pain.*

*Wring out a small hand towel in very cold
water and fold into a square large enough to
cover the abdomen. Wrap and pin a large
towel snugly around back and abdomen to
hold the small towel in place and to keep the air
from coming in around the edges. This top
towel is dry, and it is important that it be
wrapped so the air does not enter. Leave this
on for one or two hours daily or all night,
according to doctor's instructions.*

*There is a five-day elimination and
cleansing regimen, as follows: 3 days juices,
any kind, no citrus, one tablespoon of bulk 5
times daily. Next two days fruits and juices and
vegetables only; bulk 3 times daily. Sixth day
regular health and eating regimen and bulk 3
times daily until otherwise ordered. You may
drink water any time. Enemas daily. Bulk can
be purchased at any health food store.*

206

I would rather have one little rose
From the garden of a friend,
Than to have the choicest flowers
When my stay on earth must end.
I would rather have one pleasant word
In kindness said to me,
Than flattery when my heart is still
And life has ceased to be.

I would rather have a loving smile
From the friends I know are true,
Than tears shed 'round my casket
When this world I've bid adieu.
Bring me all your flowers today
Whether pink, or white, or red,
I'd rather have one blossom now
Than a truckload when I'm dead.

207

Chapter 26

Vegetarianism — the pros and cons

(The Philosophy Of Vegetarianism)

Some people think they can become vegetarians by simply giving up meat. True vegetarianism demands mental, moral and spiritual philosophy which harmonizes with the laws of Nature and God. From a moral, economic, spiritual scientific, ethical, political and health standpoint, vegetarianism is the utopian ideal. A day is coming when man may again realize a moral sensitivity which has no room for killing. He will come to realize he is his brother's keeper, and he will not feel the need to kill and eat animals or birds. For most people, this position is a difficult ideal to accept.

Consider the transition. We cannot jump instantaneously to perfect vegetarianism and expect our bodies to adjust likewise. The mind must undergo a growth period. There is much to learn. An entire lifetime may not be sufficient to develop and refine the mind to find the perfection necessary to rise above the chaos of civilization. Perfection can only flourish in a "Garden of Eden" environment.

The primary goal is to live so that we depart this world having left a better life and a better influence on our families than has been the legacy of former generations. The present generation with its white sugar, dumplings, present attitudes, supermarkets and depleted foods are not capable of promoting a better generation for the future. Those who have traveled this life prostituting and robbing Mother Earth or her natural resources will be forced to pay for those "sins." We should repent and begin to create a better place to live.

Vegetarianism — A Way Of Life

A great number of vegetarians fail to realize that a benevolent way of living must go with vegetarianism. The vegetarian world should be one of total peace. There would be no warfare. Animosities, uprisings and wars would be eliminated. Man would know better than to voice anger because he would be depleting basic vital energy. Amino acids would turn rapidly, only to be rebuilt.

The vegetarian who persists in arguing about food hasn't grasped the basic philosophy. He has much to learn. He must take his time and remain calm. He can't afford to burn or extinguish his life forces.

A man such as Gandhi, who talked smoothly and calmly and rationally and who could sit for hours in contemplative thought, could live on ordinary fruits and vegetables—on their vibratory level.

In our age of technology man is under constant and tremendous pressure. This is a day of suicides and nervous breakdowns. Highly evolved protein structures broken down and destroyed through these pressures can't be replenished "overnight." Nature and plant life are slow.

If we lived as vegetarians should, we wouldn't need such a highly evolved, live protein body. Speed and pace over-ride. We respond to a field of radiation, a pull, a vibration, electro-magnetism working in our lives. Unfortunately, we know little about these invisible forces.

The person existing under brain pressure is living a rapid vibratory rate that doesn't manifest in the vegetable kingdom. Protein values from the vegetable kingdom can't match his fast pace. The meat eater is like a lion always stalking prey. I don't believe man was intended to lead this "raging" life.

The Crux Of Survival

Man is offered a choice. We either return to the natural way of life, in tune with Nature, or continue at a deafening, destructive speed bent on destroying ourselves. Man can't survive for long this way.

Many people are returning to Nature in order to survive, to regain fine, healthy bodies with development potential. Sickness is the prevalent condition of civilization. Where is good health?

I do not advocate meat eating IF we can follow the higher path. For the majority of people in civilization, this level of consciousness has not been attained. At the present time most people in America would starve to death without meat because amino acids are so rapidly burned out. Man's strained, over-used and abused mind demands the eight essential amino acids.

Why Support Meat-Eating?

Speaking for health, I do advocate moderate meat-eating. In consideration of vegetarianism, I am attempting to show how we could live. The transition couldn't be affected instantaneously. Let us cut down on heavy, excessive meat eating. The next step is to become actively involved with fruits, vegetables and seeds — mentally, physically and spiritually. We require this slow transition, from meat consumption once or twice a day to two or three times a week.

Higher Vibration Brain Proteins

The United States is a creative and inventive nation due to the reliance on higher-vibration amino acid proteins available through animal products. Great inventions are attributed to "meat-eating" nations. Few inventions appear in agrarian nations or lands dominated by fruits and vegetables.

The question of amino acid proteins boils down to BALANCE. If we are to continue to use and develop executive abilities, we must rely on the animal products — goat's milk, eggs, leading up to fish and meat. The key is moderation.

All Proteins Originated From Plants

All proteins, including these eight essential amino acids, are constructed first by plants in the vegetable domain. If we tuned our vibrations lower, we could derive sufficient protein from a vegetative source.

Meat is a stimulating food while seeds can make us great plodders. They can sustain energy for many hours; meat energizes for only a brief time.

Cactus — High Energy Vegetarian Food

The many mineral elements necessary to sustain life can be found in the oceans, the mountains, the plains. Desert foods such as the cactus are missed by the vegetarian. It is a high energy food, "fed" from sunshine, or it could not survive the harsh arid climate. If the vegetarian learned to develop it as a food, it would be one of the best energy sources available. Cacti have strong antiresistant elements. Germ life will not attack living cactus. Sun gives life to the cacti as it does the turtle and any plant life. Foods containing the highest sun life are the most potent. They contain antiresistant elements that germ life dare not attack. The human body should build such resistance.

Where And How To Live A Vegetarian Life

There is an ideal place to live as a vegetarian, but not at the North Pole. There is a ideal region for scant clothing, free perspiration. A diet centered around fruit is possible — if you live near the Equator. The Garden of Eden did not have ice and snow. It could be under the North Pole, but I don't believe it is the North Pole. I think we were intended to live where little clothing and few fires are necessary; where sunshine is bountiful and gravity does not rob our strength. Perhaps man should study the effects of gravity to counteract the magnetic currents of the North and South Poles.

The wise man recognizes the need for other elements besides food. He sleeps with his head to the North, facing the East. He knows his herbs and the powers of certain herbs for good health. Herbs in the cold northland probably contain elements man living there requires for survival. Attempting to exist on papayas in the snows of Canada would not be utilizing the proper foods for that climate. Discovering where man lived in the past, how much sun we are capable of safely absorbing, hold keys to better living. It is impossible to move from Mount Matterhorn to the ocean in another country and adjust in twenty minutes. Our bodies don't respond instantly to such a drastic climactic shock.

The vegetarian should consider the possibility of buiding his own vitamin material within the body, providing it is working efficiently. If it isn't working in harmony with the minerals and forming proper combinations, vitamins values cannot be built. So, we are subject to vitamin C deficiencies which we can't overcome. Infections develop in the body as a result. Without vitamin B-complex the body doesn't maintain the correct heat level. A certain amount of protein is required for stimulation. Animal energy provided by lacto-vegetarianism is often necessary to coax heat into the body to build digestive abilities.

Most vegetarians resort immediately to fasting when they note an ache or pain. They fail to realize that not only a sanitary condition of the body is entailed, but also the body is dependent on strong tissue built from mineral elements derived from the earth's soil.

Vegetarian and Meat Deficiencies

The average vegetarian does not generally get enough of six of the eight essential amino acids commonly found in meat or animal products. The egg yolk and goat's milk are satisfactory sources. Seeds, nuts, avocados and other vegetarian food don't provide these amino acids. Using eggs and animal products — lacto-ovo vegetarianism — is a wise alternative to strict vegetarianism.

Meat alone is a starvation diet, using the muscle structure exclusively. Carnivorous animals have a liver capacity capable of handling animal flesh. Man does not, nor do the other primates. The large intestine in the human body is not intended for animal flesh and definitely not cared for properly. Putrefaction of flesh proteins is a serious problem due to the length of time necessary for digestion in the human body.

Fresh meat does not produce disease, but there is "diseased" meat. Also there are "diseased" vegetables, deficient in mineral elements and trace minerals. The vegetarian recognizes the lack of calcium in many soils. California oranges lack calcium as compared to Florida oranges. Sodium is lacking in New York celery and abundant in that grown in Utah.

Why Turn To Vegetarianism?

At least five reasons basically justify the trend of many people, especially from the younger generation, to vegetarianism.

1. Mystical reasons. Vegetarianism is the philosophy of several Eastern religions rapidly growing in popularity.

2. Reverence for living animals. Pacifist sympathies often reach out to include the animal kingdom along with human life.

3. Economy. Meat is costly. A low food budget survives far better and longer on the vegetarian diet.

4. Vegetarianism is healthy. Studies conducted by Seventh Day Adventists and other vegetarian concerns support better health and longer life claims. A vegetarian diet lowers cholesterol.

5. Animal feeds are drugged. Meat doesn't taste the way it once did. High-powered drugs including antibiotics, hormones and arsenicals are said to be prevalent.

A Few Words In Favor Of Meat

Meat provides balanced protein. Eggs also are a complete, well-balanced protein, as is milk. Plant foods tend toward predominantly incomplete proteins, difficult for the human body to utilize, unless served in the proper combinations.

A balanced protein source is necessary for good nutrition. Protein is composed of a blend of amino acids, eight of which are essential to qualify a protein as complete. If one amino acid of the eight is missing or in short supply, only part of the protein can be assimilated.

Lacto-Ovo Vs. Strict Vegetarianism

It is not advisable to become a strict vegetarianism — one who avoids all animal products. Eat eggs (Ovo), which contain the finest quality complete protein. All laboratory protein measurement is according to the egg standard. Eggs supply vital fat necessary to maintain body heat, especially during winter months. In primitive societies, vegetarianism is usually in a warm or tropical climate. The Eskimos are almost exclusively meat eaters to keep necessary body heat levels.

Lacto vegetarianism supports the use of milk and dairy products in the diet. Only certified raw milk, and raw goat milk are preferable because pasteurization destroys

vitamins, minerals, harms the fat content and reduces digestibility by damaging amino acids in the protein. Raw goat milk contains ten times the amount of fluorine and iron of cow's milk, is much more digestible and neutralizes overacidity by its alkalinizing effect on the stomach. Dairy products should be from raw certified milks, for best health benefits. Goat milk is a proven health builder.

Vegetarians should resist the overwhelming temptation to eat cakes, pies, sweet desserts and white flour products. They are low in protein, vitamins, minerals and loaded with empty calories.

Animal Foods In Moderation

I believe that animal foods should be taken in a very small quantity. Personally, I think we should all aim at becoming vegetarians. Studies should be conducted to find the proper way to handle nutrition requirements without meat. However, it is a fact that most people are meat-eaters today. Since most of us lead the life of a lion or tiger, so to speak, our diets have to follow along those lines. A sudden reform that took away all the past lifestyle practices would be too drastic a shock.

The first step is to cut meat intake to three times per week, including the use of fish. Prepare only lean meat — no fat; no pork. Try to limit fish to those with fins, scales and white flesh. Meat should be broiled, baked or roasted.

I advocate a diet of 60% raw food and 40% cooked. Good health will truly arrive when man's diet consists of 90% fruits and vegetables. These components are missing or lacking in the average diet. As a basic principle the daily diet should consist of two fruits, six vegetables, one protein and one starch. Also meat and all proteins are acid-forming. The diet should be only 20% acid-forming and 80% alkaline. (Starches and proteins are acid foods too.) Only fruits and vegetables are alkaline.

Elevating Consciousness A Step At A Time

Illustrating meat eating, the food-chain evolves from the grass to the grasshopper, from the grasshopper to the chicken, from the chicken to the preacher, who eats the chicken. Consciousness is built, or raised, one level at a time. It is commendable to strive upward to the higher goals.

Personally, I believe in the doctrine of vegetarianism as the ideal life mentally, physically, and spiritually. But we are far below that goal. It is feasible to teach people to take one step at a time, no more. Untimely advanced knowledge fails. The single formula for success is in approaching people at their present level of consciousness, to convince them to step up one step at a time to a better way of life than the present. People can't visualize tomorrow. They can't see what the future holds. So, we work with what is to come at the next meal or in the next month. It is the present attitude and station in life that I deal with.

The Concessions To Meat-Eating

The average American eats little fish compared to the amount of other meats. Why is this? Seafish, contains about 18% complete protein, digestible flesh, 20% polyunsaturated fatty acids, vitamins A, D, riboflavin and niacin, minerals iodine, magnesium, phosphorus, iron and copper. The appalling rate and quantity of pollutants being dumped into oceans and streams make the securing of safe, non-toxic fish difficult. Lead and mercury poisonings are especially detrimental. Buy the best and freshest fish available. Serving it once or twice a week is much healthier for the non-vegetarian than beef or pork.

In preparing fish, never over-brown, don't fry; broil or bake or use parchment paper steaming instead. Cook with low heat until the flesh flakes, and keep it moist. Try sprinklings of paprika and parsley, and top with lemon slices while preparing.

Meat Considerations

Artificial hormone injections to fatten meat animals is detrimental to health. So are the current butchering practices of aging beef up to fifteen days, the use of red dyes and adding processing and preserving additives. However, meat is a rich source of the eight essential amino acids, high in protein, fat high in vitamin A. Animals fed on rich green grasses build blood rich in B_{12}, iron, iodine, zinc and other minerals. Only organically grown beef, veal and lamb are recommended. Wild meat such as deer, rabbit, goat, antelope, bear are best. Domestic pork saturated with hard fat and insecticide residues is to be avoided. Processed pork is loaded with salt, dyes, nitrates, and other chemical additives. Avoid all processed meats.

Cook meat as little as possible, over low heat. Never fry. Bake, broil or steam using parchment paper. Remember it is a dead food and should be eaten soon after killing or frozen to protect against deterioration.

Poultry Practices

Poultry can be prepared many ways, is rich in all essential amino acids and is high in protein. Only organically grown fowl should be used, fed on natural grains, greens and free of hormones and other chemicals. Use moderate or low heat in broiling, baking or steam cooking. Again, never fry. Don't over-cook. The dark meat has the most nutritional value.

Remember Moderation

If meat is used, it should be incorporated only moderately into the weekly diet. Three times per week is suggested. Never serve it in combination with a starch. Serve with vegetables. Also double proteins are not recommended, such as steak and eggs, steak and lobster, cheese and meat.

Dangers Of Strict Vegetarianism

Dr. Arthur Vos has the following to say regarding a strictly vegetarian diet: "It will indeed be a serious mistake for a brain worker to experiment with a strictly vegetarian diet by excluding all animal foods. By doing so he would simply live on his reserve nerve force. Such a man would become prematurely old, and mental collapse and premature death would probably soon follow.

"A youthful appearance is attained by taking the brain and nerve foods (proteins), fresh fruits, fresh vegetables and little starch foods. Too many starches taken in proportion to other foods, makes the limbs stiff, and with little or no meat turns the hair gray, produces wrinkles and other evidences of premature aging appear.

"The daily use of eggs, bacon and cocoa added to a strictly vegetarian diet makes one bilous, yellow or irritable and nervous." Lucile Steele, author of *Food Science* says, "A scholarly woman of my acquaintance, who did strictly mental work, fell prey to the vegetarian age. She told me she could not understand her body's deterioration since they had been so careful of their eating; seldom touched meat but bought fruit instead. The post mortem revealed her spinal cord enlarged and large nerve trunks in a stage of degeneration, diagnosed by physicians as cancer. It was a case of nerve starvation. Fruit is an excellent food, but it cannot take the place of protein."

Professor Eddy of Columbia University states: "The next discovery was the demonstration that proteins differ in nutritive value and that not only must the body have its fifty grams of protein per day, but it is extremely fussy as to the kind of protein it demands. As a result of the studies of many chemists working in this field we know that proteins are to be thought of as mosaics made up of separate chemical pieces and that there are some eighteen of these pieces, nearly all of which are absolutely necessary to make a body-satisfying protein. These pieces are known chemically as amino acids, but the principle involved is covered if we say that not only must we be sure of the amount of protein, but we must also assure ourselves as to its quality or make-up."

In his book **Outwitting Old Age,** Dr. R.L. Alsaker says: "Lean flesh food, plainly and correctly cooked, is easier to digest than such vegetable proteins as peanuts and navy beans."

Why Is Pork An Unfit Food?

What are the objections to pork? First, hogs are scavengers; they willingly and greedily eat half-decayed poisonous matter. They are often fattened almost exlusively on corn — high in carbon and lacking essential proteins and minerals. Hog "slop" is largely fermentative and toxic. Lard produced in fattening is highly indigestible.

Secondly, hogs' flesh is often infected with parasites, particularly the Trichina spiralis, due to lacking natural antiseptics in their bodies. Dr. Royal Lee is quoted as saying the following in **Health Culture** magazine: "The United States Government has recently issued another warning against the use of pork without thorough cooking. The hog family has become so generally infected with the pork parasite, Trichina spiralis, it has been found impossible to eliminate infected animals even by the most laborious inspection and so the Government after struggling with the problem for many years, has given up the job as hopeless, and simply warns the public that if they wish to eat pork, they do so at their own peril."

The following table taken from the **Century Book of Facts** gives the relative digestibility of meats. (Wild meats are always more wholesome and easier to digest.) Note where pork ranks.

	Hours	Minutes
Venison steak, broiled	1	35
Wild turkey	2	18
Domestic turkey	2	25
Wild goose, roasted	2	30
Lamb, broiled	2	30
Mutton, broiled	3	—
Chicken, full-grown	2	45
Beef, roasted	3 (to 3 hrs. 30 min.)	
Beef, fried	4	—
Veal, broiled	4	—
Pork, roasted	5	15

(to 3 hrs. 30 minutes.)

Why Fat Meats Are Taboo

Fat meats are to be avoided since almost everyone is excessively fat-poisoned and the liver is incapacitated as a result. All fats are emulsified by the liver—cream, butter, oil or fat of meats. It is estimated that proper intake of fat is about two ounces per day. That would include all fats used in vegetables, salads, baked goods, in addition to the cream in milk and butter. The average person eats way beyond his needs in fat. Of the carbons, fat is the most difficult to work up; the body metabolizes starches and sugars first. (A pale yellowish bowel excretion often indicates lack of bile secretion and liver dysfunction due to too much fat.)

A bulletin of the U.S. Government says: "The excessive use of fats interferes with the digestion of other foods and throws a large amount of work upon the digestive organs."

The fats easiest to digest are olive oil, avocado and nonpasteurized cream and butter. After those come vegetable oils and lastly meat fats. Heating fats to a temperature from frying, produces acid poisons. Fried foods must be eliminated if health is your goal.

The Cost And Weight Reducing Vegetarian Diet

With the cost of meat so high today, a lacto-ovo vegetarian diet (with eggs and dairy products) can save you money and keep you thinner besides. For example, a small sized sirloin steak has 125 fat calories besides the 130 calories of protein. The vegetarian diet contains more bulk, so you shouldn't be hungry either. We find that in looking at the economy side (1983), pinto beans cost about 59 cents per pound and hamburger costs $1.89 a pound and up and steak can be $2.59 a pound and on for the choice cuts. Another plus is the lowered serum cholesterol in the vegetarian diet. Most can get along nicely on 1,000 to 1,100 calories a day and lose a few pounds a week if weight reduction is the goal. A woman, for instance, weighing 128 pounds needs only about 1-½ ounces of usable protein (high grade) per day. Remember variety in your foods, especially in protein, to get all the eight essential amino acids. As examples of protein content in foods, the daily requirement (1-½ oz.) could come from about 5 cups milk, 6 eggs, 12 oz. nuts, 4 cups rice (uncooked) 1-½ cups (uncooked) pinto beans, 7.5 oz. meat, etc. Cheese is about 20% to 28% protein; milk average 4%; dried pinto beans, about 23%.

Eating Plan — How To Get Enough Daily Protein On A Vegetarian Diet

4 or more servings of fruit and vegetables
(protein, 8 grams; calories 275)
For example: 1 medium banana,
1 orange, ⅔ cup broccoli and
1 medium potato

4 or more servings of breads and cereals
(protein, 10 grams; calories 280)
For example: ¾ cup oatmeal and
3 slices whole-wheat bread.

2 cups milk (protein 17 grams; calories
330; if skim milk is used, 175)

2 or more servings protein-rich foods
(protein 22; calories 225)
For example: ½ cup cottage cheese
and 1 cup legumes

Total protein, approximately **57** grams
Total calories, 1,110; if skim milk, **955.**

*Adapted from **Nutrition and the M.D.**,*
Vol. 1, No. 5, 1975.

Diet Menus

Day 1

Breakfast	Calories
¾ cup cooked oatmeal	98
with 2 T. raisins	58
½ cup skim milk	44
Coffee or tea	0
	200

Lunch	
Three Bean Salad	162
on lettuce leaf	
1 small sesame seed roll	75
with 1 tsp. butter or margarine	33
Iced tea with sprig of mint	0
	270

Dinner	
Spinach Manicotti	249
1 slice French bread	58
1 cup mixed salad greens with 2 T	20
Low-Calorie French Dressing	26
1 medium orange	73
Coffee or tea	0
	426

Snack	
Strawberry shake, blend	
1 cup skim milk	
5 strawberries	
artificial sweetener to taste	
3 ice cubes	116

Day 2

Breakfast	Calories
½ cup Granola'	177
½ cup skim milk	44
Coffee or tea	0
	221

Lunch	
1 cup Joy's Cold	
Vegetable Soup	45
English Muffin Pizza	220
12 oz. sugar-free cola	1
	266

Dinner	
1 Stuffed Green Pepper	300
½ cup bulgar, cooked as	
directed (substitute vegetable	
broth for water)	153
¼ cantaloupe	30
Coffee or tea	0
	483

Why I Am A Vegetarian (David Stry)

"SCIENTIFIC: Thomas Huxley, famous English biologist, in his book, **Man's Place in Nature,** says: "Man is biologically a primate, a fruit eater." Consult any dictionary or textbook on zoology. Any zoo-keeper will tell you that he feeds his primates (the gorillas, great-apes, chimps, etc.) fruits, nuts and vegetables and that they will not eat flesh of animals. Or, test yourself; catch a chicken and kill it with your own hands and eat it raw, (carnivorous and omnivorous animals can do it).

"ETHICS (meaning Man's relationship with fellow human beings, fellow creatures, and his universe): What is our attitude? Shall we be constructive or destructive? Life is precious to each animal — to him, his life is as important as our life is to us. Who gave us the right to snuff out other lives? If we make something, then it is ours, and we possibly have the right to destroy it; but we didn't make these lives (which manifest themselves in different body forms). 'Live and let live!' Or the Golden Rule: 'Do unto other as you would have them do unto you.' Do you just mouth these principles, or do you live them? There is a kinship of all life; we are all children of the same 'Creator.' It is true that some animals do kill and eat other animals, but our order, the primates, are not animals of prey. Other peaceful animals are: horses, goats, cows, deer, elephants, etc. (These will starve to death, rather than eat other animals.)

"AESTHETICS (meaning 'the love of what is beautiful'): would you rather walk through a fruit orchard and vegetable garden, or through the screaming, bloody, slaughterhouse (that is hidden from the public view)? Is a freshly killed animal lying on the highway a pleasant sight? It is to a buzzard, dog, tiger, or other carnivorous animal.

"ECONOMICS: Fruits and vegetables are less expensive (especially in season) than butcher-shop items pound for pound. check it, the next time you shop! One acre of land will produce ten times more food agriculturally, than when used to raise and fatten animals. Nations could support more people if their citizens were all vegetarians. Also, there is much less labor expended by the housewife in preparation, dish-washing, etc. And on greasy pots and pans.

"POLITICAL: Man is by nature a peaceful animal.

Love is the universal principle. If all human beings adopted the idea that 'All life is sacred,' then killing and War (mass murder) would be unthinkable. Why doesn't anyone pay attention to the famous commandment 'Thou Shalt Not Kill'? Instead, we are trapped in Nationalism (man-made political boundaries with flags and armies) with its traditions of War, mutual fear, runaway military technologies, and fantastic profits to vested interests. The true reformer begins with himself!

"HEALTH: Physical well-being depends upon fresh air, sunshine, exercise, right mental attitudes, rest-and-sleep, moderation, and proper nutrition (for our species). The Vegetarian diet of fruits, vegetables, and nuts in their natural, un-processed state, un-chemicalized, and tree-ripened if possible, is the cornerstone of proper nutrition. Will this diet give you enough strength? Ask any ape, gorilla, or orangutan! (They can tear a lion or tiger limb from limb.)

"WHO'S WHO: Famous Vegetarians include Plato, Plutarch, Pythagoras, Ovid, Seneca, Buddha, Ghandhi, Tolstoy, Wagner, Shelley, Voltaire, John Wesley, St. Francis, G.B. Shaw, Horace Greeley. Also, Murray Rose, 1961 Olympic swimming champion.

When asked WHY he did not eat 'meat' George Bernard Shaw once replied: "You've got the cart before the horse; WHY do you eat flesh?"

Behold, I am giving you every plant growing seed which is upon the earth and every tree in which is the fruit of a tree yielding seed; to you it shall be for meat.'
Genesis

Studies Of Vegetarianism

Anthropologists and zoologists say that the anatomy of the human body is nearest to that of the vegetarian animal — not the carnivor. About 21 pounds of ;grain is needed to produce 9 pounds of meat. The failure of one major country's crops would likely cause a famine in much of the world. Natural, pure and whole organic food is healthier. Digestion of it is easier and it is needed in smaller quantities. Much energy is needed to digest heavy meat meals. The body can remain cleaner on vegetarian diets or (dairy products and eggs) lacto-ovo vegetarian diets. Meat is very expensive, and its purity and sanitation questionable.

Vegetable Protein Ratios

Protein doesn't have to be from meat to be rich and complete. Two cups dried uncooked beans or peas is equal to 7 oz. of steak; 4 oz. uncooked rice equals 7 oz. of steak; ½ cup cooked soybeans equals 2 oz. of steak; 1 cup hulled sunflower seeds is equal to 4 oz. of steak; 2 cups unhulled sesame seeds is equal to 3 oz. of steak; 1 cup dried, uncooked garbanzos equals 5 oz. of steak.

Nature's Balanced Foods

All foods contain some protein. Nature doesn't make purely protein, starch or carbohydrate foods. Cooked or dead protein encourages toxins in the blood and putrefaction in the intestinal tract. Many researchers claim that a high protein diet can lead to cancer. According to Dr. Emmet L. Holt of New York City, meat is the most putrefactive of any food. There is no such food as only vitamin B or C, etc. Only Nature knows how to balance the living constituents of food substances. When man attempts to improve the flavor by cooking, the chemical structure is changed. All enzymes and some other elements are destroyed. Experimenters believe that much disease is linked to lack of enzymes in foods. Naturally fermented foods are rich in enzymes.

Meat and Uric Acid

Meat has uric acid, a member of the purine family, along with caffeine from coffee. They are stimulants for an immediate surge of energy but the drop has to come. Many people have claimed to control cancer by the use of raw vegetarian foods (fruits and vegetables). They are said to help in other diseases as well. Dr. Pottenger proved that meat is detrimental to cats as a cooked food and that it was highly putrefactive. Dr. Newburg, University of Michigan, studied U.S. enlisted men with hardening of the arteries during World War II. He found that by taking them off meat and adapting a vegetarian regime there was no additional hardening indicated.

Summing Up

The issue of vegetarianism versus meat eating is difficult to resolve, personally and socially, psychologically and philosophically. Given the millions of undernourished or starving people in the work, it would be best if we all became vegetarians—if the land devoted to animal raising would be converted to crops and if the crops would be shared bountifully with the hungry. Present political and economic interests prevent the latter from taking place. Wishing it were otherwise is a useless exercise. We can, however, consider it a worthwhile goal and even work toward it, to the degree that our motivation and beliefs are aligned and in balance.

From my perspective, it is better to take mankind one "real" step forward than to exhort, persuade, plead, reason, demand that they should do what they obviously will not do — at this time in history. Vegetarianism may be ultimately the best goal, but to persuade people to eat less meat for the sake of their own health is the most we can reasonably expect to accomplish in this generation.

Those born and raised in meat-eating cultures have built certain kinds of bodies and certain kinds of beliefs. When you understand that we live on what we believe, then you will begin to understand how aggressive personalities emerge through the generations from aggressive families, and how aggressive families emerge from dog-eat-dog societies. The harshness, the selfishness, the tendency to violence, go hand-in-hand with the meat-dominated diet orientation. I believe that through many hundreds of generations, genetic influences have developed which incorporate features of the hunter-warrior pattern. People who are antagonistic and hard to get along with may come from families who are that way. It will not change overnight.

Meat eating is very much a mental thing. I feel most people are starving for knowledge about the right way of living. I feel most people are starving for friendship and love. The hunger for peace lives within us, but we don't know how to feel it. One answer to the problem is education. Wise teaching will eventually lead the human race to vegetarianism, to pacifism — back to the Garden of Eden.

National leaders are much to blame for the lifestyles that dominate their cultures. Seldom are humble men raised into leadership positions. Ghandi, has long been one of my ideal heroes. Through non-violence, he led the nation of India to independence, to new laws, to a new way of life.

The Hunza people were once vegetarians, but they have become increasingly corrupted by their contact with civilization. It has been said that the Mir of Hunza died of a broken heart when he observed, over a few years, the increasing degeneration of a culture which once had no police, jails, prisons, doctors or hospitals. They didn't need them 50 years ago. But they need them now. The Mir once told me, "Our friendship means more than anything else." His priorities were right.

It is written that "God is love." When spiritual truth comes to the mental level, it begins to change the physical body. We have opportunities to know people better and better, and to love them, but instead we choose to isolate ourselves from them. We block the love and peace of God from manifesting through our own natures and from nourishing others. It is this kind of love that will eventually eliminate the destructive principle in human life. It is said, "A long life lived is not good enough, but a good life lived is long enough."

Vegetarianism, as we have said before, is much more than a meatless diet. It is a way of life, and one day the human race will discover that way.

Too many people are just living to eat. We are in an age where we want a good time all the time. Why not have a good time? Yes, you can...but not with food. Have your good time while eating and in between eating, but have foods that are nourishing to the body. Everything that goes in the mouth should be nourishing. This is one of the most important things to consider. What does not nourish is so much dross which works the digestive and eliminative organs of the body for no return. In many people, these organs are already broken down from overwork. If you are living to eat, there is a possibility your pleasure may be short lived. Better eat to live NOW.

Did you know that it is five times easier for the liver to handle goat's milk than cow's milk because the fat globules in goat's milk are five times smaller than the ones in cow's milk?

Did you know that a baby, if allowed to always sleep on its stomach, can develop flat feet?

Did you know that pineapple-guava blossoms can be used in salads?

Did you know that the trace mineral cobalt is necessary to build good blood and that the skin of almonds is very high in cobalt?

Did you know that it is the sodium in cucumbers that keeps you as cool as a cucumber?

Chapter 27

Timeless wisdom: the divine diet

Timeless Wisdom: The Divine Diet

We find that the Divine Law of the Good Book lays down specific guidelines as to what is clean and unclean — foods that should be eaten and the foods to leave alone.

One of the first important laws is this: "Thou shalt eat no manner of blood, whether it be of fowl or of beast." The Good Book implies that disease is carried in the blood and can be transmitted through the blood.

"Only thou shalt not eat the blood thereof; thou shalt pour it upon the ground as water" (Deut. 15:23).

Fat is taboo, because it is hard to digest; it is very difficult for the liver to handle.

"Ye shall eat no manner of fat, of ox, or of sheep, or of goat." (Lev. 7:23).

There is also the law that animals permitted for human consumption cannot be blemished. Consider the artificial feeds, hormones, vaccines and so on the animals raised for flesh food undergo.

We might bring out the fact that "meat" in the Good Book didn't necessarily refer to flesh food—it often meant food in general. It especially suggests solid foods. Thus, the flesh foods are referred to specifically by names, such as animal, fish or fowl.

"And God said, Behold, I have given you every herb bearing seed, which is upon the face of all the earth, and every tree, in which is the fruit of a tree yielding seed to you it shall be for meat." (Gen. 1:29).

We know that fish were an important source in biblical times. It says in Matthew 4:18, "And Jesus walking by the Sea of Galilee, saw two brethren, Simon called Peter, and Andrew his brother, casting a net into the sea; for they were fishers." And in Egypt fish were important in the diet. Numbers 11:5 tells us: "We remember the fish, which we did eat in Egypt freely." It is also interesting to bring out that broiling was mentioned in Luke 24:42: "And they gave him a piece of broiled fish, and of an honeycomb." (We recommend only broiling or baking of flesh foods — never frying.)

While flesh from some animals free from blemish was permitted under God's approval, others were absolutely prohibited.

"And every beast that parteth the hoof, and cleaveth the cleft into two claws, and cheweth the cud among the beasts, that ye shall eat.
"Nevertheless, these ye shall not eat of them that chew the cud, or of them that divide the cloven hoof; as the camel, and the hare, and the coney [rabbit]: for they chew the cud, but divide not the hoof; therefore they are unclean unto you.
"And the swine, because it divideth the hoof, yet cheweth not the cud, it is unclean unto you: ye shall not eat of their flesh, nor touch their dead carcass" (Deut. 14:6-8).

Why were the rabbit and hare forbidden? They were considered rodents, such as mice and rats. Some authorities believe the rabbit carries certain diseases to limit its population.

The swine is considered a scavenger with poor elimination and quick blood stream assimilation of foods (even filth and garbage) because it has only one stomach. Some animals have up to four stomachs or stomach chambers. Pork is also know to be susceptible to parasites, and tape worms infest the muscles. The parasite, trichinella spiralis, is well known in pork as the cause of the affliction trichinosis. Larval forms of the trichinae are found live in the pork unless it is cooked to remove every last trace of pink flesh in the center. Often this is not done.

Symptoms of trichinosis are hard to diagnose and even more difficult to effectively correct. Trichina (tri-ki-na) is a nematoid parasite worm which infests muscles of swine and human beings. Trichinosis (tri-ki-no-sis) is described as the disease produced by the presence of trichinae in the muscles and intestines. Symptoms can be abdominal cramping, nausea, vomiting and fever in the early stages of the larvae in the intestines. Later they can penetrate the intestinal walls and work their way through the bloodstream to muscles where they cause muscle pain, swelling and suffering.

In 1860 Professor Zenken, of Dresden, Germany discovered trichinae in the small intestines and voluntary muscles of a young girl who had mysteriously died. He traced the affliction to the eating of ham and sausages that were found to contain trichinae when examined under a microscope. The girl's illness had been characterized by fever, tenderness of flesh, severe muscular pains and general weakness.

Flesh-eating animals may have been prohibited partly because they also eat the blood of other animals. Hogs are know to eat other creatures, even their own young or carrion. This makes them extremely unclean.

Swine and rabbits are both producers of disease, possibly the greatest. The swine is also thought to be partly responsible for syphilis by some authorities.

The Three Abominations

We find the listing of three specific abominations in the sight of God: idolatry, the eating of humans (cannibalism) and eating swine. The "cursed" swine is intended as the land scavenger while the shellfish are the scavengers of the oceans. They have a purpose—but not as food for man.

Christ said in Matthew 7:6 that his disciples should not cast their pearls before swine because they would turn against (rend) them. And Peter likened the sinners who reverted to their former habits to female swine that wallow in the mire again as soon as they are washed (2 Peter 2:22).

God warned that if the Israelites disobeyed him and ate the unclean flesh that the diseases of Egypt would come upon them. Some things were forbidden in the diet but were not abominations as were the swine and shellfish. The swine, besides being similar to human flesh and difficult to digest, is considered the most unclean and gluttonous beast. God said that certain diseases would afflict the human race if people ate certain animals. Today many believe cancer was the "botch" spoken of as the disease of Egypt; others think the Scriptures refer to tuberculosis rather than cancer. Studies are pointing to the fact that cancer is largely due to incorrect living and wrong diets. (i.e.) the National Cancer Institute has claimed 60% of cancer in women and 40% of cancer in men lis attributed to wrong diet. The state of health in the U.S. is appalling. Degenerative diseases are growing daily.

"And the swine, though he divide the hoof and be clovenfooted, yet he cheweth not the cud; he is unclean unto you. Of their flesh shall ye not eat, and their carcass shall you not touch; they are unclean to you" (Lev. 11:7,8).

"A people that provoketh me to anger continually to my face...which eat swine's flesh, and broth of abominable things is in their vessels" (Isaish 65:3-4).

"They that sanctify themselves and purify themselves in the gardens behind one tree in the midst, eating swine's flesh, and the abomination, and the mouse, shall be consumed together, saith the Lord" (Isaiah 66:17).

In considering eating the flesh of the pig, God did not classify it as a food. It was rather one of the three abominations: 1) worshipping idols; 2) cannibalism; 3) eating of swine's flesh. This plainly removes all pork products from the food list as a diet for the human race.

As for the lard, or fat of the hog, it is just as much forbidden by the law of the divine diet. Suet, the fat that covers the kidneys and the intestines, is also expressly prohibited.

"Whosoever eateth of the fat of the beast shall be off from his people." (Lev. 7:25).

This refers to the fatty portion that can be rendered, not the fat of the meat tissue or muscle. Lard is the fat of the hog that is melted and rendered from the flesh and to eat it is considered no different than to eat the flesh itself. Moreover, we are not to eat the fat of other animals, either.

"All the fat is the Lord's. It shall be a perpetual statute, for your generations in all your houses that ye eat neither fat nor blood." (Lev. 3:16-17).

We find in Matthew 8:32 the description of Christ casting devils into the herd of swine, and the Scripture says that they ran violently into the sea.

Preparation of Food and Combinations

Many nutritionists will agree that the greatest mistake man made was the discovery of using fire for cooking foods. One story of its accidental finding was that after a fire in the forest man tasted the burned flesh of an animal and liked the taste. Thus, the firing of foods was born. This was a prime factor in the spread of flesh-eating. We know that this produces the cholesterol-prone heated oils and fats, destroys vital food elements such as lecithin and vitamins, and all enzymes are destroyed by cooking. The amount of roughage for the intestinal tract is reduced. One passage goes as follows:

"I (Jesus) tell you truly, live only by the fire of life (the Sun), and prepare not your foods with the fire of death (cooking fire), which kills your foods, your bodies and your souls also.

"With that fire of death you cook your foods in your houses and in your fields. I tell you truly, it is the same fire that destroys your foods and your bodies. For your body is that which you eat, and your spirit is that which you think. Eat nothing, therefore, which a stronger fire than the fire of life has killed. Wherefore, prepare and eat all fruits of trees, and all grasses of the fields. For all these are fed and ripened by the fire of life; all are the gift of the angels of our Earthly Mother. But eat nothing to which only the fire of death (cooking) gives savour, for savour, for such is of Satan.

"Eat always from the table of God: the fruits of the trees, the grain and grasses of the field, the milk of beasts, and the honey of bees. For everything beyond these is of Satan and leads by way of sin and disease unto death. But the foods you eat from the abundant table of God give strength and youth to your body, and you will never see disease. For the table of God fed Methuselah of old, and I tell you truly, if you live even as he lived, then will God of the living give you also long life upon the earth as was his."

(The Gospel of Peace of Jesus Christ [author unknown])

If we are what we eat, look in the mirror and decide for yourself if you like what you see. We were not intended to die of diseases, but rather to end our days like Moses, at the age of 120, "whose eye was not dim, nor his natural strength abated." he had all his faculties to the end. (Gen. 6:3; Deut. 34:7). Other members of God's creation retain their faculties and vitality into old age. Why is man different these days? We have forsaken the divine diet of the Scriptures. Perhaps the "remedy" and the only salvation is to return to the teachings of Genesis, Deuteronomy 14 and Leviticus 11.

Modern medicine and medical science have greatly reduced the number of infant mortalities, and countless lives are "saved" and prolonged among the elderly. But, the question is, why are so many of the elderly barely existing, under great pain and only half-living? Many would rather be dead and out of their misery. If strength could be accurately measured, we would find our national strength dangerously lowered. We are told that people are living longer than ever before, yet we live but a few years longer than people did in the 1800s. There is now a larger percentage of persons over 55 among the total population of the U.S., giving the false impression that people are living longer. Many of us can look back into family history and recall ancestors who lived to 85, 90 even 95 but how long will we live, *in health*, as they did? They didn't have the wonders of modern medicine to prolong life.

We find that food combining is mentioned in the Scriptures, ordering us not to "seethe the kid in its mother's milk" (Deut., Exodus, Lev.). The Lord's law stated that the people were not to eat milk and meat together at the same meal [double protein], nor cook milk and meat together [milk pasteurization] nor get any enjoyment from eating milk and meat together. (This lets out meat meals followed by pudding desserts, etc.) It specifically says that the consumption of meat and milk should be separated by six hours. Since it was forbidden to cook the meat of the offspring with the milk of its mother, it was also taboo to take them into the stomach together. Simplicity of diet was stressed over and over. How we have departed from that doctrine today!

"And Moses said, 'this shall be, when the Lord shall give you in the evening flesh to eat, and in the morning bread to the full'" (Exodus 16:8).

The Dangers of Overeating and Gluttony

"Know ye not that ye are the temple of God and that the Spirit of God dwelleth in you? If any man defile the temple of God, him shall God destroy; for the temple of God is holy, which temple ye are." (I Cor. 3:16-17).

Since our body is the temple of the living God, the Holy Spirit, we have no right to abuse, defile and destroy it with improper living and abominable dietary practices. The warnings against making the appetite our god is repeated many times. Note the following passages.

"For they that are such serve not our Lord Jesus Christ, but their own belly; and by good words and fair speeches deceive the hearts of the simple" (Romans 16:18).

"For many walk, of whom I have told you often, and now tell you even weeping, that they are the enemies of the cross of Christ; whose end is destruction, whose god is their belly, and whose glory is in their shame, who mind earthly things" (Phil. 3:18,19).

Look at Psalm 78:31 and you will find it brought out that the love of indulging the appetite lis the "second root" of evil—the cause of sickness and trouble in the physical, mental and spiritual body. (Eating beyond the needs of the body is part of the excesses also pointed to in 1 Cor. 3:17.)

"For the drunkard and the glutton shall come to poverty" (Prov. 23:21).

The American Evangelist

Billy Graham says the Bible doesn't approve of self-indulgence of the appetite and places gluttony at the same level with drunkeness. He brings out that if we become overly concerned with food we forget the importance of spiritual things. It leads to selfishness when we should be concerned with selflessness. He also points out that the Good Book forbids anything that can be damaging to the body. One of the greatest keys to life we know is temperance — even where food is concerned. Overeating KILLS!

Seafood and Fish: Clean & Unclean

Fish, like animals, were divided into the two classifications of clean and unclean, according to whether they had fins and scales (and white meat or darker meat).

"Whatsoever hath no fins nor scales in the waters, that shall be an abomination unto you" (Leviticus 11:12).

"These ye shall eat of all that are in the waters: all that have fins and scales shall ye eat" (Deut. 14:9).

Prohibited fish includes shark, dogfish, swordfish, and the sturgeon. All shellfish are forbidden because they are the scavengers of the waters. They include lobster, oysters, crabs, shrimp and clams. These scavengers live on the droppings, the offal and dead and decayed materials of the waters. Their elimination is poor, besides. The addage, "we are what we eat" is also true of the fishes and other forms of sea life as it applies to food for man. The incidence of ptomaine poisoning has been traced in about 90 percent of the cases to shellfish.

"These shall ye eat of all that are in the waters: whatsoever hath fins and scales in the waters, in the seas, and in the rivers, them shall ye eat.

"And all that have not fins and scales in the seas; and in the rivers, of all that move in the waters, and of any living thing which is in the waters, they shall be an abomination unto you" (Lev. 11:9-10).

Again:

"And whatsoever hath not fins and scales ye may not eat; it is unclean unto you" (Deut. 14:10).

To show the vital importance of observing the divine diet law of God the orders are repeated again and again throughout the Scriptures.

Allowed fish are those with *both* fins and scales: haddock, cod, whitefish, plaice, whiting, pollack, halibut, herring, sardines, smelt, anchovies, salmon, and most fresh water fish such as trout and bass.

It might be well to bring out the fact that the very appearance of the forbidden fish and reptiles is generally repulsive, often fierce, ugly, dangerous. This is intended to warn us that they are not allowed. We find that the appearance of the recommended fish is sleak, graceful, pleasant and gentle. Their fins and scales are harmless and attractive. It seems that God stamps all with a seal of either "good" or "evil."

Frogs are considered a pestilence and eels are among the creeping things with lizards, snails, etc.

The Good Book refers to fish in the diet of the disciples and mentions that Christ even prepared fish for them. Christ also ate fish, as described in Luke 24:42-43. In the feeding of the five thousand in Matthew 14 and the feeding of the four thousand, "loaves and fishes" rather than animal meat was provided. Fish, as we have pointed out, was an important staple in the diet of ancient Palestine.

Further Instructions on Meat Eating

Man was not given permission to eat flesh until after the flood, or deluge when all flesh was destroyed. Noah and his family were given specific permission to eat animal flesh in Genesis 9:3. However, it might be brought out that in only eight generations after Noah and his family began to eat meat, the life span was cut from Methuselah's maximum of 969 years to 148 years, the age of Noah's descendant Nahor.

Thus, the divine diet as laid down in Genesis was "fruits and herbs" (Gen. 1:29). The flood is estimated to have occurred about 2,000 years after the Garden of Eden creation story.

"And out of the ground made the Lord God to grow every tree which is pleasant to the sight, and good for food."

Leviticus 11 lists animals that were considered "clean" or "unclean" by the Law of the Lord. Only those that chewed the cud *and* had a cloven hoof were acceptable. Others were not.

Birds considered "unclean" included birds of prey and birds of the night. Some birds of prey fed on carrion — vulture, etc.

"These are the beasts which ye shall eat: the ox, the sheep and the goat, the hart, and the roebuck and the fallow deer, and the wild goat, and the pygarg, and the wild ox, and the chamoise." (Deut. 14:4-5).

"And every creeping thing that flieth is unclean unto you; they shall not be eaten but all clean fowls ye may eat." (Deut. 14:19-20).

Reviewing Clean and Unclean Foods

Among the clean foods we find vegetables, ripe fruits, nuts, seeds, vegetable oils, honey, milk (not pasteurized), butter, eggs, cheese, grains, beef, mutton, fish with fins and scales, venison (and other wild game) and many types of fowl.

Some of the unclean foods are pork (including bacon and ham), rabbits, hares, rodents, web-footed birds and their eggs, birds of prey, all shellfish, fish without both fins and scales, eels, snails, frogs, and all other things.

In addition to the common practice these days of eating of prohibited and unclean — or even diseased meat — we have refined, poisoned and denatured much of the rest of the food supply. Grain is milled and robbed of the life-giving elements—the bran and the germ; and almost pure starch white flour is sold to the public. The worst refined foods are white flour, white sugar and their various mixtures and products. Countless experiments have proven that life can't be sustained on this denatured, dead food. Yet the vested interests tout the value of their products and "enrichment" with synthetic vitamins and minerals.

The soil is often robbed without repayment. The God-sanctioned laws said the farmer was to allow his land to rest every seventh year. Nature and God observed the seventh period of rest. There is the fiftieth jubilee year following the seven times seven years of labor. The seventh year could be called the "sabbath" year.

The prophet Hosea says people and nations are destroyed "for want of knowledge" because they refuse to go to the source of knowledge — the law of God — and fail to put it into practice.

We believe there is still time to repair some of the diet damages from the refined foods, "dead" foods and over-cooking. A few years of an organic food regimen could revitalize the entire country. However, we find that a few more generations of foodless foods, drug taking, and chemicalized food production and processing could destroy the health of those yet to be born.

It is written that our bodies are the "temples of the Holy Spirit." This body is the temple of the living God; it's the vehicle of the soul and the spirit. Others have said, quite appropriately, that we dig our graves with our knives and forks. Don't we owe it to our higher selves to provide the best, healthiest, most efficient and productive vehicle we can? If the Divine Architect didn't care what happened to us He wouldn't have taken the time to tell us the path to take physically, mentally and spiritually.

The word "holy" comes from the word "whole," which comes from the word "heal." The Divine Dietitian is the only nutritionist to follow if you want a whole body — physically, mentally and spiritually. His nutrition classes are free to the public; his diet counseling is available at all times. The Good Book is loaded with valuable nutrition secrets if you are sincere and willing to take the time to find and apply them to everyday living.

It was in the Garden of Eden that death began — with the eating of forbidden food. How to get there from here is the problem, but the only chance for survival. Get back to the divine diet set forth in Genesis 1:29, Leviticus 11 and Deuteronomy 14. Eat from God's Garden; it's as old as the Garden of Eden. Make your diet up from the fruit of the trees, vegetables of the garden, grains and herbs of the fields, the milk of the goat and the honey of the bees. You can find the "land of milk and honey" (Deut. 8:7; (Ezek. 20) if you seek it. The tiny bee goes some forty thousand miles to make a pound of honey and predigests it for you at the same time.

The Mineral Story

Every man is the builder of a temple called his body to the god he worships, after a style purely his own, nor can he get off by hammering marble instead. We are all sculptors and painters, and our material is our own flesh and blood and bones. Any nobleness begins at once to refine a man's features, any meanness or sensuality to imbrute them.

—Thoreau

Drinking a quart of cabbage juice daily has proved the fastest cure for uncomplicated peptic ulcers, according to Dr. Garnett Cheney of San Francisco. "We have treated 100 patients with the juice and nothing else, over the last two years," Dr. Cheney said, "with somewhat surprising results. The improvement was much more rapid than is usual with more common treatments.

"Not only did symptoms disappear in the first few days, but we proved by X-ray examinations that the ulcers, themselves, disappeared in as brief a time as a week. No medicine or other diet was employed."

Chapter 28

Food history: camp fire to complexity

The Dawning Of Civilization

Twelve thousand years ago man was a relatively rare species. Nearing the close of the Old Stone Age, man's population was regulated by disease, accidents and by the scarcity of and difficulty in procuring food. In many ways he was worse off than the animals that shared his domain. He had no natural defenses such as sharp teeth, claws, speed of movement, camouflage coverings or cold-proof coats. The struggle for survival was uppermost in his mind. Survival hinged on the ability to get food and stay warm and away from predatory animals.
Stone Age Europe. Wandering tribes sought the mammals and reindeer overrunning the grassy plains. While men hunted with primitive bows and spears, the women "harvested" wild roots, fruits, berries, nuts, herbs and honey. Intuition often acted as a guide to safe edibles.

We find that many of man's inventions were accidental. So it is in the case of the advent of cooked foods. As the story goes, nomads came upon a forest fire just burning down to embers. They discovered that some animals had been trapped in the fire and their flesh roasted. The hungry people tasted the meat and found it quite pleasing to the palate. Instinct told them it was not harmful, and they soon began to build fires and roast meat on primitive spits. Until this time man subsisted largely on raw foods, and his digestive tract was adapted to this form of diet. We believe many of man's health problems began with the cooking of food.

Winter brought bitterly hard times in which many people starved to death. No herbs and berries nurtured them through the cold seasons. Some migrated to the sea shores in search of food, living on seaweed, fish and mussels. Man subsisted largely by hunting and gathering.

Gradually, east of the Mediterranean, the pattern of life began to change. As no thick forests hid plants and game life, the people learned and developed better ways of securing food. They began taming dogs to aid in snaring wild cattle, sheep and deer in natural canyons or made brush traps. This enabled them to maintain living larders and wear better clothing.

Man — The Animal Keeper Arises

About ten thousand years ago man made a revolutionary discovery. Animal milk sustained human beings.

So, man began keeping cattle, sheep and goats for milk in addition to flesh and skin purposes. Since the animals overgrazed the land quickly, they had to move the herds frequently. In time man learned to eat the grasses and their seeds, following the example of their beasts. They traveled where grasses grew abundantly, but often far from nuts, fruits and berries. The practice of scattering seeds of thanks to the gods accidentally initiated the first primitive agriculture.

The Accidental Dawning Of Agriculture

Thus, man took the first accidental step toward agriculture. In order to effect the complete transition to farming, or food production, an entirely new set of tools was necessary. None were originally suited to plowing, hoeing or reaping wild wheat and barley, man's first crops.

By the end of the old Stone Age the new Middle East farmers had successfully attuned to Nature to produce food, while their European counterparts still grappled fiercely with Nature for a bare living. Farmers multiplied while hunter-gatherers were less fortunate.

Settlements arose because the farmer could not remain nomadic and grow crops also. Early villages were seldom permanent and land was exhausted after a few years of harvesting. Unlike the previous dwellers, they had the time and need for acquiring possessions. Plows, hoes, knives, sickles, axes and spears were transformed from crude tools to beautifully ground and polished implements. Their fine finish added the name "NEW" to the final chapter of the Stone Age.

Invention Of The Ox-Drawn Plow

A wise farmer first coaxed an ox to pull his plow and his hoe. The other members of the family were freed for other types of work. The wife remained at home to prepare food, probably inventing the first "CROCK POT" of its time and the potter's wheel out of necessity. In the old Stone Age man ate raw or roasted food; now they found they could boil meat and vegetables and make cooked cereals. They learned to grind grain into coarse flour and to store food for the cold winters.

The first farming villages were self-sufficient, producing adequate food for themselves with a small surplus. With the invention of copper smelting in the Middle East, came profound changes. People began to specialize in certain vocations and activities. There were also specialist farmers. The first wars were presumed to be the result of herdsmen driven by drought and hunger into attacking the fertile valley dwellers. In Mesopotamia, which is believed by many to have housed the Garden of Eden, crops flourished. Food grew easily in the deep, dark, fertile soil of the Tigris and Euphrates river plains.

The Birth Of Trading And Transporting

Plains-dwellers had to produce excess crops to trade with tribes for masonry, timber and copper for homes and tool making. The wheel was invented to carry the products from one place to another in ox-drawn carts. Ships with sails were developed. People prospered and built larger villages, larger cities. Man began to grow fruit trees: peaches, cherries, apricots, dates. He planted herbs: leeks, endive, garlic. In time, irrigation canals were built to carry water to dry fields.

Priests Learn The Science Of Farming

Priests learned to use mathematics and astronomy to produce more food. They were able to predict the flooding of Egypt's Nile and the yearly Indus Valley monsoons. These civilizations and Mesopotamia were replaced by greater states such as Greece and then Rome. Greece developed a well-organized monetary system using coins of precious metals. Later, Rome looked to the wheatlands of Egypt to feed its populace, as the first city to compare in size and complexity to those of the modern world. Internal troubles and invasions of barbaric northern tribes finally toppled the Roman Empire in or around 300 A.D.

The Farmer's Fall From Grace

The Inca and Mayan civilizations revered and greatly respected agriculture. They had temples for maize and for the teaching of people in the agricultural arts. Farming tools were very prominently displayed in their sculptures. Maize (corn) was considered their staff of life. Agriculture was the first great step forward of all past civilizations.

Inca and Mayan farmers were very devoted to their gods. Priests were often referred to as "magicians" because they could correctly tell the people when to plant their crops. They studied the stars, knew the times to plant, were able to read and write, and kept records which increased their knowledge of agriculture. Farmers depended on them.

Today, we hear so little about the farmer. He is not revered. He is no longer considered the most important

key to our good health. Truly, however, he must be the doctor of the future. If you asked the President of the United States when to plant corn, I don't think he could tell you. I am sure he doesn't "know his onions." Who can the farmer look up to? He must be taught by his father or go to an agricultural college in order to gain knowledge for himself.

When Food Was Worth Its Weight In Gold

Central European races overcame other lands long ago, when agriculture was at its peak. They conquered other lands by trading foods. Anyone who is hungry will give up a great deal to be fed. Before money was invented servants were paid in loaves of bread, salt, other edibles or barter items.

Ships cruised the Mediterranean exchanging food and dry goods with other countries. Egyptian wheat and Mesopotamian fruits and vegetables were so abundant that their people were able to trade and export freely. For years the power of feudal nobles in Europe was in having the serfs under their authority surrender so much wheat and cattle each year in exchange for protection. The feudal lord became wealthy off his servants. Food was their greatest source of livelihood.

The lord of the manor protected the farmer but did not aid in increasing food production like the ancient priests of Mesopotamia. The peasants grew poorer while the nobles became richer. At this time spices were introduced, imported from the East. However, the peasants were fortunate to have onions, garlic and field herbs with a meager supply of salted meat. They were worse off than the farmers of the new Stone Age as they were considered part of the lord's property. The horse collar and the horseshoe were the only significant tools added during these three thousand years. The serf could no longer move when land became unproductiove.

The terrible Black Death riddled Europe in 1348-9, destroying half of England's population and throwing the feudal system into disarray. Following the ravages of the plague, many lords released their hold on their remaining serfs. The rise of trade and primitive industry led many serfs to migrate to the towns and cities. Craft guilds and merchant companies were formed, allowing more people to earn money with which to purchase food and other basic necessities of life.

The tradition of hospitality was developed in ancient times, in which food was offered to guests, friends and often strangers. The Greek and Roman cultures altered this tradition to develop orgies where lavish meals and rivers of wine were consumed by nobles and their friends. It was said that they lived to eat rather than eating to live. With the coming of newer civilizations, man found ways of preserving foods to carry him through from day to day, from season to season.

Things have changed drastically since those times. Food is no longer the primary medium of exchange. Its value has been misunderstood and lost in the shuffle of civilization and in the rise of the industrial world.

Searching The World For Spices

Through the spice trade, Venice grew to be the most powerful and wealthiest of all European cities not long after Marco Polo's return from China.

King Edward of England spent 1600 pounds a year on spices alone. Spices have always held an important place in history. Ships sailed in search of just spices alone. Persian and Arab traders brought spices from India to the Mediterranean area.

Through the ages countries have been made wealthy by foods and spices, but they have later fallen. The Turks, who imposed heavy taxes on goods removed from India, lost their identity in the struggles. Spain and Portugal spent fortunes sending ships to discover where these special foods came from.

Many of today's highly prized American foods originally came from Peru and South America. They were brought to Europe, developed there and returned to this country. World history has been made by wherever foods could travel. In fact, wars, they say were won on stomachs filled with foods. Napoleon was responsible for developing the canister for his extensive mobile war campaigns. Vasco da Gama journeyed to India in search of spices. Upon his return, he was honored as a national hero because he brought cargoes of cinnamon, cloves, nutmeg, ginger and pepper. The Spice Islands played an important part in Columbus' voyages. Magellan's ship Victoria returned with enough spices to pay for the entire expedition.

Fruits Of Travel

The first tomatoes were called "love apples." They were once used exclusively to adorn gardens. Spain first brought potatoes back from Peru. Many European vegetables and fruits came through Spain, Portugal and South America.

Civilization Breed Greed

Agriculture today has regressed from the time when everything which was grown was returned to the soil to replenish, renourish, remulch and recompost it. The modern farmer's ambition has often been to make a quick profit from the soil in order to move to the city.

Along with rapidly increasing population, certain philosophies developed that encouraged development of a conservative mind set, valuing farmlands less and depending on the fastest, cheapest methods of farming to produce the largest profits. Urban areas are more highly valued because incomes originate from the cities, from industry. During this time our agricultural system has been rapidly and steadily deteriorating from a natural standpoint. With the absence of pure, whole, high quality foods, man is degenerating his physical structure. The crumbling health of the individual affects the whole civilization as well. Civilization has planted the degenerative seeds of its own undoing. The richest person today, healthwise, is perhaps the poor farmer who is wise enough to grow and consume fresh, wholesome food. The wealthy man who has lost his health can be considered poorest. True wealth comes through right living, right thinking and a healthful life.

Man's hate and deception is unnecessary; further attacking the down trodden is senseless; robbing the poor is criminal. Health is not everything, but without it everything else is nothing.

Man Yesterday And Today

After the Stone Age, man had to struggle a great deal more than the average animal for his food. Since that time he has found ways of increasing food production until over population is a growing threat. He has to struggle to secure housing, food, clothing and other necessities of life. Today we live from year to year, not from day to day and season to season as the animals do. We've turned to the canning, storage, flavor and condiment businesses.

Yesterday's Survival; Today's Comfort

Man in the industrialized nations no longer struggles to find or grow food but is instead considering comfort and security above all other things. He has a comfortable home, beautiful car and lovely furniture. While in the 1900's the United States averaged 10 pounds of white sugar per person, today it is averaging 130 pounds per person. This is only to please our taste; a form of luxury, totally destructive from a health standpoint. We have ample heat, clothing, food, every conceivable comfort in this nation. We have developed more chronic diseases than at any other time in the history of man. We no longer catch fish one at a time or spend days gathering nuts and berries for our families. We now have modern ways of preserving and canning to allow more time for pleasurable pursuits. We have created and compounded our health troubles by learning to add chemicals to foods to give them "eternal" shelf life at the supermarket.

Eternal Shelf-Life Foods

First of all, we have come up with the commercialization of foods for profit. Foods are now developed for storage in warehouses and for the grocery shelf — so thoroughly chemicalized that they never spoil. They are unhealthy for mankind and are disease producing. Their utilization is responsible for much of our ill health today and for the development of many chronic diseases in the United States.

Farmers Move To The Cities

Today's man has emerged from his past and is making a living not from the land but from other people. Less than 6% of the United States population grows food for the rest of the country, and the government instructs these farmers what to do. No longer are natural wholesome foods easily available. Farming has been transformed into agribusiness, and food growing and processing is controlled by huge corporations, restricted to some extent by government regulations. The farmers of the past have moved to the cities.

Men Of The Soil Live Longest

During my study of longevity in nations around the world, I found that man lives best, lives longest and is happiest where foods grow throughout the entire year, where the climate is moderate, where the altitude is somewhere between 2,000 and 4,000 feet above sea level, near clean water where rainfall is plentiful, interchanged with sunshine many days.

Man lives at his best when he is close to black, rich, fertile soil. He lives best where foods grow wild such as in parts of Russia, Turkey and Bulgaria, where the longest living and heartiest people of the earth today reside. In other world localities where the centenarians live, they are happy people; they live the natural way of life on very little meat — three or four times a week at the very most and also with plenty of fruits and vegetables. A large percentage of their diet is raw, liquids are plentiful and life is close to the soil. They have lived this way for many centuries.

Processing Adulterates Natural Foods

Food producers and manufacturers rely heavily on pickling, preserving and salting the foods they sell. Manufacturers degerminate food to make it cheaper and easier to store for indefinite periods. Natural foods, as in the past, are difficult to find; but they are still necessary to maintain natural health.

I'm not advocating a return to the Stone Age, but I do believe it would behoove man to use the brains given him for the good of his body and for the prevention of disease, because with disease running rampant, we are faced with a dying civilization. The day is coming when we may find we have bodies which will not be capable of reversing disease processes to return to good health.

Man's Law Of No Return

In the beginning man worked with nature. He allowed a certain amount of materials grown to return to the soil, in keeping with Nature's laws of return. Before the advent of farming, the entire earth supported some five million people. More than twice that number now lives in New York City or London. With population figures nearing four billion, changes — drastic changes — must be executed, not only in agriculture, but in numerous other vital systems.

As agriculture developed, man began having to stay in one place in order to grow crops, develop tools and hoard certain possessions believed to be essential for survival. Today, huge tractors work the land, and society has become mechanized; man has no more time to himself than in the past, but his health is poorer than ever before.

Civilization: Regeneration To Degeneration

Man is going a degenerating way rather than a regenerating path necessary to sustain and advance a progressive civilization. The cave dweller has been replaced by the apartment dweller. I am convinced that the interim between was a relatively healthy one. While man in the past encountered disease and plagues through unsanitary conditions which developed in the early stages of civilization, today we have cleaned up everything and unsanitary conditions are not a major problem, in Western nations. Rather, our problems are degeneration of the soil, degeneration of food and polluted water and air.

Man's Divorce From Nature

As man left the natural way of life, he developed cooking and complex food processes. Cooking pots came into existence when heating foods was begun. Baskets, clay pots and crocks were made to store and preserve foods from one day to the next and to prevent them from spoiling.

One of the many health problems of today is in all the various food specialties in different countries: French sauces, Germany's pickled pig's feet, Mexico's tortillas and enchiladas; India's curry, Russia's vodka and Denmark's pastry. These are all products which must be left behind as man returns to the natural path followed long ago.

as man returns to the natural path followed long ago.

Around the turn of the century, 90% of our money was spent on food. Less than 10% of today's money goes to food. Many people argue that this gives them more time for vacations, recreation and travel. Yes, but do we want these at the expense of our health, when foods today are made so cheaply they are inferior in quality? It is difficult to understand why raw sugar should be more expensive than refined white sugar, which is detrimental to our health. Pasteurized milk, by the thousands of gallons run through an hour, is somehow cheaper than raw milk. Yet it diminishes our health gradually over a period of years. To illustrate, I've always said that if you aren't willing to pay a little extra for natural food, you will pay much more to a doctor instead.

Civilization's River To Destruction

Through the need for increasing food crops, chemical fertilizers were developed and soil quality was degraded. Quality production is no longer present. Man's scientific mind has developed gigantic agricultural machines to accomplish more work in less time. This permits a few agritechnicians to grow most of our foods.

Out of technological progress has risen greed; greed drives men to rob, steal, cheat and kill. Perhaps it all began with Cain slaying Abel. Or perhaps the reason was that someone wanted more land, more sheep, more vegetables than the other one had. Jealousy and greed have steadily increased. The philosophy for civilization's destruction was planted long ago and continues to be cultivated with fervor.

It Is Not Too Late

If man becomes a slave of his technology, he is lost; but if technology is used to serve man, there is hope in the wisdom we have gained over the past few years as we have viewed the consequences of our "progress." We need to learn to harmonize with Nature instead of trying to "conquer" her. It may take a century to reverse the harm done to much of the earth's soil, but it can be done. Historically, man has shown great resourcefulness in the face of survival crises. Surely we face such a crisis now in the deteriorating quality of foods and the disastrous consequences to health which have come. When the consumer demands healthy food, agribusiness, the food processing industries and government will respond. It is not too late.

We are — physically, mentally and spiritually — what we eat; our temperament and personality comes from what we eat. God, in His love for the creatures He made, laid out the rules for living and eating. It is to our detriment that we have deviated from these rules. (Man is self-willed and rebellious and thinks he knows best.) If you intend to be whole, healthy, hale, healed — which is what "holy" means — get back to the divine diet. You have to be clean on the inside to be healthy.

The young people say, "come clean," and they have a point. Only by a return to the divine diet can anyone become clean. What is commonly termed fat on the body is the accumulation of garbage, toxins, poisons, acids, body wastes. The ordinary "dead" food diet is not cleansing, it is putrefactive, fermentative, acid producing. Yet, we attempt to cover up these things on the outside and cleanse ourselves with soap and water. It is the cleanliness of what is put into the body, not on it, that matters. In a sense, we are trying to camouflage what's on the inside by perfuming and deodorizing the outside of the body.

health food stores for God-approved foods. Discover the lovely taste of "meat" from trees and the garden. Your body will thank you. The Lord's laws as laid down in the Scriptures weren't intended for a chosen few. They are meant for the world at large — for the race of man. It is up to us to teach others, to show them the better way. It has been said often that we get to heaven on the arms of those we serve.

Before the "Fall" man was free of sin, death, suffering, disease. Some scholars believe that before this time man was an astral being without skin, bones or blood. He consisted of vibrations — radiations of light and color.

It is well to bring out that the strongest animals in the world are not meat eaters: the gorilla, the elephant, the horse, the ox. They live on the grasses, grains and herbs of the field. The "herbs bearing seed" are for remedial use, too.

The Good Book mentions herbs some 37 times.

"I have given every herb for meat" (Gen. 1:30).

"The leaf shall be for healing" (Ezek. 47:12).

"Thou shalt eat the herb of the field" (Gen. 3:18).

"with bitter herbs they shall eat it" (Exodus 12:8).

"better is a dinner of herbs" (Proverbs 15:17).

It is in Genesis 9:3 that it says to eat the green herbs. Today we know the value of chlorophyll in the diet and so did God. Noah was told to eat of the green herbs. (He lived to the age of 950.) Herbs were the medicine provided by God and are rich in vitamins and minerals. His health laws don't include the devitalized, denatured, devitaminized and demineralized foods we have these days. His laws don't include the mining of inorganic metals and minerals from the earth to use as drugs or serums or mineral supplements.

We find many of the herbs mentioned by name: hyssop, aloe, anise, cummin, heath, mint, myrrh, saffron, mallow, etc. They all had value for health. They grew wild and some were cultivated in the valleys, mountains, marshes, deserts. The Good Book says the best diet is herbs, vegetables, fruits, seeds and nuts, and on this diet, men lived nearly a thousand years. As we survey the diet of today, the heavy meat consumption, light vegetables and fruits, refined starches, sugar and carbohydrates, pasteurized cow's milk and its products, we see how far from the divine diet we have strayed. There aren't very many divine diet "supermarkets" around either. What about the dangers of the chemicalized agriculture practices, depleted soils, eroded lands and other chemical additives and pesticides? They surely weren't part of God's divine order.

"Purge me with hyssop, and I shall be clean" (Ps. 51:7).

Hyssop is one of the oldest herb remedies for the "service of man" — for health. It was brought out by David as a purge, or body cleanser, symbolizing the cleansing of the body from sin. It is known to be a good blood cleanser. And, the Good Book says the "...life of the body is in the blood." David knew his people had to be cleansed in body, too, to rid the "temple of the Holy Spirit" of acids, catarrh, toxins. If your life, also, depends on the state of your blood stream, is your life stream fed and cleansed properly?

Remember how Daniel was described after eating water and greens for 10 days as "fairer and fatter in flesh than all the children which did eat the portion of the King's meat" (Daniel 1:15). And remember the verse, "Be ye transformed by the renewal of your mind." The physical, mental and spiritual bodies can't be separated. God links the body with the soul.

When Christ was healing people, he was often asked how he performed such might works; he replied: "The Son can do nothing of himself, but what He seeth the Father do" (John 5:19). And he said "For the Father loveth the Son, and showeth him all things that himself doeth" (John 5:20). The tremendous love that the Christ had for humanity was the healing power of God. Love is the greatest healer of all. It is significant that disease is associated with sin, death and darkness, while health is linked to righteousness, obedience to God and light. It is said that a light emanated from the Christ "brighter than the sun." Every shadow fled in his presence. We know from our experience with iridology that blackness in the iris indicates disease and light or whiteness indicates healing and health.

It is worth bringing out that the sick often tend to dwell on their sickness, suffering and misery, constantly. If we would learn to lose ourselves in helping others, we would be far better off. And we find out that even the Christ had to have faith before healing could take place — his faith and that of the afflicted. With his faith and perfect love coupled with the added faith of his followers, healing could take place. The word "therapeutics" comes from the Greek word that means to "heal."

"He causeth...herbs for the service of man" (Psalms 104:14).

In the millennium there is to be no meat, and this is where we find Ezekiel 47:12 stating "The fruit...shall be for meat, and the leaf thereof for medicine." In Revelation 22:2 we find "The tree of life" whose leaves "were for the healing of the nations." Also:

"The Lord hath created medicines out of the earth, and he that is wise will not abhor them" (Ecclesiasticus 38:4).

This indicates that we are not to search for cures, remedies, medicines outside the vegetable and fruit kingdom. An herb, the mandrake, is the first instance of herbs used as medicine found in Genesis 30:14. The good book says that the prophet Isaiah healed King Hezekiah of a boil with a pack of fig cake.

In one instance Christ applied clay to the eyes of a blind man, and his sight was restored. He used the earth, the dust from which we all came. A plant is like a biochemical factory of Nature. It "reaches out" for the "dust" (minerals and elements) that it needs for life. Our body has this laboratory that cries out for the elements it needs to make life healthy, vigorous, joyful, strong. How often we let it go "begging." Observe the animal in the wild. The dog or cat eats grass when it is ill or diseased. They have an instinctive sense of what to do; they trust Nature. All these plants are nonpoisonous. The animal also knows to fast when ill. They don't stuff like man does. The don't "feed a disease" like we do.

We find that in Deuteronomy 28 every basic cause of disease visiting modern "civilized" man is listed. The Good book says that these diseases are the result of disobedience to God. Read verses 22 and 25 to get an impression of tuberculosis and possibly cancer.

"The Lord shall smite thee with a consumption, and with a fever, and with an inflammation, and with extreme burning, and with the sword, and with blasting, and with mildew; and they shall pursue thee until thou perish."

"The Lord shall cause thee to be smitten before thine enemies: thou shalt go out one way against them and flee seven ways before them: and shalt be removed into all the kingdoms of the earth" (Deut. 28:22, 25).

In still another verse several conditions that "canst not be healed" are described (Deut. 28:27), including a "botch" that some believe refers to cancer.

The only true way to handle disease is to prevent it. Our foods have been linked to much of the disease degeneration today. We must have the Divine approval in all areas of our life — physical, mental and spiritual. If food isn't natural, pure and whole, it isn't approved by the Divine Dietician.

God creates and the prince of darkness "discreates" or desecrates. Our civilization is not regenerating or evolving, rather it is degenerating and devolving. Man has made the mystery of creation into an unnatural, degenerative imitation. With the misuse of the creative force, degeneration sets in.

When Adam and Eve fell from grace they had to shift from the "water of life" as food to the physical appetite that required earthly foods. They developed bodies of flesh and blood subject to heat and cold, suffering, pain, disease and death.

I don't believe there is disease carried in meat unless the animal is diseased. But disease conditions are often present. Some investigators say a number of our maladies may be transferred through the blood of diseased animals. Even the Good Book tells us "the life of the body is in the blood." It warns against eating the blood (and fat) many times. The blood stream carries disease to different parts of the body. Our worst malignancies are thought by many to be carried by the blood.

Fruits, Vegetables and Nuts

Many fruits and vegetables are called by name in the Scriptures. Greens, mallow, juniper roots, lentils, beans, leeks, onions, garlic, corn, barley, wheat, rye, grapes, figs, etc.

"We remember the fish, which we did eat in Egypt freely; the cucumbers, and the melons, and the leeks, and the onions, and the garlic" (Num. 11:5).

"...and lay up corn under the hand of Pharoah..." (Gen. 41:35).

"Brought parched corn, and beans, and lentils, and parched pulse" (II Sam. 17:28).

"Who keepeth the fig tree shall eat the fruit thereof" (Prov. 27:18).

"When thou comest into thy neighbor's vineyard, then thou mayest eat grapes thy fill at thine own pleasure; but thou shalt not put any in thy vessel" (Deut. 23:24).

"At that time Jesus went on the Sabbath day through the corn; and his disciples were an hungered, and began to pluck the ears of corn, and to eat" (Matt. 12:1).

"Thou shalt have olive trees throughout all thy coasts..." (Deut. 28:40).

"...and five measures of parched corn, and an hundred clusters of raisins, and two hundred cakes of figs, and laid them on asses" (I Sam. 25:18).

"...take of the best fruits in the land in your vessels, and carry down the man a present, a little balm, and a little honey, spices, and myrrh, nuts, and almonds" (Deut. 12:17).

"A land of wheat, and barley, and vines, and fig trees, and pomegranates, a land of oil, olives and honey" (Deut. 8:8).

"And a hundred summer fruits..." (II Sam. 16:1).

"And the bread and summer fruit for the young men to eat..." (II Sam. 16:2).

Many of the vegetables are mentioned in verses talking about herbs and greens. All vegetables were originally herbs. Taking oil is mentioned in Ezekiel 16:13 and other places such as I Kings 17:12 with the story of Elijah and the widow. Oil was used both as food and for anointing.

The Perfect Foods

We don't believe there is such a thing as a perfect food. But we find that according to the Good Book the perfect food of the young — milk — comes from the sheep or goat. Cow's milk is never mentioned.

"And thou shalt have goat's milk enough for thy food, for the food of thy household, and for the maintenance for thy maidens" (Prov. 27:27).

"And it shall come to pass, for the abundance of milk that they shall give he shall eat butter" (Isa. 7:22).

"Butter" in the original Hebrew means sour milk and not our conventional form of churned butter. In Judges 5:25 we find: "He asked water, and she gave him milk; she brought forth butter in a lordly dish." II Sam. 17:29 says, "And honey, and butter, and sheep, and cheese of kine, for David, and for the people that were with him, to eat...."

Hebrew 5:12 teaches, "For when for the time ye ought to be teachers, ye have need that one teach you again which be the first principles of the oracles of god; and are become such as have need of milk, and not strong meat."

It seems that God doesn't intend man to permanently continue to eat meat. But in the millennium the idea is brought out that there should not be the harming of any living things, animals included.

"In the sweat of thy face shalt thou eat bread, till thou return unto the ground; for out of it wast thou taken; for dust thou art, and unto dust shalt thou return" (Gen 3:19).

God issued this edict after the Fall and told Adam he would "till the ground by the sweat of his brow," to grow herbs and vegetables for eating. Before the Fall man didn't eat beasts, fowl, fish or vegetables.

Bread

Bread has been referred to as the staff of life since biblical times. But this was an unleavened bread, made from the whole grain, not our raised "pure" white manufactured and chemicalized "staff of death." The Good Book refers to wheat germ as the "fat of the kidney of wheat" and it is highly prized. Today it is removed along with the bran (roughage), taking the best vitamin and mineral elements with it. What remains for the white flour products is gassed, chemicalized, bleached and made into almost pure starch that is not only nutritionally worthless but detrimental (Animal experiments always show that this "pure" white anemic "bread-like" substance can't sustain life.) The wheat germ is the embryo at the bottom of the wheat berry— the "fat of kidneys of wheat."

The Christ refers to himself as "The bread of life" in the verse we find in John 6:35. "I am the bread of life; he that cometh to me shall never hunger and he that believeth in me shall never thirst."

The preparation of bread is described simply. "And Abraham hastened into the tent unto Sarah and said 'Make ready quickly three measures of fine meal, knead it, and make cakes upon the hearth'" (Genesis 18:6). Nowhere in the Scriptures was any form of refining of grains mentioned. The flour was pounded with all parts of the grain intact.

The U.S. is one of the largest alcohol consuming nations in the world. Could refining of grain have something to do with this? Our bodies are starved for vitamins and minerals and our appetite deranged and perverted into thinking alcohol satisfies and strengthens.

Bread is a symbol of higher things in many cases; it is associated with the spiritual and the soul of man. In Exodus 23:25 it says, "And ye shall serve the Lord your God, and He shall bless thy bread and thy water; and I will take sickness away from the midst of thee."

Honey

We find that the "land of milk and honey" is perhaps one of the most famous phrases in the Good Book. In Isaiah 7:22 we find, "And it shall come to pass, for the abundance of milk that they shall give he shall eat butter; for butter and honey shall every one eat that is left in the land." It would appear that goat milk and honey are the perfect foods.

"My son, eat thou honey, because it is good; and the honeycomb, which is sweet to thy taste" (Prov. 24:13).

In another verse it warns that temperance and moderation are to be observed. "It is not good to eat much honey..." (Prov. 25:16).

Spices and Wine

The spices spoken of in the Good Book were sweet spices or herbs, not the injurious and harsh spices and condiments we have today that contribute to all kinds of gastrointestinal ailments and even degenerative diseases. Mark 16:1 tells, "...Mary had brought sweet spices."

tion. It was Proverbs 20:1 that says, "Wine is a mocker, strong drink is raging: and whoever is deceived thereby is not wise." Finally, it was in Ephesians 5:18 that the command was given, "And be not drunk with wine, herein is excess...."

Conclusions for the Future

The prodigal son was in exile and even associated with swine [abominations] in a far land. But we find he came to the conclusion that it was time to return home. "I will return and go to my Father," he said. The meaning of the sentence, "Return unto Me and I will return unto you," takes on a deeper meaning. The tilme is at hand for our nation and the world to return to the divine way of life and the divine diet before it is too late. With the first show of willingness to return to the right path and higher consciousness we will be shown the way.

Nature is truly the "clock of God" and by observing the laws of Nature we can receive approval of the Omnipotent. With God and Nature on our side, "All nations shall come and worship before thee." (Rev. 15:4).

A Food/Digestion Prayer

"Give me a good digestion Lord,
And also something to digest:
But when and how that something comes
I leave to thee, who knowest best."
— found in Chester Cathedral Refectory

Why are we plagued with so many health problems today — mental, physical and spiritual? Our world today is spiritually anemic. When man began to kill and eat animals, disease grew rapidly. Meat eating led to craving alcohol, sexual excess, strong and highly spiced foods and a drastically shortened lifespan as a result. Many centuries before that time man lived hundreds of years in youth and strength and total health. He ate only natural foods, had pure air, vitalizing sunshine, freedom from oppression and compulsory labor; he lived in the tropical regions of the earth with constant summer and year round vegetation.

Many of these ancient men were giants in stature on the simple diet of natural, pure and whole foods. The sons of Anak were said to be giants living in the land of Canaan and yet we find their diet was fruits: grapes, figs, dates, pomegranates along with honey and the milk of goats and sheep. The Scriptures tell of their strength and long life, with excellent constitutions.

"And they came unto the brook of Eshcol ,and cut down from thence a branch with one cluster of grapes, and they bare it between two upon a staff; and they brought of the pomegranates, and of the figs" (Num. 13:23).

To the Jews in exile after the fall of Jerusalem, the eating of flesh became symbolic of depressed suicidal intentions. It is in Isaiah 22:13 that we find the following passage: "And behold. . .slaying oxen, and killing sheep, eating flesh, and drinking wine; let us eat and drink for tomorrow we shall die." Meat is high in uric acid and the ingredients indol and scatol that are poisonous wastes. If the animal had disease, it could be transmitted through the flesh and blood of the afflicted animal.

All God's Creatures

We should not underestimate the importance of the animal kingdom. The animals are here to serve us. But that doesn't have to be for meat. They are our gentle servants in many cases. Consider the chicken from which we get the egg and the goat that furnishes us with milk and cheese. Those who abuse and torture animal life are expressing a passionate destructive quality that could evolve to either self destruction or harming other human lives.

"A righteous man regardeth the life of his beast; but the tender mercies of the wicked are cruel" (Prov. 12:10).

The Good Book tells us that we have dominion over the fowl of the air, the beast of the field, the fish of the sea and everything that creepeth on the face of the earth.

All things that were created by the divine power have a purpose in the order of Nature. There is an evolution from the rocks or the dust of the earth to the plants to the insects to the chicken to the preacher who eats the eggs or the chicken. Nature has her own ways of balancing the populations under her domain.

Think of the child who naturally loves a cat or a dog or a horse. They don't hate or fear these animals, but love them by instinct. The parables of what the "lowly animals" could teach man are well known in the Scriptures.

A U.S. Department of Agriculture survey has shown that 20% of the population in the U.S. is deficient in iron. Of 12,000 children surveyed, 30% had iron deficiency anemia. Foods rich in iron include spinach, walnuts, prunes, raisins, eggs, lima beans, liver, wheat germ, blackstrap molasses, dandelion greens, organ meats, peas and mustard greens.

Americans should eat more poultry and fish and less meat, according to a report issued by the staff of the United States Senate Select Committee on Nutrition and Human needs.

In laboratory tests on the skeletons of 55 Romans dating back to A.D. 79, Dr. Sara C. Bisel found 84 parts per million of lead, indicating the possibility of lead poisoning in the decline of the Roman Empire. Romans used lead vessels for cooking and food storage, and the ingenious Roman aqueduct system may also have contributed to the problem.

III
The art of food preparation

The Garden of Eden Kitchen

Cookbook authors abound today, but we have attempted to add a "food planner" dedicated to a healthier family and elevated consciousness. Cooking has become an art, but it has branched out into the wrong areas. Anything that pleases a person's taste or is appealing to the eye is deemed acceptable. The demands of the consumer determine the products on the market. This is what makes finding natural, pure and whole foods so difficult.

Many foods today are causing health problems. We begin with the finest of foods and then we proceed to turn them into "foodless foods" with the vital nutrients refined out of them. A great deal of poor health and disease begins in the kitchen. Detrimental changes are taking place in our foods through preparation utilizing spices, condiments, preservatives, colorings and flavorings that are artificial. An increasing number of foods are making a living for doctors and dentists. We often forget the necessity of listening to our conscience and seeking approval of God in civilized living. Thus, we have an old saying, "Choose ye, that which is good; that ye in your seed may live."

Food preparation should be classified as work for the purpose of improving the human race. It should be an art belonging to the woman's world of knowledge. A woman's failure to possess and seek adequate health promoting facts can, and does, result in the preparation of "foodless foods." Such foods increase her children's doctor bills and keep her husband sick and home from work.

Ellen G. White wrote the following almost a century ago. She is as right today as she was then.

"Cooking is no mean science — it is one of the most essential and practical in life. It is a science that all women should learn — to make food appetizing and at the same time simple and nourishing which requires great skill. I believe the Creator knows what food is best for the creature He has created. However, man has become self-willed and rebellious, and, of course, he thinks he knows best."

Most cookbooks today are aimed at pleasing the taste rather than building good health. The home gourmet and chef has to "keep up with the Jones's," so to speak, In this process they aren't aware of depleting food to the detriment of health. Correct food preparation is an art. Healing is an art. There is immeasurably more to cooking than throwing food into a frying pan. Consider the end product — the end result. The first cigarette or first cup of coffee doesn't hurt you — but the continued use year after year does the damage. Cooking as practiced today is not the same as proper food preparation. This is what we are presenting. Common cooking today consists of frying, baking, overcooking at too high heat, adding artificial colorings and flavorings and creating questionable combinations with questionable ingredients. Harsh spices and condiments are used often, along with gravies, lavish desserts and pastries. What has happened to proper food preparation? Where did it get lost?

This book may not be popular in the realm of typical "cookbooks." It is not intended to be. Pork hide is made into "crackles;" grain is puffed or flaked, devitalized and expensively packaged; too many packaged foods are intended to be quick and easy to prepare — to get by for the moment. I don't accept or condone this philosophy. The truth has to be "laid on the line." Many foods today start out as good foods, then man handles them, destroying the life force and the natural good that may have been in them — they become "dead" foods. They become "spook food," "anemic" food and "brain-starvation" food.

We must reexamine our food philosophy and our food preparation methods. The goal of meal preparation should be to build and maintain high level well being, to bring out the best that is in us for the purpose of being physically, mentally and spiritually healthy. God has given each of us special gifts and talents to manifest in this life but there is no way we can bring them out and put them to use for mankind without the proper levels of strength, energy and vitality.

The foods for our body are made up of elements potentized by the sun, by light and by color.

Chapter 29

Equipping the health kitchen

Return to Nature Before it's Too Late

Many prison and jail inmates are there due to poor eating habits, malnutrition, lack of proper glandular and nerve foods. Cravings for abnormal foods to the point of alcoholism and drug abuse occur. Prisons, hospitals and mental institutions would not be so crowded if their diets were properly upgraded. The root of such problems can also be partly traced to the kitchens. There is a system of order laid down by the Almighty for us to obey, and this can be recognized as the system of Nature itself, the partaking of good, pure, whole foods from plants grown in proper soil.

Modern man's job in the future will be to find the diet that is most necessary to strengthen and support the human constitution. It is time to understand that our foods have been impoverished, bleached, sulphured, doped, demineralized, dyed and chemically treated. With wrong cooking methods, they have been over-heated, poisoned, scorched, pressure cooked, fried, impaired and altered in general from their natural chemistry. We now realize that many of our foods are lifeless, valueless and "dead." They have been milled down, cut up, peeled and processed to destroy vitamins, minerals, enzymes and natural molecular structure. Consider the risks we take every day. Were the foods we buy heated? How long have they stood on shelves? Have they been injured by toxins, decomposition, age, germ life? It certainly should set your mind to thinking.

Food Shop

We must also consider the percentage of our diets that consist of boiled goods, soda fountain goods, canned goods, laboratory drugs, canned fruit juices, cordials, diet stuff, preservatives, artificial colorings. We have to appraise the portion of our diets that are comprised of fried foods, overstarchy, oversugary, greasy dishes. A body molds to the nature of the food that it digests. We cannot embalm our bodies and yet expect to enjoy good health.

The abundance of white flour products, dumplings, sauces, extracts, bakery breads, cakes, pies, sweets, doped-up creams, substitute milks, substances loaded with salt, pepper and condiments is absolutely disastrous. Canned food intake must be drastically reduced. We cannot ingest rancid, stale, unsound, lifeless, foodless food materials. We must deny outselves those "crackles" cereals, salted fat-fried snacks and confectionery products. Buns soft as cake made of aerated butter, cream substitutes and artificial sweeteners such as saccharin and cyclamates have to be eliminated.

Americans must not continue to buy foods because they have fancy cartons, cans or bottles. It is essential that we read what is on those elaborate labels, beneath the brand names. We must decide that we want to live closer to Nature than to a can opener, closer to the farmer than to our commercial, packaged foods of today. Whatever goes into the mouth must be approved by God, not the palate of man. Man, before it is too late, must live closer to the Creator and recognize his good.

Utensils for a Health Kitchen

The importance of preparation cannot be overemphasized. A few basic utensils and the knowledge to use them properly are invaluable. No doubt, some or perhaps many may be foreign to you.

Keep things natural, pure and whole. A half head of cabbage placed at meal time before the family members it is not an appealing salad. On the other hand, when we pickle, spice, bring on foods which have been demineralized, devitaminized we are living in an age which is worse.k Learn not to murder foods in the kitchen. Prepare them in such a way as to simplify the present means. Do not overcook and destroy their good; prepare them so they look and taste appetizing and appealing. The average person is not satisfied by total simplicity in foods. In visiting the Hunzas, I found they no longer wanted to live in the hardships of their past. They no longer wanted to live in stone houses. They want the products and conveniences that civilization is using to commit suicide. There must be some way to prevent the natural air, pure water and pure foods from becoming destroyed and to pass along the wisdom we have acquired through trial and error.

Stainless Steel Cookware: Such utensils develop the full flavor of food and do not leave a taste or odor. Another advantage is the fact that very little water is necessary in this air-tight cookware, and the food can be prepared over very low heat. Thus, the greatest possible amount of nutritional value of foods is preserved.

Parchment Paper: An inexpensive method of preparing food has been devised with parchment paper. It is unorthodox and has not caught on as a popular feature of the art of cooking, but vegetables heated in it can be served at their very best. Moisten the paper and lay vegetables inside. Add desired seasoning. Secure the four corners together forming a bag or sack and place in a pot of boiling water. This allows putting several varieties into the same pot. Reusable parchment paper sells for a nominal price.

Steamer: Several types of stainless steel steamers are suitable for use inside regular pots and pans. These allow quick preparation of vegetables with minimal loss of nutrients.

Vacuum Cooking: Use the vacuum thermos for cooking food overnight. Take a wide mouth thermos and place cereal grain or legumes inside with boiling water overnight, tightly sealed. Slow cooking is achieved effortlessly. Solar cooking will be a useful method in the future.

Electric Frying Pan: It is a valuable aid in meat preparation due to its roasting ability. Electric frying pans are super for omelets and scrambled eggs. Also, Chinese foods are very well adapted for this type of cookware. Cook entire meals in the same pan. Many Japanese meals also work very nicely by this method.

Double Boiler: It is indispensable for gently steaming grains and cereals, in addition to numerous other uses.

Pressure Cookers: If stainless steel, they are acceptable occasionally.

Crock Pots: They are acceptable and a most worthy addition in the field of cooking.

Microwave Ovens: This means of food preparation is quite doubtful. At the present time they have not been proven to be free of radiation hazards. Much research is needed as yet to assure safety. Personally, I am not assured that food cooked by microwave radiation is beneficial to man. Also, the radiation could be absorbed by persons close to the appliance. The radiation leakage must be completely stopped and the radiation must be proven harmless to food values. Perhaps we were not meant to cook foods in a flash.

Nut and Spice Grinders: These are sometimes referred to as coffee grinders. However, lthey adapt excellently to grinding sesame seeds, almonds, sunflower seeds, flaxseed, in addition to whole nutmeg, licorice root and carob pods.

Juicer: Many models are available, according to the price range and adaptability sought. The average family can use the typical juicer often. The Acme is a fine brand; the Champion serves not only as a juicer but for making ice cream, nut butters and many other concoctions. The Norwalk is another excellent juicer, used predominently as a commercial appliance. The hydraulic press is the ideal juicer.

Blender of Liquefier: Complex models with ten or more speeds or the simplified three-speed blender are available. These types of appliances are especially useful to mix liquids, puree, chop, liquefy, etc.

Handy Kitchen Gadgets

Keep an array of wooden spoons, paring knives, chopping knives, measuring cups and spoons, mashers, strainers, ceramic teapot on hand. Pyrex, Corning Ware or earthenware are all acceptable. Most of the appliances and gadgets are available in your local health food stores where the sales personnel will gladly explain their uses. You might also want to consider an electric yogurt maker, sprouting jar kits and a roaster. Experiment creatively with flavor, color and eye appeal.

Keep your eyes open for what is available in the stores. Human ingenuity is not dead and wonderful new products come out from time to time.

Average Nutrition Loss by Boiling

According to the *Journal of Home Economics,* the average loss of the following mineral elements in boiling foods is extensive; 48% of the iron is lost; 31% of the calcium is destroyed; 46% of the phosphorus escapes; and 45% of the magnesium is lost.

The equivalent of 50% of the food value of a white potato is lost by boiling; 40% of the value of cabbage is lost; a peeled, cored and boiled apple is robbed of 50% of its nutritional value.

Use only stainless steel waterless cookware; use a minimum of water and prepare with the vessels tightly covered. Expanding steamers are handily placed in many different sized cooking utensils for steaming with a small amount of water. This is a kitchen gadget you shouldn't be without.

Cookery Processes and Health

Steaming: Whenever boiling water (in a pressure cooker or ordinary pot) is used to cook fish, meat, fruit, greens or vegetables without contact from below, through a wire container or perforated base, the process is defined as steaming. Avoid overcooking, especially of fruits and vegetables.

Broiling: When fish, meat, or other foods are subjected to direct heat from flame, electricity, coals or other heat source, the food is being broiled. In broiling fish or meat in an oven, place it on a wire rack or broiler pan with a container beneath to collect the fat drippings. Turn the food; broiling liberates the juices and destroys germ life. Slow broiling for longer periods is preferable.

Frying: Frying fish, meat or other foods with or without fat or oil is not favorable to health. The searing of meat in contact with metal has been claimed to produce carcinogens. Never eat fried foods.

Boiling: Boiling fish, meat or other foods has its disadvantages. Food becomes waterlogged by boiling;

some of the flavor and aroma passes into the water or steam. The chemistry of some food elements is altered; food elements such as fluorine may be boiled into gas, while other minerals and substances such as lecithin may be precipitated and lost. Boiling does not kill all germs. Some species of bacteria can resist being boiled for days. However, the number of bacteria is usually considerably reduced by boiling. The main disadvantage of boiling is loss of vitamins and minerals in the cooking water. The main advantage is in cooking soups and broths. Generally speaking, boiled food is soggy and lifeless.

Juniper berries contain both an oil and a resin. They are used as a diuretic, to tone up the sexual system, cleanse the liver and blood.

Cooking With Minimum Water

Vegetables especially lose vitamins and minerals when cooked in excess water, in open containers and for too long a time. The following methods can be used with very little water.

Stainless Steel Cookware: Use first quality, heavy, stainless steel cooking utensils. They should have tightly fitting covers. Fill to the brim with vegetables and use only a few tablespoons water. Steam until barely tender.

Casserole Cookware: Prepare vegetables quickly, so you retain as many nutrients as possible. (They are oxidized into the air very rapidly when cut surfaces are exposed.) Fill casserole to the top and cover tightly. Bake in moderate oven; use very little water.

Steamer: Choose a suitable size vessel with a perforated insert container and lid. Cook contents tightly covered.

Parchment Paper: Any vegetable may be cooked in parchment paper — also other foods such as fish. Wet the paper; put the vegetables in the center and secure the edges, making a closed "bag." Place the bag in boiling water. Several bags of different foods or vegetables may cook in the same pan. Put them in at such times that they will all be done at once. Save the juices inside the bag. Parchment paper is inexpensive and can be used many times.

Pressure Cooker: Pressure cooking is acceptable occasionally. Don't use this method often. Very little water is required.

Elderberry juice seems to have a special affinity for the ovaries and uterus. An oily acid in this juice vitalizes the female sex glands and organs if taken daily over a period of time.

Microwave Ovens and Pacemaker Dysfunction

We belileve microwave ovens are questionable for health at best, as we have previously stated. Research has found that battery charged pacemakers placed in the body for heart regulation were stopped by exposure to microwave ovens. So, there must also be a high-frequency radiation effect from the oven to the body in some manner. Is it safe or is this another of those processes with long-term or time-bomb effects on health? Would Nature approve it?

In a laboratory test of 15 microwave units, it was found that measurable amounts of radiation where escaping. It was also found that the same type of radiation caused cataract in test animals.

Mulberries and their juice have remarkable nerve-soothing properties. They are wonderful for reducing fevers, sedating the nerves, quieting the passions and intense emotions.

The fruit or juice from cranberries, rhjubarb or gooseberries is not recommended because they are high in oxalic acid and hard on the kidneys.

Pomegranate juice is an excellent tonic for the kidneys, an effective cleanser. A good frescade for hot summer days, it has sodium and magnesium in it.

Chapter 30

Know your magic sevens

Life and Nature Vibrate to Sevens

We have outlined a basic program for offering seven various ways of doing things; seven choices for each food category. The best elements in life and Nature vibrate to the number seven. It is a universal law.

Variety Is All Important

Variety is a diet statute. Having vegetables does not mean peas and carrots every day. Popeye made spinach famous but do not serve it every day. Potatoes are a staple but not to be used daily. Oranges are high in vitamin C, but there are many other juices. Wheat and milk are the major allergy bandits, and we should not have them as often as most do. Other grains can be substituted. Plan a different grain for each day of the week and do the same with other foods. Start over at the beginning of a new week — or, better still, use your own creativity and multiply seven times seven. The possibilities are limitless. Rearrange in multiples of seven. Offered are a few suggestions of proteins, starches, etc., arranged in sevens. Build onto those listed. Always stress variety.

There are many ways of doing anything. Remember to use natural, pure and whole foods at all times. It will become second nature before long. If what we have learned before is wront, it's time for a change. *Now.*

Seven Powerful Proteins

Many people automatically equate protein with meat. A body built on meat and potato meals alone will be no better than the quality of the meat and potatoes themselves. We mold to what the body is fed. If the material for body building is so limited, good health is impossible. Consider the following list additions. Use variety and color.

1. **Lean Meat:** No fat, pork or cured meats. Organ meats are approved; also fowl, lamb or beef.
2. **Fish:** Any white fish which has fins and scales. Halibut, trout, haddock, sole, bass.
3. **Eggs:** Soft-boiled or poached; never fried. Raw egg yolk is best.
4. **Cheese:** Any cheese which breaks, such as cottage cheese. Try a variety of raw, unprocessed or naturally processed kinds.
5. **Milk:** Unpasteurized is the best. Goat milk is better than cow milk. Buttermilk is good. Yogurt and clabbered milk can be very easily made in your own home.
6. **Nuts & Seeds:** Break these down to a more digestible form by making them into butters or drinks. Grind and sprinkle over dishes such as breakfast cereal grains or salads before serving.
7. **Legumes:** Lentils are the easiest to digest. Other good relatives are peas, beans, garbanzos and soybeans.
   Plus — Soy milk, spirulina, chlorella.

Seven Starches and Cereals

The first four of these produce the least catarrh.

1. **Brown rice**
2. **Yellow corn meal**
3. **Millet**
4. **Rye**
5. **Sweet potatoes and yams**
6. **Bananas (ripe)**
7. **Oatmeal (steel-cut)**
   The last three are weight building.
   Plus: Baked white potatoes, barley, wheat, buckwheat groats. Use crackers instead of bread. Rye crackers, Armenian crackers, rice crackers, flat breads from Scandinavian countries. If bread is served, have good bread. Add supplements to the flour such as rice polishings, wheat germ, sesame seeds. Try corn bread, sprouted wheat, nut breads and even carrot bread. We build a new body each year. Begin to build a better body for this year and every year to follow.

Seven Safe Sweets

Most sweets, especially sugars, are acid-forming and rob the body of sodium salts and calcium. This eventually leads to stomach and digestive disorders where sodium is concerned. Remember to limit the use of sweets, even the good ones.

1. **Honey:** Never use heated honey. Always buy raw, unheated honey. In cooking, baking or generally heating foods use a sweetener other than honey. Heated honey kills bees, even though it is their natural food.

2. **Date Sugar**
3. **Maple Sugar**
4. **Molasses:** It is very high in iron.
5. **Raw Sugar:** Yellow D is favored. There are others such as Turbinado and Barbados varieties.
6. **Concentrates:** These are made from whole fruit — skin, seeds and pulp. Cherry and apple are two of the best. Black raspberry and grape are also available.
7. **Grape Sugar**

White refined sugar has been manhandled extensively. The processing methods rob the natural elements and break down the remaining ones. Thus, it is void of the vital minerals and vitamins.

All sugars are acid-forming and thus should be used most sparingly. Even honey or apple sugar leaches calcium and sodium salts from the body.

Seven Selected Oils

Never use any heated oil. This factor cannot be reiterated enough in maintaining a healthy kitchen. Heating oil hardens the composition to the state where the body digestive mechanism cannot break it down. They are deposited in the body as cholesterol-forming particles. Buy raw, unprocessed, cold pressed oils. Use a variety, although I personally prefer safflower as the foremost. It is the highest of the unsaturated fatty acids. Soybean is the second best and sunflower follows.

1. **Avocado**
2. **Safflower**
3. **Soybean**
4. **Sunflower Seed**
5. **Sesame Seed**
6. **Apricot Seed**
7. **Olive Oil**

Plus: Peanut, corn, almond, linseed and pumpkin seed oils and many others.

Seven Best Drinks

Any liquid taken with meals can cause gas. If this plagues you, use drinks between meals. We do consider these to be foods, but water should never be taken with a meal.
1. **Whey:** High in sodium and a cooling food. A mild laxative.
2. **Vegetable Drinks:** Carrot, cucumber juices, etc.
3. **Green Drink:** Blend greens, strain, use liquid. Pineapple juice may be added for flavor. (Use wild greens, comfrey, beet tops, watercress, etc.)
4. **Coffee Substitutes:** PERO, Sanno-Caf, Symington's Instant Dandelion Root Coffee, Dandelion Root Tea.
5. **Herb Teas:** Cold or hot. Alfa-Mint, papaya-mint, comfrey, oat straw. Many herb teas may be used. They are also a good base for adding fruit and vegetable juices.
6. **Soy Milk, Almond Milk or Sunflower Seed Milk**
7. **Dr.'s Drink:** 1 tablespoon sesame seed butter or meal, one glass of liquid (fruit juice, vegetable juice, soymilk or broth and water), 1/4 avocado, 1 teaspoon honey (or to taste). Blend 1/2 minute.

Plus: Buttermilk, strawberry juice (high in sodium), carob drinks. Also refer to seven best teas for further suggestions.

Seven Best Cooking Vegetables

I consider the beet to be the finest of all the vegetables because it is an excellent liver and gall bladder cleanser. Many physical ailments begin with the liver. Carrots are wonderful and universally used, but the beet is king of them all.

1. **Beets**
2. **Carrots**
3. **String Beans**
4. **Zucchini**
5. **Spinach**
6. **Peas**
7. **Summer Squash and Banana Squash**

Plus: Eggplant, artichoke, green pepper, Chinese snow peas, turnips, rutabagas, kohlrabi. The tops of turnips and beets; Swiss chard, mustard greens. Sulphur vegetables which m ay cause gas disturbances can be "de-gassed" to some extent by cooking in stainless steel utensils over very low heat. These include: cabbage, cauliflower, onions, broccoli, Brussels sprouts, garlic and leeks.

Seven Chosen Salad Vegetables

1. **Lettuce:** Always use leaf lettuce instead of the head variety. The leaf is 40 times higher in iron. Head lettuce is gas forming and contains a substance responsible for retarding digestion. Romaine, Red Tip, etc.
2. **Carrots:** Raw carrots are high in vitamin A. Bland. Do not produce gas or irritate the intestinal tract.
3. **Beets:** Raw and shredded. Best for the liver as well as the bowel. A daily serving the size of a golf ball added atop various salads is beneficial.
4. **Cucumbers:** High in sodium, a summer cooling food.
5. **Parsley:** Helps the kidneys eliminate better.
6. **Watercress:** High in potassium.
7. **Zucchini:** Bland. Most people can assimilate it without difficulty or disturbance to the intestinal tract. It is suggested for a transition diet.
Plus: Try some of the wild greens, such as: malva, filiree, lamb's quarter, dandelion greens. Also use raw

some of the vegetables generally cooked, such as spinach, cauliflower, young peas, grated parsnips and turnips (much sweeter when raw), string beans. Learn how to make sprouts. Use a couple of handsful every day. Old standbys: Tomatoes, radishes, green peppers, onions, celery. Have a comfrey garden and use fresh leaves daily.

Seven Favorite Salads

Shred, chop, grate. Each imparts a distinctive flavor. Salads add essential minerals and vitamins along with enzymes the body needs. Water and bulk are brought to the body for good intestinal activity.

1. **Cole Slaw:** Cabbage, with celery seed and onions added.
2. **Fruit Salad:** With nuts and yogurt dressing.
3. **Shredded Carrots and Raisins**
4. **Potato Salad**
5. **Gelatin Salad**
6. **Guacamole:** Mashed tomatoes and avocados with chopped onion, a few drops of lime and seasoning.
7. **Waldorf Salad:** Apples, raisins and nuts.
    Plus: Take half an avocado, stuff with nut butter or cottage cheese. Try combining raw corn, coconut, lettuce and green pepper. Refer to recipe sections for further creative suggestions. Salads may be blended using liquefier for those with delicate digestive systems.

Seven Good Salad Dressings

Healthy salad dressings can add valuable vitamin and mineral supplements to balance meals more completely.

1. **Bleu Cheese or Roquefort**
2. **Vinegar and Oil**
3. **Avocado**
4. **Nut Butter**
5. **Oil and Lemon and Honey**
6. **Mayonnaise with seasoning**
7. **Cheddar Cheese with Yogurt, Vinegar and Caraway Seeds**
    Plus: Shredded beets and carrots with vinegar, oil, raw egg yolk, seasoning, (optional) honey or onion. **For children:** add the concentrates (apple, cherry, etc.) over shredded carrots. It tastes good and valuable nutrition is a bonus.

Seven Legumes and Beans

It is interesting to note that legumes are alkaline forming when fresh. Therefore, they are lower in starch formation. When dried they become acid forming. The lentil is, in my estimation, one of the finest legumes; the lima bean ranks second.

1. **Lentil**
2. **Lima Beans**
3. **Soybeans**
4. **Garbanzos or Chick Peas**
5. **Black Beans**
6. **Split Peas**
7. **Pinto Beans**
    Plus: Fava beans, aduki beans, kidney beans, blackeyed peas and horse beans. Beans provide extra nourishment for the worker whose job requires hard physical labor.

Seven Best Herbs

Herbs have been relied upon for their remedial properties since ancient times. This is almost a science in itself, and there are many books to study on this subject. However, herbs must be used in cooperation with the proper diet and nutrition for satisfactory results.

1. **Mint:** Served with fruits, lamb, vegetables.
2. **Thyme:** for meat, sauces, stocks, fish and most vegetables.
3. **Rosemary:** Noted for its flavor enhancement of lamb. Used with other meats such as duck, veal and with vegetables.
4. **Basil:** Especially good with tomatoes, fish and eggs.
5. **Dill:** With salads, vegetables, potatoes.
6. **Sage:** Used sparingly with meats, cheeses.
7. **Bay Leaves:** In soups and sauces.
    Plus: Fenugreek used as an artificial maple flavoring, onions, garlic, chives, scallions, parsley, caraway, red and green peppers, savory and marjoram.
    An herb garden outside the kitchen is ideal. Herbs also thrive indoors by the window in small flower pots.

Seven Seasonings for Health

Salt is considered a drug, for it does have cumulative effects in the body, particularly in hardening of the arteries and high blood pressure. It is wise to cut down on its use or eliminate it altogether. If salt is necessary, use a little sea salt. There is a rock salt also, called earth salt, which is natural and has not been heated to the extreme temperatures as most table salt. Vegetable broth powder is a good alternative to salt and can be purchased at health food stores. It is composed of dehydrated vegetables, protein and the natural salt taste that comes from wheat. Use cayenne pepper instead of the regular black pepper. Black pepper is $4 times more irritating to the liver than alcohol.

1. **Vegetable Broth Powder**
2. **Cayenne**
3. **Paprika**
4. **Nutmeg**
5. **Carob**
6. **Cinnamon**
7. **Ginger**

Plus: Poppy seed, allspice, mushrooms, vanilla, almond extract. Kelp and dulce from the sea are tasty. Remember to add any salt at the end of cooking time. In this way its use is diminished. Never use honey in any baked goods; it forms an acid when warmed to high temperatures.

Seven Good Soups

A protein soup does not require meat as the main ingredient. A tablespoon of a nut butter or seed butter added just before serving transforms any soup into protein soup. Egg yolk may also be added after cooking. Never cook any of the creams, oils or butters as heat destroys lecithin and vitamin E; add to cooked dish while warm. Always simmer soup instead of boiling. Meat cooked for long periods of time is hard on the kidneys. Soups can be made from the joints of meat or the bones and cooked with the jelly. The uric acid present in the meat is not there.

1. **Vegetable Soup**
2. **Borsch**
3. **Onion Soup**
4. **Split Pea**
5. **Potato Soup**
6. **Miso** (soybean paste)
7. **Barley and Mushroom**

Seven Nifty Nuts to Use

The almond is the undisputed ruler of the nut kingdom. It is the most alkaline. The Missouri black walnut is the second challenger to the throne because of its high manganese content which feeds the brain and nervous system. (Good for the memory.) Nut butters lend themselves readily to easy digestion. Use nut milk drinks such as almond nut milk.

1. **Almond**
2. **Missouri Black Walnut**
3. **Cashews**
4. **Pinenuts or Pignolas** (they are 44% fat)
5. **Pecans**
6. **Coconut**
7. **Hazelnut**

Seven Great Seeds

Nothing matches the rejuvenation powers of seeds. Every life component is encased in their hulls. Sesame is the finest of all.

1. **Sesame**
2. **Sunflower**
3. **Squash**
4. **Melon:** Blend them with equal amounts of water and strain; use only the liquid, add fruit juice for flavoring.
5. **Chia Seed**
6. **Alfalfa Seed**
7. **Fenugreek Seed**
   Plus: Sprouted seeds (see sprout section)

Seven Fresh Fruits

The ones listed below are high in vitamins, especially vitamin C, and additionally have laxative powers. Fruits provide a balance for water for the system.

1. **Peaches**
2. **Bananas**
3. **Apples**
4. **Pears**
5. **Berries**
6. **Pineapple**
7. **Apricots**
   Plus: Nectarines, avocados, papayas, mangoes, cherries, persimmons, grapes, plums, melons.

Seven Dried Fruits

Dried fruits listed are very concentrated, eat sparingly. Always revive before eating. Eating dried fruit without reviving encourages gas.

1. **Black Monnuka Raisins**
2. **Prunes**
3. **Figs**
4. **Dates** (Reviving is not necessary because they are semi-dried).
5. **Apricots**
6. **Peaches**
7. **Pears**
   Plus: Apples, pineapple, bananas.

Seven Best Teas — and Then Some

Herb teas with a touch of honey or mint are very pleasing to the taste. Prepare tea by bringing water to a boil and pouring it over leaves into a heated teapot. (Heat by filling with boiling water while tea water is boiling). Do not boil tea with the exception of oat straw tea which is simmered for 5 to 7 minutes to capture the essence from the stalk. Teas may be mixed in any combinations desired.

1. **Alfalfa and Mint**
2. **Comfrey**
3. **Lemon Grass**
4. **Oat Straw**
5. **Camomile**
6. **Papaya**
7. **Cornsilk**

Mint and sassafras are used to flavor other teas. Mint is also an effective gas propellent. Orange and lemon peel provide additional flavoring.

Plus:

1. **Hawthorne Berry Tea:** For the heart.
2. **Parsley Tea:** For kidney disturbances.

3. **Blueberry Tea:** For low blood pressure.
4. **Fenugreek Tea:** For catarrhal buildup.
5. **Comfrey Tea:** Along with Fenugreek tea, mixed together for catarrhal disturbances; comfrey is also used for intestinal disturbances.
6. **KB 11:** A kidney tea; a mild diuretic.
7. **Shave Grass Tea:** For silicon and for the kidneys.

And:

1. **Licorice:** Aids digestion.
2. **Sage:** For colds.
3. **Valerian:** A natural tranquilizer.
4. **Uva Ursi:** For kidneys.
5. **Flaxseed Tea:** For the bowel.

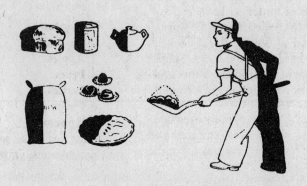

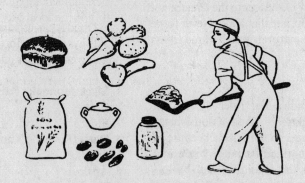

HALF A LOAF—HALF A BODY

In this illustration, we have pictured foods in black and white showing only a certain percentage of the foods we eat are chemically balanced properly so that the life we get from these foods gives us all that is necessary for a strong, healthy body.

Chapter 31

Food shopping made easy

Vital, Live Foods Build Life

Live foods are the architects of life. They are the tissue builders, containing the embryo, the germ, and they are the sparks which start the body toward the repair and rejuvenation we desire. Live proteins are necessary to execute the body's life principles. The soul or spirit cannot build a good physical body using dead foods. Eve wasn't equipped with cooking utensils, drying pans, electric appliances. Doctors and drugstores were unheard of in the Garden of Eden. The Lord our God said: "Behold, I have given you every herb bearing seed, which is upon the face of all the earth, and every tree, in which is the fruit of a tree yielding seed; to you it shall be meat." (Gen. 1:29)

lives during the biblical era? Is it any wonder men as tall as cedars and as strong as oaks walked the earth? Man cannot live without live foods. Foods which spoil are the only healthy foods. To appropriate the principles of life, we must learn how to prepare natural foods, not always relying on cooking, baking, boiling or otherwise changing the original state. Cooking, and especially overcooking, destroys and disorganizes vitamins, enzymes and minerals. Many essential nutrients are drained off in the cooking water.

Today's foods are producing convalescents, weak children, feeble women and aged men. Is this the manner in which you choose to exist? Get closer to the Creator and recognize His good to appropriate that good. Never forget that in God's garden grow natural, pure, whole foods.

Don't Substitute Good Health

Any food ingested will become "bricks" in the living temple, our body, as working material for bones, muscles, tendons, ligaments. Thus, we must reach for the finest building material money can buy. The wise individual selects the very best for himself because he deserves the very best. Superior elements are necessary for the transition to new and higher horizons. Take care of others as you would want them to care for you. Don't reach for substitutes. The single exception is in the substitute which is better than the original product. Substitute only the "real" and natural products.

Labor Is the Greatest Cost

We pay for man's labor in the canned, wrapped, specially packaged items. In most cases we pay additionally for man's tampering with Nature's perfection and in all cases we pay for the package or can. As a rule, the simpler the food, the healthier. Labor escalates the price of food. For example, tomatoes purchased from a farmer cost very little as compared with the price of canned tomatoes. We pay for the growing, harvesting, shipping, storage, heating and canning; we pay for the container and the factory, distributor and retailer profit. Only a fraction of the cost is for the food itself. The cereal grains used in most dry breakfast cereals cost about one third or less of the finished product. Novelty packaging, preservatives and fancy advertising zoom consumer cost. The person who expects "something good" for nothing usually gets something "good for nothing."

Why Not Prepare Food Fresh at Home?

We can make many foods from scratch at home. We are prone to depend on ready-made, premised, prepared foods, even precooked, rather than to create our own. These homemade foods are nutritious and inexpensive. Fresh is the ideal way to serve food. Any commercially packaged food is adulterated by preservatives. When you buy such items you often pay double — once for what is in the package and again for the adverse effects it has upon the body. Effects range from irritation, to stimulation, to depression — all precursors of ill health. The payment for most prepared foods doesn't cover the doctor's fee.

Beware of Misleading Labels

It is critical to understand the labels and especially to recognize "coal tar" additives and the thousands of other additives. As a rule, the simplest pure, whole and natural foods are best. Many additives require a knowledge of chemistry to understand, deceiving the simple minded into thinking that they are all right. If they are not natural, they are not all right.

Advertising Is a Consumer Cost

A product may cost a few cents to concoct, while $2.00 to $2.50 is spent in advertising and promotion. The consumer absorbs the advertising budget of of manufacturer and retailer. It has been reported that many drug companies will expend 50-60% of their budget in sales promotion.

Land of the "Dollar Foods"

Countless commercial food companies are on the stock market. People invest large sums of money in these products with the intention of deriving profits. The basic quality and nutritional content of such products is of little or no concern to the investor. They are classed as "dollar foods" or "commercial foods," which make two classes of people rich: investors and doctors. For instance, milk substitutes are realizing tremendous profits as compared to very little revenue from the original "organic" milk.

Natural substitutes are the only safe, health-promoting foods to trust. Natural, pure and whole foods are the law. Sacrifices must be made to attain good health these days. We cannot live on taste alone. The table is a place of wisdom as well as pleasure. The idea is to dine in joy in such a manner that the joy continues after the feast, and future maladies and miseries are prevented.

The Land of Milk and Honey

In a wonderland of such abundance and wide arrays of tantalizing alternatives, foods confuse and misguide the senses. Unnecessary substitutes should be replaced by natural foods.

Living in a land of plenty encourages limitless gorging. Take only the portion you need from the plentiful supply God has provided and Mother Earth has produced. Moderation benefits the body most.

Don't contribute to the billions of dollars spent to build new hospitals to accommodate sick Americans during the years ahead. Build an individual temple to house good health, not illness. You are the master of that temple, the body you walk in. The wise man recognizes the difference between the temple of health and the temple of sickness.

Food Additives To Be Careful Of

People today are beginning to see that we must have fresh air and pure water. But as for food, it's the neglected stepchild. We find pollution there, too. Some 3,000 food additives should be tested for safety. There are two basic criteria I would recommend. The additive should be a natural substance that can be digested and used by the body or it should be a substance that passes through the body without harming or irritating any organ or tissue. It should be totally excreted. It should not be a product which accumulates in any organ or tissue with the potential of contributing to disease, discomfort, catarrhal discharge or a growth.

Some of the most prevalent food additives for flavoring and coloring are:

Amyl Alcohol: It is used to imitate brandy flavor in numerous bakery products. Medical tests prove 30 cc can cause death. Smaller dosages can damage kidneys. Labels only say "artificial flavoring." Industrially, the chemical is used as a varnish solvent.

Allyl Isothiocyanate: Adds artificial mustard flavor to sauces. It was used industrially in the making of poison gas in World War I. It is capable of producing slow-healing ulcers.

Amyl Acetate: It adds a butter flavor to baked goods. It is used as a solvent in oil paint.

Butyric Acid: It is also used to impart a butter flavor to baked goods. Industrially, it decalcifies hides and is an ingredient in varnishes.

Ethyl Formate: It gives baked goods a rum flavor. It is a tobacco fungicide and a solvent for nitrocellulose.

Ethyl Acetate: It gives bakery goods a pineapple taste. It is used in the manufacture of a smokeless powder, photographic films and in textile cleaning. Medical findings state it is a poison which can cause liver and heart damage.

N-Butyl Alcohol: This additive gives baked goods a whiskey flavor. It is also employed in the manufacture of detergents and for preparing paraffin imbedding. It is known to cause headaches, dizziness and drowsiness.

Diethylene Glycol: It has induced cancer in test animals. Though manufacturers are well aware of this fact, they continue to use it. It is present as additives in breads, rolls, ice cream, shredded coconut, jelly-like candies, marshmallows and chocolate.

Sodium Benzoate: It appears in the manufacture of margarine, jellies, carbonated drinks, jams, fruit juices, candy, mincemeat and pickles. According to medical literature, it can cause nausea, and a therapeutic dosage can prove fatal to a sensitive person.

Sodium Nitrite and Sodium Nitrate: They are common dyes used to make cured meats "pinker." The government ban on the use of sodium nitrite in fish is largely ignored.

Triphenylmethane Dyes: One of the most common is light green SF and also fast green. They are known carcinogenic products.

Other Dangerous Dyes

Many dyes are profusely used in coloring candies, cordials, biscuits, essences, cakes, maraschino cherries, jellies, frozen desserts.

Findings have reported Brilliant Blue as a cancer producer. It is a prevalent additive in icings, inc cream toppings, milk-bar syrups, candies, soft drinks, cake decorations, bakery products and puddings.

Coal Tar Manufacture Is Big Business

Numerous colorings have disappeared from the list upon discovery of their evident danger. Countless others, known to be dangerous, still remain certified and approved. In 1941, approximately 2-1/4 million pounds were certified. by 1959, the figure had increased to 6 million pounds. Testing takes time, and long range effects often not evident. Ideally, a ban should include all untested and unsafe colorings. Safety rechecks should be repeatedly administered. Very few colorings could quality as safe, at least initially. These triflings with coal tar products are openly inviting carcinogenic conditions. Coal tar products should be eliminated entirely.

Lastly, we should eat foods as they occur naturally — void of artificial colorings and additives.

Are You a Wise Food Buyer?

The food shopper should always keep in mind several principles. Food should be as natural as possible. It should be as whole and pure as possible — uncooked, unpreserved, unpolished and undevitalized. Insist upon foods raised in Nature's garden, not made or manhandled by man.

We know that the majority of supermarket foods have traveled many miles from field to storage and distribution destinations. Often they have become acid forming
or vine or bush. The great majority of market fruit is picked green. The stomach is sorely distressed at the quantity of green acids it must try to take care of. Reactions such as joint stiffness and aches are often the result. The stomach has trouble in breaking down the chemical elements and extracting the vitamin values needed to run a healthy body from fruit picked green. for total sun ripened benefits and to get the life force.

It is extremely difficult to obtain perfectly sun ripened fruits in the supermarkets. It is highly advantageous to visit a farm to secure fresh fruit naturally ripened on the tree or vine or bush. The great majority of market fruit is picked green. The stomach is sorely distressed at the quantity of green acids it must try to take care of. Reactions such as joint stiffness and aches are often the result. The stomach has trouble in breaking down the chemical elements and extracting the vitamin values needed to run a healthy body from fruit picked green.

The maturity date for fruit is critical, unlike that of vegetables. It is okay to eat young or old beets, for instance, and young or old asparagus. Vegetables retain food value at almost any age to feed the body well. But this is not true of most fruit. This explains the basis in my recommended diet for six vegetables per day and only two fruits. This proportion is especially stressed due to the unlikelihood of being able to purchase sun ripened, mature fruit. Body balance is dependent on the proper diet proportions.

Specific "Orchard and Garden" Buying Tips

Apples, for example, should have a finished flower end. A red apple should be red completely to the flower end; the same applies to yellow apples. This signifies ripeness.

An avocado should be squeezed gently inside the entire hand and fingers. If the avocado moves from the seed, it is ripe and ready.

In buying pineapple, pull out a leaf or two. If they respond to the pressure easily, the pineapple is ripe and sweet.

Look for the female species in melons. Indented stem ends signify a female. Those narrowing to a sharp point are the male variety and not as sweet.

Corn should possess a completely browned and dry tassel. Thus every kernel has been nourished. Each silk fiber is the sunshine life line to each kernel on the cob.

Find a dry stem in selecting grapes. When it begins to dry, the grapes are ripe. If the stem and the little stem ends entering the grapes are not dry, the grapes are not finished, not completely ripened. They will lack sweetness.

When buying certain kinds of greens, such as beets, use the greens first and allow the beets a couple days more to mature. Try to find unsprayed greens, though it is increasingly difficult. Follow this suggestion especially at the beginning of the season when the producer is likely to rush foods to market early.

Most beet greens are not sprayed. Neither is watercress or endive. Watercress is one of the highest potassium-yielding greens known.

Always buy leaf lettuce, the large, soft type, such as the Romaine variety. It contains many times the amount of iron as head lettuce.

Select cheese that breaks. Buy raw cheese when possible. Aged cheeses are better and easier to digest. Avoid cheese spreads.

Buy plain natural yogurt and add your own fresh fruits and juices to it.

Choose bottled juices over the canned juices. The metal container can adversely affect the juice. However, don't purchase sugar-laden bottled juices. Read the labels.

Frozen foods are superior to those packed in preservatives, salted down or put up with any unnatural chemical additives. Invest in plain frozen foods. They are packed at their peak in order to be good when thawed. Organically grown foods, of course, are the best.

Buy nuts or seeds whole and grind them yourself as needed. They should be finely ground and eaten in flake form, or better yet, made into nut or seed butters. Hard shelled nuts contain the highest amount of rich oils. Soft shelled pecans, almonds and the like allow the oils to dry out in the meats. Oils are vital for the brain and nervous systems.

Select the smallest hull legumes, such as peas, beans, lentils and garbanzos. Lentil hulls are finer and easier to handle in the delicate digestive tract. Use the smallest beans possible.

Likewise, use the smallest seeds. They are the most vitally packed. Chia, sesame and alfalfa are prime choices.

A health food store product is available that aids in breaking down harmful sprays. However, it is impossible to rid the fruits and vegetables of all the spray. It was applied liberally many times during the flowering stage. The apple core, for example, contains 75% of the spray residue.

grind it yourself, if you can. Grind freshly just prior to using it. Millet is one of the finest cereal grains known.

Every kitchen should use health teas. Alfalfa Mint tea is great for digestion. Dandelion tea soothes liver disturbances. Try hybiscus flower tea. The choice is infinite.

Remember one axiom for shopping: Never try to skimp and save money. Pay a little extra to insure getting the vital elements the body must have. Money saved foolishly today on foods may be spent ;many times over on doctor bills tomorrow.

We are idealists; without ideals we sicken and die. Know which foods are best; we must study to gain the knowledge necessary to survive.

Foodless Food for Illness

During the past 50 years Americans have consumed increasingly tremendous quantities of artificial food products. Supermarkets are crushed beneath the load, yet more are heaped onto their shelves daily. It is estimated that some 15,000 "foodless" foods line the supermarket lanes.

More and more food is man-handled in preparation for shelf-life durability; more transportation and storage is required before reaching the often unsuspecting consumer. Public ignorance and apathy allow the abominable and detrimental practices to continue unchallenged. In guarding and promoting family health, isn't natural, pure and whole food preferable to man-handled, adulterated products?

Questionable Commercial Foodlist

Below is a listing of commercially-handled food products. Some could be transformed to health-style foods; others are questionable; the majority are to be avoided. Above all, learn to be an avid label reader, bearing in mind that labels don't always tell the whole story.

Acetic Acid	Hot Biscuits
Ale	Diabetic Biscuits
Alkaloids	Light Biscuits
Almonds (sulphured)	Puffed Biscuits
Allspice (adulterated)	White Flour Biscuits
Apple Butter (doped)	Boric Acid (used in foods)
Apple Dumplings	Bouillon, canned
Apple Snow	Bread with Alum
Apricots (sulphured)	Baking Powder
Apricot Sauce	Baker's Bread
Baker's Eggs	Short Bread
Baking Powder	Bread, White
Barley Drinks	Breakfast Foods, scorched
Batter Cakes	Broths of Meat
Beans in excess	Buns
Beef, dried	Butter Preservatives
Beef, fried	Butter Preserves
Beef Extracts	Butter, rancid
Beef Juice, canned	Butter, doctored
Beef Soup, canned	Baker's Cakes
Beef Teas (made to sell)	Griddle Cakes
Beet Sugar	Layer Cakes

Fish broth has remarkable nerve-restoring vitality. It is not a stimulant but a vitalizer to brain and nerves.

It is possible that injury-prone athletes may not take care of themselves as well as they should, allowing a combination of fatigue and inherent weaknesses to take them out of the game.

Cinnamon, a popular flavoring is antiseptic, drives gas and is said to be good for flu.

Johnny Cakes
Candy
Candied Fruit Peel
Candied Walnuts
Candied Food not in glass containers
Caramelized Foods
Catsup of all kinds
Cereal Coffees
Cherries, red, canned
Chili Con Carne
Chili Sauce
Chili Chips
Chocolate Cake
Chocolate
Chocolate Candy
Cider
Cocoa Drinks
Cocoa Butter
Cola Drinks
Codfish Balls
Coffee Cereals
Coffee
Coffee Cake
Coffee Rings
Coloring Matter
Cookies
Compound Lard
Condensed Milk
Condiments, adulterated
Conserves
Commercial Consomme, canned
Corned Beef, drained
Corn Flakes
Corn Flour, processed
Corn Starch
Crackers
Cream Adulterants
Creamed Candies
Cream Pies
Cream Puffs
Creamed Potatoes
Instant Whips
Cupcakes
Crullers
Custard Powders
Diabetic Bread
Dried Sulphured Fruits
Doughnuts
Drinks with Glucose
Malted Drinks
Soda Fountain Drinks
Salty Drinks
Sweet Drinks
Drop Cakes
Drugs
Dumplings

Dye Stuff
Egg Substitutes
Extracts and Essences from the laboratory
Fancy Cakes
Figs, sulphured
Fillings
Fish and Vinegar
Fish, preserved
Flours, enriched
Fluorine, in drinking water
Foods, adulterated
Food, inferior
Food Substitutes
Foods, decomposed
Foods impoverished or injured by manufactureres
Foods, fried
Foods, bleached
Foods left standing uncovered
Foods with artificial sweetings
Foods, lifeless
Foods chemically altered from original
Foods, stale
Foods containing oxalic acid
Foods containing alum, dyes, glues, formaldehyde
Foods generating excess gas
Foods fried in fat
Foods highly seasoned
Frostings
French Rolls
Fritters
Fruit Juices, Flavorings and Essences (manufactured)
Fruits which are green
Fruits which have been spiced, peeled, candied,
    preserved
Sweetened Fruits
Fruit Syrups
Blanched Fruits
Very sour Fruits
Fudge
Ginger Bread
Ginger Snaps
Glucose foods such as table sugar, candy, dainties,
    bakery goods, syrups, jams, jellies, molasses,
    beverages, fountain drinks, confectionery, pies,
    puddings, sweet drinks, adulterated maple syrup,
    man-made sweeteners
Grape Drinks other than grape juice, punches
Grape Juice, over-sweetened
Grape Preserves, over-sweetened
Griddle Cakes
Canned chemically-smoked Hash
Hominy
Hot Cakes
Ice Cream, doped and containing "ethereal" flavors,
    glucose, coal tar dyes, artificial colorings and
    made from pasteurized milk

Icings
Infant Formulas
Infant Foods, containing cheap sugar
Invalid Foods, most of them devitalized foods
Lady Fingers
Lard
Lard Compounds
Lard, imitation
Layer Cakes
Lemon Extract
Adulterated Lemon Pie, fillers from laboratory
Drugstore Lime Water
Liquors
Macaroni
Macaroons
Malted Milk (due to excess of glucose)
Maple Sugar, imitation or adulterated
Marshmallows
Meat unclean, unsafe, canned, deviled, old, gouty,
    embalmed, fried, burned, smoked with chemicals,
    man-made, drained or from diseased animals
Meat Soups which are business soups
Milk pasteurized and chemically altered in its
    molecular structure or vitamins, killed by boiling,
    or doctored, or containing disease or bacteria
Milk from old cows
Milk that has been condensed, badly soured, contain-
    ing drugs to alter taste
Milk which has been sweetened, preserved with for-
    maldehyde or milk which is laden with dirt and
    impurities
Milk Powders
Minced Meat, commercial
Mustard Drinks
Noodles
Noodle Souffle
Obesity Drugs
Oils that are cooked or heated
Oleomargarine
Orange Ade
Oyster Crackers
Pastries
Rolls
Peaches, if bleached
Peanut Butter, heated
Pickles
Piccalilli
Pie Crust
Pigs Feet
Plain Rolls
Pineapple Essence, from the laboratory
Plums, canned
Popovers
Pork and Beans
Potato Puffs
Potato Rolls

Potato Fritters
Preserves
Pretzels
Puddings made from white flour, tapiocas, rhubarb
Rice Flour, polished
Saccharin
Salt
Sauces, commercial
Sausage, canned
Scones unless made with natural materials
Short Bread
Snaps
Soda Drinks
Soda Biscuits
Soda Crackers
Soup Meat
Spaghetti
Sponge Cake
Sugar (all kinds)
Sugar Buns
Sugary Foods
Sweeteners, artificial
Syrups, except maple
Sweets
Tapioca, impoverished
Tea Biscuits
Tea
Tea Cakes
Tonic Drugs
Vinegar and vinegar soaked foods
Wheat Muffins
Wafers made of devitalized flour
Water which has been minerally charged
Hard Water
Fluorine Water
Weiners

Diet Substitutes — Condemned and Condoned

Not Recommended	Recommended
Soda Pop	Fresh Fruit Drinks
Candy	Dried Fruits, Nuts
Milk Shakes	Sesame and Nut Whips
Lard, Heated Oils	Natural, Cold Pressed Vegetable Oils
Pastry	Graham Cracker crusts, un-fired ground raisins and nuts, carob meal, whole grain
Tea	Herb Teas

Not Recommended	Recommended	Not Recommended	Recommended
Coffee	Dandelion Root Coffee	Sugar Prepared Gelatins	Unflavored Gelatin or Agar — add fruit and vegetables
Vinegar	Lemon Juice, Apple Cider Vinegar (aged in wood)	Cocoa	Carob
Black Pepper	Capsicum, Red Peppers, Herbs, Horseradish, Cayenne	Chocolate	Carob, Stuffed Dates, etc.
Catsup	Natural Tomato Sauces	Potato Chips	Fresh Raw Nuts, Sunflower and Pumpkin Seeds
Pickles	Herbs, Fresh Vegetables and Fruits	Salted Nuts	Fresh Raw Nuts, unsalted
Pies	Fresh ripe Fruits, Fruit Whips, Puddings	Hamburgers	Sprout and Cheese Sandwich, Nut dishes and loaves
Bread	Whole Grains, Baked Potato	Beer	Vegetable Cocktails
Cakes	Unfired Fruit Squares	Ice Cream	Fruit Sherbets, Sour Cream and Fruit desserts
Doughnuts, Crullers	Whole Grain Cookies and Cakes, Stuffed Celery, Fruits	Mayonnaise	Health Mayonnaise, Yogurt-based dressings
White Rice	Unpolished Rice	Cornstarch Custards	Yogurt and Fruit, Arrowroot custards
Cornflour (starch)	Arrowroot	"Quick Desserts"	Egg Custards, fresh and dried fruits
White Bread	Whole Grains, whole grain breads, slice raw eggplant with avocado dressing, etc.	Artificial Flavorings and Colorings	Concentrated Fruit Juices, chlorophyll, beet juice, etc. to color; pure flavor and color
Corned, canned, preserved meats	Fresh young lean meat, veal (no fat or pork) soybean products, tofu	Tranquilizers	Herbs, Valerian, Warm Milk and Molasses
Antacids	Peppermint Tea, Alfalfa Tea	Cough Mixtures	Honey and Warmed Minced Onion (see recipe)
Aspirins, Drugs	Elimination Diets, Water Treatment, Herbs	Dumplings	Steamed Potatoes in Jackets
Cathartics	Blackstrap Molasses, Flaxseed, Yogurt, Apple Concentrate, Whey	White Flour	Whole Grain, Stone Ground Flours
Canned Fruits	Fresh Fruits	White Flour Macaroni, Spaghetti	Soy and Whole Grain Spinach Macaroni and Spaghetti
Salt	Vegetable Broth Powder		
Commercial Cereals	Steamed Millet, Muesli, Whole Barley, Rye, Yellow Cornmeal	Crumpets	Whole Grain Waffles
Sugar	Honey, Dried Fruits, Date Sugar, Fruit Concentrates	Pasteurized Milk	Fresh raw milk (goat milk preferred), nut, soy and seed milks

Not Recommended	Recommended
Spread Cream Cheeses	Aged, Raw Natural Cheeses, Goat Cheese, Tofu
Head Lettuce	Romaine, Endive, Watercress, Beet Leaves, Leaf Lettuce, Spinach
White Flour Gravies	Arrowroot, Rice Polishings for Thickenings, no grease or fat; add a little soy sauce

Selecting the Best Coconut

Shake the coconut vigorously to make sure it is full of rich milk. Avoid coconuts with moldy surface or no liquid.

Pierce the outer layer or shell with a sharp instrument such as an ice pick in one of the eyes. Drain milk through the hole.

Pare off the brown shell. Grate coconut a piece at a time. The blender can be used.

Be sure the milk can be heard to swish in selecting fresh coconuts. The more milk, the more tender the meat will be. When the milk is hardened, the meat is drier.

Coconut milk is an excellent companion to fruit juices; mix 1 part coconut milk to three parts fruit juice. The coconut is richer than other nuts and an excellent oil comes from it. It is almost free of starches, and its sugar is the finest. The water in coconut is rich in minerals.

Many coconuts are preserved in glycerine; many are highly sugared. Avoid these where possible. Buy unflavored shredded or fresh coconut without additives and sweeten ;it yourself if needed; add your own natural flavors.

What Do We Pay for Food Processing?

In 1983 at a West Coast supermarket, 20 pounds of potatoes cost 7 cents per pound; a pound from the vegetable bin cost 24 cents. Canned and sliced potatoes were 52 cents, frozen French fries were 69 cents and instant mashed potatoes $1.05 per pound. A well-known brand of potato chips cost $2.96 a pound.

How about the nutritional value lost in processing? What does that cost? What does it mean to your health? It seems that increased price in a product can be an indicator of how much processing has been done and of how much more of a health hazard the product has become.

Convenience foods are defined as those that "take less work or the adding of fewer ingredients in the home and in homemade recipes." Industry still insists that these foods are as cheap or cheaper than homemade varieties.

What about nutritional content? They avoid that subject.

Economical Food Practices

Buy food when you can store it easily during the period of seasonal abundance (lowest price). Learn to home freeze and home can. Live on a few basic foods daily and learn to add to your diet by sprouting. Become your own organic gardener even in the window box or flower pots. Never discard the tops of greens such as beets, carrots, radishes, turnips and what not.

Liquefy greens in the blender and then thermos cook them in boiling water.

Store such foods as apples, barley, yellow peas, goat milk products, cheeses. Dry foods during the season they are produced for use during winter months. Good winter foods are persimmons, pomegranates, sun dried olives, apricots and others that dry well.

Use cabbage often. Save the valuable outer leaves because they contain 40% more calcium.

Pick your own fruits and vegetables and buy them by the crate or bushel. Potatoes, carrots, turnips, beets, onions to name a few, store well in a root cellar or buried underground.

Make nourishing soups from beans. Ask markets for beet tops and turnip greens they discard. Use these for rich broths. (Try a cornmeal broth.)

Watch for store bargains due to over stocking of ripe fruit or vegetables. You should be alert for such sales.

Use lima beans, garbanzos, barley, green kale for soups and other dishes. Whole peanuts are difficult to digest; use them only occasionally in butters, raw. Try nut and seed butters such as cashew, sunflower, sesame, walnut, almond. Make your own and use in drinks and dressings.

Many so-called weeds are very nourishing and pleasant tasting. Malva, nasturtium, lemon grass, dandelion, comfrey, hibiscus may be growing in your field or yard. Grow at home or pick wild.

Cultivate a garden in a vacant lot, with permission, of course. Pay in vegetables and exchange what you grow with others for variety. Switzerland's people have their own gardens. This tiny country is isolated from the outside world from all sides, especially during times of world conflicts. They were forced to learn to take care of themselves. The Swiss people attribute their strong, healthy bodies to the rocks they are forced to move around. They deal physically with the land.

Shopping the "Thrifty Way" Supermarket

Following are a few handy suggestions for grocery shopping. With the cost of food so high and health so dependent on it, we can use all the help we can get.

Make a shopping list before you leave home. Shop less often.

Don't ever shop on an empty stomach.

Shop for the specials, especially for the big items in your food budget.

Return bad merchandise always.

Don't be tempted by the displays at the end of aisles or loose and disarranged displays. They are not there by accident.

The more expensive items are placed purposely at eye level. The cheaper ones are on bottom shelves.

Watch the dating of items for freshness.

Compare sizes and prices to get the best buy. Generally the larger size is a savings. Also read the weights.

Refer to nutritional information when given.

Check ingredients and remember that they rank in order of the largest percentage contents first. Beware of chemical or laboratory terms you can't even pronounce. Avoid other additives and sugar.

Pass up "empty calorie" snacks and convenience foods. Buy natural, nutritious snacks such as fruits, nuts, vegetables, cheese, yogurt, whole grain cereals and juices.

Start cutting down on the amount of meat you purchase. Buy only the leanest meat, white fish with fins and scales. Leave pork alone. Also leave alone processed meats and luncheon meats.

Buy food in quantity to save money when possible.

Buy as many natural, pure and whole foods that are not preserved and processed with additives as you can. Try to find organically grown fruits and vegetables. Try country stands and farmers. Learn to sprout.

Buy as many raw foods and unpasteurized milk products as possible.

Buy cold-pressed oils (unhydrogenated) and butter or polyunsaturated margarine made from soy and safflower oil in a health food store. Use less. (Do not heat these.)

Look for a source of fertile, non-caged chicken eggs. The birds should be allowed to run free and obtain green food.

The Healthy Budget Technique

One way of budgeting for health suggests dividing the weekly budget into fifths for each of the following:

— a fifth or more for milk, milk products, cheese, butter

— a fifth or less for meats, fish, eggs, meat substitutes.

— *a fifth or more for cereal, grains, other starches and breads (limited bread)

— a fifth or more for fruits and vegetables

— a fifth or less for miscellaneous additions and supplements.

*Consider this to include potatoes, bananas, hubbard squash, etc.

The milk and cheese group is the protein source for the one serving of protein per day. Cottage cheese is a very good protein source and aged, hard cheeses that break. Try making some of your own using raw milk and some of our recipes. Use buttermilk, powdered skim milk and nut and seed milk substitutes. Soy milk powder can be used in many ways. These substitutes are cheaper than regular milk. All pasteurized milk products should be avoided, because they are much more costly to health in the long run.

The meat and meat substitute group is the other protein source. If not a vegetarian, use fish in place of red meat, since it is cheaper and lower in fats, often. Don't forget the value of sardines for RNA — the anti-aging factor. Use tuna, packed in water. The meat budget is the best to cut down on. Use eggs often; average up to one or even two a day per person. Use dried beans such as soybeans, lentils, garbanzos, red and kidney beans and pinto beans, etc. The lentil is the best choice and along with the garbanzo, they make excellent binders ;and extenders. Try souffles.

The cereal and grain group are the starch source for a serving a day. Use only whole grain products, especially cereals served steamed. Have very little bread and include cornbread in this occasionally; serve cornmeal cereal a couple of times a week. Brown rice is a good starch. Have baked white potatoes and sweet potatoes along with other starchy vegetables such as corn, bananas (baked), winter squashes. If you must have bread occasionally, make it the whole grain variety and try making it yourself the slow-baking method.

Fruits and vegetables are very important, though not considered so in the average food budget. Two fruits a day and six vegetables are suggested, or more vegetables in raw salads. Fruits are an excellent source of vitamins and vegetables have more of the minerals. Raw, these both furnish valuable bulk for the intestinal tract. Learn to sprout for one of the best sources or live bulk foods and wonderful nutritional additions. Remember that fruits have a maturity date and vegetables do not. This is one reason for using more vegetables; fruit is often picked green. Find your own good organic source of produce, even in the field. Choose these for color; avoid the bleached, white ones because they lack nutritional value. Don't buy head lettuce. If you use dried fruits, make them the unsulphured kind.

The miscellaneous items can include seasonings such as dulse, kelp, broth powder, sea salt; sweeteners such as honey, unsulphured molasses and dried fruit; vegetable oils that are cold-pressed; supplements of rice polishings, wheat germ, flaxseed meal, sunflower and sesame seeds (meal); use only unprocessed nut and seed butters. Omit all refined and "junk" foods such as cola drinks, sweets, pastries, pickles, coffee, tea (common) and syrups. Replace foodless foods and drinks with herb teas and natural, pure and whole foods.

Foods can be cheap, but if they're not natural, pure and whole they will be expensive in the long run. You'll spend your money on doctors and dentists if you don't get the best food — even if you have to pay extra. Learn to use the health food store; you'll save a lot in the long haul. (Buy in bulk, even with neighbors if necessary.)

The "Unexpected Company" Shelf

Keep foods on hand that can be whipped up for emergency guests, large crowds or unexpected parties. The freezer is a good storage place for some foods that can be easily prepared without much time or fuss. Soups and casseroles freeze well. Freeze some appetizers.

Also have canned, (preferably home canned the correct way) foods available such as fruits and vegetables, juices, sauces and relishes.

Have canned pimentos, tuna, salmon, ripe olives, sardines on hand. Keep a supply of dried fruits. Canned soup stock, vegetable broth powder and natural bouillon cubes can be a saver for soups and other dishes.

Eggs are always welcome for emergency meals. Make omelets or souffles with interesting ingredients — fresh or frozen.

Waffles can be an easy meal. Have a canned fruit sauce with them. Or use other ingredients in them—fruit or vegetable or cheeses for top garnish.

Fruit and cheese can be a simple and easy meal.

Remember that these need to be "keeping" foods — freezer, root cellar or canned. Some can be bought on sale.

A few handy items to depend on are eggs, milk, whey, nuts, nut butters, cheeses (also parmesan), onions, garlic, carrots, tomatoes, fruit, lettruce. These are the "perishables."

Here are some storage staples:

Boullion cubes and soups such as tomato, mushroom, vegetable bouillon, split pea soup, vegetable broth powder.

Frozen and canned vegetables such as mushrooms, tomatoes, tomato sauce, tomato juice, peas, Jerusalem artichokes, carrots, beets, corn (home canned).

Canned fish such as tuna, anchovies, salmon, herring, sardines.

Frozen fruit such as apples, pears, peaches, apricots, pineapple, cherries (Also these keep frozen.)

Canned fruit juices such as pineapple, apple, grape, raspberry, black cherry. Also have fruit juice concentrates.

Rice, spinach or whole wheat noodles and spaghetti.

Have salad dressing materials, homemade relishes, homemade sauces and jams. Also have dried fruits. Good fruits are dates, raisins, apricots, figs, prunes.

Dried beans, legumes, cereal grains, nuts and seeds.

"It is estimated that one half of the fatal cancers in women and one third in men may be attributed in part to diet habits."
—Dr. Paul A. Marks, Director Cancer Research Center
Columbia University's College of Physicians & Surgeons

Did you know there are over 300 varieties of avocados?
Did you know Tupelo honey can be used by some diabetic people?
Did you know many dentists do not believe in using lemon juice steadily and heavily because of its direct deteriorating effect on the teeth?
Did you know millet is a seed cereal and that it is one of the most vital and potent breakfast cereals we can use?
Did you know there is 40% more calcium in the outside leaves of cabbage than in the inside?
Did you know that nasturtium flowers and rose petals can be used in salads?
Did you know copper (a trace mineral) is needed to keep us from becoming anemic and its highest food source is apricots?
Did you know those men working outdoors in the sunshine are more likely to have girls in the family than those who work inside?

248

Chapter 32

How to shop in a "health food" store

What Are Health Foods?

Dr. Hugh Sinclair, professor of nutrition at Oxford University in England, says we are "told" the present world is better fed than at any time in history and healthier besides. Yet, he points out that tooth decay and hardening of the arteries are found everywhere in Western nations. About ¼ of the people in "civilized" countries suffer from diverticular disease (bowel pockets) of the colon. "It may be nutritional in origin," he says. He adds that other chronic diseases, degenerative diseases in particular, are more and more evident in the Western countries. These diseases are: cancer, heart disease, diabetes, arthritis and numerous others.

We shall for the present define a health food as any food that retains all its nutritionally desirable constituents and has not had added to it any substance that is harmful. This definition allows the inclusion of nutritionally valuable compound foods, such as margarine that retains a high proportion of the original vegetable oils; and has added to it the legal amounts of synthetic vitamins A and D.

What Foods Are in a Health Food Store?

Based on this definition what will we find in a health food store?

1. Unprocessed cereal grains and their products: Whole grain breakfast cereals, breads and flours. They have no additives or preservatives.
2. Seeds and nuts in the raw natural state: Peanuts, sunflower seeds, squash seeds, chia seeds, almonds, sesame seeds, etc., and nut and seed butters. All are unprocessed and without additives.
3. Special diet foods such as low sodium foods, foods low in sugar, low in gluten, low in cholesterol, such diet foods as are prescribed by physicians.
4. Naturally sweet foods: honey; carob powder, syrup and flour; maple sugar and syrup; dried fruits, raw sugars, fruit concentrates.
5. Herbs, herb teas and other tea and coffee substitutes: The leaves, seeds and blossoms are unprocessed parts of trees, shrubs and plants. Coffee substitutes are often made from cereal grains.
6. Fruit and vegetable juices and fruit juice concentrates. These are unsugared and unprocessed. They should contain no additives or preservatives.

7. Vitamin and mineral supplements and herb remedies. Also miscellaneous supplements such as protomorphogens, chlorophyll, whey, algae, amino acids and so forth.
8. Organically grown fruits and vegetables produced without the use of chemical fertilizers and pesticides. (Found in some health food stores, not all.)

What Foods Aren't in a Health Food Store?

Processed foods, "convenience" foods, mixes, artificial fruit drinks, snack foods that are made mostly of air, salt and sugar along with artificial ingredients are taboo. These line the shelves of the supermarket lanes.

Standard Products in Your Health Food Store

alfalfa seeds	milk, cow, raw
almonds	milk, goat, raw
apples	molasses
baking powder (Royal or cream of tartar type)	mung beans
	nut butters
beans, dried	oils
bone meal	peanuts, peanut butter
brewer's yeast	peas
butter	pecans
carob chips	pumpkin seeds
carob powder, flour, syrup	raisins
	rice, brown
cashew nuts	rice, wild
cheese	rose hips, powder
chick-peas	sea salt
coconut	seed butters
dates	sesame seeds
dulse	soybeans
eggs	tofu
Swiss muesli	soy margarine
filberts (hazelnuts)	soy milk and products
fruits, dried	miso (soy bean paste)
granola	sunflower seeds
herbs and herb seeds	tahini
honey	vegetable broth powder
kelp	vegetable and herb
lecithin	seasonings
lentils	whole wheat berries
maple syrup	yeast
millet	

There are usually many more products than these, varying with the type and size of the store and the food philosophy of the owner.

Seeds, Grains & Legumes

Alfalfa Seed — Use untreated seed for sprouting and teas. It is high in minerals.

Arrowroot Starch — Use it in place of corn or tapioca starch. It is said to have an alkaline ash and contains calcium.

Hulled Barley — It is natural barley, not pearled or polished; only the very outer chaff is removed. Use in soups, cereals, casseroles and other dishes. (Barley is a winter food.)

Barley Grits — They are made of whole, hulled barley by cracking and removing flours. Add barley grits to soups, loaves, cereals, casseroles, burgers and patties as an extender for meats and other proteins.

Barley Flour — It is a finely ground hulled barley that blends well with other flours for baking breads, muffins, cakes, cookies, pancakes, and so on. It is a good substitute for restricted wheat diets.

Buckwheat Groats — They are made from whole, roasted buckwheat. Use them for cereals, stuffing, soup and puddings. Buckwheat groats are used in many Jewish dishes.

Buckwheat Flour — It should be pure with no additives. It makes good pancackes and waffles and can be used in other recipes also.

Carob Powder — It may be referred to as "St. John's Bread," "Honey Locust," "Locust Bean" and many other names. It is delicious and ideal as a replacement for chocolate and cocoa for confections, cakes, frostings, milk drinks, syrup, cookies, candy, etc. It is alkaline, high in calcium, natural sugars, low in starch and fat.

Corn, Whole — Yellow is the best. Grind your own meal at home or use in hominy and for parching.

Corn Meal — Yellow is preferable. Stone ground is best because excess heat is not applied. The grinds can be from fine to coarse. All the corn germ and flour is left intact, so other flour should be added to prevent crumbling in making cornbread. Use it for cornmeal cereal, cornbread, hotcakes, waffles, tamale pie, etc.

Corn Flour — Again, yellow is the best. Whole corn is ground by the cool method. Use it as flour in breads, cakes, hot cakes, waffles and many other dishes; add to other flours.

Hominy Grits — They are usually made from white corn; hulled and degerminated. Add to other dishes as an extender.

Popcorn, Yellow — Popcorn can be made without the use of heated oil. Pop in hot container.

Flaxseed — It should be untreated. Add to cereals before cooking, grind for adding to cooked cereals, make into a tea for intestinal disturbances. Add small amounts to many recipes.

Flaxseed Meal — Whole flaxseed is ground to a medium meal consistency. Blend with cereals, flours, drinks and other recipes.

Garbanzos (Chick Peas)—They should be untreated land large sized for cooking. Use in soups, casseroles and loaves, or sprout them. They are alkaline usually.

Lentils — They should be untreated. Sprout or add to soups, loaves, casseroles. They tend to be alkaline.

Hulled Millet — Untreated, freshly hulled millet is best. It is alkaline forming, easy to digest and one of the four best starches or cereals. It absorbs 3 to 4 parts of water when cooking. Use in casseroles, puddings and as an excellent hot cereal alone.

Millet Meal — It is ground to medium consistency from hulled millet. Use with corn meal in equal parts for many dishes. Use as a cereal. It has an alkaline ash and is high in protein and lecithin.

Millet Flour— It should be made from pure, hulled, untreated millet. It is alkaline, easily digested and excellent for breads and wheatless diets. It is high in B-2, potassium, lecithin, silicon, iron, magnesium, calcium, phosphorus and some amino acids.

Mung Beans — They should be untreated, select quality. Use for sprouting or in cooking. They are excellent for sprouting because of their high content of vitamins C and B. Add sprouts to salads, omelets, soups, sandwiches and many oriental dishes.

Steel Cut Oats — They are natural, unrefined and make an excellent hot cereal. Blend with other cereal grains such as millet, wheat, rye for variety.

Rolled Oats — They cook into a flaky cereal and should be steamed slowly for best results. Use in cookies, bars and alone as cereal.

Oat Flour — Use in combination with other flours in baking breads, muffins, cakes, hotcakes, or for thickening. Use in infant feeding. It is good for wheat restricted diets.

Green Split Peas — They should be untreated, natural green peas. Use in soups.

Potato Flour — It can be used in soups, breads, gravies, hotcakes, waffles, muffins, etc. To prevent lumping, blend with other flours before adding liquids.

Natural Brown Rice — It should be specially hulled to prevent loss of germ. All the bran and polishing should remain for maximum nutrition. It is one of the four best starches.

Brown Rice Flour — Natural brown rice is reduced to flour; use by blending with other flours in baking. It is good in hot cake and waffle batters.

Rice Bran — It is the outer layer removed from brown rice, a by-product of polishing and refining. Use as rice polishings or wheat germ.

Rice Polishings—They are the inner layers from brown rice, obtained from the refining and polishing process of white rice. Add to any foods as you would wheat germ. They are good in health "cocktails."

Rye, Whole — Use for home grinding and cereal. It one of the four best starches.

Rye Grits — Use as other grits or as a cereal alone.

Rye Meal—It is the consistency of coarse cornmeal. Blend with other meals or flours for baking. Use as cereal or alone.

Rye Flour — Use for bread, rolls, muffins, waffles. Mix with other flours. It is great for wheat restricted diets.

Hulled Sesame Seed — It should be untreated and ground cool to retain the oils. It is high in lecithin, protein, vitamins and minerals. Add to cookies, cakes, candies, other cereals, cooked vegetables and desserts; add to salad dressings. Blend with liquefied drinks. Keep refrigerated for best results. It is made into "tahini" or sesame butter.

Soy Beans — The soy bean is power-packed with protein. It contains all the essential amino acids, lecithin, low carbohydrates, low fat, is rich in vitamins and has an alkaline reaction. Use it in place of meat as a protein. Serve them cooked, baked, sprouted, as soy milk, in soups, casseroles and loaves. Tofu, miso and soy sauce are made from the soy bean.

Soy Meal — Use as an extender for all kinds of loaves and casseroles. Use as cereal.

Soy Flour — It is toasted or untoasted soy bean flour. If toasted it has a nutty and sweet flavor that adds richness and smoothness to many dishes. It can be used to partly replace other flours, one part soy flour to five parts other flour.

Soy Powder — It is like soy flour, except more finely ground. Use as milk substitute or powdered milk.

Hulled Sunflower Seeds — They can't be beat for energy-giving food additives or as a wholesome snack. Raw sunflower seeds contain rich oils and many vitamins and minerals. Add to cereals, cookies, cakes, salads, soups or almost any recipe. They can be ground into meal and added easily to many solid and liquid foods. They are excellent as a supplement in cereals.

Sunflower Seed Meal — It can be bought, or you can grind your own. It is rich in oils and nutrients. Blend with many dishes and drinks. Add to flours in baking, up to 50% replacement. It is quick baking. Add to soup after cooking.

Wheat Grits — Use them for cereals, loaves, burgers, patties, etc. Use as cereal alone.

Whole Wheat Flour — It should be stone or cool ground. Nothing should be removed — all bran and germ should be intact. Use where ever white flour is called for — baking breads, rolls, thickening, hotcakes, waffles, etc. Where pastry flour is called for, a whole wheat pastry or unbleached whole wheat flour is available.

Graham Flour — It is a whole wheat flour with the inner part of the kernal ground to fine flour and the bran layers are left flakey and coarse. Use for bread, cakes, rolls, etc.

Pastry Whole Wheat Flour — It is made of finely ground whole, soft, white pastry wheat. Use in place of all white flour in pastry baking such as pies, cookies, waffles, cakes, etc. Extra sifting may be desirable for lighter cakes.

Bran Flakes — Bran is from the outer layers of hard, red wheat. Use flakes in muffins, cereals, breads, health drinks and teas, etc.

Wheat Germ — It should be natural, untreated and vacuum packed for freshness. Refrigerate to keep freshness; to prevent rancidity always make sure it is carefully packaged. Use in omelets, breading fish and other meats, in drinks and cookies or candy. Add to nearly any food. It is a basic supplement for every diet.

Wheat Germ Flour — It is made from finely ground, pure and raw wheat germ. About 2% wheat germ flour adds the germ to flour that has been refined. Add to cakes, pies and health "cocktails."

"Unbleached" White Flour — It is a refined flour made without bleaching, additives or chemical preserving. It is still a "live" food, cream colored with much more flavor than regular white refined flour. It is between commercial refined flour and whole wheat flour. Use in breads and other dishes except for cakes.

"Unbleached" White Pastry Flour — It is a refined flour made from soft wheat. Use for cakes, pies and general pastries.

Gluten Flour — It is a low starch flour made by washing the starch from high-protein wheat flour. Gluten is dried and ground. When using gluten flour, more soya, rye or other specialty flours can be used in baking breads, hotcakes, waffles, etc. It makes a good thickener.

Making the Most of Your Health Food Store

A number of foods have always been equated with health in general. They symbolize the "health food" philosophy. They include yogurt, blackstrap molasses, wheat germ, powdered skim milk and brewer's yeast. Add sprouts, whey and vegetable broth powder and seasoning to the family for their highly nourishing qualities and versatility, plus their natural goodness. Nutrition is a serious business, but it should also be enjoyable and enlivening.

To derive the utmost from nutrition, stress sense appeal of taste and sight in order to stimulate the flow of digestive juices and cause the "mouth to water."

Make these foods an indispensible part of any dietary regime. Remember the adage: "Variety is the spice of life." Listed are a few extra health ideas with which you may not be acquainted.

Acidophilus Culture: A wonderful aid for the bowel.
seaweed.

Arrowroot: A good thickening powder — high in calcium and alkaline in reaction.

251

Bran Water: An extract of minerals from simmering common wheat bran.

Carob: Chocolate-flavored powder with none of the disadvantages of cocoa and with higher nutritional value.

Dandelion Root Coffee: Has a "coffee taste" — made from roasted root of dandelion. Good for the liver.

Desiccated Liver: For building the blood.

Dulse: A powdered seaweed very high in iodine and manganese. A good supplement for underactive thyroid. Can be used as a salt seasoning.

Flaxseed Meal and Tea: Healing for intestinal tract; good natural laxative.

Fruit Juice Concentrate: Pure concentrates of whole fruits prepared by a special vacuum method, without high heat application. Cherry, apple and grape are usually available.

Gelatin: Use 100% pure gelatin. Gelatin is a valuable protein supplement, handy to reducing and normal diets.

Herb Teas: Healthful drinks made from steeping various herbs in boiling water.

Kefir: A wonderful "liquid-yogurt" type drink, easily digested, good for the bowel.

Molasses: High in iron and sugar. Use unsulphured blackstrap variety.

Oils and Fats: Use only cold pressed, unrefined varieties. Avoid fats.

Raw Cheeses: (aged and unprocessed)

Rice Polishings: High in silicon, good sources of B-complex vitamins.

Soy Milk: A milk substitute, non-catarrh forming.

Soy Sauce: Flavoring derived from the soybean. Use in broths, in cooking vegetables, in gravies and vegetarian loaves, in place of salt.

Sprouts: High in B-complex vitamins; add to soups just before serving, use in salads or eat them plain.

Unsulphured Dried Fruit

Vegetable Broth Powder and Seasoning: Excellent seasoning to replace salt. High in organic minerals.

Vegetable Bouillon or Vegetable Stock or Vegetable Broth: Juices in which vegetables have been cooked, free from meat stock. Rich source of minerals.

Whey (Powdered): A high sodium food, good for arthritis and reducing diets, in handy powder form, made from fresh raw milk.

Yeast: Excellent source of B-complex high in protein and RNA. Brewer's or primary grown yeast may be sprinkled on cereals, fruits, added to drinks.

Yogurt: Contains "friendly bacteria," good for the bowel. Good protein source.

Calcium and Women Over 25

Major surveys show that the average woman's diet only provides 450-500 mg of calcium per day, when they actually need 1000-1500 mg. One expert says that women over 25 need to start increasing their calcium intake, and not wait until deficiency symptoms appear.

Vegetarians and Deficiencies

Researchers have found that a strict vegetarian diet nearly always results in a shortage of the amino acid methionine, found commonly in animal proteins but seldom in vegetable sources of protein. Methionine is needed for growth and tissue repair, and a chronic shortage can lead to liver degeneration and cirrhosis.

Critical Amino Acids

Lysine and tryptophan, essential amino acids, are easily destroyed by heat. Lysine is important in metabolism and is found in raw milk (but not pasteurized or powdered milk), wheat germ, green peas and soybeans. Tryptophan is a precursor to niacinamide and is converted in the brain to serotonin, necessary for normal relaxed sleep. Nuts and seeds are high in tryptophan.

Chapter 33

Seasonal foods: summer and winter

Foods Should be Eaten in Season

Nature offers different foods during the various seasons, and foods eaten in season are healthiest. More fruits appear in spring and summer for elimination and body cleansing. Fall and winter supply the necessary fattening and heating foods to accommodate cold weather. Warm days are intended for more fruits and salads. Heavier starches and proteins are reserved more for colder seasons.

Summertime Is Preparation Time

To prepare for winter, we need calcium and tissue tone to prevent disease and flu from viruses. Summer sunshine fixed calcium. Recreation, outdoor exercise, vacations, swimming, lighter clothing and outdoor activities build firm tissues, make better circulation, repair broken-down tissue, remove chronic settlements, replace old tissue with new. Take every opportunity in summer to build a strong body for the harsh winter season.

Doctors see fewer patients in the summer because Nature is exerting extra power to build reserves for the winter cold. Winter brings heavy clothing, less activity, especially outdoors, and many ailments begin to appear as a result.

"Cool as a Cucumber" Summer Suggestions

When the mercury soars upward, a vegetarian diet is your best assurance for coolness and equilibrium. During the summer season, Nature showers fresh fruits and vegetables lavishly upon us. These cooling foods assist the body in regulating body temperature with reduced energy demands. The homemaker should enjoy much liberation from the stove and cooking pots.

Fruits are a natural blood thinner for summer, adding more liquid to the diet, which aids elimination processes such as skin perspiration.

Raw vegetables are the most cooling. Create a variety of salad combinations. Green mixture salads: leafy greens and tops, romaine, endive, watercress — use your favorites in whatever proportion you desire. Make protein salads such as celery and pecan tomato baskets or stuffed cucumber. Add protein salad dressing using honey with cream cheese, yogurt, avocado, nut butter.

Good summer foods are strawberries, cherries, peaches, apricots, fresh figs, fresh pineapple, all melons, cucumbers, squashes, all greens, including parsley, celery, beet tops and watercress.

Light starches are best — found in carrots, beets, turnips, millet and bananas. Avoid barley, cranberries and concentrate on more fresh than dried fruits. Many liquefied combinations in the form of juices, punches, cocktails, are beneficial. Liquefy many vegetables and have soups and broths. Use vegetable broth powder in preference to salt. Drink whey and celery juice freely for their high sodium content known for its body cooling ability. Lime juice and whey cools the blood and lowers blood pressure.

Special Summer Outdoor Tips

Avoid excessive sun and head exposure, expressly. Protect the skin. Sleep outdoors in a sleeping bag, on pine needles when possible. Wear thin clothing, no hose, go barefoot and wear a hat to guart against strong midday sun.

Most Common Summer Mistakes

The most common mistake is eating ice cream, which is strictly a winter food. It heats the blood more than any other food. Commercial ice cream is a villainous calcium robber due to the ingredients white sugar, pasteurized milk, artificial coloring, coal-tar flavors, foodless fillers and the cheapest of gelatins.

The worst cold drink is ice water, which shocks the warm stomach tissue.

Never let a cold wind dry your skin after swimming. Don't play or work hard during the heat of the day. Avoid extreme glare from sunshine reflection.

Winter Is Dormant "Be-Careful-Time"

Good health built during the summer months can be rapidly depleted through careless winter habits. We naturally stay indoors more, wear heavy clothing, are subjected to longer hours of artificial lighting, extreme temperatures, eat less fresh foods and have less variety in our foods. Unless we are winter sports enthusiasts, exercise is largely curtailed, or confined to indoor forms. Systems can become sluggish, developing poor circulation, lower digestive ability, poor skin elimination, bowel stasis, toxic settlements and, eventually, chronic diseases.

atives, cold shots, suppressants for fevers, bronchial and flu remedies. If we had lived well during the summer months, we should have built up energy reserves to help carry us through the more trying winter months. Providing summer reserve building was stressed, winter ailments should be avoided or thrown off quickly, including those "flu" viruses that sweep through entire unprepared populations.

Doctors make a better living on catarrhal conditions through the winter months than any other time of the year. Flu is a winter ailment. March finds more people dying from pneumonia. At this time all energy reserves carried from the summer season are exhausted. The body is depleted. The two times during the year to see a good nutritionist are the beginning of summer and the beginning of winter. See your doctor and prepare for the long winter with additional vitamin supplements if needed. Eat more starches and proteins during the wintertime. (Summer is the time for thinning, elimination foods, blood thinning foods.)

For those living in foggy weather with little outdoor activity, vitamin A or cod liver oil could be helpful. Swedish doctors send arthritic patients to the sunny Sahara Desert during the cold, foggy months. Compensate for lack of sunshine with vitamin A or cod liver oil.

Winter Food Suggestions

Take hot drinks made of vegetable broth powder at least once a day. As the seasons change, add a small amount of cream to soups and broths, at the table, not while cooking. Use more butter and oils through the winter, especially in northern climates. But do include greens with them to help the liver process fats. Combine eggs with green vegetables, green juices, or high iron foods like black cherry juice to avoid cholesterol deposits.

More natural sweets are allowed to maintain energy at high levels; such as maple sugar, date sugar and dried fruits. Sweeten cereals with revived (soaked) dried fruits and raisins. Carob flour is an acceptable winter flavoring.

Winter teas should include Buchu Leaf, oat straw, boneset, blue violet and chamomile. Blackstrap molasses is a good iron source and natural laxative.

The average person gains weight during winter months. Make sure you gain with natural foods only. The three best hot winter cereals are: barley, yellow cornmeal and whole wheat; also, unpolished rice and millet are assets. Rye builds muscle but is less heating. Legumes are to be used more generously during winter months. Choose from lentils, garbanzos, soybeans, red kidney beans, navy beans and others. Salads and greens combine well with beans. Split peas aid those people who have digestive difficulties with bean hulls. Barley is the best winter heat producer, nerve and muscle builder. Buckwheat is also good, and moderate amounts of oatmeal can be taken.

I would suggest cream over butter since it aids the manufacture of lecithin necessary to every body cell. It is anti-arthritic. Dried figs (soaked) are a good energy source and laxative. Nuts are heat-producing and nutritious, but fattening. Many digestive systems aren't efficient enough to utilize them. Almonds, black walnuts, and sprouts are wintertime foods. Use sprouts when greens are scarce for salads.

Important Winter Supplements

Winter supplements should build blood. Use vitamins A and C, bone marrow capsules, cod liver oil, liquid chlorophyll, bonemeal and lecithin. The body is more likely short of vitamins and minerals during the winter hibernation. A good multiple vitamin/mineral supplement can be fortifying.

Many people suffer winter fatigue symptoms due to excess toxin accumulation in the body. Insure against a lack of foods rich in balanced winter minerals. The sports boredom, lassitude and lack of energy, encourage vague aches and pains. The stress of exposure and temperature extremes uses up excessive heat energy, forcing the body to work overtime. Recuperation takes longer and additional sleep is often necessary.

Winter Foods and Alternatives

Search for fruits and vegetables in season during the winter. These foods contain vitamins and minerals essential for colder months. Consider using at least 60% seasonal foods and supplements with the remaining 40% non-seasonal. The ideal out of season fruits and vegetables are those lending themselves to freezing. Higher caloric foods are advisable during winter for body heating properties.

Decayed teeth are a disease solely of civilization. Whether a native lives on fruit and vegetables in the tropics or raw meat in the Arctic Zone, his teeth do not decay because he doesn't eat devitalized foods.

Chapter 34

Be your own organic gardener

A Revolution in Food Concepts Is at Hand

It is time for a revolution in food concepts. The last revolution, the junk food revolution, should have taught us a valuable lesson by now. We have been killing ourselves with our own inventions. Now we are beginning to wake up to the fact that Nature knows best.

There were no French chefs in the Garden of Eden, no can openers, cans or prepared foods; there was no stove; there was no sickness. Disease came in with man's departure from godly ways and godly foods. Now, food pollution problems are ignored while water and air pollution get all the attention. The psychiatrist works with polluted minds, drug addiction, criminal habits, but no one seems to be taking care of the nutritional evils.

The current trend is to just get by on any food, especially convenience foods and fast foods. Less than 6% of the U.S. population raises food for the other 94%. We should take care of these people and our foods as well as the soil they grow in. The farmer, transporter, storage concerns, preservation industry should work together. There is much work to be done to ally these factions for the good of our food supply. The farmer and the food industry must combine forces for the good of all.

We find out that the sea is the soil for sea foods and sea vegetation just as the earth is the soil of land foods. However, the sea is generally constant in its quantity of minerals while the soil varies greatly according to locality and how heavily it has been farmed. So sea foods have a more balanced mineral content than land grown foods. We should look to the sea for some of our foods such as fish (white fish with fins and scales), especially sardines, dulse, seaweek of all kinds. We find the foods from the sea have a better range of essential trace minerals than land foods. Land soils vary too much.

The Dangers of Chemicalized Agriculture

Research has found that the use of chemical fertilizers and other inorganic materials in the soil produces food with more carbohydrate and less protein values. The protein value of wheat, for example, is diminishing as soils are depleted and not replenished. It is a fact that chemical residues remain in the soil up to 10 or 15 years after their use.

Drugs are commonly used to hasten the growth of animals for market. A noted example is diethylstilbestrol (DES), a proven carcinogen (cancer-producing agent), widely fed to cattle and sheep a few years ago. It is used to lessen the feed needed for the animals. The FDA banned it from feeding but allows it to be injected, providing it is stopped a few weeks before slaughter. The weight gain the hormone stimulates is in fat, not protein. Hogs have been fed penicillin and other antibiotics for fast and increased weight gains.

What can we do? The only solution is to buy only organically grown products — animal and vegetable or fruit; or better still, grow your own. People must demand safe sources of food before we will get them.

Chemical sprays and pesticides are another problem. Not only do they kill undesirable insect pests but the beneficial ones as well, including the bacteria and other microorganisms that make soil healthy. Poison residues on fruit, vegetables and other crops end up in our bodies.

Many older pesticides are not as harmful as the new ones they are developing. Yet we are told they are better and less dangerous than the ones just discontinued. Do you stop to think that the residues of these poisons remain in the soil for 10 years or longer? What about the possibility of lethal combinations of so many different sprays and pesticides? It's something to think about.

It is estimated that disease and degeneration cost Americans over $100 billion each year and are steadily on the increase. That does not include the cost of lost worktime or lower efficiency on the job due to poor health and frequent sickness.

Earthworms — The Humble Chemists

Earthworms are the unrecognized heroes of the soil kingdom. They enrich, nourish, aerate and balance the soil for man. It is said that we owe our very existence to them because without them there would be no plants, organisms, animals or humans. They can convert waste to rich compost material or loam within two to three weeks, generally. Chemists don't know how they convert wastes into the elements essential for life; the earthworms are the master chemists. The tunnels they form by squeezing through the soil plow and cultivate the earth and distribute plant food. Rich soil has some 26,000 worms per acre. Earth worm castings have been analyzed and found to be seven times higher in potash (potassium), five times higher in nitrogen and three times higher in magnesium than the soil they ingest and live in; they enrich the soil for plants.

From healthy, rich soil come hardy plants, and they bear the best and most balanced fruits and vegetables. Without these we can't expect healthy bodies.

A vegetable can't be any better than the soil from which it comes. The man can't be any better than the vegetable from which he receives sustenance. We need to take care of the soil first. As we are built from the dust of the earth, we must have all the necessary elements present in that dust or soil. The earthworm business is not just a fly-by-night idea or a myth. The present is a time when many nations suffer from loss of good topsoil. We must protect and attempt to reclaim the soil and rebuild it, and earthworms are one of the best answers to this problem.

Fertilizers and Balanced Soils

The U.S. Dept. of Agriculture says topsoil composition is 25% air, 25% water, 5% organic matter and 45% minerals. Fertile topsoil is vital to man's health and survival. A healthy and balanced soil has organic matter and billions of molds, yeasts, bacteria, fungi, worms, protozoa, algae, insects and other microorganisms. They live mostly in the top few inches. Soil is made up of chemical elements, living organisms and organic matter made up of dead plants and animals.

Organic matter is called humus, and the more the soil has, the healthier and more completely balanced it is. The soil organisms' digestive action produces humic acids and changes inorganic elements to organic, making them more easily assimilated by plant roots. Humus holds rain and prevents damage from runoff. Humus conditions the soil, feeds its organisms, aids in aeration and makes the soil temperature more uniform. Humus is most often lacking in unbalanced soils. Minerals can be present and not be broken down so the plants can assimilate them. Humus is essential for soil fertility and balance.

Fertilizers can be classed in two groups — organic and inorganic. Inorganic fertilizers are either ground or crushed minerals in their natural state or chemical fertilizers manufactured for quick growth results. Organic fertilizer has been discussed elsewhere. Chemical fertilizer was never intended to restore the lost fertility of the soil. Today's farmer is encouraged to believe that chemical fertilizers are his panacea, his salvation and quick profit insurance. What has been the ultimate result? As Dr. William Albrecht found, plant life has been invaded by pests, insects, parasites and disease. Industry has had to provide an arsenal of over 50,000 chemical insecticides and poisons to fight them.

It has also been found that too much nitrogen weakens the plant, and disease is then attracted. Nitrogen-fixing bacteria in humus-rich soil don't force the plants to grow; they nourish as the plants need it. Professor Albrecht has shown that more carbohydrates and less proteins are found to exist in such plants. Insect pests find artifically fertilized plants easy prey. Albrecht also says that the purpose of insects is to return weak and sickly plant life to the soil, to destroy them.

Lab research has found that inferior seeds are often incapable of germinating or reproducing. Something is missing!

Some seven million tons of nitrogen fertilizers were used in a recent year in America. Nitrate pollution of air, water and food is a very real problem. Nitrogen, carbon, hydrogen and oxygen make up most of living tissue, but man has upset the nitrogen cycle balance. Nitrate poisoning is a risk to human health. The nitrate level in many farming areas is above the safety level for public health; there is an additional hazard from nitrogen oxides from cars and industry. Nitrate residues found in vegetables and fruits are the result of heavy nitrogen fertilizing, research has found. Some of the nitrate pollution in the atmosphere comes from agriculture, experts say.

Man can't continue to rob and deplete the soil without having to pay for it. Organic farm practices are the only answer. Famine and poor health await us if we don't reeducate farmers and change the current farming methods to rebuild the soil. Less than 6% of the population raises food for the U.S. There must be a trend toward the return of the small farmer. That's why we say "Be your own organic gardener."

According to the *Countryside and Small Stock Journal,* 3.7 million acres, or almost one half of the available farmland is under the ownership of 45 corporations.

Simple Guide to Planting by the Moon

The moon cycle goes from the new moon through the quarters to the full moon and returns again to the new moon. It has an important effect on planting and growth.

New Moon to First Quarter — The first three or four days following the new moon are very fruitful; you should plant and transplant on these days. Plants following this phase show good top growth, especially when it is during the rule of a fruitful astrological sign. Those plants most suited to this time are annuals, leafy herbs and leafy greens. Garden vegetables such as summer squash, peas and other top-fruiting plants can be put in, also grasses and cereal grains. The final days of this cycle are for weeding and growth control.

First Quarter to Full Moon — Don't plant or transplant on the first two or three days of this phase. Plant on the three or four days before the full moon for best results. This is the second best phase for planting leafy or above ground fruiting vegetables. Sow annual vegetables that bear large fruits above the ground such as tomatoes, melons, and so on. Also plant flowering herbs or seed fruits (tender) and graft or divide in this period, for perennial roots.

Full Moon to Last Quarter — Sow perennials that have to have a hardy root development during the first three or four days of this phase. Such vegetation includes all fruit and nut trees, vines, shrubs, berry bushes, flowers and many herbs. This is the time to begin perennial house ornamentals from slips, cuttings; divide and trim roots. This is also a good time to harvest seeds. Three or four days prior to the quarter beginning is the harvest time of the lunar cycle. Pick roots and fruits for storage, canning or drying during this time.

Last Quarter to New Moon — Trim and cut trees and clear ground at this time. This is the end of the cycle and it is time to regenerate or begin over again with the new. Decay sets in at this time. Fertilize and compost during this phase. Near the end of this cycle only a few crops can be planted successfully. Onions, potatoes and garlic do well sowed at this time. Plant those crops intended for seeds.

Fruitful and Barren Astrology Signs

The most fruitful and productive astrological signs are Cancer, Scorpio and Pisces. The second choices are Taurus, Capricorn and Libra. Third choices are Aquarius, Aries and Sagitarius. The barren signs are Leo (most unproductive), Virgo and Gemini. Choose the correct seasons for various seeds and plants and use the days and moon phases indicated for best results.

The Astrology of Farming and Gardening

Aries: (the ram — Mar. 20 - Apr. 18) Barren, not the time for planting. Moderately good for destroying unwanted and harmful growths. Dig potatoes. Spray for pests.

Taurus: (the bull — Apr. 19 - May 19) Moderately productive sign; better for root crops. Plant potatoes, flower bulbs and hay, field corn, cabbage, lettuce, etc. 3rd quarter of moon good for pruning grape vines; 3rd and 4th quarter for planting potatoes, beets, etc.

Gemini: (the twins — May 20 - June 20) Barren; not good sign for planting or transplanting. Good for cultivation and destroying weeds and other harmful growths. Good time for attacking pests, vermin, rats, etc., (especially during the 3rd and 4th quarter of the moon).

Cancer: (the crab — June 21 - July 21) Very fruitful and the most productive sign of the zodiac. Plant all seeds, irrigate. Never dig potatoes at this point. Plant hay, grain and cereals during the 1st quarter and 2nd quarter; 2nd quarter for planting above the ground vegetables; flowers; bud, transplant and graft. 3rd quarter for planting potatoes, carrots, etc. 3rd and 4th quarters prune plants and trees.

Leo: (the lion — July 22 - Aug. 22) Least productive sign. Best time for destroying weeds and unwanted and harmful growths. Plow soil to turn up undesirable roots. Attack rodents and pests (especially when the moon is in the 3rd and 4th quarters). 3rd quarter, dig potatoes; prune grape vines.

Virgo: (the virgin — Aug. 23 - Sept. 21) Barren and unproductive. This is not the time for planting or transplanting. Cultivate during this time and destroy obnoxious weeds, growths, pests (especially during 3rd and 4th quarters).

Libra: (the scales — Sept. 22 - Oct. 22) Fairly productive sign. Plant hay, grain and cereals during the 1st and 2nd quarters. Plant flowers for fragrance and beauty during the 2nd quarter. During the 3rd quarter plant fall crops of hay, field corn, cabbage, lettuce, etc.

Scorpio: (the scorpion — Oct. 23 - Nov. 21) Very productive sign and excellent for all types of planting; irrigate, also. Don't dig potatoes then. Plant hay, grain, cereals during the 1st and 2nd quarters. Plant above ground vegetables, abundant growing flowers; bud, transplant and graft during the 2nd quarter. Plant below the ground vegetables during 3rd quarter; also fall hay, grains and cereals; prune grape vines in this quarter. Prune trees and plants during the 3rd and 4th quarters.

Sagittarius: (the archer — Nov. 22 - Dec. 20) Barren. Moderately good time for seeding hay, grains and onions. Moderately good time for destroying weeds and other unwanted growths. Prune grape vines in the 3rd quarter.

Capricorn: (the goat — Dec. 21 - Jan. 18) Moderately productive. Favorable for potatoes and root crops; plant flower bulbs. Graft trees during the 1st and 2nd quarters.

Aquarius: (the water-bearer — Jan. 19-Feb. 16) Barren. Good time for cultivation and destroying weeds and other harmful growths. Exterminate mice and rats (especially when the moon is in 3rd and 4th quarter).

Pisces: (the fishes — Feb. 17 - Mar. 19) Very productive. Excellent for all plants; good time to irrigate. Don't dig potatoes at this time. Plant hay, grain, cereals during the 1st and 2nd quarters. Plant corn and all above the ground vegetables, abundant growing flowers, bud, graft and transplant during the 2nd quarter. Plant vegetables yielding below the ground, hay, grain and cereals, etc. during the 3rd quarter. Prune plants and trees, pick apples, pears, etc. at the time of the 3rd and 4th quarters; also develop bulbs for planting during these phases.

What Is Hydroponic Gardening?

Hydroponics is basically a water culture method of growing plants without soil. Seeds sprout and grow to maturity in a liquid nutrient medium. The solution can be pumped for daily feedings into tanks or trays where the plants grow, or used to irrigate the gravel in the plant containers with essential growth nutrients.

In most modern dictionaries or encyclopedias

hydroponics is defined as the science of growing plants without soil by feeding them on a solution of water, mineral salts and other nutrients necessary for growth, rather than relying on the traditional methods of cultivating the soil as most gardeners and farmers do in producing crops.

What Can be Grown by Hydroponics?

Hydroponics can be applied to large commercial operations to grow fruits, flowers, house plants and vegetables; professionals or amateurs can be successful with this method.

The term hydroponics is from two Greek words, hudro, water, and ponos, work. Together they mean "water-working." This is a reference to the use of solutions of water and fertilizers for soilless "farming." (Geoponics is the normal method of caring for the earth.) The same basic principle applies to earth farming and hydroponics — that of cultivating plant life, but the difference is in the growing medium. The beauty of the concept of hydroponics is that we don't have to depend on worn-out or deficient soils. Plants could be grown in desert wastes, with suitable allowance for heat and humidity effects.

How Did Hydroponics Originate?

Nearly three centuries ago John Woodward, of England, began experiments to find how plants derived their food from the soil and/or water. He was greatly hampered by lack of proper testing equipment as were those after him until the 19th century. At the opening of the 19th century, research methods were vastly improved, pawrtly by the advances in the field of chemistry. In 1904, Nicolas de Saussure published findings showing that plants needed mineral substances for satisfactory growth. Much later (1859-65) Julius Von Sachs of Germany proved that it was possible to develop a laboratory soil-less culture. Soon other scientists around the world took notice, and by 1920, hydroponics was universally known and accepted.

In 1929-30, Dr. William F. Gericke of the University of California, decided to adapt it to practical use. It was Dr. Gericks who coined the term "hydroponics." His experiments were highly successful; one of them resulting in 25-foot-high tomato plants. He raised fruits, flowers, grains, root vegetables and other vegetables. News soon spread his findings all across the U.S. and around the world.

The U.S. armed forces used hydroponics during the second World War at their military bases. The U.S.S.R. is studying and experimenting with it, as are many countries of the world. The American armed forces are still using hydroponics today in the Far East and in many parts of the world. Hydroponics is used in the Canary Islands, Puerto Rico, Mexico, India, England, Switzerland, France, Germany and the Netherlands. (The latter five use it extensively in the flower industry.) It is also in current use in Australia, New Zealand, South Africa, Spain and Israel to name a few other countries. This gives some idea of the wide range of cultures and climates where it is used. Almost every country on the globe is represented.

Commercial hydroponics is quite successful, with amateur and hobby interest rapidly growing.

How Hydroponic Principles Work

Hydroponics supplies three of the five essential requirements for plant growth as they are supplied in orthodox cultivation. Air, water and sunlight are Nature's contributions. Mineral salts and root system support are the two other requirements. The soil must be plowed and fertilized, but the chemically inert root base in the hydroponics system does not, and the liquid solution provides nutrients to the desired balance. Besides oxygen and carbon dioxide, some 11 mineral salts are known to be essential to good plant growth: nitrogen, potassium, phosphorus, calcium, magnesium, sulphur, iron, manganese, zinc, boron and copper. The soilless farmer or gardener takes the guesswork out of soil balance by using a specially prepared mixture or formula plant food. It is rapidly assimilated by the plants for fast, hardy growth.

Root supporting material is available in many forms to anchor the maturing plant life. Simple growing units can be made from household containers such as pots, small barrels, bowls, old sinks, shallow boxes, etc. The growing medium can be such things as sand (especially the coarse variety), gravel, crushed bricks, cinders, peat and many other substances.

Soilless Food for the Future

There is extensive research to be carried out in the future, but the implications of hydroponics for the future supply of food is encouraging. I can say from personal observation that experiments in which sick animals were fed hydroponic foods were most encouraging. The animals improved rapidly. This does not mean that they were completely well, that they were brought to the highest level of health. But we might think about such things in considering the future use of hydroponics.

Composting The Organic Way

Organic composting has numerous advantages — and no disadvantages. First, it improves the soil quality greatly; and it allows earlier planting. Early planting is important to get the most out of the garden and beat some of the summer heat. If the climate in your area tends to be dry, compost lessens the watering requirement. The soil is noted as darker and richer, and this helps it warm to the sun's rays earlier in the year. It improves the quality of the harvest greatly. Earthworms are attracted to composted soil. They help break down organic matter, increase soil fertility, aerate the soil and distribute minerals better. The idea of improving the soil and its yield naturally has built in safeguards for farmer and consumer. Both sandy, porous soil and hard or clay-like earth are improved in nature.

When, Where And How To Build The Compost Pile

It's never the wrong time of year to begin a compost pile. Start now. Spring or fall is the time for laying out the compost pile, but material can be gathered for it all year. Collect piles of cut grass, weeds, plants, leaves, soil, constantly. Nearly anything can go into the compost pile — egg shells (for lime and sulphur), tea and coffee grounds, vegetable discards, corn cobs, fruit peelings, nut shells, leftover table scraps—anything that will rot.

Place the compost pile in a secluded area, protected from the wind, close to both the garden and kitchen for easy reach, and near a water hose. When the compost pile is built it should be well watered; then keep it spongy moist, not overly wet or dry.

It is well to have several compost heaps going at once, as material is added. Decide on the size it is to be and then organize in layers. Bacterial starter is often used for uniformity in fermentation. The pile may be turned with pitchfork to encourage aeration. Opening the inside to oxygen hurries the decomposition process along. However, the heat can become too intense, and watering down is required. Sheet composting or digging compost directly into the soil is often used but without best results, and decompostion time is lengthened. Barrel composting uses an open bottomed barrel with a tight lid. It is filled with kitchen waste and other materials in layers. When full, the barrel can be removed by lifting.

Cow, horse, chicken, rabbit or goat manure is excellent for compost piles. They should be included in the compost material, along with straw. Moderate weather requires about six months for compost maturity, longer for colder weather or shorter time in heat. The compost is ready when it appears as rich, dark topsoil and has an earthy odor. All the material should be decomposed. If the heap was built on normal soil, not hard-packed, earthworms will have made their entrance. It is then time to transfer the compost to the garden for maximum benefits.

before harrowing for good results. Also spread it in the fall before spading. Scatter it over the ground before plowing, spading or harrowing.

Livestock manure may be used alone, but should be allowed to "age" in covered heaps. Otherwise, if used too soon, it will chemically burn the roots of new plants. It is best used with other compost material. Putting fresh manure directly on soil takes much longer to decompose. Livestock manure is essential for the best quality compost.

Sprout Sense

Seeds and sprouts are undoubtedly the finest food in all the vegetable kingdom. They are the freshest, most "alive" food you can eat. They are natural, pure and whole, offer adequate bulk for the system, and most sensitive digestive systems welcome them.

Living foods are undergoing a revolutionary phase. Sprouting, which has been in practice for centuries, is becoming a necessity. The present escalated cost of foods and the mounting trend toward adulteration and devitalizing of foods, makes sprouting a means of "survival."

The most "alive" foods are sprouted seeds. Soaking seeds in water awakens enzymes from their dormancy, and the nutritional values of the seeds are increased from 10 to 2,000% in some varieties. The sprouted seeds also become much more easily digested. Vitamin B increases greatly, vitamin E increases up to 20 times and vitamin C is introduced where none was previously. Sprouted seeds and beans are quite tasty, providing a source of safe, poison-free food.

Purchasing Seeds And Beans For Sprouting

When selecting seeds be sure to buy the best available. These may be purchased from your health food store or a reliable garden supply house. Beware of seeds that have been sprayed or treated by poison chemicals to inhibit fungus growth or kill rodents. Make sure the seeds or beans are pure, chemically untreated, especially if you buy from an agricultural supply outlet, garden supply store, hardware store or nursery.

A partial list of seeds and beans for sprouting include: Alfalfa, barley, buckwheat, fava, mung, lima, pinto, soy beans, corn, cress, clovers, caraway, celery, dill, flax, fenugreek, garbanzos, kale, lettuce, lentils, millet, parsley, purslane, pumpkin, peanuts, onions, oats, radish, red beet, safflower, sunflower, wheat, etc. Some of the best are soy or mung beans, alfalfa and buckwheat.

Sprout Garden Tools

Use a large wide-mouth glass jar (quart canning jar is excellent) and a piece of cheesecloth, screen or nylon hose, secured over the mouth with the jar ring or a rubber band. Other containers such as perforated collanders may also be used.

259

"Planting" The Sprout Garden

1. Place ½ cup seeds or beans in a quart jar. Mixtures are permissible. (Use 1 tablespoon for alfalfa seeds.)

2. Cover the jar with screening material and fill with water; agitate and pour off water. This washes the seeds. Fill the jar half with water and soak seeds 12 to 24 hours. Pour off water and save for green drinks or soups and broths. After the jar has drained, place it in a warm, dark place. Rinse and drain twice daily with tepid water (to avoid chilling). When the leaves begin to show (such as alfalfa) place the container in indirect sunlight to improve chlorophyll content. (Note: if your city water is fluoridated or contains other chemicals, alfalfa may not sprout easily.)

3. Once sprouting has begun, the entire sprout can be eaten. For optimum nutrition allow lentils and mung beans 3 days; garbanzo-chick peas 2-3 days; alfalfa, clover, radish and fenugreek 3-6 days; and wheat 2 days.

4. Drain well and store in refrigerator in a ventilated container. Refrigerator life is 2-4 days, sometimes a week. Sprouts are most nutritious eaten in the raw state. Incorporate into salads, soups, drinks, other dishes and use as snacks. Sprouts bring oxygen to the system, acting as an energy booster.

Growing Beansprouts In Your Kitchen

1. Wash 4 tablespoons of beans 3-4 times.

2. Soak overnight in a cup of lukewarm water.

3. Rinse again the following day until the water runs clear.

4. Spread two layers of cheesecloth or paper towels over a flat container or pan with perforated bottom for drainage.

5. Spread the rinsed beans (or seeds) over the cheesecloth.

6. Sprinkle with ¼ cup lukewarm water.

7. Cover with a clean, wet cloth.

8. Place in a dark, warm place.

9. Once a day, for approximately 3 days (germination depends on bean variety), pour lukewarm water over the pan. (Mung bean sprouts are ready in 3 days; soybeans take 6.)

Sprouts Have Multiple Uses

Chop sprouts into any salad such as cole slaw, tossed greens, gelatin with fruit or vegetables. Use for breakfast with cream or milk cultures or raw milks over cereals. Add to yeast breads along with the final flour. Chop and add to soups or stews just before serving. Use as a green in drinks or salads. Add crisp freshness to lunch boxes and sandwiches in place of lettuce. Gently steam and add to vegetables. Use in omelets, toppings for soups, dressings. Start sprouting!

Further Notes On Sprouting

Alfalfa is the king of sprouts; the mung bean sprout follows. Then, or course, there are others which are very good. Consider these which come from the smallest seed the best. The sunflower seed sprout should not be overlooked. (Much has been written about sprouts in many other books: *Survive This Day; Health Magic Through Chlorophyll; Seeds and Sprouts for Life.*) They may be of interest to those who want to go into sprouting more deeply.

Harvesting Your Sprouts

Seeds	Sprouting time	Best length
1. Sunflower	2 days	¼ inch
2. Lentils, dry	3 days	½-1 inch
3. Alfalfa seed	3-5 days	1-2 inches
4. Garbanzos, dry	3 days	1 inch
5. Fava beans	3 days	½-¾ inches
6. Mung beans, dry	2-3 days	2-3 inches
7. Soy beans	3 days	½-¾ inches
8. Wheat, whole	2 days	¼-½ inches
9. Flaxseed	2-4 days	¾ inch
10. Sesame	2 days	¼ inch

Sprouted Soybean Analysis

Analysis	Dry	Sprouted
Protein	38%	48%
Fat	20%	14%
Carbohydrates	38%	37%
Vitamin A	90 IU	800 IU
Thiamine (B)	1.2	1.6
Riboflavin (B)	0.35	1.5
Niacin (B)	2.4	7.0
Vitamin C (Ascorbic Acid)	0	100

The above is taken from the USDA Handbook No. 80 on the composition of foods. It is listed in percent or grams per 100 grams of dry weight. Other sprouted seeds and grains show similar gains in nutritional value when sprouted.

Hope Springs From Harmony With Nature

Man will one day become a farmer of the sea. He will be forced to seek food at the bottom of the ocean. We must learn to live in harmony with Nature and with each other. Mankind's philosophy determines the goodness of his food, beauty and joy on this earth.

Replacing butter with heated oils and margarine is a suicidal course to follow. Coal-tar derived vitamins and additives replacing Nature's foods are poison. Artificial colorings are killing us just as coal tar flavorings are destroying us. Consider margarine made from coal, beefsteaks from oil and sugar from wood. At the same time, mind processes and faculties are slowing and deteriorating. Are we thinking fast enough to survive?

Where Has Man's Purpose Failed?

Foods have not been studied sufficiently to ascertain their relevance to disease, if any. Disease is spreading in plant and animal life as it is in the human race. Sick, unhealthy animals and plants produce unhealthy foods. We haven't found the keys to quality as yet.

Artificial milk was developed to fill the void on inadequate land quality and insufficiency in cow's milk. This single example will bring a rapid physical decline to man. England's dairies are discovering that cows bred to the height of milk-production efficiency have little resistance to diseases, many of which cannot be successfully treated. What has destroyed this resistance? Where does it come from? Is it in the feeding? Are these animals cared for properly to ensure their health and ours also? Are fish today becoming unfit to eat because of polluted waters, radiation, strontium 90?

The Cycle Leading To Nowhere

America has sent millions of dollars worth of vitamins and drugs to India when what they really needed was hoes, rakes, shovels and the knowledge to take care of their soil, their crops and how to grow foods conducive to improving their national health. We "fix up" rather than getting to the base and the cause of the problems. We gave white flour to the Italians after World War Two, and it developed gas in their children's stomachs. One of these days there will be revolution produced by the foods we eat. In the Amazon region of Brazil, the first sight which greeted me was a soft drink sign. Thailand street cars extol soda pop as do Fiji Islands umbrellas. Where are the foods they really need? We are methodically destroying ourselves.

We find ways of producing more to keep man constantly laboring earning more money. We don't seem to care what kinds of foods we move, just as long as we move them in large quantities. The food quantities transported from country to country are the greatest of all commodities. The French and the Australian aborigines no long remember their natural foods or natural state of living.

Science Could Be Too Late

We haven't found a norm. Doctors are arguing over how much protein we need, how many starches, yet we don't have a norm, a guideline, in quality, quantity or in varieties. The study of man has been left until last. This should be our first interest today. If we are to survive, we must become interested in our preservation. Next week may be too late.

Modern inventions allow more and more men to be removed from agriculture than ever. Refrigeration keeps foods longer than ever. Preservation, through cooking, canning, additives, artificial flavorings, is allowing people to do everything overnight. These inventions alone spell disaster.

In the past, as countries began to trade foods, they had to devise ways of preserving food through cold, storehouses, salt, sun drying. We've added sugar to jams and vinegar to pickles and salted foods until they are no longer natural foods. The door has opened to poor health as a result. Perhaps too late we will discover we cannot detour from natural, pure, whole foods.

One of the most horrendous crimes is the introduction of fluorine to water supplies, making the water a carrier of one more toxic substance. These and other destructive patterns weren't initiated by medical doctors or those responsible for national health. Those promoting these habits haven't the faintest idea what actual relation this bears to health.

We are currently using infrared and microwave cooking. We may think we are emerging from the age of primitive food preparation methods, but taste and appearance are poor criteria for judging the quality and value of foods. Natural wholeness and purity make much more sense. Vegetables and fruits may be large but lack minerals; TV dinners may be filling but are "foodless" foods.

Salvation For Our Civilization Or . . .

I am not against civilization, it is a wonderful way to develop. We should have everything to afford us comfort and with it beauty and joy. We must have our pleasures, but they must be those expressed consistently with the good of our fellowman. Brotherhood is at stake today. Our lives are at stake and those of our families, as well as the future citizens of the world.

Can we say we are fit and fearless? Can we say we are strong? DDT residues are still being found in human bodies. Do we know about the after effects of drugs, the cumulative effects of chemical sprays, of artificial fertilizers used on the soil today? How many of us can reckon with the after effects and the cumulative effects of the plain chemical fluorine found in many local water supplies today? These and countless other dangers confront us **now**... **Not** in the future.

Are Proteins The Answer?

Frederick Gowland hypothesized that if animals were not fed properly, they would develop deficiency diseases. He termed the needed substances "accessory food factors"—we call them vitamins. Vitamins and minerals regulate the living processes of our bodies. Proteins are the chief body building foods. "Protein" comes from the Greek word meaning, "first." Life, plant or animal, cannot exist without protein. Enzymes break down the amino acid patterns which make up the protein in our hair, flesh and blood. As soils are depleted, so is the protein content of foods grown on them.

Calories Aren't The Answer

It is claimed that 4500 calories a day is reasonable for a farmer or a coal miner; 3000 for a less active man or a nursing mother; 2100 is adequate for most adult women. However, four tablespoons of some foods may equal 2100 calories but may not be the right kind of sustenance. Meals cannot be measured by calories alone.

Poisons Are Cumulative

The accumulation of poisons daily, even in tiny amounts, will inevitably cause disease and ultimately death. This is what is happening today. Innumerable experiments point to dangers. Poison is noted for bringing slow death as well as a rapid demise. Did the Almighty Creator intend such a horrible fate for his children?

Nature's Not always Merciful

We have pitied people who starved to death: the ten million who died in the 1796-70 Bengal famine; the nine and one half million who perished in the 1800's North China famine; the 1942 Bombay rice crop failure, more recent famines in Bangla-Desh and North Africa. These people were pitted against the ravages of rainstorms, drought, floods, fires, earthquakes and other natural phenomena. To survive, we must use our intelligence to develop many alternative methods of food production.

We Are Our Brother's Keeper

No one today should be forced to starve if we truly were our brother's keeper. We have enough food. If food were evenly distributed, the third world countries would not be starving. Nature balances weather conditions to compensate for "lean" years in certain areas. The real threat to America's future is civilization itself. Famine has followed those people who have had a bad harvest. And, it is most clear we are having it now.

Man Must Rebuild What He Destroys

Another Sahara Desert could be produced through continuous abuse and misuse of our lands. It is time to awaken to the point of action. Rains will no longer come to the proper parts of the world. Man is becoming so neglectful of self-preservation and health that he will one day soon reach the "point of no return."

The Good Book Holds A Prophecy

It is foretold that in the last days man will die of pestilence and famine, among other things. I believe that day is approaching. Look at what is going on in the pantry and in the kitchen. Intelligence is in direct proportion to the quality of the food supplied, experiments show.

Belligerence And Violence Caused By Food

It is not by happenstance that we have a belligerent nation today. A certain percentage of criminality is attributed to food habits from youth. I am convinced criminals are sick people, malnourished people. Violence, crime and antigovernment movements are linked to unhappy childhoods brought on by poor feeding. Recent experiments carried out with prison inmates showed great improvements in behavior, dramatic drops in violence, when prisoners were given nutritionally balanced meals and were deprived of candy, soft drinks and other sugary products.

Blessings Are The Rewards Of Service

I believe good health starts when the mind is set on the right path, in the direction that God intended it to be. The best harvest comes from the maximum effort. The world and Nature, owe no one a living. Refusing to work and expecting a check is a condemning attitude. If everyone wants to be on the receiving end, the end is quite near.

When Civilization Is No More...

Today, food supplies are no threat to man. We have plenty. Steps to curtail the multiplying population will not be needed. As we are killing the wild animals and vegetation, so we are killing ourselves. During the next 20 years the results will become increasingly evident. America has more sterility than ever, largely due to improper food processing and inferior food. In the future we will see multiplying cases of "childless parents."

Man is degenerating to the point where Nature will have to return to civilization and man to the dust. The abnormal, impure, unnatural foods today are encouraging man's decline. They are encouraging his "ungodly" philosophies.

Man's Misguided Destiny

Man has learned to bathe every day, but he is still unclean from within. Beneath civilization runs a black current of destruction. As Sai Baba, an Indian master, once said, "There are many who are wearing the yellow robe, but they are dark on the inside."

During the last days, we are going to have to be careful of man's inventions. Those people who lived in the countries where the best foods were grown and the best soils existed had to go through more wars than those in other countries of the world. Those who are in the most remote places, who don't live the longest, have had the fewest wars. On the other hand, who wants the countries where there is difficulty in finding food or making a living?

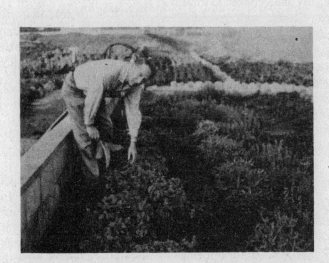

AMERICAN FARMERS
The average American farmer produces 375,000 pounds of food per year as compared to 30,000 pounds produced by the average Soviet farmer. The American farmer grows enough food for 68 people, and that food creates nine jobs in the food industry.

FOOD FOR ALL
Only 2.3 percent of the U.S. population grows the food used by all the people in the country, with surpluses that are sold or given away to other nations.

Chapter 35

Home drying, freezing and storage

General Freezing Tips

Use only top quality food in freezing, as foods for freezing must be at the peak of freshness and ripeness. Speed from the garden to freezer is the prime secret to conserving nutritional quality and taste. Frozen foods must be properly packaged, accurately labeled, (contents, date, serving number). Leave an inch head margin in freezer containers for freezing expansion. Soups and juices may be frozen in ice cube trays and repacked later in plastic bags. Freeze cooked dishes slightly undercooked to finish "just right" when reheated. Season with restraint, especially with herbs. Salt loses flavor.

Freeze foods in season. Don't stock up on foods available all year round. Rotate food in storage. Keep a food inventory listing. Of course, use food stored the longest first. Purchase in bulk to save money.

The plastic container is the ideal. Plastic bags are also useful in freezing. Wax paper does not hold up well in the freezer.

Nutritive Values Of Freezing

Freezing seems to protect nutritive values of foods the most satisfactorily of all preserving methods. Fruits and vegetables to be frozen should be prepared and frozen with all possible speed to prevent loss of vitamin C. Uncooked fruit should be cut sufficiently to pack solidly without air spaces. Crushed or pureed fruit retains more vitamin C than whole or halved fruit because it packs more solidly.

In purchasing fruits and vegetables for freezing rather than growing your own, buy in the early morning and prepare immediately. Pick or gather your own in the early morning when nutritive content is at its highest. Loss of vitamin C begins to take place when food is thawed.

Freeze freshly picked food promptly, seal to exclude all air and eat soon after defrosting to make the most of vitamin C in it.

If vegetables are cooked in minimal water and if the liquid is served with them, there is almost no loss of minerals and very little loss of vitamins. (Vitamin F is destroyed by the freezing process.)

Rules For Freezing Success

Drop the temperature of food rapidly to 10° F. below zero or lower. Use relatively thin packages or freeze in open trays and package afterward. Place packages in direct, flat contact with a metal freezer plate. Make sure the food is not allowed to rise above 0° until ready to use. Do not refreeze thawed food.

Recommended Fruits For Freezing

Apples, juicy, barely ripe, tart, fall varieties
Apricots, ripe, juicy, flavorsome
Berries, blackberries, boysenberries, loganberries, raspberries (red and black), youngberries, strawberries (well ripened, freshly gathered).
Cherries, sweet, sour; ripe and freshly picked
Grapes, Concord and Red
Grapefruit & Oranges, fully tree ripened; use soon after picking
Guavas
Papayas
Persimmons
Plums, any varieties
Tomatoes, well ripened, deep in color, sound fruit only
Pineapples

Guide To Freezing Fruit

Berries, such as strawberries, raspberries, blueberries, etc., should be handled as little as possible. Wash well in ice water, pick out any damaged berries, allow to drain and freeze loosely on a tray. Bag in plastic for future use; or freeze in puree form.

Any melons can be cut into balls and frozen or juiced in a liquifier and frozen for later fresh drinks.

Dice pineapple in chunks, sticks, or slice; place in container and freeze. Defrost one hour prior to use.

Fruit may be frozen whole, (peaches, plums, apricots, etc.); place a single layer directly on freezer plates or coils; store in plastic bags when completely frozen; or other containers. Slice and use as fresh fruit when thawed. To serve partially frozen, hold under cold water and remove skin if desired.

Dried fruit conserves space. Pack into trays or into containers and freeze. Defrost; peel and use as fresh fruit.

Treat fresh fruit the same way, except for first dipping in boiling water and removing peel. Dip in lemon juice; chill; package and freeze.

Honey is suitable for sweetening fruit. Use only the best fruit. Freezing fruit in all-honey syrup doesn't require use of vitamin C or ascorbic acid to prevent discoloration. Honey syrup may be prepared in quantity and refrigerated until needed. White clover honey is the best flavor.

Direction: Boil 1 quart water; remove from heat; stir in 1-½ to 2 cups honey. Pour ¾ cup cold syrup into each container. Wash peaches or other fruit in cold water; slice or peel and slice into syrup, working rapidly to reach 1 inch from the top. Cover with piece of crumpled vegetable parchment to keep fruit under syrup while freezing. Seal tightly with cover and freeze.

Thaw fruit in unopened container in the refrigerator or at room temperature.

Best Freezing Varieties Of Vegetables

Asparagus	Mary and Martha Washington varieties.
Green Beans	Stringless Green Pod, Kentucky Wonder, Refugee, Egyptian
Lima Beans	Fordhook, Baby Potato, Henderson Bush
Beets	Detroit, Dark Red, Crosby
Broccoli	Italian Green, Calabrese
Brussel Sprouts	Long Island Improved, Green Sprouting
Carrots	Red Core, Chantenay, Nantes Corless
Cauliflower	Snow Ball, Forbes, White Mountain, Sunrise, Perfection
Corn	Golden Cross, Bantam, Eight Row Bantam, Aristogold
Eggplant	Black Beauty, New York Improved
Kohlrabi	Early White, Vienna
Mushrooms	Cultivated Agaricus Campestris
Okra	Dwarf Green
Peas	Thomas Laxton, Strategerm, Worlds Record, Gradus, Little Marvel
Pumpkin	Kentucky Field, Small Sugar
Spinach	King of Denmark, Nobel, Long Standing, Bloomdale, Hollandia
Squash	Summer: Yellow Crookneck, Zucchini; Winter: Buttercup, Green Cold, Golden Delicious, Hubbard
Sweet Potato	Jersey (for slicing); Puerto Rico (yams for pies)

Guide To Freezing Vegetables

Generally, vegetables are prepared for freezing as for cooking. Then they are blanched, chilled, drained and packaged. Cauliflower and a few others need the addition of ascorbic acid to retain color. They may be blanched or unblanched, according to preference. Remember, most vegetables are blanched too long. All vegetables should be dry, as moisture in the bag or container spoils them.

Buy onions at their cheapest; slice and chop; freeze in small packages. Do likewise with green peppers. Freeze mushrooms raw. Don't even wash. Whole, unshucked corn freezes beautifully. Tie tassel end with a string and freeze quickly. Transfer to bags. Use within 6 weeks. Packages of mixed vegetables are handy for later use.

Vegetable Blanching List

Asparagus. Preparation: Leave whole or cut; wash. Blanch 2-3 minutes, according to size; chill; drain package.

Lima beans. Preparation: Blanch before shelling. Blanch 1-2 minutes according to size; shell; drain; package.

Green beans. Preparation: Leave whole or slice; wash. Blanch 2 minutes; chill; drain; package.

Broccoli. Preparation: Immerse 1/2 hour in salt solution; cut lengthwise. Blanch 3-4 minutes, according to size; chill; drain; package.

Corn on the Cob. Preparation: Shuck; remove silk. Blanch 4 at a time 6 minutes (small)—8 minutes (large); chill; drain; package.

Cut Corn. Preparation: As above. As above; remove kernels after blanching and cooling; drain; package.

Peas. Preparation: Shell. Blanch 1 minute; chill; drain; package.

Spinach and Greens. Preparation: Wash leaves gently; Blanch 2-1/2 minutes, using 8 quarts of water to 1 pound greens; chill; drain; package.

Freezer Storage Time Limits

Lean Fish and Lamb	6-8 months
Beef, Veal, Poultry	9-12 months
Fruits	10-12 months
Vegetables	10-12 months
Eggs	6-10 months
Butter	6-8 months
Cheese	4-5 months
Cream	2-4 months
Ice Cream	1-2 months
Milk	½-1 month
Baked Products	6 months
Pies	2-4 months
Breads and Cakes	4-6 months
Unbaked Products	2 months
Cookie Dough	4-6 months
Stews and Meat Dishes	3-6 months
Vegetable Casseroles	6 months
Corn Pudding	4 months
Salad Dressings	3 months
Salads made with Gelatin	1 month

Cakes frosted keep less than one month. Unfrosted cakes will keep several months. Pies baked and unbaked should not be kept any longer than 2 months. Fruit cakes keep up to a year. Unbaked cookies keep up to 8 and 9 months.

While many foods will keep for months, it is not economical, as you are not getting the most from your freezer.

Almost Any Food Freezes Well

Salads: Even salads can become part of your quick frozen meals. Salad greens tend to become limp when thawed, but other fruit and vegetable combination salads can freeze well. Thaw salads in refrigerator. Individual salads take about one hour. Use within two to four weeks of freezing.

Fish: The main requirement is speed. Freeze the day they are caught or pack in ice and freeze as soon as possible. Never permit fish to become warm. Clean and prepare for cooking. Small fish can be frozen whole and large fish should be cut in steaks.

Defrosting: Meat, poultry and fish may be cooked in the frozen state. But for more uniform preparation, defrost first.

Dairy Products: These are economical and easy to freeze. Buy when plentiful. **Butter:** Freeze in waxed carton, or for long storage, overwrap with freezer paper or foil. **Cheese:** Wrap hard cheese in quantities to be used at one time. Place freezer wrap between cheese slices. Uncreamed cottage cheese freezes safely longer than creamed. Freeze cream cheese in its original wrapper for short periods of time; wrap in freezer paper or foil for longer storage. Cheese grated freezes well. **Whipped cream** or left-over whipped cream frozen in small dollops sealed in plastic bags is ready for garnishing.

Milk Substitutes: Make as usual and freeze in trays.

Ice Cream: Use rich cream for the best product. Recipes containing egg yolk and gelatin are recommended. Prepare according to directions. Place in well sealed container and freeze to allow ripening with age.

Eggs: Stir eggs enough to mix. Place in ice tray (same number eggs as tray dividers). When eggs freeze, remove from tray and put in plastic bags and store in freezer. Each square is equivalent to one egg. Hard-cooked egg whites are non-freezable; freeze grated. Extra egg whites or yolks may be frozen for future use. Leave head space for whites. Add 1 tablespoon raw sugar or maple syrup or 1 teaspoon vegetable salt per cup of yolks. Use later for custards, sauces, dressings, vital drinks, scrambled eggs and omelettes.

2 Tbsps. Egg White is equal to 1 Egg White
1 Tbsp. Egg Yolk is equal to 1 Egg Yolk

Soups: Concentrated soups freeze best to conserve freezer space. Make thick soup to be thinned later. Make purees of vegetables and freeze for soup later. Don't overcook vegetables. Cool rapidly and pour into air- and liquid-tight containers. Store up to 2 months.

Casseroles: The frozen casserole dish is a life saver for the busy homemaker. When making casserole dishes, make at least twice the needed amount and freeze for later use. Freeze most casseroles before or after baking. Cool; package in shallow casserole; wrap tightly in foil or slip into plastic bag. Freeze.

Sandwiches: All kinds of bread freeze. Prepare filling ahead and refrigerate. Don't use mayonnaise in filling, as it separates upon defrosting and makes bread soggy. Wrap sandwiches as soon as made and cut. Plastic sandwich bags are especially handy for freezing. They thaw 2 to 4 hours, so place frozen sandwich in lunchbox. Use sandwiches in 2-4 weeks.

Lunches; Allow a special section in your freezer for "lunches" and let children choose their own. Wrap in moisture-proof paper if freezing for more than 4 days. Freeze individual fruits; nut breads, health cakes; vegetarian loaf; baked potato; burgers, etc. Add lettuce, celery and other salad ingredients fresh.

Pies: Pies and pastries freeze well, baked or unbaked, keeping about 4 months.

Cakes: Cake batter freezes well if double acting baking powder is used. Plan to use within 2 weeks. Baked cakes freeze more efficiently. They store up to 6 months. Wrap in freezer paper and freeze, if unfrosted.

Cookies: Unbaked cookies, rolled, unrolled or drop will freeze. Place freezer paper between each rolled cookie. Baked cookies freeze more efficiently. Unbaked store for about 3 months; baked for up to 6.

Bread: Freezing keeps bread perfectly fresh, and actually improves freshness. Freeze it either baked or unbaked. Allow dough to double in bulk; place as for baking (in bread tins or rolls on trays), grease well, wrap and freeze; or freeze rolls and wrap afterward. Store one week only. Thaw at room temperature. Let rise to double bulk and bake as usual. After baking, cool bread; wrap in freezer paper or plastic bags and freeze. Baked breads store for up to 12 months. Keep two plastic bags of breadcrumbs, one plain, one buttered for hasty topping or casseroles or breading burgers. Cool and wrap baked biscuits for freezing; keep 1-4 weeks.

Pancakes & Waffles: These freeze excellently and need only to be heated in a 350° oven before serving. Frozen waffles can be reheated in a toaster. For moistness, package waffles warm.

Nuts: Chopped or ground nuts may be frozen. Freeze nuts in pint plastic containers. Defrost at room temperature. Leftover nuts are safely refrozen.

Cereals: Pour hot, cooked cereal into a loaf pan or round can rinsed in cold water. Cool, chill, remove from pan. Wrap for freezer and freeze immediately. Hot cereal may be poured into custard cups. Freeze. Rice freezes well.

Drying: Preserving Foods Naturally

Seeds are the classic example of drying to preserve them, indefinitely for some varieties. Dried food kept free from moisture can be stored for long periods of time. The advantage in drying is that the moisture is removed so the food isn't attacked by microorganisms that cause spoilage; mold, yeast and bacteria have to be in the presence of moisture to thrive. Also the food isn't actually heated enough to cook it and destroy many of the nutrients. Dried foods have concentrated flavor; thus it is sufficient in small quantities. It can greatly add to food variety in the winter months when fresh fruits and vegetables are likely to be scarce.

Prepare foods for drying as though you were going to use them fresh; wash, drain and remove the parts that aren't to be eaten. If the foods are cubed or sliced small or thin, drying is faster and easier.

Simplified Drying Methods

Oven Drying. This is one of the easiest methods and faster than some other methods. A wood cook stove can be an excellent dryer if the temperature can be kept low and uniform. Your electric or gas range oven is less difficult to use however, especially when drying will take five to six hours or longer. Very shallow trays or cookie sheets work nicely for placing the food on; line it with waxed or parchment paper first. Most drying is started at a temperature of about 130° F. (If the heat is too low the food can sour and if too high it can cook.) It is usually turned at least once during the drying process. A pound of dried food yields as little as one ounce when dried; this is an average figure. When is drying finished? Fruits should be like softened leather and vegetables should be crisp like potato chips.

Sun Drying. This method is best suited for warm, dry climates. Pieces of food are usually placed on trays that the air can circulate through, even wooden trays. Cheesecloth often lines the trays and a covering of the same is on top or screen wire to keep insects and so forth off. There is more work involved because the trays have to be taken indoors at night to protect them from the dew; or the trays must be covered with waterproof material, such as plastic. The vegetables or fruits should be turned several times during drying. Drying time takes from one day to weeks, depending on the food, moisture content and weather.

Air Drying. The attic or summer kitchens are often used for this method. Air drying is less bother than sun drying because you don't have to worry about the weather or night dew. It is handled basically the same as sun drying, otherwise. An easy way to handle sun and air dried foods is to string them on a strong, thin cord rather than using trays. A darning or carpet needle can be threaded; spear the food one piece at a time and tie the ends in a necklace fashion. Hang them on pegs or nails to dry.

Easy Storage Of Dried Foods

If quantities for storage are small, use cans with plastic lids or canisters or fruit jars with lids. Plastic bags may also be used; press out the air before securing the top with wire twists or bands.

How To Use Dried Foods

Drying should be used more; the commercial method of sulphuring dried fruits is not recommended for health. Use dried fruits and vegetables revived in soups and liquefied drinks. Always revive dried fruit before using to free it of any organisms or debris. Dried foods can take the place of fresh foods in recipe ingredients.

Of course, foods should be tree ripened, organic and the most perfect you can find. Drying does not improve the quality. A tip for keeping the cut fruits white is to dip them in lemon and water right after cutting. (Apples, pears, etc.) Apricots make a delicious revived compote or combine with other fruits or nuts or seeds. Strawberries, raspberries, blackberries and other berries make delicious liquefied drinks (revive first). Even though the dried fruits may not be as appealing as fresh, they can be used where fresh are called for. They make excellent marmalades, sauces, jams, syrups, toppings, health candies, sweeteners for cereals, energy snacks, etc. Give them to children instead of candy and other sweets. Use your imagination and refer to some of the recipes in my book *Vital Foods for Total Health*. Many fruits can be dried such as apples, pears, peaches, apricots, bananas, pineapple, berries, plums, grapes, cherries and currants.

Drying vegetables are leafy vegetables, tomatoes, corn, green beans, onions, zucchini and summer squash, cucumbers, garlic, mushrooms, carrots, cabbage, celery, broccoli, beets, parsnips, peas, pepper and turnips.

Use them in liquefier drinks, soups and broths; powdered and whole as seasonings and garnishes.

Don't forget the herbs; they dry very well, too. Try comfrey, nettles, malva, plantain, lambs quarters, parsley; cultivate your own herb garden with bay leaf, thyme, chervil, oregano, sweet basil, red pepper, dill, tarragon, sage, marjoram, lovage, chives, etc. They grind or crush well for storage. (They are often dried in paper bags or in the open air, with little effort.) Use mixtures of spices as seasonings or garnishes, in soups, drinks, vegetables, casseroles, eggdishes, etc.

Drying is discussed a great deal more in my book, *Survive This Day*.

Storing Vegetables At Home For The Winter

You should know how to store vegetables in their natural state along with canning, freezing and drying at home. Potatoes, carrots, beets, parsnips, turnips, salsify, celery, onions, cabbage, sweet potatoes, dry beans and peas may be stored successfully.

If you have a house heated by a furnace in the cellar, partition off a small space to make a storage room. One outside window at least is suggested for best results; this lets you regulate temperature. Store potatoes, parsnips, carrots, beets, salsify and turnips in this room. Place them in bins or wooden boxes, baskets or barrels. Harvest the vegetables when the soil is dry and allow them to lay outdoors until all moisture has evaporated and they are dry. (Remove the tops from the beets, turnips, carrots and salsify to use as greens if they aren't too tough.) Store them without the tops.

If you want to store the vegetables out of doors, dig a pit 6 or 8 inches deep and as large as needed in a dry, well drained place. Line the bottom with straw, leaves or similar debris. Put the vegetables on top of the lining piled in a conical formation. Cover the vegetables with more straw and enought soil to prevent them from freezing. It is well to make several smaller pits rather than a large one; because when a pit is opened the entire pile should be removed. This form of storing is good for potatoes, carrots, beets, turnips, parsnips, cabbage and salsify. For a suggestion, it is well to store several varieties in each pit. This is convenient and will encourage you to use variety.

Dig a long, narrow pit for cabbage. Lay cabbages in a row with the heads down; cover them with dirt. They can be removed a few at a time without harming the keeping quality of the remainder. Or store cabbages in the cellar in boxes, barrels, soil or sand.

In storing celery by the pit method, the plants are set side by side as close together as you can get them and wide boards placed along the outside of the pit. Bank them with soil and cover with corn husks or similar material.

An outdoor cellar is an ideal storage place. In cold climates this should be partly underground. A side-hill location is easier for handling the vegetables. To build your own cellar dig a suitable size hole; make a frame by setting posts in rows near the earth walls. Saw the posts off at matched heights and put plates on their tops. Place rafters atop the plates. Board this structure up completely except for the door space. Cover the whole building with soil and sod. In the colder regions add fodder, straw and similar materials. The floor should be dirt for the best results; this lets some moisture in. A small opening in the roof may be made to allow air when necessary; you should be able to open or close it according to the weather. This storage setup is suitable for several families.

Cold-frames may also be used to advantage in storing vegetables providing the drainage is adequate, or thorough. After the frames are filled the sash should be covered with boards and the outside banked with soil or manure. If the weather becomes severe, straw or matting should be added as a covering. The covering must be heavy enough to avoid freezing.

If cauliflower is not mature yet, plant it in shallow boxes of soil after taking it up from the garden, in a corner of the cellar. If it is well watered, it will mature for winter use.

Store onions in a cool, dry place. Cure, dry and remove the tops before storing. Keep them in baskets, trays or other vessels to allow air to circulate around them.

Potatoes store well in a cool, frostless cellar in boxes, baskets or long narrow bins sectioned into two or three bushel sizes. Sand or soil used to cover them will keep the moisture intact. After they are harvested don't expose them to much light or wash them; it will cause them to turn green. If they begin to sprout, rub the sprouts off. Look at the contents of the bins once in a while to remove rotting potatoes to keep the rot from spreading.

Sweet potatoes and squashes are sensitive to cold and moisture; so they should be stored in a dry place with a temperature of about 50 degrees F. Pile squashes on a dry floor and cover with rugs or carpeting; make sure they are not bruised before storage.

Sweet potatoes may be packed in layers with dry sand, wheat chaff or charcoal in a warm cellar. A good place for them is near the furnace in a basket.

Peelings Most Valuable
"The average housewife peels her vegetables, thus throwing away the part directly underneath the skins containing the most plentiful amount of mineral salts; then the remaining portion is boiled and the water which has also dissolved out more minerals, is thrown away."

—*Dr. Charles H. Mayo*

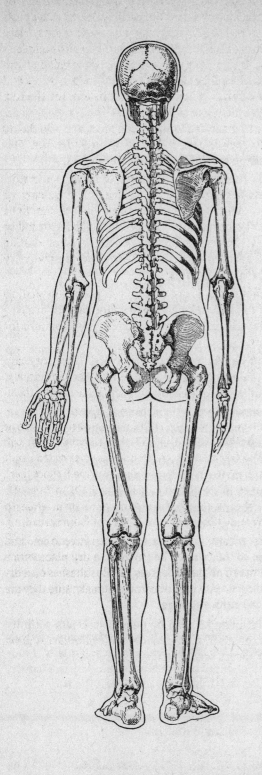

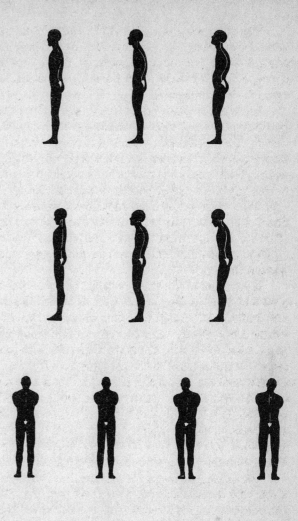

Posture is dependent a good deal on the calcium development in your body. Calcium gives the tone, energy and power to work with a positive stance. Good posture is dependent upon how much calcium we get in our foods and our daily diet routine.

The skeleton is made up of a good deal of calcium. It needs this chemical for its maintenance. Many mothers, during their pregnancy, did not give the child all that was necessary for its body growth. Many ailments of the body develop. When the skeleton degenerates, look to the chemical balance and your nutrition.

Chapter 36

Restaurant, travel and camping foods

Dining Out Successfully

Restaurants do not seem to be aware that many people are ailing and must take care of their health — for instance, in the use of salt. Why not leave the salting of foods to the diner himself? In many cases the only alternative for those with special diet needs is in abstaining from restaurant dining completely.

Most restaurants fry food abundantly. Cholesterol permeates the fried food, or at least its surface, while the lecithin that balances cholesterol is destroyed by heat. Most people today make enough money to buy some meals in restaurants. Many of today's meals are bought by people who are "restaurant minded." Get away from this conception. Foods cannot be health building if they are fried. Desserts are also great offenders. If you must have desserts occasionally, be sure they are made with natural sweeteners, not refined sugar and artificial flavorings, colorings and additives. Cut down on the frequency of having sweets and the amount of sweetening agents used in those desserts. Try to compromise by making "health desserts."

In buying a $2.98 dinner, 2 cents goes to the dishwasher, 4 cents goes for the butter, another 3 cents for the seasoning. We realize that in selling that meal that cheap the proprietor wants to cut down the cost as much as possible. The cheaper food has the highest profit. We cannot stay healthy on cheap foods. The health-minded person needs the best for himself. There is no reason why food can't be fresher, show greater variety, be unpreserved and not artificial. We are looking for fewer condiments, fresher salads and more of them, less salt and pepper, fewer artificial ingredients, colorings and flavorings. This does not border on the unreasonable or "nutty" ideals. There is no reason why restaurants, at least some of them, couldn't comply by slanting more of their foods towards the natural, pure, whole foods, that could be served to the public patronizing the restaurants of today. Herbs make excellent substitutes for many of the condiments used so indiscriminately.

Herb teas could be substituted for the coffee and regular teas served in the average restaurant. Alfamint or papaya or garden mint teas could be served. More people are becoming aware that caffeine and tannic acid are harmful drugs in the body. They are looking for cleaner bodies and better health. At least a few restaurants should be more receptive to the ideals of persons seeking the best in health.

The Bircher-Benner Sanitarium in Zurich, Switzerland has inspired many of the local restaurants to serve a small loaf of bread according to their specified recipe. Also, muesli, their popular breakfast cereal, is found in many eating houses. Muesli is made of untoasted oats, almonds, raisins, flaked nuts, filberts, dried apples and other ingredients; it is not cooked.

American restaurants could serve these dishes; but the patron wants the easiest, fastest, snack dishes available. It is all part of our industrialized system today; it is part of all commercial ventures. We are not against the restaurant business unless it keeps the husband home from work and the children away from school by contributing to poor health; this personally affects each and every one of us. Many cheap, poorly prepared foods produce future doctor bills, sickness and hospital stays.

I do not advocate the extreme measures of altering menus completely, but just the addition of more natural, pure and wholesome foods. Baked potatoes could replace mashed and fried; meat prepared by roasting and broiling could be offered. More fruit desserts could be available along with herbal teas, vegetarian and dietetic dishes. More variety might be offered so that the patron could have a better selection. Healthier foods could very easily be added to any menu.

Some airline flights have added vegetarian and Kosher dishes to the usual bill of fare. You must inquire 24 hours before flight time to be sure of their availability. Ships and trains are adding more natural foods. Begin to make inquiries and suggestions.

Natural foods restaurants are beginning to crop up in many areas of the country. There is no reason why they should not, but we should be able to order "health" foods in any restaurant, to replace head lettuce with leaf lettuce, to order broiled dishes instead of fried foods.

Foods That Travel With You

Consider the importance of special foods taken along when traveling. Leave your troubles at home. Think of traveling to relieve tensions to break the monotony, change the scenery, the climate and perhaps the altitude. Don't let the hum of wheels, other drivers, fears of accidents, noise, wind or moisture upset a happy mood.

A food basket is easily taken along. Remember that the body will not respond as it does in its own setting at home. The metabolism changes, the heart quickens and the thyroid metabolism increases. These are all good changes. Do not mar a trip with unsavory or unhealthy foods eaten in restaurants.

Eating in "hamburger joints" is not the way to treat your body while traveling, no matter how short the trip. Take foods in their freshest, most natural state possible—life giving, filled with natural essences. Take foods packed in jars; teas, nuts, marmalades, honey, sauces, fruit, vegetables, cheeses, snack bars and cookies. Include dates, figs, prunes, raisins, natural breads, hard cheeses, honey nut cakes, dried apricots, pears, apples, pineapple, persimmons, peaches and all juices. Pack foods in an ice chest to keep cool and use thermos bottles for hot and cold foods. Take juices in concentrate forms such as cherry, raspberry, apple and add prune, fig, huckleberry and other fine juices. Flaxseed meal can be beneficial as a mild laxative when riding for long periods and where the system may be upset. It might be wise to take along distilled water to make drinks and use alone. Add flaxseed meal to drinks or cereals.

Take sun-dried olives, spring water, raw vegetables such as beets, turnips, carrots, parsnips, potatoes and fruits such as apples, pears, dates, raisins, figs. Use only unsulphured dried fruits. These are excellent energy sources for the hiker or cyclist, also.

Stop at roadside markets for fresh fruits and vegetables and other fresh, wholesome, natural and pure foods and beverages. Be able to live on raw foods alone for periods of a week or perhaps more. Eat raw tomatoes, celery, okra, spinach and other vegetables if necessary. The person who can and will do this is well ahead in retaining good health. He can meet any unusual or adverse traveling circumstances.

Locate health food stores and markets, health ice cream parlors and restaurants. Refer to travel guides to locate the establishments you wish. Ask other friends who travel and relatives or friends in the areas you will be touring. Know how to order in a conventional restaurant. Leave sandwiches alone, especially if on reducing programs. Eat raw salads, baked potatoes. A restaurant meal can be a welcome change from the packed basket foods. Take your own tea bags (herbal) and ask for boiling water or mix cream with the water for Cambric Tea.

For the steady brown baggers, include breadless meals, soups, salads, liquid drinks and fresh raw vegetables and fruits.

Serious Camping And Hiking Foods

Camping out is one of the most glorious adventures a person can possibly experience. The open air is invigorating to compensate for the less than perfect foods taken along. Hiking, swimming, fishing, boating and other physical exercises are beneficial and help burn off food and calories, especially lacking in freshness or fiber.

However, don't depend on the air and water and mental attitude to compensate for lack of the proper foods. Do take them along.

For an outing fill a basket with fresh and healthy foods to carry along. An abundance of canned foods can lead to bowel disturbances, diminished blood count, kidney upsets and weakened heart to name a few. There is no reason to neglect a balanced meal program during outing expeditions.

At times we may be placed in unusual or inconvenient circumstances such as mountain hiking or glacier treks and cannot obtain fresh foods. If foods taken along can be concentrated and dried for stamina and endurance such as nuts and dried fruit, the outcome may be better. My wife and I trekked with a group of glacier travelers into the Hunza Valley a few years ago. It was no easy trip by any means. While some members of the company packed saltine crackers, we took rye crackers. We weren't along for just a good time where food was concerned. We took care of our bodies.

When we arrived in the valley, the Hunzas themselves were truly "camping out" so to speak. These dwellers of the valley could only get out two to three months of the year. They depended entirely upon themselves approximately ten months of the year. They live on dried fruits, vegetables, but they are all natural. They make drinks from dried fruits. They use whole grains in cereals and make bread called, "chapati." They take care of themselves well into the cold season. Many of these people live to 110 and sometimes 120. Problems of the teeth were unheard of; dying with every tooth intact was common. They did not need doctors or dentists. This proves what good food can do for people. Now a new road has been built into the Hunza Valley, and the effects of civilization are beginning to show up in deteriorating health. It is often true that mankind does not appreciate a good thing until it is gone. However, we should know better by now.

The privilege of climbing mountains, hiking and engaging in physical sports should be enjoyed and experienced by all. The physical body is a servant to the mind, to follow and obey, but only when it is nourished and treated properly.

Travel, Picnic, Vacation Food Basket

Russian Rye Bread	Almonds
Blueberry Sauce	Cashews
Prune Juice	Pecans
Raspberry Sauce	Sunflower Seeds
Dried Figs	Walnuts
Huckleberries	Raw Prunes
Raw Honey	Dried Apples
Nut Cake	Dried Apricots
Strawberries	Dried Pineapple

Raisins	Celery	Cottage Cheese	Sesame Crackers
Currants	Peaches	Flaxseed Meal	Raw Hard Cheeses
Blueberries	Pineapple		
Spice Cake	Carrots		
Angel Food Cake	Onions		
Raw Cheeses	Radishes		
Plums	Cucumbers		
Dates	Tomatoes		
Canned Olives	Distilled Water		
Sundried Olives	Rye Crackers		

To eat in restaurants, on trains, aircraft, ships never favors health for long. It is better to fill and refill a food basket and/or ice chest with good food. Use vacuum thermoses.

Mountain scenery gives impetus to blood, heart and impulse; journeying by sea often affects the sense of equilibrium and produces seasickness, requiring essence of peppermint or pumpkin seed extract.

What wants a cancer diet? Avoid all food additives and refined foods. They may be carcinogenic. Is it worth the chance and waiting through years of research for inconclusive conclusions?

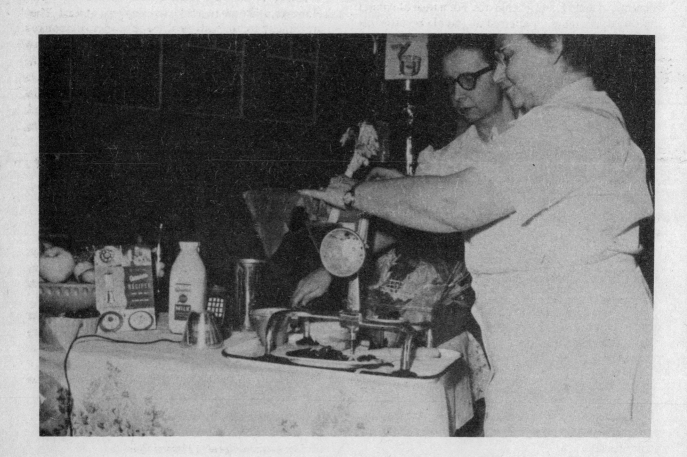

There are many ways of preparing foods. Equip your kitchen with the tools for shredding and preparing your salads properly. Have stainless steel equipment in your kitchen. Learn the best methods in cooking to preserve vitamins and minerals, but above all, remember half of your food each day must be raw.

Chapter 37

Keeping foods natural, pure and whole

Preparing Cereal Grains

It is better to prepare whole grain cereals in a double broiler or use vacuum cooking. Drying, flaking and puffing cereal grain is not beneficial nutritionally. Cereals are vital to bone and teeth growth of children. They should be cooked very slowly to preserve life force.

To prepare cereal by the thermos method, cooking the night before, bring water to boil and then place in tightly capped and preheated thermos with the cereal. The cereal will be ready the following morning. Heat to warm and serve.

Never heat cereal above 212 degrees F. (boiling or steam temperature) to prevent destruction of chemical elements, vitamin E and lecithin oils. For a treat of natural dry cereal, use muesli, preferred to granola because it is not cooked or toasted. Try to use a variety of grains — other than just wheat. Waffles are allowable occasionally or corn cakes; the aim of our program is not the extreme. It is not what we do once in a while that tears down the body, but what what we do on a regular basis.

Granola Becomes Civilized

Granola started out a good compromise food. Do you know what the latest "improvement" is? They are puffing it! Man has managed to make granola into a civilized food too!

Ideal Cheeses And How To Use Them

1. Cheese adds tang and diversity to any menu. Raw, aged & unprocessed cheeses are best for health.
2. If mold appears on cheese, don't discard. Cut off the moldy portion.
3. Grate or grind extra cheese and refrigerate in a tightly capped glass container. Time and effort can be saved.
4. Cheese souffles should be placed in a water filled pan to avoid excessive heat. Bake long enough to assume a firm texture.
5. To melt cheese, place it in the top of a double boiler. Heat must remain below boiling point.
6. Excessive heat makes cheese tough and difficult to digest. Add it as a topping at the end of baking and melt only slightly.

7. Use hard cheese for grating. It makes an excellent garnish for salads or oven-browned vegetable dishes; in omelettes, sauces or soups for zesty flavor.
8. Hard cheeses that break are best. Try Cheddar, Swiss, Jack, etc. Use cottage cheese in menu planning, too. Add liquid whey to cheese meals as a natural laxative. Cheese is binding to the bowels.

Right To A Fair Trial

Eggs are condemned for their high cholesterol, which is known to coat the arterial walls in arteriosclerosis. However, there are two sides to every egg, at least. They are difficult for the body to digest only when overcooked especially in the case of frying. Takes as nearly raw as palatable, they are assimilated well. Eggs are also the highest lecithin food available, and lecithin balances cholesterol in the body, preventing it from coating arterial walls. Therefore, Nature has balanced eggs for our good, and only through man-handling, through overcooking and frying, are they troublesome.

Proper Use Of Eggs

Because eggs are a rich, fatty food, we should always make sure that we eat them with high iron foods to carry them easily through the liver. Recall Grandma's "poached eggs on spinach," a very nutrition wise combination.

Eggs require gentle cooking for easy digestion. Never fry. Use a double boiler or stand baked dishes in a pan of water. **Remember:** overheating destroys lecithin, necessary for preventing high cholesterol.

Eggs should be fertile, from chickens allowed to run free and fend for themselves.

Deadly Kitchen Enemy: Heated Oils

Heavy use of oils and fats in the diet is not advisable. They are unnatural and highly concentrated; this places extreme hardship on the liver. Overindulgence in fats and oils can result in high blood cholesterol and triglycerides.

The body needs these in moderate amounts but when intake is too high, cardiovascular problems can result.

Vegetable oils — sesame, safflower, avocado, soy and corn — are preferable due to the polyunsaturated fatty acids present. Don't use heated or hydrogenated oils; never fry or cook foods in oil. If oil is desired for extra flavoring, add after cooking, only in small amounts. Heated oils are the deadliest kitchen enemy. They are responsible for much of today's poor health.

High heat hardens and changes the chemical structure of oils and fats so that the body can't handle them. We don't have the digestive juices to take care of hard fats and oils; acids aren't strong enough to break down these substances. Fried foods have an accumulative effect in the body; they act as a drug, due to the fact that the chemical structure is altered during heating. High cholesterol is the result over a period of time, and one of America's most serious problems. Thus, we advocate the use of cold pressed, unheated oils and those sparingly. Heated oils have no place in the healthy kitchen.

Brewing Herb Teas The Easy Way

Add 1 to 1-½ teaspoon dried herbs such as clover, comfrey, alfamint, papaya, to each cup rapidly boiling water. Remove from heat and allow to steep 3 to 5 minutes or longer according to individual preference. Strain and serve with honey and/or lemon if desired.

Oat Straw Tea

Oatstraw tea must be boiled to extract the silicon essence from the stalk. Cover ordinary clean oat hay, oatstraw or chaff with cold water; bring to boil. Boil gently or simmer for about 20 minutes. Strain carefully and serve warm.

Heating Is Taboo

Heating changes the natural chemistry of honey and destroys some of its food elements. Thus, it is not approved or wise to use honey in cooked dishes. If the rule is broken only occasionally, it is not serious.

Generally, when substituting honey for sugar in a recipe, reduce the amount of liquid called for. As the consistency of honey varies, no exact rule applies. Remember that honey is approximately two-and-one-half times sweeter than sugar. Allow one-third cup honey for each cup sugar. Reduce liquid one-quarter to one-half cup. A dash of salt or a little extra salt enhances the flavor of honey. Lower the baking temperature 25 degrees to prevent overbrowning.

Honey Canning

When canning with honey, avoid the use of honey syrup. Can fruits unsweetened and add honey at the time of serving.

Honey Storage

No refrigeration is required. Place it in a readily accessible dry area. Freezing does not impair the flavor or color but may speed granulation.

Raw Vs. Heated Milk Products

Clabbered milk is the ideal cultured milk. Also include yogurt, kefir, cottage cheese and all cheeses that break. Aged cheeses are the easiest to digest.

Clabbered Milk

Clabbered milk is superior to yogurt because yogurt has been cooked or heated. The application of heat possibly reorganizes the chemical structure of the food. Throughout history raw milk has surpassed pasteurized milk in promoting better health. Use yogurt as a supplement—don't depend on it as a major source of calcium or other nutrients. Depend instead on the good healthy way of life—close to nature. Include clabbered milk as part of your basis for diet guidelines. Yogurt is not complete (whole), or natural and pure because it is heated. Classify all foods on the basis of natural, pure and whole. This is the basis of the philosopy set forth in this text.

Cottage Cheese And Yogurt

Cottage cheese comes under the same classification as yogurt, as it has been heated. Cheeses can be made without heating. Aged raw cheeses are the best. The bacteria produced by aging fermentation can be conducive to good health. They encourage the development of "friendly bacteria" in the intestinal tract. Have raw, whole milk and raw cheeses for best health.

Reviving Dried Fruit

Reviving is the term used to describe reconstituting dried fruit to its nearest original fresh form. It is more than merely soaking. The cleanest appearing dried fruit is likely to contain insects and their eggs. In addition, dried fruit is difficult for the digestive system to handle effectively, due to the lengthy time necessary to complete digestion —

about ten hours. Thus, we do not get the full benefit unless they are first revived and presoaked. Reconstitute raisins, dates, prunes, figs, etc.

There is an art to reviving fruit properly. Cover the fruit with cold water; bring to a boil slowly. Remove from heat and allow to stand overnight or from 8 to 12 hours, tightly covered. The parasites are destroyed and the fruit regains a juicy plumpness. The recipe section refers to "revived" fruits often.

For flavor add the juice of a lemon, a little rind, a whole clove or two, a stick of cinnamon or a dash of nutmeg to provide a tangy taste variation.

Seeds You Shouldn't Throw Away

What do you do with watermelon seeds? You spit them out. You could make a nutritious watermelon seed drink. Liquefy the seeds with a small amount of water in the blender. Strain off the hulls, sweeten with honey if desired for a good kidney cleansing drink.

We also throw away the white part of the watermelon rind. This is higher in sodium. You know sodium keeps joints young and limber. The very outside green peeling is high in chlorophyll. The watermelon was created as a whole food. The secret of surviving today and in the future is in whole foods.

For a whole watermelon drink add the white part to the blender with seeds. Use a little maple sugar, honey or date sugar. Also use some of the green peeling for chlorophyll. Whirl until blended and strain. You have a whole drink; this can build a whole body. It is lovely for the kidneys and glands. Canteloupe seeds make an excellent drink. Also, soak chia seeds and whirl them in the blender with a little water for a great drink. Do the same with flaxseeds or alfalfa seeds. Seeds contain the vitamin E that everyone is chasing after today. Alfalfa seeds are the best for arthritis. Make a tea or a drink from them.

Proper Care Of Vegetables And Fruits

Wash vegetables as soon as they are brought home from the market. Soaking for a short time in water to which a small amount of bleach has been added can help remove chemical spray and pesticide residues. However, much of the chemical sprays have penetrated the cores and seeds of fruits, such as apples or pears. Refrigerate vegetables and fruits not to be immediately used to keep them fresher.

Rub fruits with a small amount of lemon juice or dip them in water and lemon juice to prevent the cut edges from turning brown. Make sure all salad ingredients are washed and then dried well before using in salads.

Nutritional Salad Dressings.

Salad dressings should add to the nutrition of the salad. What kind do you use? You shouldn't use the prepared and bottled dressings. They are likely to contain numerous food additives and chemicals. Oils used in salad dressings should be kept to a minimum because this concentrated oil, cold pressed or not, is difficult for the liver to handle. When using salad oils pay attention to the linoleic acid content because it is believed to be the most important of the unsaturated fatty acids in preventing cholesterol buildup and hardening of the arteries. Safflower oil contains more of this acid than any other oil. Wheat germ oil is the highest in Vitamin E. Try many of the dressings made with buttermilk, sour cream, yogurt, avocado, lemon juice, egg yolk (raw), tomato sauce and numerous others. Use oil dressings sparingly.

Creative Salad Ingredients

Serve salads every day! Encourage your family to order salads when dining out. Rabbit food, some doubters call it. But so far as we know, rabbits, especially wild rabbits, are extremely healthy. They don't suffer from hardening of the arteries, constipation, diabetes, heart trouble, nerve tension, headaches, varicose veins and a host of other human afflictions.

Salads can serve as complete meals. Add such ingredients as cheeses of many kinds, hard cheeses that break, cottage cheese, and so on; add poultry, fish, eggs, ripe olives, avocados, nuts, seeds and other proteins. Include whatever vegetables you have on hand: radishes, scallions, raw turnip or cauliflower, or broccoli, celery, avocado, peppers, pimento, raw peas, garlic, green onions, herbs, tomatoes, carrots, raw shredded beets, squash, zucchini, parsnips; the ingredients are endless. Make sure the salad is fresh; vegetables lose vital nutrients rapidly from cut surfaces. Enzymes combine with oxygen to hasten the loss of vitamins. Make salads colorful for eye appeal.

Most people don't eat enough raw foods, especially salads. Raw food is essential for good health. Enzymes contained in raw food are destroyed with the hint of heat. Vitamins and minerals are lost in the cooking process, also. The fiber content of raw food is necessary for good elimination and for bowel bulk.

We have mentioned mostly tossed salads. Any raw vegetables can accompany meals alone. Use radishes, carrots, scallions, raw broccoli, peppers, cucumbers and so on. If you pack lunches, always include raw vegetables. Wrap whole vegetables for packed lunches carefully.

275

Chapter 38

Basic and special nutrition programs

"Not what we eat, but what we digest counts."

Diets Belong To Doctors

Diets belong to hospitals and to doctors. Some people who are always on a diet — watermelon, tea, grapefruit — or on some remedy, from a health standpoint or not, will eventually get into trouble. Many are developing chemical shortages in the body that will eventually have to be treated by a doctor. About 30 million Americans lose and regain weight more or less regularly. Most are overweight by 10 or 15 pounds. We find that the body chemistry is drastically upset by this "routine," and experts say such "see-saw" eating practices encourage hardening of the arteries, heart disease and increased blood cholesterol.

We need to realize that food patterns along with exercise habits have changed very much in the past few generations. In grandmother's day, half the protein intake came from meat and half from vegetables, while the amount of walking and physical activity was much higher, keeping digestion, elimination and weight distribution at a healthier balance. Today, animal proteins make up 70% of the average family's protein intake. Fresh vegetables are more neglected, as are whole grains and other complex starches. An extra 100 calories a day adds up to 8 to 10 lb. in a year's time. The way out of these ups-and-downs in weight is to follow a few common sense procedures; avoid fried foods and do not cook in hot oils; broil, braise or roast meats; avoid gravies made from fats; trim excess fat from meats before cooking; prick the skin of poultry to let out fat; roast at lower temperatures to let out more fats; use skim milk and whey in cooking instead of whole milk; use water-packed tuna instead of oil-packed; don't cook more than those who'll be eating should consume; remember, the average person eats over 1,000 meals a year — a little more or a little less at each meal can make a great deal of difference.

Every housewife should learn about fruits, vegetables, berries and flavorings for meals. In order to get well and keep well, we need to learn how to leave our sickness behind. From a physical standpoint, I believe bad eating habits are one of the primary roots of poor health. We must take good care of this physical body if we expect it to take good care of us.

Each person should know how to buy proper foods, how to freeze them, how to store them, how to dry or preserve them properly. The simple methods are always the best. We should find out how to prepare foods for optimum health benefits. Let food be your health insurance.

My patients are sick of being sick. They are tired of living in fear and misery. They want to know what to do, but few seem to know how to make things better. It is time to return to the garden of Eden, to Nature, to a better way of life. It is to this end we are striving.

A health revolution is necessary, and it is at hand. Our stomachs are revolting; our arterial systems are rebelling against crippling cholesterol deposits. Our hearts are resisting and resenting the extra work forced on them. Acids are developed through our refined and sweet foods, "empty calorie" foods and pickled foods. The body is often unable to maintain the balance between the acid and alkaline elements; there are more acids built through wrong living than the body can possibly neutralize. The entire body is thrown into a state of revolution through the mental, industrial, environmental situations man has placed himself in.

Rich, Sweet And Greasy Diets

It is sometimes alleged that America is the healthiest and best fed nation in the world, but well informed people know better. Little do the proponents of these assumptions realize that our television advertised snick-snacks and "good" living habits are based on deception and illusion — sugary desserts, biscuits, shortcakes, breakfast cereals, doughnuts, soda pop, coffee and alcohol. These foods can't build sturdy, vital bodies. Soda pop on every other billboard and in neon signs on every street corner make us the sweetest nation in the world but not the healthiest. French fries and hamburgers don't build healthy bodies; neither do hot dogs and potato chips.

In traveling the world over I found the Indian, though generally short on protein, is willing and able to do more work than those trying to survive on degenerated, devitalized, foodless foods in the U.S.A. Our diet is rich and refined, white sugar foods, fried foods, greasy and fatty foods. I am certain the digestive system has to eventually revolt when bombarded with these atrocious concoctions and rich refined dishes. The average person today never knew the meaning or feeling of good health. They don't know what it is like to have a body that feels wonderful.

My Health and Harmony Regimen

The following general daily diet regimen should become an integral part of every life style. When adhering to the suggested program, supplements, vitamins, minerals or calories are automatically balanced beautifully.

The general concept is to have, each day, two different fruits, at least six vegetables, one protein and one starch, with fruit or vegetable juices as between meal snacks. Include at least two green leafy vegetables daily. 50% to 60% of the daily intake should be in raw food, as an important dietetic statute.

Rules Of Eating

1. Do not fry foods or use heated oils.
2. If not entirely comfortable in mind and body from the previous meal, miss the following meal.
3. Do not eat unless you have a keen appetite for the plainest of foods.
4. Do not eat beyond your needs.
5. Thoroughly masticate all food, even liquids.
6. Miss meals if in pain, emotionally upset, not hungry, chilled, overheated, during acute illness and crises.

Food Healing Laws

1. **Natural food** — 60% of the food eaten should be raw.
2. **Your diet should consist of 80% alkaline and 20% acid foods.** Refer to the Acid/Alkaline Chart, page .
3. **Proportion** — 6 vegetables daily, 2 fruits daily, 1 starch daily, 1 protein daily.
4. **Variety** — Vary proteins, starches, vegetables and fruits from meal to meal and day to day.
5. **Overeating** — Eating beyond needs is a waste of energy and an aging pastime.
6. **Combinations**—Separate proteins and starches; have one at lunch and the other at dinner. Have fruits for breakfast and at 3:00 pm. Don't combine fruits and vegetables at the same meal.
7. **Cook without water** — Cook with low heat. Don't allow air to contact hot food while cooking.
8. **Bake, broil or roast** — If meat is included in the diet use only lean meat, no pork. Use unsprayed vegetables if available and prepare as soon after picking as possible.
9. **Use stainless steel, low-heat cookware** — It is the modern health engineered method of safely preparing food.

Acid/Alkaline Chart (pH values)

A pH value of from 1.0-7.0 is acidic, with 1.0 being the most acidic and 7.0 being neutral, neither acidic nor alkaline. A pH value from 7.0-14.0 is alkaline, with 14.0 being the most alkaline. Many fruits and vegetables, acid to begin with, become alkaline in the process of digestion.

Apples	2.9-3.3
Apricots (dried)	3.6-4.0
Asparagus	5.4-5.7
Bananas	4.5-4.7
Beans	5.0-6.0
Beer	4.0-5.0
Beets	4.9-5.6
Blackberries	3.2-3.6
Bread, white	5.0-6.0
Butter	6.1-6.4
Ginger Ale	2.0-4.0
Gooseberries	2.8-3.0
Grapefruit	3.0-3.3
Grapes	3.5-4.5
Human Milk	6.6-7.6
Jams, fruit	3.5-4.0
Cabbage	5.2-5.4
Carrots	4.9-5.2
Cheese	4.8-6.4
Cherries	3.2-4.0
Cider	2.9-3.3
Corn	6.0-6.5
Crackers	6.5-8.5
Dates	6.2-6.4
Eggs, fresh white	7.6-8.0
Flour, wheat	6.0-6.5
Potatoes	5.6-6.0
Raspberries	3.2-3.6
Rhubarb	3.1-3.2
Salmon	6.1-6.3
Sauerkraut	3.4-3.6
Shrimp	6.8-7.0
Jellies, fruit	3.0-3.5
Lemons	2.2-2.4
Limes	1.8-2.0
Maple Syrup	6.5-7.0
Milk, cows	6.3-6.6
Molasses	5.0-5.4
Olives	3.6-3.8
Oranges	3.0-4.0
Oysters	6.1-6.6
Peas	5.8-6.4
Peaches	3.4-3.6
Pears	3.6-4.0
Pickles, dill	3.2-3.6
Pickles, sour	3.0-3.4
Pimento	4.7-5.2

Plums	2.8-3.0
Pumpkin	4.8-5.2
Spinach	5.1-5.7
Soft drinks	2.0-4.0
Squash	5.0-5.3
Strawberries	3.0-3.5
Sweet Potatoes	5.3-5.6
Tomatoes	4.0-4.4
Tuna	5.9-6.1
Turnips	5.2-5.5
Vinegar	2.4-3.4
Water, drinking	6.5-8.0
Wines	2.8-3.8

pH Values Of Biologic Materials

Blood plasma	7.3-7.5
Spinal fluid, human	7.3-7.5
Saliva, human	6.5-7.5
Gastric Contents, human	1.0-3.0
Duodenal Contents, human	4.8-3.0
Feces, human	4.6-8.4
Urine, human	4.8-8.4
Milk, human	6.6-7.6
Bile, human	6.8-7.0

Before Breakfast

Upon arising, and one-half hour prior to breakfast, take any natural, unsweetened fruit juice, such as grape, pineapple, prune, fig, apple or black cherry. Liquid chlorophyll, 1 teaspoon to a glass of water, can be used.

Substitute a broth or lecithin drink if desired. Take 1 tablespoon vegetable broth powder and 1 tablespoon lecithin granules in a glass of warm water.

On doctor's advice citrus fruits such as orange, grapefruit, lemon or tomato are allowed.

Between fruit juice and breakfast, follow this program: Skin brushing, exercise, hiking, deep breathing, playing. Shower. Start with warm spray; cool water until breath quickens. Never shower immediately upon arising.

Breakfast

Stewed fruits, one starch and health drink or two fruits, one protein and health drink. (See list of acceptable proteins and starches, also health drinks.) Soaked fruits such as unsulphured apricots, prunes, figs; fruits of any kind — melon, grapes, peaches, pears, berries or baked apple; use fruit in season, if possible. Sprinkle baked or stewed fruit with ground nuts or nut butter.

Suggested Breakfast Menus

Monday — Reconstituted dried apricots, steel-cut oatmeal — supplements, oat straw tea. Add eggs or cottage cheese for protein; supplements, herb tea.

Tuesday — Fresh figs, cornmeal cereal, supplements, shave grass tea. Add eggs or nut butter if desired, or raw applesauce and blackberries, coddled egg, supplements, herb tea.

Wednesday — Reconstituted dried peaches, millet cereal, supplements, alfalfa tea. Substitute with eggs, cheese or nut butter or sliced nectarines and apple yogurt, supplements, herb tea.

Friday — Slices of fresh pineapple with shredded coconut, buckwheat cereal, supplements, peppermint tea or have baked apple, persimmons, chopped raw almonds, acidophilus milk, supplements, herb tea.

Saturday — Muesli with bananas and dates, cream, supplements, shave grass tea or cantaloupe and

Sunday — Cooked applesauce with raisins, rye grits, supplement, shave grass tea or cantaloupe and strawberries, cottage cheese, supplements, herb tea.

Preparation Hints

Whole grain cereal should be cooked over very low heat, tightly covered; use a double boiler or soak overnight in boiling water in widemouth thermos.

Supplements are to be added to cereal or fruit. Use sunflower seed meal, rice polishings, wheat germ, flaxseed meal (about 1 teaspoon of each). Dulse may be used also and sesame seed meal.

10:00 a.m. is juice time, vegetable or fruit, or substitute vegetable broth.

Lunch

Raw salad, or as directed, one or two starches, as listed and a health drink. If following a strict regimen, use only one of the starches each day. Vary the starches from day to day.

Raw salad vegetables: Tomatoes, lettuce (green, leafy only such as romaine), celery, cucumber, bean and seed sprouts, green peppers, avocado, parsley, watercress, endive. Onions and cabbage are sulphur foods.

Four Best Starches & Others

1. Yellow cornmeal; 2. Rye; 3. Brown rice; 4. Millet; Others: barley (winter starch); buckwheat, baked or dead

ripe banana, winter squashes, baked potato, baked sweet potato.

For variety include steel cut oatmeal, whole wheat cereal, shredded wheat, rye crackers, bran muffins, bread (whole grain, rye, soy, corn bread, bran breads preferred).

Best Health Drinks

Vegetable broth, soup, coffee substitute, buttermilk, raw milk, goat milk, oat straw tea, alfalfa mint tea, huckleberry tea, mint tea or whey.

Suggested Lunch Menus

Monday — Vegetable salad, baby lima beans, baked potato, spearmint tea.

Tuesday — Vegetable salad with health mayonnaise, steamed asparagus, very ripe bananas; or steamed unpolished brown rice, vegetable broth or herb tea.

Wednesday — Raw salad plate, sour cream dressing, cooked green beans, corn bread and/or baked hubbard squash, sassafras tea.

Thursday — Salad, French dressing, baked zucchini, okra, corn-on-the-cob, rye krisp, buttermilk or herb tea.

Friday — Salad, baked green pepper stuffed with eggplant and tomatoes, baked potato and/or bran muffin, carrot soup or herb tea.

Saturday — Salad, turnips and turnip greens, baked yams, catnip tea.

Sunday — Salad, lemon and olive oil dressing, steamed whole barley, cream of celery soup, steamed chard, herb tea.

Salad Vegetables

Use plenty of greens; choose four to five from the following: Leaf lettuce, watercress, spinach, beet leaves, parsley, alfalfa sprouts, cabbage, young chard, herbs and any green leaves; cucumbers, bean sprouts, onions, green peppers, pimentos, carrots, turnips, zucchini, celery, asparagus, okra, radishes, etc.

3:00 P.M.

Have a health cocktail, juice or fruit.

Dinner

Raw salad, two cooked vegetables, one protein and a broth or health drink if desired.

Cooked Vegetables

Peas, artichokes, carrots, beets, turnips, spinach, beet tops, string beans, Swiss chard, eggplant, zucchini, summer squash, broccoli, cauliflower, cabbage, sprouts, onions or any vegetable other than potatoes.

Proteins Suggested

Once a week: Fish — use white fish, such as sole, halibut, trout, or sea trout.

Vegetarians: Use soy beans, lima beans, cottage cheese, sunflower seeds and other seeds; also, seed butters, nut butters, nut milk drinks, eggs.

Two to three times per week: Meat — use only lean meat; never use pork, fats or cured meats.

Vegetarians: Use meat substitutes or vegetarian proteins.

Twice a week: cottage cheese or any cheese that breaks.

Once a week: Egg omelette.

If you have a protein at this meal, health dessert is allowed, but not recommended. Never eat protein and starch together. (Note how they are separated.)

The noon meal may be exchanged for the evening meal, provided the same regimen is upheld. Exercise is necessary to handle raw food; generally more exercise is applied after the noon meal. Sandwiches should be combined with vegetables at the same meal.

Dinner Menus

Monday — Salad, diced celery and carrots, steamed spinach (waterless cooked), puffy omelette, vegetable broth.

Tuesday—Salad, cooked beet tops, broiled steak or ground beef patties, tomato sauce, cauliflower, comfrey tea.

Wednesday — Cottage cheese, cheese sticks, apples, peaches, grapes, nuts, apple concentrate cocktail.

Thursday — Salad, steamed chard, baked eggplant, grilled liver and onions, persimmon whip (optional), alfamint tea.

Friday — Salad, yogurt and lemon dressing, steamed mixed greens, beets, steamed fish — with slices of lemon, leek soup.

Saturday — Salad, cooked string beans — baked summer squash, carrot and cheese loaf, cream of lentil soup or lemongrass tea, fresh peach jello, almond-nut cream.

Sunday — Salad, diced carrots and peas, steamed tomato aspic, roast leg of lamb, mint tea.

Vegetarians—Use vegetarian dishes to replace meat dishes.

See *Vital Foods for Total Health* for other recipes and ideas.

A Closer Look At Meal Planning And Timing

Some people seem to think three meals a day are a necessity. Many individuals could get along nicely on just two. At the end of the day be able to look back on a balanced day with six vegetables, two fruits, a good starch and a good protein.

If you have just one meal a day, have a good proportion of all these food groups. The idea of the large "healthy" breakfast is possibly a myth, also. Many peoples of the world believe that you should "earn" your breakfast. Still other groups don't "break" the night's fast until noon the next day, especially in some of the tropical islands.

The food we ate yesterday gives energy for today. The food we ate in the morning often stimulates us at the time we should be turning in for the night. About 18 hours is necessary for the food to be digested and to reach the tissues of the body for building, repairing and energy; it has to be carried through the blood stream. A large amount of vital energy is used to digest food. We should eat according to the type of job we have to do. For example, physical workers need extra starch and the mental worker needs protein for the brain and nervous system. Growing children need starches and the over 40 age group needs more protein.

The noon meal reaches its destination the following morning. Breakfast gives energy in the evening. For some, protein is stimulating and this meal is better taken at noon, and the starch meal helps them get to sleep easier. However, several hours should separate meals and the evening meal should be taken early, many hours before retiring.

A Good Mealtime Philosophy: *"Eat like a prince for breakfast, a King at noon and a Pauper at night."*

Breakfast

The strength we feel in the morning is from lunch the day before. When the nervous system, the "response" part of the body, is fed and repaired we have strength. Breakfast begins to react at the time we should be retiring for the night. For this reason, we don't advise a heavy breakfast.

Breakfast comes from the root "break-fast" that means to break the night's fast. In the morning digestive juices flow slower; the whole body is functioning slower. So I suggest you break the fast with a fruit juice or light drink. Fruit makes an ideal meal to break the fast. A little protein is acceptable with it. Also dried fruits and carbohydrates together are all right. The practice of having fried foods, biscuits, muffins, bread, French toast and other heavy foods is not good.

Lunch

Eat a healthy and hardy lunch for energy the next morning. We follow the starch idea at lunch since most people have the sandwich habit for lunch. If you must have sandwiches, make them of thinly-sliced whole grain breads; stuff them with a good filling and lots of vegetables, even sprouts. A few ingredient suggestions are avocado, grated carrots, celery, cottage cheese, lettuce, alfalfa sprouts, lentil sprouts, leaf lettuce, olives, nut and seed meal and butters, health mayonnaise, health cream cheese, yogurt, mashed or sliced banana and honey. (See the midday meal section for more ideas.) Season with broth powder and dulse. Add raw vegetables and salads. The possibilities are endless.

Very ripe bananas make a good starch; try baked potatoes, steamed brown rice, banana or hubbard squash, corn on the cob. Wild rice, millet or cornmeal make good changes. They don't have to be for breakfast. Never forget variety. If you pack a lunch use a thermos for hot and cold foods and soups or health drinks.

Noon is the time for a large green salad, using as many vegetables as you can. Many foods you usually have cooked make great raw salad ingredients. Use summer squash, asparagus, Jerusalem artichokes, okra, cauliflower, turnips, zucchini, beets to mention a few.

Have a cooked low-starch vegetable with the meal if you want. Remember to serve a "top" growing vegetable when a root vegetable is served. The negative and positive balance one another. (Negative is the root vegetable.) On colder days a soup is welcome. Cool raw soups are good in the summer.

Add a health beverage to the meal such as herb tea, buttermilk, whey, raw milk or clabbered milk.

Dinner

Dinner should be a happy family affair at the end of the day. Now is the time to make sure you balanced the day nutritionally. Did you have two fruits? Did you skimp on or skip the large noon salad? Make up for it now if you did. Did you have four to six vegetables, including the salad? Did you have a noon starch? Dinner can be your protein meal and should be. More exercise is needed for a starch meal; that's why I suggest having it at noon.

Plan your dinner around this basic formula: a small raw salad, two cooked vegetables, one protein and a health beverage. For those not vegetarian, have meat, including fish, two or three times a week. Never fry meat and avoid pork and fat meats. Fish once a week is a good protein choice. (It is high in phosphorus and iodine.) Choose fish with fins and scales; steam, grill, broil or bake it. Have a cheese dish two nights a week. Cheese and fruit make a good evening meal especially in the summertime; have it a couple of times a week if you want. Cheese that breaks or cottage cheese makes a wonderful combination with fresh fruit. (It is better not to mix acid and sweet fruits.) An egg dish such as an omelette or souffle can round out the week's menuis; have poached, soft boioled or scrambled eggs.

Nuts are a high-protein food. They are difficult to digest and should be soaked several hours in honey, fruit juice or tea before eating for this reason. Nut butters are an ideal food. Make sure the nuts or nut butters are raw, not roasted and not old or rancid. Rancidity and roasting destroys valuable vitamin E and lecithin oils. The almond is the king of nuts and alkaline in reaction. Hard-shelled nuts are best to preserve oils, vitamin E and lecithin. The sesame seed is the best of the seeds; sunflower seeds are a high-grade protein also. Nut butters and seed butters make excellent health drinks and additions to dishes.

The legumes are good protein sources. Beans can be baked, used in roasts, casseroles and patties. Tofu (soy bean cheese), is a good and versatile vegetarian protein. Lentils, garbanzos, split peas, lima, navy, pinto beans make good dishes and casseroles. Soy meat substitutes are all right occasionally.

Serve a small raw salad with the protein meal. Vary the ingredients. A sulphur vegetable is a good addition to the protein meal to help drive the nerve fats to the brain (cabbage or onion family vegetables are sulphur foods.)

A beverage can be broth, soup, herb teas, whey, buttermilk or raw milk.

If a health dessert is permitted once in awhile have a protein-type dessert or fresh fruit. Dessert is not recommended. Limit it to twice a week. Fruit desserts such as gelatin molds, fruit whips, sherbets, yogurt and fruit concentrates or fresh fruit are much better than the average dessert — pies, cakes, ice cream. The starchy dessert should be for an occasional indulgence at the noon meal — after a large salad.

Menu Exchanges

If the noon and evening meals are exchanged, follow the same regime. Starches make you sleepy; proteins are stimulating. If insomnia is a problem the meals may be switched for better results. Starch meals are for physical labor; proteins for mental work.

Never eat when emotionally upset, chilled, over tired, over heated, ill or lacking the keenest desire for the simplest of food. Missing a meal will do you more good.

The "Big Four" Supplements

Most people who have subsisted a number of years on poor diets find they are short of biochemical elements. They have lived on devitaminized, demineralized foodstuffs. For this reason we recommend four main supplements for rebuilding and revitalizing. They are not necessary to the person who has been living correctly, not burning up chemical elements faster than they can be replaced, under normal circumstances and under the proper diet. These are needed to make up what we especially lack in the "average" American dietary habits.

Four supplements should be encouraged in the diet daily. Serve them at the dining table, especially adapted to the morning meal. They help counteract the shortages found in the common diet today. Also add them to liquefied drinks, salads or even desserts.

Dulce: The highest source of iodine needed for proper thyroid gland function. (My patients always lack iodine.) Use ½ tsp. daily.

Sunflower Seeds & Sesame Seeds: The vegetarian's best protein sources and valuable gland and nerve foods. Grind into a meal.

Rice Polishings: Very high in silicon—for skin and hair health, general vitality; the nerves and brain receive B-complex vitamins.

Wheat Germ: Vitamin B and Vitamin E rich — heart and muscle vitamin. Use it raw and refrigerate for freshness.

Additional Supplements:

Add sesame seed meal to the sunflower meal.

Include flaxseed meal for bowel bulk and good elimination.

Use 1 teaspoon (heaping) of each supplement daily; add to cereal.

Flaxseed meal is a wonderful addition to the cereal bowl, specifically for children too, to keep their bowels regulated. Flaxseed is also high in vitamins E and F, a bowel lubricant, regulator and bulk source.

Supplements don't have to be given in pill form. A person has to be in good health to assimilate "pill" form supplements. The supplements just discussed can be assimilated by anyone, even though they are concentrated. Use them in cereals, tonics, drinks, dressings and almost any recipe. However, heat and baking destroys vitamin E and lecithin.

General Reducing Diet Guide

It is best always to consult your doctor before going on any reducing diet.

Meats approved are lamb, fish, lean beef, turkey, chicken. Never use fats or pork. Bake, broil or roast fish and meat. The fish should be a white fish which has fins and scales. Tomatoes (sliced, ripe — canned in emergency) or grapefruit must accompany meat or fish meals.

If you are vegetarian, then use other proteins: eggs, cottage cheese, gelatin mold, skim milk, soy tofu, low fat yogurt. All vegetarians should utilize the 5% carbohydrate list (see below).

Drink in-between meals, only; one hour before or two hours following meals. Use KB 11 or Cleaver Tea (two cups daily).

Five Percent Carbohydrate Vegetables

Artichokes
Asparagus
Beet Greens
Broccoli
Brussels Sprouts
Cabbage
Cauliflower
Celery
Chard
Chickory
Cucumber
Dandelion
Eggplant
Endive
Escarole
Leeks
Lettuce
Mushrooms
Mustard Greens
Okra
Radishes
Sauerkraut (not canned)
Sea Kale
Sorrel
Sprouts (alfalfa, mung, etc.)
Spinach
String Beans
Swiss Chard
Tomatoes
Turnip Tops
Vegetable Marrow
Watercress

Regular Reducing Diet

Suggested eating plan for a week:
Breakfast: Fresh fruit (1); 1 or 2 eggs or cottage cheese
Lunch: Brown rice; 1 vegetable and salad
Dinner: Meat or fish with tomato or grapefruit; 1 vegetable
Additional suggestions for Regular Reducing Diet:

Skim milk, 1 tablespoon of sesame seed meal, one-third avocado and 1 fruit; liquefy.
Skim milk, watercress or romaine lettuce (liquefy) and salad with fish and tomato.
Fruit and cheese.
Apples and cottage cheese.
Rice cakes or rye crackers, are allowed occasionally.

Strict Reducing Diet

Use this menu only:
Breakfast: Fresh fruit (1); 1 or 2 eggs.
Lunch: Vegetable; salad.
Dinner: Meat or fish with tomato or grapefruit.

Vegetarian Reducing Diets

Always consult your doctor before going on any reducing diet.

Vegetarian Reducing Diet

Suggested eating plan for a week:
Breakfast: Fresh fruit (1); 1 or 2 eggs or cottage cheese.
Lunch: Brown rice; (1) vegetable and salad.
Dinner: Protein (see list) with tomato or grapefruit; (1) vegetable if desired.
Additional meal suggestions:
Soy milk or skim milk, 1 tablespoon or sesame seed meal, ⅓ avocado and 1 fruit. Liquefy.
Fruit and cheese.
Apple and low-fat yogurt.
Skim milk, watercress or romaine lettuce (liquefy); salad with fish and tomato (or use 4-6 watercress tablets per meal).
Rice cakes or rye krisp are allowed occasionally.

Vegetarian Strict Reducing Diet

Use this menu only:
Breakfast: Fresh fruit (1); 1 or 2 eggs.
Lunch: Vegetable Salad.
Dinner: Protein with tomato or grapefruit.

Additional Diet Directions

Both Diets: Drink in-between meals only; one hour before meals or two hours after. Use KB 11 or Cleaver Tea (2 cups daily).

Both Diets: Use tomato (sliced, ripe — or canned in emergency) or grapefruit with protein at dinner.

Proteins: Fish, eggs, cottage cheese, gelatin mold, soy tofu, low-fat yogurt (fish used should possess fins and scales).

Both diets: All vegetables should be taken from the 5% Carbohydrate List outlined on page 282.

The Bland Food "Building" Diet

Have 3 to 5 vegetables daily. Prepare by cooking/and liquefying, pureed, raw or cooked only. Cook vegetables in soft water. Boiling extracts valuable mineral salts.

Vegetables — String beans, beets, beet tops, cooked, liquefied or pureed if not tender. Swiss chard, spinach, cooked (don't cook long). Carrots, summer squash, zucchini, yellow-neck squash, chayote; pear, cooked, as is or pureed. Escarole, endive, romaine lettuce, watercress, pureed or liquefied. Sprouts, without seed shells on ends, liquefied. Okra, celery, parsley, liquefied or pureed. Jerusalem artichokes, yams, sweet potatoes. White potatoes, cooked and mealy. Asparagus and asparagus soup, split pea soup, corn soup with no hulls in it, liquefied, Vital Broth (potato, celery, carrot, parsley).

Fruits And Fruits Juices — Juices: Grape, prune, papaya, pineapple, black cherry and fig. Fruits: Nectarines, peaches, apricots, sapota, watermelon, honeydew, casaba, grapes, no peels no seeds; ripe strawberries without seeds. Papayas, mangos, raisins, prunes (may have to be pureed due to peels), fresh seedless figs, dates, bananas, persimmons, all stewed fruits except pears, apple, sun dried or regular olives.

Revive all dried fruits by soaking 20 minutes in water brought to boil.

Fruits are suggested alone and between meals.

Proteins — Scrambled or lightly boiled eggs, fish, meat — lean, no fat or pork, gelatin, cheese, any kind allowed, fresh goat milk, buttermilk, yogurt, tofu, cream soups and nut and seed butters.

Milk should be taken immediately after it is drawn from the cow or goat.

Drinks — All teas are considered bland. Mint tea is the best gas-driving aid. Bran tea is good. Oat straw, huckleberry, mint, papaya, are the four most recommended teas. Soy milk drinks — whey drinks, Acidophilus milk. Sesame seed milk with dates, rice polish or carob flour.

Starches — Breakfast cereals such as rolled oats, rice, millet, rye meal. (Have one starch daily.)

Gruels — Agar agar can be mixed with cereals; barley soup is good (does not cause excessive gas).

Sweets — Maple syrup, honey, date sugar are suggested.

Juices — Vegetable juices with milk or flaxseed tea (half and half), or use liquid chlorophyll (1 tsp. to a glass for water) in place of fresh juices.

Supplements — As necessary. Springgreen tablets, Whex (goat's whey), liquid chlorophyll, slippery elm food, okra powder, acidophilus culture, flaxseed meal, Veico 77, yogurt, apple concentrate.

Patients adhering to this diet should be taking a bulk as found in most health food stores.

Foods very hot or too cold are to be shunned. Pureed and soft foods are easy to digest and produce less gas. Soy toast is a good bland food. Hot foods and drinks weaken the mucous membranes, result in spongy gums and undermine the stomach. Cold foods contract the glands of the stomach, thus harming the flow of hydrochloric acid necessary to digestion. Cold foods prevent digestion, produce irritation and oppression.

Bland foods serve to deter gas and minimize irritation in the stomach and intestinal tract. Roughage present in many bland foods causes irritation to the intestinal tract. Always liquefy or puree in advance.

Gas-Producing (sulphur foods) — cabbage, cauliflower, onions, broccoli, Brussels sprouts, are to be eliminated from the bland diet. Bland foods are taken to alleviate gas symptoms and reduce irritation. when foods cooked or not cooked contain much fiber, strings, peelings or seeds, the result is irritating. Liquefy or puree.

Variety — Daily variety is important. The danger of this diet is in failing to supply the necessary variety as in a healthy diet. Have 6 vegetables daily; 2 fruits daily; 1 starch daily; 1 protein daily; with juices or liquids between meals.

Menu

Breakfast: Juice, fruits; protein or starch.
10:00 a.m.: Liquid or fruit.
Lunch: Two vegetables, one starch, tea or drink.
3:00 p.m.: Fruit juices, tea or fruit.
Dinner: Two vegetables, protein; tea or drink.

Enemas — These diets usually call for enemas. Flaxseed enemas are best.

Practical Weight Loss Tips

Many people can gain weight on the food they eat. Overeating is one of the major causes of obesity. Personally, I know that I live on past food memories. When the meal was over and dessert was passed, I couldn't refuse it. As a child I was taught that I paid for the food and therefore I had to eat it. Often children aren't allowed to leave the table until the food is all eaten. Maybe a reassessment of the food values and habits we have is necessary.

A successful trick is to eat only half the portion placed on the plate, no matter what the serving size. If a child's portion is placed in front of you, eat only half of it. If you are overly fond of such things as butter, take only half the usual amount. Get to the place where food is not god; don't let it rule your life. By practicing the half portion method each time you go to the table, it becomes increasingly easier to eat less. The "tune" gets better as any tune on a piano does with practice. The first few times are rough. The normal reaction is, "Why should I throw away food I paid for?" and especially in the case of dessert favorites. George Bernard Shaw, the well-known vegetarian author, once said the following when his housekeeper tried to coax him to eat more so she wouldn't have to throw it out: "You can't make a garbage can out of my stomach!" I will never forget that comment.

It is much better to throw away the best food if it is over what the body can use, if it over-taxes the digestive system, forcing it to work over-time and beyond its capaci-ty. Ill health is produced by over-use of the digestive system, forcing it to work overtime and beyond its capacity. Ill health is produced by overuse of the digestive system and by forcing the vital energy to be squandered in digesting, storing, assimilating and eliminating excess food. Some 30 miles of veins and arteries exist for every five pounds of flesh. The vital forces must work extra hard and abnormal cravings are set by excess tissues. The only way to win is to autosuggest the best principles to live by and to stick to this philosophy. Use harshness, if necessary, for you are being good to yourself in the long run.

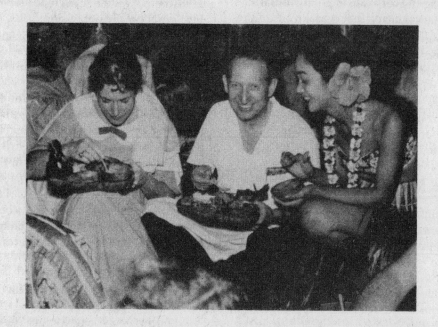

To relax a bit is necessary. Food should be a happy time in life, but make sure that what you eat is nourishing. Fruits and vegetables are noncatarrhal-forming foods.

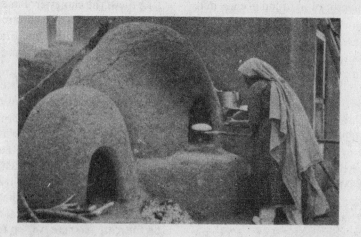

Many times, the primitive ways of handling food was much more proper than the ways foods are man-handled today. This is one of the Taos Indians baking bread from a natural wheat that was stone ground, giving all the elements that are necessary for your health.

Chapter 39

The truth about eggs

Now that the dust is settling on the controversy over the link between eggs and coronary heart disease, scientists are once again recognizing that eggs are one of the finest foods available to man. In fact, eggs contain more of the nutrients needed by man than any other single food, and I believe they are very important in the diet.

The controversy began in the 1940's when many doctors became convinced that the high cholesterol content of eggs was contributing to atherosclerosis, hardening of the arteries. Authorities recommended cutting down to two or three eggs per week, and in 1973 American egg consumption dropped 5% from the previous year.

It all started when Russian researcher Nikolai Anichkov in 1913 showed that rabbits fed a high cholesterol diet quickly developed hardening of the arteries. A flurry of subsequent experiments with rabbits and chickens by other researchers supported Anichkov's results, making cholesterol into one of the greatest food villains of our time. Only a few scientists had the presence of mind to point out that rabbits and chickens were natural vegetarians, not used to handling animal fats in their systems, unlike human beings. It didn't matter. Heart disease had reached epidemic proportions in the United States, and officials were looking for something to blame. They blamed cholesterol — found in eggs, milk products and meat.

A 20th Century Disease

Heart trouble, atherosclerosis in particular, was not a big problem in the United States or other countries until the 20th century. It is still not a problem in many primitive cultures, including some where milk and eggs are eaten. But for the most part, coronary heart disease is highest in areas where a great deal of dairy products and beef are eaten, such as New Zealand, Finland and the U.S.

Atherosclerosis is believed to be caused by one or more chemical substances in the bloodstream that attack arterial walls. To protect the lesions, calcium deposits create rough spots, on which smears of cholesterol and saturated fats begin to appear. The build up of atherosclerosis plaque in the walls of arteries and other blood vessels can become so severe that the blood is seriously impeded in circulating through them. The danger, however, is that a chunk of plaque will break off and block blood flow to the heart, causing death or severe heart damage.

What could cause the original damage to blood vessel walls? Dr. Kurt Oster, M.D., believes that the enzyme xanthine oxidase enters the bloodstream via homogenized milk particles assimilated through the bowel wall. Xanthine oxidase is known to attack the plasmalogen lining heart and artery walls and has been found in arterial plaque deposits. Dr. John Yudkin believes that consumption of too much refined sugar is linked to coronary heart disease. He points out that sugar intake in Great Britain, the U.S. and many other developed nations has increased fivefold in the past hundred years. There are other theories, none of them proven.

The fact is, doctors and scientists do not know what causes heart disease. Dr. Michael De Bakey, a world famous heart surgeon, has written "An analysis of cholesterol values by usual hospital laboratory methods in 1,700 patients with atherosclerotic disease revealed no definite correlation between serum cholesterol levels and the nature and extent of atherosclerotic disease." Dr. Roger Williams, discoverer of pantothenic acid, has said "I believe the cholesterol in eggs will take care of itself if the other foods you eat are good." Dr. Carl C. Pfeiffer, author of *Mental and Elemental Nutrients*, recommends two eggs per day and believes that cholesterol alone is not the problem.

Chemical imbalance is a major problem in every disease. I believe that cholesterol was meant to be balanced in the body by lecithin, but overcooking destroys lecithin, leaving only cholesterol. Excessive use of salt on foods, smoking, drinking, obesity and lack of exercise are all factors contributing to atherosclerosis. So is a toxic, underactive bowel, which reabsorbs cholesterol from bile salts through the bowel wall when wastes are not moving fast enough. Dr. Dennis Burkitt found no evidence of atherosclerosis among rural African natives whose average bowel transit time was twice as fast as that of most Americans. Dr. Burkitt believes that bulk and fiber in the diet are a key factor, and recommends a tablespooon of wheat bran every day to add fiber and speed up waste transit time.

The World's Oldest Man Eats Eggs

Ibrahim El Korimy, claimed to be the oldest living person on earth at the age of 160, eats up to ten eggs per day and is unaware of the cholesterol debate in the United States. Ibrahim, an Egyptian, lives in a hut without electricity or plumbing and walks six miles to a store twice a week to buy his food. He has no idea that some health authorities in the United States and elsewhere would consider his diet extremely dangerous. However, others would approve his diet.

A Purdue University study of 156 men by Dr. A.J. Ismail, a fitness expert, showed that a supplementary egg diet did not increase blood cholesterol levels. One group of men who exercised regularly over the 4 month period of the test had lower blood cholesterol levels at the end, the older men's levels being lowered the most.

"Instead of telling their patients to beware of eggs, doctors should tell them to eat more," said Dr. George Briggs, professor of nutrition at the University of California at Berkeley.

A study at the Weizmann Institute in Israel shows that an "active lipid" in eggs helps keep brain membranes soft and pliable, preventing the deterioration of brain function usually associated with aging. "This rigidity is why older people react more slowly when they try to recall names, places and facts," said Dr. David Samuel, director of the Center for Neurosciences and Behavior Research at Weizmann Institute. "Active lipid appears to fluidize this membrane so oxygen and various brain chemicals and enzymes can penetrate from cell to cell." Dr. Samuel believes the new discovery about eggs will make it possible to add 5 or 6 useful years to the average person's brain.

The overwhelming evidence of recent years is that eggs belong in a well-balanced diet. We should eat plenty of fresh fruits and vegetables, 60% of them raw, and whole grain cereals as well. But of the basic protein foods, eggs are second only to mother's milk in total nutritional value. The nutrients from eggs feed every cell in the body — brain and nerves, bones and ligaments, muscles and membranes, organs and glands.

One unanticipated bonus of the attack on cholesterol in eggs has been increased effort in producing higher quality eggs. Darrell Bragg, head of poultry research at the University of British Columbia, has found that adding the unsaturated fat linoleic acid to chicken feed produced eggs with twice the normal level of unsaturated fats. Such eggs may help reduce cholesterol deposits in arteries. Keep in mind that the cholesterol and lecithin in eggs work together nutritionally, and both are needed by the brain and nerves.

The Nutritional Value of Eggs

I believe it is significant that the United Nations Food and Agricultural Organization has selected the egg as the ideal food to compare other foods with. My greatest teacher, Dr. V.G. Rocine believed eggs were one of the finest foods because they contained vitellin, a high-phosphorus brain food. Vitellin is mostly composed of lecithin. Most importantly, a single egg has all the ingredients necessary to form a complete baby chick.

The average egg of 50 grams contains 6.5 grams of protein, about half a gram of carbohydrate and 5.8 grams of fat. The protein contains all 10 amino acids essential to human nutrition. The egg has 1.7 grams of saturated fatty acids and 3.3 grams of unsaturated fatty acids. Total cholesterol is about 230 grams.

Chemical Elements and Vitamins in a 50 Gram Egg*

Calcium	27.0 mg	Vitamin A	590 IU
Iron	1.2 mg	D	25 IU
Magnesium	5.5	Thiamin	0.06 mg
Phosphorus	102.5 mg	Riboflavin	0.15 mg
Potassium	64.5 mg	Niacin	0.05 mg
Sodium	61.0 mg	B6	0.13 mg
Sulphur	67.0 mg	B12	0.14 mg
(slighty more in white		Biotin	10.0 μgm
than in yolk)		Pantothenic acid	0.8 mg
Zinc	0.7 mg	Choline	253.0 mg
Inositol	16.5 mg		

* Trace amounts of selenium and flouride have also been found in eggs.

All About Egg Factories and Eggs

One of the interesting things about eggs is that healthy hens lay the most eggs, so we find there is a built-in incentive for egg farmers to treat their hens well. The most nutritious eggs are produced from free roaming hens, allowed to scratch and peck on real dirt. The practice of keeping hens caged to lay eggs is not the best procedure, since chickens need the sunshine to develop vitamin D in their bodies and need to scratch and move around to keep their hearts, muscles and nerves toned.

The best feeds for chickens are made of whole grains, vitamins, minerals and cultures, and are produced by health conscious egg ranchers who want to be sure that their hens are getting the best.

Shell color, brown or white, makes no difference in the nutrient content of the egg. Rhode Island Reds and Plymouth Rocks lay brown eggs, but they are bigger chickens and more expensive to feed than White

Leghorns, the chickens responsible for white-shelled eggs. That's why brown eggs cost more.

Some nutritionists claim that fertile eggs are more nutritious, and these can be obtained at the health food store, if desired.

Yolk color varies with feed. Chickens with access to greens, corn and alfalfa lay eggs with darker yolks. A wheat-fed chicken produces light-yolked eggs, although they are just as nutritious as the darker-yolked kind. In wheat producing areas of the U.S. and Canada, most people believe a dark-yolked egg is inferior.

To slow loss of carbon dioxide through the porous shell, eggs are dipped in mineral oil to seal them. Fresh eggs can be kept in the refrigerator up to five weeks without loss of quality, but California law requires that commercial eggs refrigerated for over 30 days be classified as Grade B. Older eggs are flatter and runnier when broken, and are best used for scrambling or baking. Few people buy Grade B eggs, and they are not widely sold in stores.

Hard-boiled eggs are difficult to peel if the eggs are very fresh, because layers of the white stick to the inner shell. Storing eggs in the refrigerator a few days before boiling makes them easier to peel. To make peeling easier, put hard-boiled eggs in cold water right after cooking them. Begin peeling at the big end of the egg and hold the egg under cold running water to remove the shell.

Blood and meat spots in eggs do not prove or indicate fertility, since they occur in about 1% of all eggs. Most of these are removed during grading. While blood spots don't affect the nutritional value of the egg, some consumers feel they are a sign of something wrong, so they are usually not marketed to stores.

Egg carton language. The letter grade on an egg carton (AA, A or B) indicates how fresh the eggs are, the AA eggs being the freshest and the B eggs being refrigerated for at least 30 days. Higher grade egg yolks stand higher and their whites are thicker. As for size, eggs are officially considered by the weight per dozen, so mixed individual sizes may be found in the same carton. Egg producers recognize six classes of size: Jumbo (30 oz.), Extra Large (27 oz.), Large (24 oz), Medium (21 oz), Small (18 oz) and PeeWee (15 oz).

Some Final Thoughts

Eggs have not been proved to have any affect on coronary heart disease one way or another, except possibly in those whose fat metabolism is out of order. Eggs are a balanced food, and if poached or boiled, the lecithin remains intact and balances out the cholesterol.

Because eggs provide protein, carbohydrates and fats, they are a whole food. Untampered with by man, they are also pure and natural. I recommend whole, pure and natural foods as the best health-builders. About the only things eggs lack are adequate calcium and vitamin C, easily obtained from other foods.

When we stop and think about it, eggs are the best protein buy per pound for the money; they keep well and can be quickly and easily prepared.

Eggs feed the brain and nerves. One of the best nerve tonics I know is a egg yolk in black cherry juice, and raw egg yolk can be added to many blender drinks to build up the protein value.   strange but true.

Strange But True

A chicken developed by the U.S. Agriculture Department laid an egg each day for 448 days. The average chicken lays 275 eggs per year, 17 times its body weight.

A University of Missouri researcher has patented a "chicken bra" to prevent chickens from bruising or blistering their breast meat.

The biggest chicken on record weighed 22 pounds.

Researchers are testing red-tinted contact lenses for laying hens to reduce fighting and pecking in cages. It seems to help, and has increased egg production.

Chicks hatched under green incubator lights are most likely to be deformed, while blue lights increase hatchability.

Baby chicks begin cheeping while still in the egg and will respond to clucks from the mother hen.

The largest chicken egg on record was 9 inches in diameter around the short way and over 12 inches around the long way.

How to Substitute for Table Salt in Recipes
An unheated earth salt or sea salt can be used in equal or slightly less quantity; or use a genuine vegetable salt. It is difficult to make a yeast bread without salt, but where color in your other products allows it, the very best substitute is a naturally salty vegetable seasoning.

Chapter 40

What we know about milk

In the 1930's, I had the pleasure of visiting Randleigh Farm in Lockport, New York, owned by William R. Kenan, Jr. Randleigh Farm was a dairy farm, the most scientific and future-minded farm of its kind in the United States at that time. They carried out a great many experiments designed to find out the healthiest foods for their dairy cattle and to discover the best means of producing "the most nutritious and safe milk for mankind," as the owner put it.

William Kenan found out what the best milk was, and he produced a book to document his findings. The book, *History of Randleigh Farm,* recorded many of the experiments done there. And, he showed that raw milk was superior nutritionally to milk treated in any way — pasteurized, boiled or condensed.

Americans And Milk

A few years ago, a government survey showed that over 25% of the average American's diet is composed of milk and milk products — cream, butter, cheese, cottage cheese, yogurt and the thousands of food products containing milk. Allergy specialists find that milk is one of the most common allergens, so we must realize that milk has its problem side. I believe most Americans are milk-logged, in need of greater food variety in their diet, but I also believe that the only kind of milk truly fit to drink is raw milk. We will soon discover why.

Where It All Starts

No matter where we start on the food chain, we always end up with the dust of the earth — the basic chemical elements needed to build the structures of life. Even the plants and creatures of the sea require the dust of the earth to live, grow and thrive in their watery environment.

Without good soil, we cannot have healthy, vital plantlife. And, without healthy plantlife, we cannot have healthy cattle and healthy milk. So, we recognize at the outset that we must have high quality soil, grass, alfalfa and other food supplements (such as grain) to get high quality milk from dairy cattle.

Experimental Tests With Milk

In 1941, Mr. Kenan, owner of Randleigh Farm, conducted an experiment in which several groups of young white laboratory rats were fed diets of milk supplemented only with a mineral salt mixture. One group was fed raw milk, another pasteurized milk, a third group boiled milk and a fourth group was fed sweetened condensed milk. Two control groups of rats were raised for comparison, the same starting age and weight as those fed on the milk diets. The first control group was obtained from Ohio State University and was fed stock feed supplied by the University. The second control group was from New York Breeding and Laboratory Institute. They were given stock feed supplied by Allied Mills of Peoria, Illinois.

When the rats had been on their diets about 4½ months, they were shipped to Francis M. Pottenger, Jr., M.D., for analysis and comparison. Dr. Pottenger had done many experiments of his own on diets, and was very interested in the nutritional value of foods and their effects upon the body.

Findings Of Dr. Pottenger

Since the rats of control group number 2 arrived later than the others, they were about 1¾ months older when inspected, so allowances must be made for some differences due to the additional age.

Raw Milk-Fed Rats. The muscle tissue of the 27 rats in this group was more highly vascular than that of any of the other groups. There was moderate abdominal fat and excellent tone. Lung lesions were found in two of the rats, one male and one female. One male showed a kidney lesion and three females showed mottled livers suggestive of pathology. Activity was excellent, the fur in good condition.

Pasteurized Milk-Fed Rats. Hemorrhagic areas were found on the inner surface of the skin ext to the muscle layer. Skin was dirty white, rough, irregular. There was dilation of the intestinal tract and a moderate amount of soft, white fat on the inner skin surface. Of the 27 rats in this group, 4 males showed gross pulmonary pathology. Two showed evidence of heart injury and 2 others appeared to have kidney disturbances, 1 of these also showing lung pathology. Three had gross liver disturbances, 2 of which had lung pathology. Three females had pulmonary disturbances, four had liver disturbances and three showed kidney disturbances.

Boiled Milk-Fed Rats. The 14 animals in this group had rougher fur than the raw milk rats and were not as clean. There was more of a pink hemorrhagic quality to the skin. There was marked dilation of the intestines, especially the cecum, as compared to the other groups. Muscular tissue was slightly lighter than that of the controls but less vascular, and some areas appeared anemic. Four animals had lung lesions, two had liver disturbances.

Sweetened Condensed Milk-Fed Rats. The 12 rats in this group, 5 males and 7 females, were larger than any of the other milk-fed rats. Fur was dirty, with patches of alopecia in the males. Muscle tissues were soft, gelatinous and watery. A great deal of white fat was found in the pelt. Dilation of stomach, cecum and colon. Females appeared in better condition than males, but most of these animals had soft, rose-colored livers instead of the normal mahogany color. Three had kidney lesions, three showed lung disturbances and four were found to have gross liver pathology. All had excessive fat.

Control Group #1. The 6 Ohio State University rats had clean, creamy white fur and showed no gross pathological lesions which could be associated with diet.

Control Group #2. The 12 New York controls had whiter fur than those in Group #1. Skins were thicker and fattier, flesh was more vascular and the skin showed purplish cast. All viscera had a peculiar chocolate brown cast. Considerable pathology was apparent. Four males had lung lesions — infectious lung abscesses and bronchitis — and three females had the same condition. One kidney lesion was found. In nine of the twelve, hemosiderosis of the spleen was apparent. One had acute interstitial myocarditis and a positive fat stain for the heart. Another showed moderate liver fat stains.

Comparative Organ Weights. The smallest livers were found in the raw milk rats. The kidneys of the condensed milk rats were heaviest in proportion to body weight of all male groups. The adrenals of the condensed milk male rats were smallest in proportion of body weight of all male groups. The hearts of the condensed milk females were heaviest in proportion of body weight of all female groups.

Summary of Results: 1. Of milk-fed rats, the least number of lesions were found in the raw milk-fed animals. 2. The greatest number of lesions on gross examination in milk-fed rats occurred in the pasteurized milk-fed group. 3. Under microscopic examination, the number of lesions increased in the following order: raw milk group, pasteurized milk group, boiled milk group and sweetened condensed milk group. 4. The pasteurized milk fed rats showed a greater number of

organs involved than any other group on microscopic examination. 5. The femurs of the raw milk males were the heaviest, longest and greatest in diameter of all milk-fed males. 6. The weight of the femurs of the boiled milk rats, male and female, was the least. 7. The percentages of calcium and phosphorus, respectively, in the femurs of the raw milk males, exceeded that of all other milk-fed groups. 8. Raw milk-fed males and females, under X-ray, had larger thoracic cavities than other milk-fed groups, but less than Control #1 (for the males) and less than both control groups (in the case of the females). 9. Based on activity level, bone calcification and muscle tone, the raw milk-fed rats in this experiment showed a physiological superiority over all other milk-fed rats.

Considering that the analysis of the rats was conducted by an experienced medical doctor with a strong background in nutrition, we must take the results of this experiment seriously. Raw milk was demonstrated to be superior to the usual types of processed milk that people drink. Of course, we must realize that a strict milk diet is not a balanced diet for any animal, and no one should go on a raw milk diet, excepting possibly under a doctor's supervision. I had a patient with an extremely sensitive gastrointestinal system whose main food was raw goat milk for many years, but that was an unusual case.

Reseachers have found that significant losses of vitamin B-6 occur during the processing of milk. During pasteurization, enzymes are killed and 10% of the vitamin B-12 is lost. Evaporated milk loses 40%-90% of its B-12. Condensation of milk can cause losses of 10%-33% of vitamin C, 14% to 27% of thiamine and 10% of niacin. With the enzyme and vitamin losses, the protein, fats and minerals are less well digested and assimilated. Boiled milk is almost nutritionally worthless.

Other Randleigh Farm Experiments

In another experiment at Randleigh Farm, laboratory rats from the same litter were selected and fed milk diets over 6½ months. At the end of that period, the rat fed on raw milk weighed 206 gm. and the rat fed pasteurized milk weighed 146 gm. The quality of fur on the pasteurized milk rat was poor as compared to the fur of the other rat.

Comparisons of litter mates always showed greater weight gain for the rats fed raw milk over rats fed any other type of milk. Many such comparisons were made.

Dr. Pottenger's Experiments

Dr. Pottenger selected two groups of cats, about the same size and age, and gave the first group raw milk and raw meat, while the second group was given pasteurized milk and cooked meat. By the second generation, the

GROUP XXIV — BOILED

Rat No.	2-11	2-18	2-25	3-4	3-11	3-18	3-25	4-1	4-8	4-15	4-22	4-29	5-6
1	40	55	74	93	96	107	108	118	112	114	116	118	120
2	43	67	76	94	103	115	120	131	137	137	148	142	135
3	34	43	53	61	67	76	75	85	83	85	87	86	90
4	42	47	74	68	73	82	80	82	92	92	98	93	100
5	46	53	63	78	83	92	93	106	108	106	112	110	118
6	56	67	82	92	107	116	127	140	146	154	168	168	160
7	48	47	75	92	102	107	110	112	112	116	123	118	118
8	54	67	78	93	97	108	108	106	116	116	122	115	105
AVERAGE	45.4	55.7	71.9	83.9	91	100.4	102.6	110	113.3	115	121.7	118.7	118.3

GROUP XXV — EVAPORATED CONDENSED MILK

Rat No.	2-11	2-18	2-25	3-4	3-11	3-18	3-25	4-1	4-8	4-15	4-22	4-29	5-6
1	27	35	43	54	58	61	68	78	90	105	106	110	116
2	40	50	61	78	80	87	93	95	104	122	118	122	128
3	48	64	72	92	94	97	105	114	120	134	137	137	140
4	47	57	67	83	90	95	103	107	115	130	132	120	130
5	53	63	76	78	82	85	93	97	103	124	122	116	127
6	57	65	68	83	92	93	103	112	107	124	134	120	142
7	50	53	63	72	76	78	82	87	92	105	105	95	102
8	47	57	57	65	70	76	78	89	96	106	104	100	106
9	44	57	62	73	78	73	80	85	91	104	104	98	102
AVERAGE	45.9	55.7	63.2	75.3	80	82.8	89.4	96	102	117.1	118	113.1	121.5

GROUP XXII — RAW

Rat No.	2-11	2-18	2-25	3-4	3-11	3-18	3-25	4-1	4-8	4-15	4-22	4-29	5-6
1	41	53	67	73	73	84	91	100	108	122	128	130	145
2	44	58	75	92	100	108	115	117	118	137	125	119	132
3	30	48	58	78	84	94	102	106	116	131	137	136	165
4	42	63	73	97	93	96	95	104	106	114	120	120	136
5	42	57	67	87	88	96	98	105	112	122	130	127	135
6	57	82	91	111	117	129	138	150	160	175	187	190	218
7	52	67	76	87	97	103	114	130	142	162	168	168	180
8	47	75	73	82	88	102	106	118	120	132	133	130	146
AVERAGE	44.4	62.9	72.5	88.4	92.5	101.5	107.4	116.3	122.7	136.9	141	140	157.1

GROUP XXIII — PASTEURIZED

Rat No.	2-11	2-18	2-25	3-4	3-11	3-18	3-25	4-1	4-8	4-15	4-22	4-29	5-6
1	42	53	80	92	102	111	116	122	125	122	127	110	103
2	45	55	67	75	88	97	104	112	115	114	118	118	122
3	40	54	73	92	95	106	108	112	120	116	122	115	110
4	48	63	83	99	98	113	120	135	135	138	138	130	134
5	42	67	84	110	117	132	140	154	161	167	175	167	170
6	47	62	70	80	88	98	104	112	123	128	127	125	130
7	52	67	73	81	83	92	93	104	105	104	105	102	104
8	57	68	82	97	107	118	121	137	145	147	152	140	140
AVERAGE	46.6	61.1	76.5	90.7	97.3	108.4	113.3	123.5	128.7	129.5	133	125.9	125.9

Litter mates 1-2 (3-22) 1/18/41.
Litter mates 4 (3-24) (3-25) (5-22, 5-23, 5-24) 1/17/41.

Litter mates 6 (5-25) (7-22) 1/16/41.
Litter mates 8 (7-23, 7-24, 7-25) (9-25) 1/14/41.
¾ weight after feeding milk.

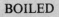

BOILED

Rat No.	Litter	2-3	2-10	2-17	2-24	3-10	3-17	3-34
1	1	75		104	102	104	115	115
2	2	50		78	78	80	85	82
3	2	54		87	92	94	101	102
4	2	54		90	82	83	83	86
5	3	60		73	92	107	112	118
6	3	47		66	78	82	82	93
7	3	49		68	80	78	83	87
8	4	57		67	97	97	102	108
9	4	77		90	118	125	137	147
10	5	dead — malformed — Zenthalmia.						
11	5	50		65	90	86	97	102
12	5	50		67	87	83	96	99
13	6	53		78	96	97	106	112
14	6	61		72	100	104	114	116
15	7	74		67	118	123	128	132
AVERAGE		57.9		76.5	93.5	95.9	102.9	107.

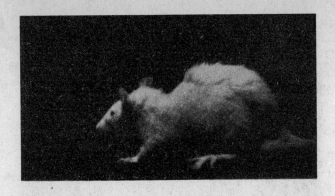

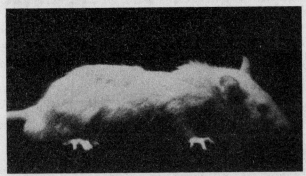

Two rats—condensed milk.

PASTEURIZED

Rat No.	Litter	2-3	2-10	2-17	2-24	3-10	3-17	3-34
1	1	80		92	92	130	141	145
2	2	57		64	97	109	126	134
3	2	60		78	92	104	118	122
4	2	62		78	106	115	128	134
5	3	53		88	92	100	107	115
6	3	48		68	80	87	97	103
8	4	48		74	83	93	97	103
9	4	70		104	102	110	121	122
10	5	45		74	74	75	91	91
11	5	48		84	84	96	106	111
12	5	44		74	74	90	104	109
13	6	58		100	108	107	121	131
14	6	55		78	81	87	106	102
15	6	38		68	68	75	87	93
AVERAGE		54.7		80.3	88.	98.4	110.7	115.3

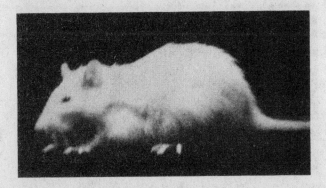

Two rats—Randleigh Farm milk.

RAW

Rat No.	Litter	2-3	2-10	2-17	2-24	3-10	3-17	3-34
1	1	82		102	124	135	143	154
2	2	54		74	86	95	103	112
3	2	62		76	93	105	104	109
4	2	52		45	86	120	132	142
5	3	50		80				
6	3	65		85	102	120	132	140
7	3	40		65	84	80	82	122
8	4	57		75	95	112	122	132
9	1	80		104	97	94	133	136
10	5	48		65	83	94	103	115
11	5	45		67	76	94	104	116
12	5	45		68	76	95	103	87
13	6	53		70	83	127	87	94
14	6	50		70	102	89	93	100
15	7	72		97	115	125	126	138
AVERAGE		57.		76.2	93.	104.6	111.9	121.2

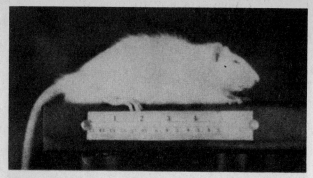

Fed Randleigh Farm raw milk; 7 months; weighed 288 grams.

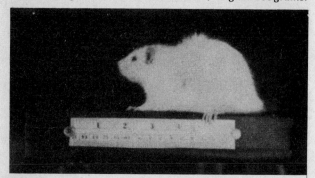

Fed Randleigh Farm pasteurized milk; litter mate; weighed 174 grams.

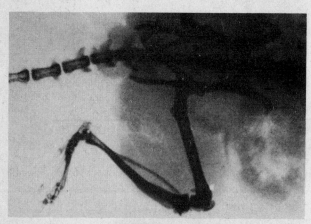

X-Ray section.   Raw

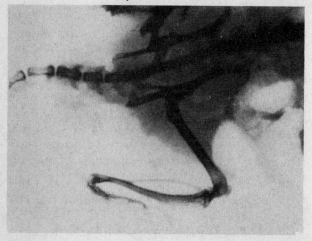

Pasteurized   Note: Gas pockets.

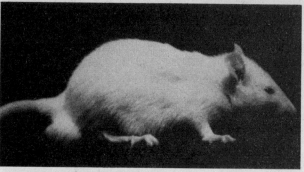

Randleigh Farm raw milk; initial weight 46 grams; final weight 175 grams.

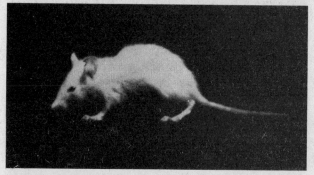

Condensed milk; initial weight 46 grams; final weight 124 grams.

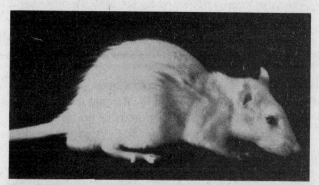

Randleigh Farm pasteurized milk; initial weight 42 grams; final weight 122 grams.

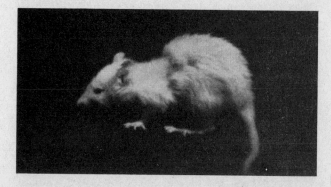

Farm boiled milk; initial weight 42 grams; final weight 106 grams.

cats fed pasteurized milk and cooked meat were unable to reproduce.

The effects of processing foods were further shown by Dr. Pottenger in another experiment. Using a clay soil (in which navy beans grow poorly) in two pots, to one he added excreta of cats fed pasteurized milk and cooked meat, and to the other he added excreta of cats fed raw milk and raw meat. Then he planted navy beans in both pots. The beans that grew in the pot fertilized by the excreta of the cats on raw milk and meat were healthier, larger, more uniform in size and greater in number.

Cow Milk vs Goat Milk

Despite the popularity of cow milk and dairy products in the United States and Western Europe, it is said that 65% of the milk used in the world is from goats. Goat milk is comparable to cow milk in flavor (when both are fresh) and in nutrients, but is much more digestible, possibly because the fat particles are much smaller.

Goats tend to be more disease resistant and more economical to keep than cows. In fact, a milk goat is sometimes referred to as the "poor man's cow"; but the milk it produces is superior to cow's milk, in my view, in terms of its effects on health. I have seen fresh, foaming, warm goat milk practically bring people back from the dead. (Keep in mind that the vital force in the milk diminishes rapidly from the time the animal is milked and is gone in 4 hours.) All milk should be taken as fresh from the animal as possible.

Although I have seen many adverse reactions to cow milk, I have observed only a few problems with goat milk. In fact, most children and adults who have trouble with cow milk do very well with goat milk. Anyone who has an allergy problem or catarrhal problems of any kind will do better on goat milk. Because goat milk is deficient in folic acid, a 100 microgram supplement should be taken per quart of milk or per day.

On many occasions when babies could not breast feed and were not tolerating cow milk or formula well, goat milk has been used with great success. Dr. Charles Parry, nutritionist, states that goat milk with 5-10 milligrams of niacinamide, will often bring infant diarrhea under control within 24 hours.

V.G. Rocine, my greatest teacher, recommended goat milk for the sexual system. He believed it was charged with vitality and was good for people suffering from low vitality. We find that goat milk, buttermilk and whey contain important cell salts and can be used to great advantage in any drink. Goat milk is germ resistant, a strengthener of the body's immune system and an excellent source of protein.

For babies, invalids and indeed for anyone who can get it, goat milk is invaluable. As a remedy for diseases

Comparison of Nutrients in Milk

ITEM All Items Per Liter		Breast Milk	Goat's Milk	Cow's Milk
Energy	Kcal	710	670	660
Protein	gm	11	32	42
Fat	gm	38	40	37
Carbohydrate	gm	68	46	49
Calcium	mg	340	1290	1430
Phosphorus	mg	140	1060	1120
Sodium	meq	7	15	27
Potassium	meq	13	46	45
Iron	mg	5	1	0.5
Zinc	mg	3.5	2.4	3.5
Chloride	mg	375-450	1200	1050
Magnesium	mg	46	100-145	120

Vitamins

A	i.u.	2000	2074	1500
B-1	mg	0.160	0.400	0.440
B-2	mg	0.360	0.1840	0.2100
B-3 (Niacin)	mg	1.47	1.9	1.0
B-6	mg	0.100	0.70	0.640
B-12	mcg	0.3	0.6	4.3
Pantothenate	mg	1.84	3.4	3.5
Folacin	mcg	52	6	55
Diotin	mcg	8	39	31
Choline	mg	90	150	121
Inositol	mg	330	210	110
C	mg	43	15	21
D	i.u.	22	24	14*
E	i.u.	1.8	—	0.4
Essential Fatty Acids, per 100 gm of Milk Fat			4.1	2.6
Percent Fat Globules Less Than 3 dram			63	43

* Not Fortified

such as tuberculosis, malnutrition, rickets, anemia and stomach troubles, goat's milk holds a unique place.

As a tonic for the weak, for the aged, and for growing children, it is unexcelled, building strong teeth and bones, also firm tissues with the power to resist disease.

Dr. Carl Wilson, of Palo Alto, California, says: "After careful study on the subject of goat's milk, and after considerable experimental work and practical demonstration of the value of goat milk as a food for infants, invalids, and for home consumption, I have arrived at the following conclusions:

1. Goat milk is a far better emulsion than cow milk.
2. The oil globules are one-fifth the size of those in cow milk.

3. The reaction of goat milk (cow milk gives an acid reaction) is alkaline, the same as mother's milk. I have yet to find a case where it did not agree.

4. Goat milk is approximately one-third richer than cow milk.

5. The curd in goat milk is small and focculent, hence easily attacked by the digestive organs. In cow milk the curd is large and dense.

6. When using goat milk there is only 2 per cent curd, which precipitates in the stomach, compared with 10 per cent when using cow milk.

7. A goat is an exceptionally healthy animal, immune from tuberculosis, consequently gives a healthful milk of uniform consistency. Goat milk has been proved of untold value as a food for infants, and invalids who are unable to retain or digest cow milk.

8. The goat is a very particular animal. It likes to eat only the top or honey leaves.

If you must drink cow milk, try to get the raw milk from a high quality dairy farm. But, use goat milk whenever possible.

WHICH DO YOU CHOOSE?

RAW CERTIFIED MILK	PASTEURIZED MILK
A. Cleanliness Regulations	**A. Cleanliness, California State and County Law**
1. Tested daily at an independent laboratory for the Certified Milk Commission.	1. Tested once a month by the Health Dept.
a) Bacteria count for standard plate count:* 10,000 per ml** maximum for Certified Milk or Cream.	a) Bacteria count for the standard plate count: 50,000 per ml maximum before pasteurization; 15,000 per ml maximum after pasteurization for milk, 25,000 per ml maximum for cream.
b) Coliform*** bacteria count may not exceed 10 per ml.	b) May not exceed 750 Coliform per ml in raw milk before pasteurization, taken at farm pick-up.
	Coliform bacteria count may not exceed 10 ml after pasteurization.
2. Streptococci test once a month.	2. No regulation requires test for Streptococci.
B. Herd tests in Los Angeles County, CA	**B. Herd tests in Los Angeles County, CA**
1. All dairy cows in a certified milking herd are vaccinated for brucellosis between the ages of 2-6 months.	1. All dairy cows are vaccinated for brucellosis between the ages of 2-6 months. All dairy cattle moving within the state must bear evidence of official calfhood vaccination.
2. Each certified cow is blood tested for brucellosis before entering the milking herd and receives a blood test at least once a year; thereafter reactors are removed.	2. All dairy cattle must be blood tested for brucellosis if imported into California.
3. All raw certified milk is ring tested at least 4 times a year for brucella. If the ring test is positive, then the entire dairy herd is blood tested for brucellosis and any positive reactors are removed.	3. The milk from all dairy herds is ring tested at least 4 times a year for brucella. If the ring test is positive then the entire dairy herd is blood tested for brucellosis and any positive reactors are removed.

* Total count of all bacteria in the milk.
** Milliliter

*** Bacteria which is normally foreign to the cow's udder.

294

RAW CERTIFIED MILK	PASTEURIZED MILK

4. TB skin test is performed annually on all cows in the certified milking herd by a state veterinarian. If reactors were found they would be removed from the certified herd. All certified milk dairy herds are free and are maintained free of TB because of constant vigilance and testing.

4. TB skin test is performed on all cows by a state veterinarian at intervals longer than one year. If reactors are found, additional tests may be required. Reactor cows are removed.

5. Herd sanitarian from the County Medical Milk Commission visits the dairy weekly or more often. A health inspector from the county visits the dairy at least monthly.

5. Health inspector visits dairy monthly.

C. Employee Health Examinations

C. Employee Health Examinations

1. Once a month examination of each employee at certified farm. All new employees have a complete physical examination and tests when starting to work on a certified farm.

1. Examination required at time of employment.

2. Once a month throat culture and examination for streptococcus.

2. None required.

3. During the year other tests are made at regular intervals. Another step to insure disease-free milk.

3. None required.

4. Stool specimen is required from each employee bi-annually.

4. None required.

5. Chest X-ray or skin test for TB required annually.

5. None required.

D. Nutritional Values

D. Nutritional Values

1. Enzymes, catalase, peroxidase and phosphatase are present.

1. Pasteurization destroys the enzyme phosphatase.

a) Phosphatase is needed to split and assimilate the mineral salts in foods that are in the form of phytates.

a) absence of phosphatase indicates that milk has been pasteurized.

b) Wulzen Factor (anti-stiffness) available.

b) Wulzen Factor destroyed (anti-stiffness nutrition factor lost).

Wulzen and Bahrs reported that guinea pigs fed raw whole milk grew excellently and at autopsy showed no abnormality of any kind. Guinea pigs fed pasteurized milk rations did not grow as well and developed a definite syndrome, the first sign of which was wrist stiffness.

c) X Factor in tissue repair available.

c) No evidence of alteration by pasteurization.

RAW CERTIFIED MILK	PASTEURIZED MILK
2. Protein — 100% metabolically available; all 22 amino acids, including the 8 that are essential, for the complete metabolism and function of protein.	2. Digestibility reduced by 4%, biological value reduced by 17%. From the digestibility and metabolic data it is concluded that the heat damage to lysine and possibly to histidine and perhaps other amino acids destroys the identity of these amino acids and partly decreases the absorbability of their nitrogen.
3. Vitamins — all 100% available.	3. Vitamins
a) Vitamin A — fat soluble	a) Vitamin A — destroyed
b) Vitamin D — fat soluble	b) Not altered
c) Vitamin E — fat soluble	c) Not altered
d) Vitamin K — fat soluble	d) Not altered
e) Vitamin B — complex Vitamin B-1: Thiamin Vitamin B-2: Riboflavin Vitamin B-3: Niacin Vitamin B-5: Pantothenic Acid Vitamin B-6: Pyridoxine Vitamin B-12: Cyanocobalamin Folic Acid Biotin Choline Inositol	e) Vitamin B complex — pasteurization of milk destroys about 38% of the vitamin B complex.
f) Vitamin C	f) Vitamin C is weakened or destroyed by pasteurization. Infants fed pasteurized milk exclusively will develop scurvy.
g) Antineuritic vitamin	g) Testing of pasteurized milk indicates destruction of this vitamin.
4. Minerals — all 100% metabolically available. a) Major mineral components; calcium, chlorine, magnesium, phosphorus, potassium, sodium and sulphur. b) Vital trace minerals, all 24 or more, 100% available.	4. After pasteurization the total of soluble calcium is very much diminished. The loss of soluble calcium in regards to infants and growing children must be a very important factor in growth and development, not only in the formation of bone and teeth, but also in the calcium content of the blood, the importance of which is now being raised.

RAW CERTIFIED MILK	PASTEURIZED MILK
5. Carbohydrates — easily utilized in metabolism. Still associated naturally with elements (unstable).	5. Carbohydrates — no evidence of change by pasteurization.
6. Fats — all 18 fatty acids metabolically available, both saturated and unsaturated.	6. Pasteurization harms the fat content of milk.

E. Possible Damage to the Health of Consumers from Drinking Pasteurized Milk

1. Dr. J.C. Annand has written a series of articles in which he has advanced the theory that the increase in the incidence of heart disease was proximately related to the onset of pasteurization of milk. Different population groups were studied in various parts of the world. His theory is that the heat process of pasteurization alters the protein found in milk and as a result heated protein is responsible for the large increase in the incidence of heart trouble in citizens of western civilization, during the course of the past generation.

2. Dr. Kurt A. Oster has advanced the theory that homogenization of milk is proximately related to the atherosclerosis which is so prevalent to citizens in developed countries of the western world. The reduction in the size of the fat particles caused by homogenization permits them to be assimilated into the stomach lining in a manner that was not contemplated by nature. When these fat particles along with xanthine oxidase get into the bloodstream the human system sets up a defense mechanism which results in the scarring of arteries.

Vitamin C Helps Cancer of the Bowel

Dr. Jerome Decosse of the Sloan-Kettering Institute reported that in experiments with animals, vitamins were effective in preventing precancerous conditions from developing into cancer. Dr. Decosse also cited supplementary vitamin C as effective in preventing bowel cancer in patients with bowel polyps.

Fiber Vs. Heart Disease and Cancer

Reports from Holland show that people on natural high-fiber diets have less heart disease and cancer. The greatest protection was evident for those taking more than 30 grams of fiber per day. In taiwan, dietary fiber intake from pea pods, bamboo shoots and Chinese lettuce was compared with fiber from cucumbers, tomato and asparagus. Cholesterol was reduced more by the Oriental fiber foods. A West Virginia fiber study showed that high-fiber foods can significantly lower cholesterol in only four days. Bran-supplemented diets were not as effective as diets using natural fiber foods such as whole wheat bread, fruit, salad greens, brown rice and beans. Individuals are cautioned to increase dietary fiber slowly to avoid cramps and diarrhea.

297

Chapter 41

Raw juices, tonics and special broths

Liquid drinks occupy a useful and pleasant niche in any health building program. By and large, they are more easily digested and assimilated than solid foods. Specific juices, tonics and broths can be taken for specific purposes, such as to supply more of one or two needed chemical elements or to bring in a concentrated array of vitamins and enzymes. Some are acid forming; others are alkaline forming. We can make heating drinks or cooling drinks, laxative drinks, blood-building drinks. We find that our health drinks can be vitalizing, sleep-promoting or thirst quenching — or they may have combinations of the preceding qualities.

It is useful to understand what the various raw juices, tonics and special broths will or will not do for us. For example, in a catarrh-laden body, raw fruit juices will stir up acids and toxins but are of little help in eliminating them. Citrus juices are the worst offender in this area, and I do not recommend taking them. Use vegetable juices for elimination and fruit juices for their vitamin values. The advantage of juices is that they contain concentrations of ingredients found in the whole fruit or vegetable but without the cellulose and fiber. Keep in mind that fiber and bulk are needed in the diet to promote a clean and properly toned bowel. It is not wise to rely too much on liquids alone for long periods of time without being under a doctor's supervision.

Juices, excepting in cases of juice fasts, are best taken between meals. If taken with meals they may dilute the digestive juices and interfere with digestion. Juices taken with meals, however, should be sipped, never gulped down. It is best not to take any liquid either ice cold or boiling hot.

Some Qualities Of Juices

Drinks that elevate the body temperature and help sustain body heat are called thermades, while drinks that reduce body heat and temperature are called frescades. All fruit juices that contain cooling acids such as formic, citric and acetic acid are wonderful hot weather drinks. In climates where the heat becomes oppressive, there are usually local fruits available from which to make cooling drinks. We will also find certain herbs, plants and leaves that enhance this effect. The dwarf nettle and duckweed are useful in replacing the formic acid lost through perspiration on hot days, and limes are also high in formic acid. If too much formic acid is lost through perspiration on hot summer days, illness often follows. When plants lack formic acid, disease quickly overtakes them.

Vegetable juices high in potassium may be useful for their laxative effects but may promote digestive problems if taken over a long period of time. Blackberry juice, high in iron, can be constipating. Fruit juices tend to contain more vitamins than the vegetable juices, and we call them vitalizing juices. Various juices have mild antiseptic properties to help us battle against bacteria and viruses. It is important to remember, however, that bacteria and viruses seldom cause trouble in the body unless there are pockets of unmoving toxic waste for them to grow and multiply in. Keeping the body clean is important to health.

Most mineral waters available at the store contain carbonic acid and sodium. Drinks made with them are alkaline and can be favorable to the body when the stomach is overacid, particularly if used with alkaline foods. Chamomile tea is a mild tonic to the stomach and is used much by the German people. It should not be used to excess because it acts as a stimulant, and often the stomach needs rest, not stimulation.

Chemicals And Properties Of Juices

Blackberries are rich in iron, tannin, fruit acids and mineral salts. Blackberry juice, antitoxic and sanative (cleansing) to the body, is a good blood builder but can be constipating. Loganberries and raspberries are high in fruit acids.

Wild blackberries, found in Oregon, Washington, Northern California, Virginia, Michigan and Tennessee, contain more iron than the domestic variety, and, like domestic blackberries, are constipating.

Wild cherries contain the same acids as blackberries, phosphoric, tannic and tartaric. They are high in potassium, sodium and iron salts, beneficial in cases of anemia. If the stomach is acid, it is better to leave them alone. Domestic cherries, both light and dark, contain a gum good for the bowel. As in the case of wild cherries, the domestic types contain many salts needed by the tissues, especially potassium. They are laxative to an alkaline stomach.

Prune juice and plain water are laxative to most but not to all people. Prunes and plums contain potassium, phosphorus, calcium and sodium.

Mulberries and their juice have remarkable nerve-soothing properties. Mulberry drinks are wonderful for cooling and calming hot-blooded young people, for reducing fevers, sedating the nerves, relaxing an overheated brain, quieting the passions and intense emotions. We find that mulberry drinks, with moraxytic acid, reduce body heat without bringing on perspiration.

Barberries (or berberries) and their juice are bitter to the taste and constipating, yet tonic to the stomach and bowels. Similar in its effects to blackberry juice, it affects the system differently.

Tamarinds are cooling and laxative and are good in sultry weather.

Quince is high in fluorine, gum, glucose and several chemical salts but because it requires cooking to be palatable, the fluorine is usually lost. Raw quince can be peeled and put in a blender, or run twice through a Champion juicer (without the screen), and a little honey can be added for sweetening.

Strawberries are mildly laxative, containing malic acid, sodium, potassium, calcium, phosphorus, sulphur, iron and a small amount of evonymin.

Sebesten plums, grown primarily in Asia, are soothing to the mucous membranes and laxative to the bowels.

Whortleberries are found in many varieties, some more acid than others. They contain valuable fruit acids and salts and make a nice summer drink. Shadberries (Juneberries, Serviceberries) also make a good juice.

Black huckleberries have much the same qualities as blueberries. The juice makes a wonderful drink.

Hackberry juice, high in iron and tannic acid, is constipating.

Cowberry juice provides a cooling, refreshing, acidic summer drink for the hot sultry days of July and August. In Russia a decoction called "Brovsnika" is prepared from cowberries, red whortleberries and others, and used for rheumatism. It may give some temporary relief but complete healing requires much more than this.

Elderberry juice seems to have a special affinity for the ovaries and the uterus. An oily acid in this juice vitalizes the female sex glands and organs if taken daily over a period of some time, relieving menstrual difficulties in many cases and apparently attracting an increased blood flow to the pelvic area.

Blueberry juice contains phosphoric, tartaric and tannic acids, and is high in potassium, calcium and magnesium. It makes a good drink diluted with distilled water.

Pineapple juice may be used freely in throat ailments. It has an ether of value for this, plus several fruit acids and sodium, calcium, magnesium and iodine.

Bilberry juice, mixed with distilled water, makes a good frescade or cooling drink in hot, sultry weather. In it we find citric and quinic acids.

Currant juice, both black and red, holds many valuable chemical salts and fruit acids, especially citric acid. Red currants are slightly more acid than the black. The acids and salts in currants seem to exhibit germicidal properties and also act as detoxicants. Black currant juice, tolerated nicely by an acid stomach, builds the bloodstream.

Mangoes contain gallic acid, binding to the bowels and a mild disinfectant. Mangoes and their juice counteract perspiration, reduce excessive body heat and act to eliminate bad odors from the body. Potassium, calcium and chlorine are the main elements.

Coconuts contain an oil-rich white meat with caproic and other acids in it. The oil, easily assimilated by the body, becomes rancid quickly. Coconut milk is a good drink but should not be used when the gastro-intestinal tract is known to be toxic laden.

Pear juice makes a sweet bland drink but quickly ferments in an acid stomach. When the stomach is acid, we should leave sweet drinks alone.

Peaches and nectarines, also bland when juiced, contain potassium, phosphorus, sodium, calcium, magnesium and sulphur. They are laxative.

Pomegranate juice is an excellent tonic for the kidneys, an effective cleanser. A good frescade for hot summer days, it has sodium and magnesium in it.

Persimmons, high in calcium, phosphorus and a gum of value to the bowel, can be used in summer drinks.

Dewberry juice contains almost the same acids and salts as blackberry juice. It makes a pleasant tasting drink, good for bowel ailments and anemia since it is high in both iron and an aromatic essence which appears to act favorably on the bowel.

Hot lemonade is excellent for colds, especially if mixed with clam broth. This tonic stimulates perspiration and moves the blood, but can be binding to the bowel in some people.

Apple juice makes a good drink, hot or cold. It contains potassium, sodium, magnesium, phosphorus and several fruit acids, including malic acid. When juicing apples, do not run the core, which may contain pesticide residues, through the juicer. Apple juice can be mixed with many other juices, especially those that are too sweet, too bitter or too sour to the taste by themselves. Apples and apple juice are not good for an acid stomach.

Watermelon juice is a good kidney cleanser and is especially effective when the pink meat, seeds, white and outside green skin are juiced together and strained through cheesecloth. The white rind is rich in sodium, wonderful for the stomach and bowel, while the outside green skin is rich in chlorophyll, a blood cleanser and detoxifier. The seeds act as a mild diuretic while the pink meat contains silicon, calcium and enough fruit sugar to supply energy to the body. Watermelon or watermelon juice should not be taken within one-half hour of other foods (nor should any of the melons).

Apricot juice or nectar is high in potassium, phosphorus, iron, silicon and copper as well as several fruit acids. Apricots, both fresh and dried, were one of the mainstays of the Hunza diet, and the people of the Hunza Valley were among the healthiest in the world before "modernization" began to make inroads there. They also ate apricot kernals, but only the sweet ones.

Grape juice is high in magnesium phosphorus and, if grapes are juiced with the skins, very high in potassium. It has some iron. Grapes should be run through the juicer with the seeds and strained through cheesecloth. This juice is good in catarrhal conditions, as a blood purifier and also acts as a laxative.

Tips On Fruit Buying

Although most vegetables can be picked and eaten before they are mature, fruits cannot. Fruits are dependent upon the sun for the maturing of their sugars, acids, enzymes, vitamins and mineral salts, and if picked and eaten green many fruits can upset the stomach, causing pain, bowel spasms and diarrhea. We should only eat sun ripened fruit, which means it is best to find your own source of supply from farms surrounding your area and to buy direct from the farmer.

Fruits in our grocery stores and supermarkets are often shipped from long distances away, which means that considerable time, sometimes weeks, elapse between the time the fruit is picked and the time it reaches the store. Most fruits, if picked ripe, would spoil during shipment. Soft, ripe fruit — such as strawberries, peaches, pears and so on — bruise easily during transit. For these and many other reasons, fruit is often picked green for the market.

Citrus fruits, wonderful if picked when tree-ripened, are not good for the body when picked early, as most are for shipping to market. Oranges, tinted and spotted green when picked, are run through a "gas chamber" and come out a beautiful ripe-looking orange color, while the inside fruit remains unripe. This is done before shipping. I do not recommend citrus fruit, except for ripe, sweet oranges eaten in sections, not in juice form, excepting where the citrus can be purchased tree ripened. The habit of so many Americans of drinking orange juice with every breakfast is a poor idea, healthwise. There are many other juices to choose from, and we should have a variety.

Buy fruits at the peak of ripeness, direct from the farmer, if possible. Eat the whole fruits in season, and make juice for between meal refreshments. Most fruit juices can be frozen in ice cube trays then stored in plastic bags in the freezer for later use.

Special Tips On Fruits And Juices

Many fruits and juices can be eaten in combination with one another, excepting for melons which should be eaten separately. It is occasionally permitted to have watermelon or cantaloupe pieces in a mixed fruit salad but it should not be a regular practice. Have fun experimenting with combinations.

We should eat fruit and vegetables in season to get the most good out of them. Fruit, especially, is meant to cleanse the body after a season of winter foods, more time spent indoors and layers of clothing on the body, inhibiting the release of toxins through the skin. We should not be alarmed if we have a few days of diarrhea after eating fruit, for this is often a natural cleansing action of the body. If cramps or pains develop, reduce the amount of fruit used.

Fruit juices can be diluted with water or mixed with herbal teas. We discuss herbs in a different part of the book, so only a few recipes will be given here. The best water is obtained from reverse osmosis distillation processes. I do not recommend any of the commercial soda waters.

I have not recommended fruit or juice such as cranberry, rhubarb or gooseberries, because they are high in oxalic acid. Oxalic acid in its white powdered form is an ingredient in some commercial cleansers. It is a powerful bleach and stain remover, and it is also hard on the kidneys. Oxalic acid, when taken internally, is known to reduce blood clotting time, which can make it useful in treating hemorrhage or jaundice. If eaten or juiced, cranberries, rhubarb and gooseberries should be taken along with a calcium supplement or high calcium foods to make them more compatible with the body chemistry. They should also be mixed with other fruit juice to reduce tartness from the oxalic acid.

Always wash fruits well before using. Toxic sprays are so widespread these days that it is unwise to assume any fresh fruit or vegetable is clean. The skins of most fruits should be eaten to get the valuable cell salts there, but of course do not eat the skins of pineapples, oranges or bananas.

In many health food stores you will find apple, cherry and grape concentrates, which can be added to water to make a wonderful, fresh-tasting juice. They can also be used as flavorings or syrups.

Vegetable Juices — The Builders

While fruit juices are cleansers, vitalizers, coolers and great sources of vitamins, vegetable juices are builders, toners and wonderful sources of the chemical elements. We must realize that these roles are mixed, however, because fruit juice has chemical elements and exerts some building activity, and vegetable juice contains vitamins and has considerable cleansing power, especially the green leafy vegetables. Chlorophyll from green leaves is one of the most effective, safe and powerful detoxifiers known to man.

Iceburg or head lettuce, I have found, has so little nutritional value that I do not recommend it. Leaf lettuces are much higher in chlorophyll and various vitamin values, along with iron, potassium, calcium, phosphorus, silicon, magnesium and chlorine. There is simply no question concerning where the better value lies.

Onion water or juice stimulates the kidneys, lungs and throat. Onions contain an oil called allyl sulphide, potassium, calcium, phosphorus, iron, sulphur and silicon. Garlic and leeks belong to the onion family and have similar constituents. Garlic is a natural antiseptic and antibiotic, a wonderful aid taken raw for colds, if family and co-workers can stand the resulting body odor. For those who cannot take garlic raw, an alternative is to chop it up into small pieces and put it into gelatin capsuls, available at most health food stores. Garlic can be put in a juicer or blender, but its oil tends to coat the metal surfaces for some time before wearing off. The sulphur in garlic, leeks and onions is a stirring element, going deep into the cell structure.

Celery and parsley, both, contain a small amount of apiol, a principle that acts on the sexual system. When these juices are taken liberally over a period of time, the nervous system is toned and sexual function is substantially improved. Apiol is considered an aid in overcoming some menstrual problems. Whole parsely can also be mixed with celery juice in a blender. Celery juice, high in sodium, has proven to be of great value in taking care of stomach and bowel problems. It is alkaline, and this property, together with the high sodium content, has assisted many people in getting rid of rheumatism and arthritis, for which most doctors say there is no cure. It is often taken along with whey, also high in sodium, to help restore chemical balance in the joints.

Carrot juice, sweet to the taste, is very high in pro-vitamin A, the carotene that is transformed into vitamin A in the body. The juice of carrots contains potassium, silicon and chlorine salts. Most of the salts needed by the body can be supplied by a combination of carrot and spinach juice, which is high in iron and other salts. We find that most people can tolerate carrot juice very well, including those who are allergic to many other substances, and it has been a wonderful aid to many people who have used it to work their way out of chronic and degenerative conditions. We sometimes hear of warnings about the yellowing of the skin caused by taking too much carrot juice. In my experience, this yellowing is part of a natural cleansing process by the body, and it disappears as the chemical balance of the body is restored. A new product derived from carrot juice is now

being prepared for marketing and promises to be a wonderful health aid.

Spinach, I believe, is the queen of the greens. The ash of spinach is: 39.9% potassium, 9.4% sodium, 2.6% calcium, 2.2% magnesium, 2% iron, 2.2% phosphorus, 12.2% sulphur, 8.4% silicon, 11% chlorine, 0.3% fluorine, and a trace of manganese. The total ash content of spinach is 2.1%.

In tomato juice we find potassium, phosphorus, calcium and many fruit essences. The tomato is a fruit, not a vegetable, but it is often classed among the vegetables. Its juice is good for the blood, cooling and refreshing.

In cucumber juice we find potassium, phosphorus, sulphur and a little colocynthin. Cucumber juice is mildly tonic, a refreshing frescade for summer and strongly sedative. It promotes healing, is antiseptic and an effective blood purifier. Bitter oils are in the rind, so always peel before juicing. Tip: before peeling, cut off a small piece near one end and rub the two cut surfaces together vigorously in a circular motion. A foam will usually build up, eliminating bitter oils from the inner lining and leaving a sweeter fruit. Then peel and juice.

Dandelion greens are high in iron and have tonic and laxative qualities.

Hop water promotes circulation, is a mild diuretic and soothing to the stomach. It contains lupulin.

Beet juice is very strong and should be diluted with water or other milder vegetable juices. It contains a small amount of ergot and betin, and its solvent property makes it a good liver cleanser. Beets contain potassium, sodium, phosphorus, magnesium and a trace of iron.

Horseradish, high in sulphur, also contains potassium and silicon. It is a strong kidney stimulant (diuretic) and can be used in drinks and tonics for this purpose.

Coffee and tea are high in caffein, whose effects on the body are largely destructive, so I recommend against using them. Common tea contains gallic, tannic, phosphoric, carbonic and boheic acids and a potent alkaloid. Coffee contains quinic acid. Habitual coffee consumption has been linked to higher incidence of heart disease, and it encourages excess acidity in the stomach.

Rye water is bland and laxative.

Asparagus juice is found to have potassium, phosphorus, sodium, calcium and silicon. It is laxative.

Rice water is mucilaginous, comforting to a weak or inflamed stomach.

Cabbage is comparatively high in many organic salts and in brassidic acid, which is good for asthma. The entire cabbage family includes cauliflower, kale, sea kale, broccoli, savoy, sprouts, kohlrabi, shallot and red cabbage. All are rich in the organic salts, especially potassium. Their juices can be combined with those of other vegetables to improve the mineral values. Some of the cabbage family have a great deal of sulphur, which can produce stomach gas.

Juice can be pressed from salsify, cress, endive, nasturtium, romaine, clover blossoms and any edible greens, or these same things can be added to a basic juice, such as celery, in a blender and mixed until fine.

Flavor can be added to vegetable and fruit drinks by using grated orange rind, lemon rind, apple peelings, cloves, banana, vanilla, lavender, pineapple, juniper berries, mint, peppermint, sassaparilla, cardamon, cinnamon, spearmint and honey.

Almonds, sesame seeds, sunflower seeds, pumpkin seeds and other raw seeds and nuts can be blended into many vegetable and fruit drinks. They should, however, be soaked overnight in apple or pineapple juice first. Many nuts and seeds contain linoleic acid (which helps dissolve cholesterol off artery walls) but also protein, vitamins, enzymes and vaulable salts. The oils from seeds and nuts feed the nerves and glands.

Herbal Teas

Peppermint tea contains pimenthol, good for the nerves and for fermentation gas generated from starches and sugars.

Catnip tea, rich in potassium, is a gas driver and expulsion agent. Stomach gas from a diet high in milk, such as in children and some elderly persons, will often yield to this tea.

Sage contains salviol and tannin. It is generally binding to the bowels, but its tea is a good tonic, especially mixed with hot clam juice with a little lemon juice.

Spearmint or plain mint (also dill) can be made into soothing, gas driving teas, or mixed into salads. These gas-driving foods are needed, generally, only for discomfort and excessive gas.

Wintergreen juice is binding but tonic, counteracting uric acid gout.

Thyme juice is bacteriocidal, tonic, calming and helps overcome itch. It can be added to other juices.

Clove water, with caryophyllin and eugenin, is good for infection and toothache, is tonic, and rids the body quickly of some types of bacteria.

Vanilla, a common kitchen flavoring, is nerve calming, tonic and heat reducing.

Red pepper can be added to drinks to counteract bloating. It is a diuretic and overcomes undesirable bowel flora, but it is somewhat irritating to the tissues.

Sarsaparilla drinks are good for stimulating the kidneys and bowel, and for moving the lymph. Several saponins, a volatile oil and a resin are found in sarsaparilla.

Lavender reduces bloating and can be added to juices and drinks.

Cardamon drives gas, is aromatic and makes a good addition to other drinks (as all the aromatic spices and herbs do).

Nutmeg contains a mild narcotic and myristic acid, of value in calming the nerves, and is aromatic.

Ginger is aromatic, gas driving and is beneficial to the stomach.

Cinnamon, a popular flavoring for mild fruit juices and drinks, is an aromatic containing tannin, cinamic aldehyde and sodium salts. It is antiseptic, drives gas and is said to be good for flu. Reportedly, it helps counteract tuberculosis and cancer in the early stages.

Anise, a good aromatic flavoring agent, is mildly effective in getting rid of gas.

Sassafras is made from a bark that contains tannin and an aromatic oil. It makes a pleasant tea which helps eliminate catarrh, purify the blood and aids digestion. Insects reportedly abhor sassafras. A chicken breeder once told me he used sassafras poles for his chickens to roost on to prevent lice.

Caraway adds flavor to juniper beverages so widely used in the U.S.S.R. and Sweden.

Juniper berries contain both an oil and a resin. It is used as a diuretic, to tone up the sexual system, cleanse the liver and blood. Father Kneipp would start with one or two berries a day, build up to 15 on the 10th day, then reverse the order until he was back to one or two berries — for cleansing purposes. It is hard on the kidneys to take juniper berry drinks often.

Ways To Use Raw Milk

We have covered milk in other places, so I will only briefly review the subject here. First of all, cow's milk and its various products make up such a large portion of the average American diet that it has become allergenic to many and produces excessive catarrh in a great many more. Pasteurization is one of the main problems since it kills enzymes, eliminates or reduces the vitamin content and renders the milk no longer whole. The fat particles in cow's milk are large and somewhat difficult to digest. Those for whom cow's milk is not a problem are encouraged to use whole raw milk, if available. Homogenization possibly creates other problems, and Kurt A. Oster, M.D., believes it may be the main cause of arteriosclerosis, so I do not recommend homogenized milk.

Seed And Nut Milk Drinks (Milk Substitutes)

The great advantage of the seed and nut milk drinks is that they are non-catarrh forming and generally non-allergenic. While most people benefit from goat milk, there are some who can't take it, and there are vegetarians who want to stay away from all animal products.

Viable seeds carry the life force necessary to germinate in the soil and grow into a complete plant. They are "live" foods — whole, pure, natural and uncontaminated. Seeds thousands of years old have been found in Egyptian tombs, and when planted, they still grew. The life force in seeds is a wonderful thing.

The following recipes will demonstrate how to make the basic nut and seed milk drinks most often used. The same approach, of course, can be applied to other nuts and seeds.

Sesame Seed Milk: The sesame is the king of seeds, used a great deal in Turkey where strength is valued in men and where a healthy sex life in marriage is considered very important. The oils in sesame seeds feed the glands and nerves. Sesame seeds make a wonderful drink for gaining weight, for lubricating the bowel and for providing protein, calcium, phosphorus and other minerals and vitamins.

Add ¼ cup sesame seeds to 2 c. water or apple juice. (Raw cow milk or goat milk can be used if they do not constitute a problem.) Place in blender and run for 2 minutes. Strain through fine wire strainer or 2-4 layers of cheese cloth to remove hulls. This is the basic seed milk drink.

For flavor or added nutritional value, any of the following may be used. One tbs. carob powder and 6-8 dates. Or banana, stewed raisins, apple or cherry concentrate, date powder or grape sugar. Various salad dressings can be made with it as the base, with the imaginative addition of herbs and seasonings.

Almond Nut Milk: I consider the almond the king of nuts, but any other nuts may be used also. It is highly alkaline, high in protein and easy to assimilate. Soak nuts overnight in apple or pineapple juice or honey water to soften. Put 3 oz. of soaked nuts in 5 oz. water and blend 2-3 minutes.

For flavor, add honey, fruit, apple or cherry concentrate, strawberry juice, carob powder, dates or bananas. Or vegetable juices can be added.

Sunflower Seed Milk: Perhaps second only to spirulina and chlorella algae, sunflower seeds are the vegetarian's best protein. Soak ¼ c. whole sunflower seeds in apple or pineapple juice overnight, and proceed as in directions for almond nut milk. The same flavorings and additives can be used.

Soy Milk: Add 4 tbs. soy milk powder to 1 pt. water. Sweeten with honey, molasses or maple syrup, and add a pinch of vegetable salt. For flavorings or additions, see the previous milk drinks. Refrigerate to keep. You can use this in any recipe where cow's milk is called for. It closely resembles the taste of cow's milk (and will sour just as quickly). It is wise not to make too much at one time.

My Drink: Sometimes when I need an energy boost or don't have time to eat a meal, I just say, "Bring me my drink". Here's what is in it: 1 tbs. sesame seed butter or meal, 1 glass fruit juice, vegetable juice, soy milk or broth and water, ¼ avocado, 1 tsp. honey. Blend ½ minute.

Mixed Drinks, Broths And Tonics

I am sometimes asked, "Why go to all the trouble of making juices? Why not eat the foods, raw or cooked, as necessary?" For one thing, cooked food has undergone chemical changes and loss of nutritional values. Discarded liquid from cooked vegetables is often loaded with vitamins and minerals. Some elements, such as fluorine — the resistance element — are lost in cooking. Complex substances such as lecithin, a brain and nerve food, can be diminished or lost in cooking when it is needed to balance cholesterol, which is not lost in cooking to any appreciable extent.

Liquids represent the "essence" of the solid they are derived from, the most vital part. I have often said, "It isn't what we eat that counts, it is what we digest and assimilate." Liquids require less work on the part of the gastro-intestinal system to make their way through the digestive processes and into the bloodstream. This distinction is critical when we are talking about raising the health level of those with greatly weakened bodies and systems.

I don't exactly like to talk about "basket cases", but we all encounter patients in such a low state of energy, will and ability to move that we can't tell whether or not they have bought their ticket to the other side. What can you do for these people? Every bit of energy they have is being used to keep that body alive one more day. All sick people are fatigued, and a fatigued body cannot digest well. We must realize that digestion takes energy. We have to burn some energy in the digestive processes to gain energy back from the foods taken in. Warm liquids of certain kinds take the least energy to digest and produce the most strengthening energy in return. I have remained with bed-ridden patients and have spoon-fed them broth every half hour, a teaspoon at a time, until that subtle change in skin color, the spark in the eye, told me they were coming back. I know these things work because I have used them in my sanitarium. I have waved goodbye to patients walking out with spring in their step when they had to be carried in, some weeks or months before.

Certain juices work well in combinations, others do not work so well. As we have said, there are hundreds of possibilities. We recommend water distilled by the reverse osmosis process for dilution. In extreme cases we have used the juice pressed from raw meat, and you must have a press of some kind to do this effectively. We use a Champion juicer at the Ranch because of its versatility of operation in making nut butters as well as juices. The Acme is also good, particularly for carrots, celery and other non-leafy vegetables. And there are others, I am sure. We also use a blender to make nut milk drinks and various combinations. There are many high-quality blenders available in the stores.

Additives to Drinks: From the following drinks and combinations, you will come up with some of your own ideas for combining things, but here are some basics. Use honey as a sweetener, as needed. Cayenne pepper may be used to add tang to vegetable drinks, as can other herbs. A raw egg yolk adds an excellent balanced protein to any drink and feeds the glands and nerves. Whole fresh raw eggs contain many needed elements such as phosphorus, sodium, potassium, calcium, chlorine and sulphur, as well as many vitamins. Leftover cooking water from steaming vegetables can be blended into vegetable juices. Seeds and nuts can be added, or a tablespoon or so of the seed or nut butter. Ripe avocado or banana can make a wonderful contribution to a drink. We can add sprouts, parsley or cilantro to add a fresh taste. I do not approve of adding sea water to drinks, but it is certainly all right to add dulse, algae or other such substances to bring in the trace elements. Spirulina or chlorella microalgae powders are potent, high protein supplements which can boost the nutrient value of most vegetable juices; one teaspon to a glass may be taken. Fresh clam juice or fish broth is also good. We can also use apple or cherry concentrate, date powder, carob powder.

In the pericarp of oats, we find a valuable principle (avenin) which is of value to the nerves and sexual system as a tonic and mild sedative. Oat water or oat extracts, rightly prepared, can be mixed with juice from lettuce, celery, parsley, raw meat juice, and flavored with aromatic herbs. An egg yolk or grated almonds may be included for protein and oils. Silicon, potassium, phosphorus, sodium, calcium, iron and many valuable essences are found in such a drink.

Raw meat juice contains many different properties, potassium, sodium, phosphorus, iron are found in the ash of meat juice, which can be mixed with many drinks. Juice from the meat of a healthy young steer is highly alkaline and vitalizing, increasing the bile function and counteracting constipation (if used over several days). It is an excellent drink when the muscles have been overworked or when a person suffers from muscular prostration, ulcer, fatigue or stomach trouble.

Fish and fish broth are high in phosphorus, potassium, calcium, sodium, chlorine and also iodine and many trace elements if they are ocean fish. Fish broth has remarkable nerve-restoring vitality. It is not a stimulant but a vitalizer to brain and nerves. Its oil is soothing to the nervous system. This is also reportedly true of the broth of clams, oysters, lobster, crab and sea mussels. Mussels, however, can be very toxic in polluted water or during certain times of the year.

Protein Drinks

Protein drinks can be made in considerable variety to please a range of tastes. I believe the people of the United States eat too much protein, but to make a graceful transformation to a less stressful way of life, we must still use some protein to get there.

The following ingredients are recommended for protein drinks:

soybean milk powder
egg yolk
gelatin (without pork products in it)
wheat germ (or wheat germ oil)
vegetable broth powder
Brewer's yeast
dried raw milk powder
dried whey
lecithin (fresh)
skim milk (raw)
yogurt

Any two, three or four of the preceding can be used in a base of tea, pineapple juice or almost any other juice daily. They can be sweetened with honey, maple syrup, or concentrates of apple, cherry or grape juice, as found in your health food store. Use a tablespoon of any of the solids, excepting the vegetable broth powder which should be used only a teaspoon at a time, and yogurt, two tablespoons. Raw milk or pineapple juice or other liquid should be about ¾ glass, while fruit concentrates and sweeteners should be about a tablespoon.

Recipe #1
1 tbs Soy milk powder
1 tbs Gelatin
1 Egg yolk
1 tbs Grape concentrate
¾ glass Water

Recipe #2
¾ glass Raw milk
1 tbs Wheat germ oil
1 tbs Lecithin
1 tsp Vegetable broth powder

Recipe #3
½ glass Pineapple juice
½ glass Skim milk
1 tbs Brewer's yeast

Recipe #4
¾ glass Tomato juice
1 tbs Wheat germ
1 tbs Gelatin
1 tbs Brewer's yeast

Broths

There are two broths I have used that have often brought about such spectacular results with patients that I recommend them with great enthusiasm.

Vital Broth (Potato Peeling Broth)

This high potassium broth has brought many people out of their beds and on their feet again. It is highly effective in any heavy catarrhal, acidic condition.

Basic Recipe

Peel 2 medium-sized potatoes and simmer peelings only in a pint and a half of water for 15 min. Strain and drink broth only. Repeat once or twice a day for over a month.

For a more elaborate but equally potent broth for elimination try:

2 c. potato peelings
2 c. carrot tops
3 c. celery
½ tsp. veg. broth powder
2 c. celery tops
2 qts. distilled water
Add a carrot or onion for more flavor if desired.

Finely chop or grate vegetables and greens, add to water. Bring slowly to boil, simmer about 20 min. Strain off broth and drink one or two cups per day.

Veal joint broth is another potent broth, rich in sodium and excellent for rheumatism, arthritis and catarrhal elimination. It is good for the glands, stomach, bowel, ligaments and joints, and helps keep the body young.

Get a clean, fresh, uncut veal joint and wash thoroughly in cold water. Put in large cooking pot, cover half with water, and add the following vegetables and greens cut up fine.

1½ c. apple peelings (½ in. thick)
2 c. potato peelings
½ c. okra, fresh or canned or 1 tsp. powdered okra
1 large parsnip
1 onion
2 beets, grated
½ c. chopped parsley
1 stalk celery

Simmer all ingredients 4-5 hrs. and strain off liquid, throwing solids away. There should be about one and a half quarts of liquid when done. Drink a cup hot or warm, store remainder in refrigerator. Soy sauce can be added for flavor.

Broths may be made of any meat, fish or bones, provided they are fresh, with the addition of many combinations of vegetables and grains. To give more of a fruit flavor add apples (or peelings), plums, prunes, lemons, limes.

Tonics

Tonics have had a "bad press" over the past two decades because unscrupulous manufacturers have made false claims about relatively worthless liquids they were selling. Even before, during the frontier days of America and the medieval and renaissance periods in Europe, worthless tonics have been sold by traveling quacks. Any honest nutritionist, however, knows there are honest food drinks with the power to invigorate, strengthen, restore, purify and build up the body. A tonic is not fit to be called a tonic if it doesn't accomplish some good for a person's health.

As life goes on and youthful vitality gradually fades, our work, attitudes, habits, dispositions, eating, drinking, ailments and various other conditions may draw upon our body chemistry in such a way that serious deficiencies creep up on us, affecting our comfort, well being and health. To supply that which is needed is often the purpose of a good tonic.

A tonic is basically a restorative of lost energy, and there are many good ones with special names and purposes.

Blood Stir: Extracts cooked from garlic, leeks or onions seem to have a beneficial effect on the lungs and general circulation in times of colds, coughing, sore throats and tender upper respiratory tracts. We do not consider this a cure but a tonic, a substance for building the body so it can heal itself. It should be taken steaming hot, with honey.

California Sun Glow: Two or more egg yolks, tbs. grated almond, juice from 2-4 oranges, tsp. concentrated parsley juice, tsp. honey. Blend and serve.

Hormone Stir: 1 tsp. sarsaparilla, juniper berries (two), tsp. wintergreen, 10 dandelion flowers, 15 red clover buds, per cup of water, served steaming hot upon retiring. Add a little honey for sweetening. This cleanses the blood and tissues, improves assimilation and rejuvenates the glands if used several times a week for two or three weeks.

Health Puff: Two-thirds cup wild blackberry juice, 1 egg yolk, one third cup concentrated oat water (simmer clean, whole oats in water for 10 hours, use liquid). Add tablespoon honey.

Laxades are cleansers. The juice of beets, celery, limes, tamarinds and thyme have solvent properties. Juniper berry drinks are laxades to the kidneys. Elderberry juice is a laxade to the sexual system. A mixture of whipped egg white, water and celery juice is a laxade to the stomach. There are many types and combinations of laxades.

General Laxade: One cup prunes, 1 c. raisins, 1 c. figs, 1 c. orange (with peelings), ¼ c. senna leaves. Cover with water in saucepan, simmer 20 min., strain. Add 2 tbs. honey, boil again for 10 min. Take ½ cup before retiring.

Cooling Laxade: Juice from 6 limes and 1 grapefruit, 1 tbs. cucumber juice, ½ cup distilled water. Add ice, shake and serve.

Calming Laxade: One cup mulberry juice. Add ice, shake and serve. Calms the whole system wonderfully.

Solvent Laxade: Three-fourths c. tomato juice, 1 tsp. lime juice, juice from one orange. Shake with ice, serve cold.

Alkaline Laxade: One-half cup pineapple juice, ¼ c. raw spinach juice, ¼ c. distilled water, add wintergreen juice to flavor. Shake with ice, serve cold.

Digestive System Laxade: One-half cup rye water (from 3 c. whole clean rye covered with water, brought slowly to boiling point, removed and strained); add ½ c. lettuce juice, 1 tbs. goat whey (Whex). Mix well, drink warm or cold.

Bowel Laxade: Add 1 tbs. goat whey to 1 cup hot water upon arising. In 15 min. or so drink a cup of coffee. This acts energetically upon the bowels of some.

Blood Laxade: A few leaves each of leaf lettuce, cabbage, beets, watercress, dandelion, endive, run through juicer. (Or, blend with small amount of water in blender, strain off enough liquid for ½ cup). Add juice from 1 asparagus and 1 medium carrot. Mix and drink fresh.

Cleansing and Vitalizing Laxade: One-half c. raw beet juice, ¼ c. green pepper juice, ¼ c. raw meat juice. Season with vegetable broth powder. Add 1 tbs. grated almonds, run through blender and drink.

Sleep Restorer: Equal parts hop buds, lettuce juice, mulberry juice. Flavor with nutmeg.

Pickup Tonic: Extract pericarp essence of barley by soaking barley bran in cold water until an oily substance floats to the top, then skimming it off. Add to fresh raw juice of celery, parsley, thyme, beet greens and spinach. Drink.

Portland Special: Combine juices from 1 bunch parsley, 3 stalks celery with 1 cup raw meat juice, 1 tsp. oat extract, ½ cup sarsaparilla, 1 can clam juice. Drink warm to hot for a fast pick-me-up high in iron, chlorophyll, sodium and many trace elements.

Skin Food: One c. oatstraw, ½ c. dandelion buds, 1 green pepper, handful of nasturtium. Cook 40 minutes, strain and drink. Helps clear up and build new, chemically balanced skin.

It is suprising how easily the coffee-and-donut habit can be replaced by a raw juice habit, with wonderful benefits to health. Raw juices can be prepared the night before, kept in a thermos and taken to work the next morning. At work, we can take a juice break while others are taking their coffee break.

Raw juices are not miracle cures for anything, nor will you experience a dramatic change in health overnight when you use them. But, over a period of time, little by little, the cells and tissues are revitalized, rebuilt, rejuvenated, by nature's own biochemical formulations.

Juices contain the life essence of the plant, chemical elements in their most potent, most easily assimilated form. Their nutrients are assimilated into the bloodstream faster than solid food, and juices do not require the considerable energy expenditure required to digest solid foods. Juices, then, are ideal for conditions in which body energy needs to be conserved or devoted to eliminating toxic substances from the body. There are times when our digestive system can benefit from a rest.

Unlike drugs, there are no undersirable side effects with raw juices. Only desirable ones. They benefit people of all ages equally, from babies to centenarians, and they are much superior to the cola drinks, fruit-flavored sugar water drinks and ades, caffeinated drinks and various other beverages mankind has invented in imitation of Nature or in an attempt to surpass Nature's ways. Raw juices build health. Most commercial drinks either tear down health or fail to build it, at best.

Use of juices in fasting or extreme diet therapies has been effective in numerous cases of chronic and degenerative disease, but it must always be done under a doctor's supervision. In one case, a man remained on a strict carrot juice diet for over a year after his doctor told him he had terminal cancer. When he went back for his checkup, it was gone. A woman with open running leg ulcers who had been to some of the top medical clinics and specialists in the United States was healed only after she turned to raw, fresh juices from green leafy vegetables. No other medication helped.

We are made of the dust of the earth, but the greatest part of our body weight is liquid and the liquids of our bodies carry vital nutrients to the cells, carry out wastes, lubricate, protect and serve in many life-giving capacities in the body. Raw juices, tonics and broths strengthen and vitalize our body liquids because of the "life essences" they carry from plants nourished by soil, air, sun and water.

Extreme raw juice fasts and diets may occasionally be necessary to correct some extreme imbalance in the body, but they are not the ultimate goal on the path to health. Our goal should be a balanced body chemistry and the high level well being that goes along with it, which comes only when we get away from diets and extremes and into the variety of foods and drinks that we find available in God's garden.

Garlic

We have found that many people have sores that will not heal well on the outside of their body. If they will take a clove of garlic and crush it into a paste, put it over the sore just once, a scab will form. Leave it on until it falls off. Many of these external sores have healed up beautifully. The garlic, when mixed with lanolin makes a wonderful salve in many skin diseases and blemishes. We have used apple cider vinegar very successfully, by applying it to skin blemishes and external sores. However, when there are any sores which do not heal, it might be well to be under a doctor's care, so he may watch and follow through with these conditions.

There is a wonderful liquid chlorophyll. Use this as a nasal douche: 1/4 tsp to 1/2 C of water. Sniff this into the nose. also drink 1 tsp in a glass of water three times a day. We have found this very effective in sinus disturbances and inflamed nasal membranes.

There are three foods that dietitians, as a rule, say are not good for us; these are cranberries, rhubarb and prunes. It is said they are not good because of the acids they contain. Personally, I don't believe that rhubarb and cranberries should be used more than once or twice a year—at Thanksgiving and Christmas—we all try to have meals on those days that practically kill us! (In fact, my busiest days are the days after these holidays; the same with almost every doctor. It is because of the crazy combinations we eat.)

Rhubarb is a laxative, very high in oxalic acid. Cranberries are also high in acid. I don't advise using these two. But prunes, while high in acid, may be eaten along with some of the alkaline foods because they have a nerve salt that is especially good for the nervous system and brain. If we would take prune juice and mix it with celery juice, which is very alkaline, we would have a splendid combination, a wonderful cocktail for the nervous system, one which would neutralize the nerve acids and feed the nerves at the same time. These liquefied cocktails, with a little imagination, can be concocted into fascinating combinations that will do wonders for our body and more than satisfy our taste buds. In a mixture like beet juice, coconut milk and a little celery juice, we have an excellent food for the stomach—one that is soothing and can be taken care of very nicely.

Chapter 42

Special and specialty foods

We find that Nature has provided an array of healing foods that are almost astonishing in the results they produce. Some of these are honeybee pollen, aloe vera, ginseng, malva (or mallow), microalgae, chlorophyll, herbs such as evening primrose and lady slipper and the vitamin A carotene combination. My experinece shows that there are no panaceas provided by Nature or modern science, yet we find that certain individuals may respond to a particular food with dramatic results, often to the equal surprise of both doctor and patient. Not all "miracle cures" through special foods or diets are myths. I have witnessed some amazing healings in the past 50 years. Yet, it is so often true that what brings wonderful results for one patient brings little or no relief to another (with the same symptoms), that we cannot enthusiastically promote any one food, herb or procedure to everyone with a certain disease like, for example, diabetes. The varying body chemistries of people make this impossible.

The special foods in this chapter have been tested in some cases by health researchers, nutritionists and doctors. Repeated verifications of certain healing powers (such as bee pollen's ability to build up the red blood cell count) indicate the reliability of the information but do not guarantee the same results for everyone.

Nevertheless, the foods in this chapter are very impressive, and all health professionals and serious students should be familiar with them.

The Carotene-Vitamin A Issue

Deficiency of vitamin A is at the root of more health problems than most people, even in the health professions, generally realize. A study by one doctor revealed that 70% of his patients were deficient in vitamin A, and I believe this deficiency is widespread throughout the general population.

Vitamin A is the anti-infection vitamin, protecting the integrity of all epithelial tissue — the skin and the surface layer of all mucous membranes and serous membranes. Deficiency causes dryness of the nasal and sinus passages, loss of cilia, impairment of secretion of the mucous membranes of the lungs and elsewhere and even interference with salivation. The result is vulnerability to infection and inflammation, the initial stage from which all chronic diseases develop. Vitamin A is needed to form visual purple (rhodopsin), necessary for vision, and night blindness is the best known vitamin A deficiency symptom. In severe cases, eye disease and blindness can result.

Tests have shown that animals deprived of vitamin A do not grow due to the halting of bone growth. When tissue reserves of vitamin A are completely gone, the animals die. Acne, and other skin diseases, commonly arise when this vitamin is short in the body, while tissue in the ovaries or testicles atrophies to the point of loss of reproduction capability. There is some evidence that steroid hormone production is impaired by vitamin A deficiency, possibly because of the body's inability to convert cholesterol into the steroids without it.

The liver is the great detoxifier of the body, and vitamin A deficiency affects it in several ways. When this vitamin is lacking, inflammation and infection in the body generate toxins which must be handled by the liver. If the quantity of toxins becomes excessive, the liver is overloaded, and its function is impaired. Ironically, one of its most important functions is storage of vitamin A (also stored in kidneys, lungs and fatty tissue). Excessive use of alcohol and drugs can destroy liver tissue, reducing its capacity to store vitamin A. Diseases like hepatitis and cirrhosis can do the same thing. Since vitamin A circulates through the body bound to a plasma protein manufactured by the liver, there is a limit to the amount of damage the liver can take without creating a chronic vitamin A deficiency, an extremely dangerous condition. With the liver already impaired, the deterioration of epithelial tissue due to lack of vitamin A allows airborne toxins, heavy metals, bacteria and viruses to penetrate tissue and cause infections with little to stop them from the body's natural immune system.

It is evident that vitamin A should be given at the onset of any infection, cold or flu. Excessive amounts of vitamin A are recognized as toxic, but pro-vitamin A carotene is safe in any quantity.

While most commercial preparations of vitamin A come from fish liver oils, vegetables such as carrots, yellow squash, corn, spinach and all green, leafy vegetables are excellent sources of carotene or provitamin A. Carotene is an excellent source of vitamin A.

Many doctors caution against drinking too much carrot juice because of possible carotenemia — yellowing of the skin. This condition has no harmful effects and disappears when the intake is reduced. It can be due to an undersize or hypoactive liver. Carrot juice taken in small doses throughout the day can be tolerated by anyone.

At my sanitarium in Escondido, California, we grew 3,000 pounds of carrots per month to provide juice for our patients. I believe carotene as combined with vitamin A in nature is best and I have found carrot juice to be the most effective form. While I have used heavy doses of fish oil vitamin A with some patients, it was generally for skin disorders. Use of large amounts of vitamin A should always be under a doctor's supervision.

I have seen many patients helped greatly by vitamin A in carrot juice. One study has shown that adequate daily intake of vitamin A keeps cholesterol down.

The famous 19-year Western Electric study showed that those who used foods high in beta-carotene (the most common carotene in foods) tended to have a lower risk of lung cancer. In fact, the most carotene taken, the lower the cancer incidence was. The National Cancer Institute has stated that the risk of certain cancers can be reduced up to 40% when the diet is high in beta-carotene, and a Cancer survey in Norway has confirmed these findings. Harvard University has started a 5-year study with 200,000 participants to see how effective beta-carotene is in reducing a variety of types of cancer.

Why do people become deficient in vitamin A? The most obvious reason is that they do not eat enough foods rich in vitamin A, green, leafy vegetables, yellow vegetables and fruits, organ meats and egg yolk. Another reason is that cooking vegetables at high heat without a lid can cause loss of vitamin A. It can be destroyed at high heat in the presence of oxygen. Impaired liver function reduces the amount of this vitamin in the bloodstream, as does imbalance in fat metabolism. One doctor found that 70% of his patients were borderline or deficient in vitamin A.

In my experience, carotene is assimilated much more easily than vitamin A from fish oil capsules or organ meats. Raw carrots and carrot juice are the best sources.

Vitamins A and D are thought to interact by some researchers, affecting the calcium metabolism. It is known that lack of vitamin A results in lack of bone growth, which is generally considered to be affected by vitamin D. But calcium has many other functions in the body besides bone growth. It is needed by the nerves, muscles and to some extent, all cells of the body (along with phosphorus). Calcium stimulates iron absorption, and anemia is often accompanied by low calcium. To the extent that vitamins A and D work together to normalize calcium metabolism, vitamin A can be said to have an indirect role in counteracting simple anemia. Low calcium is also found in asthma, many upper respiratory conditions, severe menstrual cramping, slow healing of broken bones, brittle fingernails and osteoporosis. Vitamin A might be the answer to bringing up the calcium level in many of these cases.

Other conditions associated with deficiency of vitamin A include canker sores, dry mouth, hay fever, sinusitis, ringing of the ears, enlarged or infected tonsils, skin rashes, gallstones, high blood cholesterol, leucorrhea, headache, diabetes, hair loss and cataracts.

Because so many of the problems resulting from vitamin A deficiency are accompanied by a sluggish, toxic or hypoactive liver, we must consider the easiest assimilable form of this vitamin under such conditions. Carrot juice is the best choice at present. In the near future, we may see the development of micronutrient suppliments which make carotene-vitamin A available in a high potency, highly-assimilable form.

Foods high in vitamin A include:

Apricots	Whole milk
Peaches	Liver
Carrots	Eggs
Sweet potatoes	Cod liver oil
Watercress	Carotene
Butter	Peas
Cheese	Spinach
Cream	Parsley

Malva Or Mallow

Malva (or mallow, in English) is an herb of many uses. It is called eibish in German, gui mauve in French and its Latin name, recognizable by all herbalists and botanists irrespective of nationality or mother tongue, is Althea Officinalis.

Most of us are familiar with marshmallows, the white, sugary pellets bobbing and melting in a cup of hot chocolate or impaled on sticks to be roasted over the coals of a campfire. Originally, however, marshmallows were made from the mucilage obtained from the root of the malva plant (or mallow) combined with eggs and sugar to be made into a soothing poultice used on a patient's sore chest as a cure.

In Europe, the flowers and root of Althea Officinalis are used for many purposes. In America, only the root is usually used. The ingredients of Althea Officinalis are as follows: 37% starch, 11% pectin, 1.25% fat, 25-30% mucilage, 11% sugar, 2% asparagine. The root contains a mucilage-like substance which has a soothing effect on the intestines. It is often made into a decoction to alleviate the inflammation of mucous membranes and is effective as a demulcent. It may be taken as a tea or as an enema.

The leaves, flowers and root of malva may be crushed or powdered to make a poultice which will take care of the most obstinate inflammation. As a decoction, it has been helpful as a vaginal douche, an eye wash or a sitz bath for rectal irrigation. Taken internally, it is said to help heal ulcers and colitis.

Hollyhocks are in the malva family. They were often grown around the farm house as much for medicinal purposes as for their lovely tall stalks with broad fan-like leaves and cheerfully colored flowers.

The order Malvaceae which includes the previously mentioned marshmallows and hollyhocks also includes other herbs in the mallow family. All of them are known for their soothing and demulcent properties and are not toxic. They should not be used, however, when there is a bowel obstruction or any other serious bowel disorder.

The order Malvaceae has edible leaves and flowers which may be added to soups or prepared as ingredients for syrups, teas and wine. The tops of the plants may be eaten in soups and salads, and the purplish flower of the mallow can be used as an edible decoration of fresh-cut salads. The flowers may be harvested in August and September and have a mild, pleasant scent.

Mallows have healing, softening and soothing effects. Root infusions are reported to be good for urinary tract infections. Mallow is also good for the lungs, kidneys and bladder. The liquid from boiled leaves and roots may be drunk by nursing mothers to increase milk flow. This potion helps speed delivery also and eases painful urination. Eating the leaves and stalks of malva is said to relieve the pain of gonorrhea.

When the roots and seeds of malva are boiled in white wine and the resultant ointment is massaged into the breasts, it eases swelling and inflammation. The seeds may be steeped in vinegar and used as a skin wash. In order to relieve itching, bruise the leaves of malva and lay them on itchy, inflamed skin or insect bites. Boil the juice of malva stalks and leaves in oil and apply gently to the skin to alleviate roughness; rub it into the scalp to help prevent hair from falling out.

There is a lot of mucilage in malva's leaves and stalks, and it is known to be a soothing extract. You can boil the flowers in oil or water, add honey and a pinch of alum to use as a gargle. The American Indians were probably the first to apply the leaves as a poultice.

To make cough drops (lozenges) for hoarsness and coughing, use malva as follows: 1½ oz. powdered marshmallow root, 4½ oz. brown sugar and enough gum tragacanth mucilage to make drops of the mixture on a waxed paper. Orris root or orange flower water may be added to give a pleasant scent for the lozenges.

It is useful to know that malva may be used in conjunction with other herbs after being soaked overnight in cold water. It should be strained before adding a small amount to any other herb tea. Honey may be stirred in to suit taste. The tea made from malva has a tendency to seem slimy and somewhat unpleasant to the eye and taste buds, which is why it is a good idea to use it in mixture.

Some years ago, I visited the Hunza Valley and stayed with the King. The Hunzans were a hardy, healthy people who often lived to be over a hundred years of age, some considerably longer. But at the time I was there, a problem had come up and the King asked my advice.

He told me that many Hunzans of all ages were developing painful eye problems, dryness of the eye surface, with ulcers and some cases of bleeding. A few had gone blind. This was a classic case of vitamin A deficiency, but in the primitive Hunza Valley, no vitamin pills were available. What could be done? I told him I would do what I could, and I began thinking about what foods and herbs with vitamin A were available in the area.

As often is true, the solution lay right beside the problem. Malva grew everywhere in the Hunza Valley, but no one there realized it could be eaten. I brought some to the king and showed him what malva looked like. "Tell the people to pick it and eat it while they're outside working or going somewhere," I suggested. "They can eat as much as they want. It has no toxic effects." The king was delighted.

Within a short span of time after I left, I was informed that the problem had been brought under control.

Malva is certainly an herb of many uses, an herb for all seasons and many reasons.

Honeybee Pollen

Honeybee pollen is the only nutritionally complete food known to man. Each grain is an incredible storehouse of the vitamins, minerals, enzymes, co-enzymes, hormones, amino acids, carbohydrates, fatty acids and trace elements identified as being needed by the human body. Of all the natural foods, bee pollen is claimed to be the most complete and the most complex. Chemical analysis reveals the presence of certain unidentified mysterious compounds that may account for bee pollen's ability to correct the chemical balance of the body and restore normal functions, thus helping the body to rid itself of any abnormal or unhealthy condition.

Bee pollen is not only said to be the most potent and richest food in nature, its composition is unequalled by any other food. It is a pure, live vegetable source of all nutrients and is actually richer in protein than any animal source. Bee pollen is reported to contain 5 to 7 times more of the essential amino acids than meat, cheese or eggs of equal weight, plus all other nutrients in abundance.

Studies have shown that subjects fed only bee pollen and water under controlled fasting conditions were actually in better health at the close of the lengthy experiment than at the beginning, proving bee pollen to be not only nutritionally complete, but the perfect survival food as well.

Many "old wives tales" attibute the prevention or cure of just about every common ailment, from arthritis and allergies through colds, sore throats and stomach upsets, to be a spoonful of honey taken regularly. It is important to remember that in olden times, all honey was taken right from the comb and was loaded with pollen particles. When modern researchers attempted to find out whether there was a scientific basis to these old stories, they used the honey commercially sold today. This honey is usually clarified by heating and straining, reducing its quality to that of only a sweet. With the pollen particles removed no curative properties were observed.

Analysis of Bee Pollens

Keeping in mind that bee pollens differ from area to area, the following analysis of the main ingredients of bee pollen made from clover gives some idea of its nutritional power.

Moisture	23.9%
Solids	76.1%
Protein	20.2%
Ash	2.7%

ENZYMES AND COENZYMES

Disstase	Phosphatase
Amylase	Catalase
Saccharase	Diaphorase
Pectase	Cozymase
(and others)	

CARBOHYDRATES
Sucrose
Levulose/Fructose
Glucose

FATTY ACIDS

Caproic	Caprylic
Capric	Lauric
Myristic	Palmitic
Palmitoleic	Stearic
Linoleic	Oleic
(and others)	

MINERALS

Calcium	Potassium
Phosphorus	Magnesium
Iron	Manganese
Copper	Silicon
Sulphur	Sodium
Zinc	Iodine
(and others)	

VITAMINS
All of B complex, C, D, E, K, biotin, choline, inositol, rutin.

AMINO ACIDS (percent)

Arginine	5.3	Methionine	1.9
Histidine	2.5	Phenylalanine	4.1
Isoleucine	5.1	Threonine	4.1
Leucine	7.1	Tryptophan	1.4
Lysine	6.4	Valine	5.8

Plus Cystine, Tyrosine, Glutamic Acid, Glycine, Serine, Proline, Alanine, Aspartic Acid, and others.

MISCELLANEOUS
Fats and oils 5%
Carotenoids and other pigments
Waxes, resins, steroids, growth factors, guanine, lecithin (about 15%), nucleic acids, flavenoids, various amines, phenolic acids and many more.

Health Research And Pollen

In France, pollen has been tested for value in taking care of a number of disease conditions and physical problems. Pollen was judged to be helpful in raising the red blood count, killing bacteria and other harmful microorganisms, stimulating appetite and growth in sickly children and aiding many bowel conditions.

Children in tuberculosis sanitariums were given a teaspoon of pollen per day in a glass of juice at breakfast. Within a month the red blood cell count increased by as much as 800,000. Bee pollen is considered one of the best ways to get rid of anemia.

The effectiveness of pollen in bowel conditions is well tested. Constipation, diarrhea and spastic activity disappeared when pollen was taken every day. It has proven effective in taking care of many cases of colitis. In one case of diverticulosis, bouts of diarrhea, constipation and bloody mucus in the stools stopped two weeks after taking two teaspoons of pollen per day. Fevers stopped, and the patient, who had been losing weight for eight months, gained two pounds in one month. Two cases of chronic constipation not helped by the usual laxatives were completely relieved with bee pollen. Pollen appears to restore natural bowel regularity in those who use it.

The Russians have reported success in treating nervous and endocrine disorders with pollen.

A young teenager with rheumatism in the joints and neck vertebrae was given cortisone and was sent to a sanitarium for recovery. He had catarrh problems, fatigue and no appetite, and he stopped growing in weight and height for eight months. Given a tablespoon of pollen each day, his appetite returned and he gained

311

15 pounds and 2 inches in height during the next six months.

Allergies treated with pollen have shown excellent response. Dr. Leo Conway of Denver, Colorado, using pollen gathered from botanists, gave oral doses to his allergy patients instead of the usual shots, at one-third to one-half the usual cost. Of 6,200 early cases, 94 percent became completely free from symptoms. The doctor later compiled a total of 60,000 documented cases.

Acne has been treated with pollen with considerable success.

Weight reduction can be achieved with bee pollen by taking it before meals. It depresses the appetite while providing plenty of energy. Pollen itself is only about 90 calories per ounce, which makes it ideal for weight control without requiring special starvation diets.

Bee pollen can't be heated or used in cooking without destroying the enzymes that make it such a powerful supplement. It can, however, be stored in the refrigerator or freezer to protect its potency.

In the U.S., Dr. Kilmer McCully of Harvard Medical School discovered that heart disease is often initiated by a deficiency of pyridoxine (vitamin B_6) and an increase of methionine. Foods with a high B_6 to methionine ratio may prevent some types of heart disease. Carrots have a ratio of 15 to 1, bananas have a ratio of 40 to 1, but honeybee pollen has an incredible ratio of 400 to 1, the best of any known food substance.

German researchers used pollen on patients receiving radiation treatments. Pollen was taken three times a day with meals for three days before treatments, during treatments and afterward. The usual side-effects from radiation, such as hair loss, did not occur. Patients who took the same treatments but without pollen supplements experienced the usual side effects.

Bee pollen was tested on prostate conditions by a German and Swedish urology team, with excellent results. It has been reported that pollen contains a hormone similar to the pituitary hormone that stimulates the sex glands.

Former Russian Olympic coach Remi Korchemny studied the effects of bee pollen on athletes, showing that regular use improves the recovery power of athletes. Those using bee pollen were able to equal or better their running time for a given distance soon after the previous run. A control group of athletes on placebos remained fatigued and did poorly on a repeat run under identically the same conditions.

Lars-Eric Essen, a Swedish dermatologist has researched the beauty benefits of pollen. He has reported that pollen prevents premature aging of the skin, protects against dehydration and smoothes away wrinkles.

Many reports of bee pollen restoring sexual potency have been published. It is said to have been successful in a number of persons in their 70's and 80's. Pollen is 15% lecithin, which makes up most of the male semen.

Pollen is best when it is fresh and natural, since it can lose up to 76% of its nutritional value in a year. The only completely satisfactory method of preserving fresh pollen is flash-freezing at zero degrees. Some researchers recommend 130 mg of pollen per day to prevent disease and enhance well being.

Propolis And Royal Jelly

Propolis is made from a resin gathered by bees from the buds of trees and is formed into a kind of glue-varnish for coating the interior of the beehive and sealing all the cracks. It is about 5 percent pollen, 30 percent wax, 55 percent resins and balms and 10 percent oils. Propolis is also loaded with vitamins, minerals, amino acids, flavinoids and ferulic acid. Scraped from the insides of hives, propolis has been found to have a potent effectiveness against germlife and viruses, a natural antibiotic effect.

The Russians have been using propolis for over seventeen years to treat bowel and kidney conditions, allergies, hypertension and vascular problems.

Royal Jelly is a highly potent nutrient fed by nurse bees to the queen bee, who may lay several thousand eggs per day and who lives five or six years as compared to the life span of the worker bees who live from 28 to 42 days. It is said to prolong life, build up the sex glands and restore vitality more rapidly than any other food.

Summary

Bee pollen is one of the most potent foods we can find to assist the body in throwing off disease producing conditions and in building the health toward high level well being. Along with propolis, it appears to have a natural antibiotic ingredient which kills germlife. It contains high quality proteins and sugars, and normalizes bowel funciton. In my experience, a sluggish bowel is one of the greatest contributors to disease conditions in the body, and any food which exerts a cleansing, toning and stimulating effect on the bowel is a wonderful thing to use.

Pollen has been found to be an excellent source of protein, as is royal jelly. Taken before meals, it aids in weight loss; taken after meals, it aids in weight gain. Experiments in many countries have shown that it is effective in assisting the body to get rid of many disease conditions.

Aloe Vera

The aloe vera plant (aloe barbadensis) has been used for thousands of years for healing purposes, and its

312

benefits have been repeatedly verified by modern researchers, some of them doctors. However, the stories of its miraculous power to cure everything should be disregarded. There is no such thing as a panacea, and the effectiveness of aloe vera for the cases we know of should be taken at face value and no more.

Aloe vera is a succulent with long, pointed leaves growing outward from a central stem. Along the edges of the leaves grow sharp rubbery barba, and it is inside the thick leaves that we find the fleshy gel used for healing purposes. Although aloe vera has been analyzed carefully, it contains so many biochemically active ingredients — enzymes, vitamins, minerals, amino acids and other chemical compounds — that no researcher has been successful in explaining how it works. It is fair to say that different combinations of its ingredients probably go to work on different conditions on and in the body. Aloe vera has no known toxic side effects.

Estimates of the number of chemical ingredients in aloe vera have gone as high as 75. The rind is known to produce a cathartic action, and it is most often peeled off when the aloe vera is to be taken internally. Chemical elements in aloe vera are known to include calcium, chlorine, manganese, potassium, sodium and sulfur. Vitamins are B-1, niacin, B-2, B-6, vitamin C and choline. Eighteen of the known amino acids are found in it, along with fourteen anthra quinnones which are believed to kill germlife, relieve inflammation and perhaps reduce itching. Amino acids, of course, are the protein building blocks which form new tissue. Sugars found include glucose, mannose, rhamnose, pentose, and aldonentose, which provide energy for healing, movement and fuel for cell processes. Saponins were found, which have antiseptic and cleansing properties. There may be as many as 30 enzymes, but only 5 have been identified. Enzymes are living, biologically active substances that trigger chemical reactions and speed up the repair and building of tissue. Researchers say there are around 900 enzymes in the human body.

To summarize, there are a great many possible combinations of healing components and properties in aloe vera, and we don't need to know exactly how they work as long as we know they get results. We may simply note that calcium, manganese, amino acids and enzymes are always involved in any healing process. Other components no doubt assist.

Conditions Helped By Aloe Vera

Aloe vera has been taken internally for stomach ulcers, colitis, arthritis, respiratory conditions and muscle cramps. The colitis is taken care of faster when aloe vera gel is used additionally in enemas. With arthritis, external applications also speed up relief. Some dramatic results have been reported in the healing of respiratory conditions. As a preventative tonic, aloe vera may be taken daily with meals, from one tablespoon to two ounces, depending on the condition and preference of the user. Many persons have said their general feeling of well being was much improved after using aloe vera as a tonic. It seems to act as a general cleansing agent in the internal organs, helping the body throw off toxins. It is also good in getting rid of worms and has been used by people of all ages for this purpose.

All sorts of digestive problems are helped by aloe — acid indigestion, food allergy reactions, gas, heartburn, stomach ills and ileitis. Of course, all of these conditions need to be taken care of by appropriate diet changes as well.

External: Because aloe vera relieves pain, reduces inflammation and swelling, soothes the skin, kills germlife and fungus, and stimulates healing, it is very effective for a broad array of external conditions. Sunburn, burns, cuts, bruises, infections, boils, bedsores, acne, insect stings and bites, eczema, psoriasis, dandruff, athlete's foot, ringworm, cold sores, shingles, hemmorhoids, vaginitis, skin ulcers and other external problems have responded well to applications of aloe vera gel or lotion. For any condition expected to take a week or longer to heal, it is best to take the aloe vera internally three times a day as well as applying it externally.

Infections and boils. A poultice is often best, made out of freshly ground aloe vera leaves. Cut off the spurs along the side of the leaf, chop leaf up fine (or put in a blender briefly), and heat in saucepan or double boiler until it is as hot as the person can take it. (Do not boil.) Apply hot and leave on an hour or longer, if possible. A gauze bandage can be placed over the poltice to hold it all day. Change it every 12 hours.

Dandruff, ringworm, athlete's foot, fingernail fungus: Full strength gel is used in direct application. For dandruff, apply gel liberally and allow to remain on hair for half hour, then shampoo. Do this daily until dandruff is gone. For ringworm on the head, cut hair short, if possible; shampoo head, rinse and dry (ringworm is contagious, so towel used to dry head must be laundered before use by others); massage in gel, comb the hair and leave the gel on. Repeat daily until cured. If the ringworm is on another part of the body, wash it daily and put on the gel. Athlete's foot, "jungle rot", or fungus under the fingernails can be killed by daily full strength applications of aloe vera gel. Use at least twice a day for athlete's foot and more often for "jungle rot" and fingernail fungus. Stubborn cases may linger more than a month, but the fungicidal properties of aloe vera are proven and will eventually do the job.

Sunburn, cuts, insect stings and bites, mild burns: Aloe vera lotion or gel relieves pain and prevents itching, also disinfects. For bee stings, *do not remove with tweezers,* or poison will be forced into wound; instead, scrape the stinger out sideways with the edge of a knife blade, then apply aloe vera.

Serious burns: Always consult a doctor first when the skin is broken or damaged by a burn. In most cases, however, the burned area should be washed in cold water, patted dry and covered with applications of aloe, which is famous for its effectiveness with burns. Vitamin E can be put on top of the first layer of gel, before other layers are added. Healing often takes place without scars. In one case of terrible burns to a person's feet, healing did not take place, despite the use of antibiotics and everything in the usual medical arsenal, until gauze bandages soaked in aloe vera were put over the burned areas. This, however, was done under a doctor's supervision, and it should not be attempted by nonprofessionals.

Bruises and oozing scrapes (strawberries): Athletes and others who get deep bruises and those painful skinned spots called strawberries will reduce pain and speed up healing by applying aloe gel.

Vaginitis: This can be caused by fungus, bacterial infection, toxic condition due to underactive colon, or physical irritation. Aloe gel helps in all cases. (I don't know if it has been tried on Herpes II, but it appears to help in Herpes simplex cases.) Dilute aloe gel for use as douche, and make suppositories of full-strength gel using capsules available at health stores. Take aloe internally 3 times daily, as well.

Colitis, hemorrhoids: Aloe has been shown to be very effective with both. For colitis, enemas are recommended with aloe added to enema water, plus taking aloe with meals 3 times daily. For hemorrhoids, aloe suppositories have helped trememdously, and application of the gel stops itching right away. Many have reported that hemorrhoids have been healed entirely over a period of time with aloe. The effectiveness of the suppositories is improved by taking small enemas first to cleanse the inside area.

Cold sores, Herpes simplex, sore teeth and gums, shingles: All these have responded well to aloe vera. Shingles can be relieved dramatically, and rapid healing has been reported. Aloe used as a frequent mouthwash gets rid of most cold sores and helps sore teeth and gums. Herpes blisters respond fast to aloe. Use repeat applications.

Acne, eczema, psoriasis: These three conditions need long-term diet changes for complete healing, but aloe vera has given dramatic results in many cases. Must be taken internally 3 times daily as well as applied externally for best results.

Bedsores and skin ulcers: When these refuse to heal, problems with chemicals lacking in the body are evident. Usually, it takes a long time to acquire a bedsore (generally these are at the end of the spine), and they are found most commonly in invalids and elderly persons confined to bed. However, I knew of a three-year-old girl who had a sore from birth which resembled a bedsore and stubbornly resisted healing, as bedsores do. Applications of aloe vera, again, can aid in the healing process. Skin ulcers, especially when they are oozing putrid matter, often indicate kidney problems, poor circulation to the legs and toxic blood. Aloe vera, taken internally and applied externally, can bring surprisingly rapid healing to these difficult ulcers. It may well be worth applying poultices the first two days before using the gel directly on the ulcers.

How To Prepare Aloe Vera

You can get aloe vera preparations in most health food stores, and these are very good, but most have stabilizers added. For this reason, I advise using fresh aloe vera wherever possible. Make sure it is aloe barbadensis, the true healing plant.

There are two ways to prepare aloe vera leaves for taking the plant internally. The green part of the leaves has strong laxative properties and is not needed for most internal applications. To prepare an infusion, take 8 ounces of aloe vera leaves, wash them and with a sharp knife trim away the sharp stickers along both sides and throw away. Slice thin sections of the leaf and put in a clean quart glass jar with lid. Add enough distilled water to fill the jar, put on the lid and refrigerate overnight. The gel will seep out of the cut sections of leaves, but the green outer covering of the leaf will not dissolve. Always stir the liquid before taking from one teaspoon to 2 ounces with each meal. The taste is mild to most people but it can be added to apple juice or grape juice if desired. When the jar is half empty, you can fill it full one more time with distilled water. When the latter is used up, make a fresh batch. Another way is to peel the leaves carefully with a potato peeler or thin paring knife, then liquify the clear inner part in a blender with some distilled water, if desired, for dilution. The more concentrated you make it, the less should be taken per dose.

For external application, we can use the full strength gel liquified in a blender as previously described, or we can cut off part of a new leaf and just rub the gel over the area of the body to be taken care of. Some people take a leaf, split it open and scrape the gel out with a spoon or knife to get as much as they want to use.

To make a poultice, the aloe skin can be used as described in the previous section on Infections and Boils, or it can be cut away and discarded. A bandage of sterile gauze soaked in aloe gel can be applied to the area instead of applying the thin mash of aloe directly. Poultices draw out toxic materials more efficiently when they are heated.

Suppositories are made from the large size gelatin capsules found in drug and health food stores. Refrigerate both capsules and aloe gel before filling capsules, and keep refrigerated afterward. To lubricate suppositories before insertion, simply dip into a little fresh aloe gel.

When applying aloe gel to cuts, burns, abrasions, etc., several coats are best. The thin film that builds up acts as a bandage.

Ginseng

Ginseng, so the story goes, was discovered in Manchuria perhaps four or five thousand years ago. The Chinese began to use it and carried it along their trade routes to India, Iran and Korea, where it became popular as a folk medicine and tonic. The Russsians most likely encountered it in Manchuria, and it is now one of the most widely researched herbs in that country. The Japanese, of course, picked it up from their Chinese neighbors. Ginseng has, in the past three decades, attracted a wide following in Europe and the United States.

The powers claimed for ginseng are nothing less than phenomenal. Its name comes from two Oriental words, "man" and "plant", or "man-plant", because the shape of the root (the only part of the plant that's used) looks something like the human form, and Chinese folklore says it promotes long life. Li Chung Yun, its most famous user, is said to have lived for 256 years.

Russian Research

Russian research, the most advanced so far, has established that ginseng strengthens the natural immune system and increases the body's resistance to disease and stress. Physical and mental efficiency are increased, blood sugar is reduced in diabetes and blood pressure is normalized. It is capable of revitalizing a fatigued person with a stimulant effect but without interfering with sleep. That is, it doesn't act like caffeine or other stimulant drugs. Ginseng stimulates the glandular functions, such as the pituitary, adrenals and sex glands. However, there are different kinds of ginseng with somewhat different properties.

Panax ginseng is the classic Asiatic species, while *panax quinquefolius* is the kind found in North America. *Panax notoginseng* from the mountains of southern China is a third type of ginseng, noted for its effectiveness in taking care of bleeding, from wounds to conditions like bleeding ulcers, menstrual problems, hemorrhoids, childbirth problems and others. American ginseng is reported to be good for fevers and stomach acidity, while the *panax ginseng* is most often used as a preventive tonic and a blood cleanser. It is not wise, however, to take ginseng for a specific condition unless a herbalist doctor is consulted.

The Makeup Of Ginseng

The ingredients of ginseng are known but not entirely understood. From its six glycosides, four saponins have been derived with known effects: Panaxin — improves circulation, panacene — improves digestion, panaquilon — stimulates endocrine glands, panaxapogenol — raises metabolism rate. The functions of two others panaxadiol and panaxatriol are unknown. One ginseng expert has suggested that the steriod substances in ginseng may help regulate the body's rate of burning of energy. Biochemicals in ginseng include aluminum, copper, cobalt, iron, manganese, silica and sulphur, while vitamins include B-1 and B-2. Like so many herbs and bioactive plants, the combined enzymes, sugars, vitamins and minerals together may be assumed to have healing and regulating effects in combination that simply can't be tested adequately when they are separated.

Ginseng's effect on the stress response of humans and animals is very specific. Normally, if stress is created by fright (for example), adrenaline is released from the adrenal glands to prepare the body for emergency action. Blood sugar goes up, the heart rate increases and so forth. If repeated "fright" situations are presented, adrenaline becomes more and more depleted. If ginseng is taken, however, the adrenaline remains high for a much longer period of time, allowing a more effective stress response.

Researchers believe that ginseng's reputation for promoting longevity may be due to one or more ingredients which neutralize harmful catabolic waste products that accumulate in the body as we grow older. If the body can be kept reatively clear of toxic substances, including metabolic waste products, cell regeneration and rejuvenation can continue indefinitely provided the necessary nutrients are supplied. Many of the long-lived Russians of the Caucasus Mountain region have taken ginseng all their lives.

The potential effect of ginseng in promoting longevity is consistant with French research in which elderly persons troubled with memory lapses, slow thinking and difficulty with most mental information processing showed some improvement after a week of taking ginseng and remarkable improvement after two months. (However, vitamin and mineral supplements were also given.) What this research may show is that toxic processes that interfere with brain function and contribute to aging are the same, or similar enough to be counteracted by the same substances — ginseng, vitamins and minerals, for example.

Korean and Russian research on the effect of ginseng on the stress response may have further implications as well. I do not doubt that stress plays a significant role in aging, simply because we know it plays a part in bringing on certain diseases, and it seems obvious that the wear and tear of stress and disease on the body accelerate aging. On the other hand, I believe peace of mind promotes peace and harmony in the body which contribute to long life. Both ancient Chinese tradition and modern research support the notion that ginseng contributes to peace of mind.

No doubt the properties responsible for cleansing the blood, stimulating protein metabolism and reducing fatigue also contribute to longer life and better brain function, which are closely linked. The brain controls and correlates physiological functions, and as gravitosis, anemia and nerve deterioration increase in the brain, the body goes downhill. The brain is the symphony conductor and the organs, tissues and glands of the body are the orchestra. Ginseng appears to keep the symphony conductor "on his toes," so to speak.

Heart and Circulation

Chinese research on the effects of tienchi-ginseng (panax notoginseng) on the heart and circulation has turned up some interesting results. At Wuhan and Kumming Medical Colleges, 89 heart patients with angina pectoris were given tienchi-ginseng powder orally. Of these 40 showed a good deal of improvement, 19 showed moderate improvement, 22 were slightly better and 8 were unchanged. Electrocardiograms and blood pressure checks verified reports of subjective improvement.

Chemical analysis revealed two sterols which reduced fats, cholesterol included, in the blood and also disclosed flavonoids which directly affected the heart and circulation.

Atheletes were tested with tienchi-ginseng, and it was found after hard exercise that the pulses of those taking the ginseng returned to normal (60/minute) after a 3-minute rest, while the pulse rates of the control group still averaged 120/minute. The morning resting pulse rates of the test group also dropped from an average of 55.8/minute to 50.5/minute, while the resting pulse of the controls was relatively unchanged.

How to Take Ginseng

Ginseng in capsules or liquid concentrate can be found in most health food stores, while the actual ginseng root may usually be found only in herb stores or in health food stores with large herbal sections. Experts warn that there is a wide range in quality of ginseng, and the potency of the root or its powder is directly related to the quality. Poor quality ginseng has little beneficial effect. The most consistently high quality ginseng is said to come from Korea. Buy ginseng from stores in which the people know where their ginseng comes from.

We find that ginseng should be taken in small doses. A little of the liquid concentrate, which looks like dark syrup, in a cup of herb tea twice a day is sufficient. Or, if capsules are selected, try one capsule morning and evening for one month, then two capsules morning and evening for one month to compare the difference. The object is to test the subjective response of the body. For best results, do not take fruit or vitamin C for 12 hours after using ginseng. Of course, that means it is best to take it in the evening.

Those who buy the raw root will take ginseng in a somewhat different manner. Dr. H.M. Wu, a California herbal doctor, advises that ginseng should never be cut with a metal knife. Instead, it should be steamed for 5 or 10 minutes to soften it enough to be cut by a nonmetallic implement. It can be eaten raw or steamed. Two small pieces of root (1 oz.) are enough, taking both morning and evening.

Tea can be made by heating 4 small ginseng pieces (1/8 oz.) in 3 cups of water in a double boiler. Cook over low heat until water is reduced to 1 cup. Then throw the ginseng pieces away and drink the tea. (The ginseng is worthless after the beneficial ingredients have been dissolved in the water.)

Unlike the American ginseng (panex quinquefolius), the tienchi-ginseng (panax notoginseng) should *not* be taken for colds and fevers. Pregnant women are also advised not to take the tienchi-ginseng.

We find that Nature has many remedies in her garden, and ginseng has been found to be one of the best. However, we must learn how to use the herbal remedies properly, and care must be taken when using even natural remedies in combination with one another. If in doubt, seek the advice of a qualified herbalist.

Chlorophyll

Chlorophyll is the pigment that makes plants green and allows them to synthesize food using the energy from sunshine. It is a powerful cleanser for the body when taken in foods, purifying the bloodstream, detoxifying the liver and building up the beneficial bacteria in the bowel. All green leafy vegetables are good sources of chlorophyll. It is found in generous amounts in microalgae such as chlorella and spirulina, and a liquid chlorophyll extract can be purchased in most health food stores.

The interesting thing about chlorophyll is that its porphyrin molecule is almost identical to the hemoglobin molecule of the blood. The difference is that chlorophyll has a magnesium atom at its center while the hemoglobin has iron. This may explain why chlorophyll is such an excellent blood builder, since it is almost always accompanied by iron in green plants. When we eat greens, then, we are getting the essential constituents of hemoglobin.

Many years ago, I took care of a young woman from Canada with an extreme case of anemia. She was a vegetarian, opposed to getting iron from such rich animal sources as liver, so I put her on an intense supplement schedule with liquid chlorophyll. In less than three months her red blood count was above normal. I have a great deal of respect for chlorophyll.

It has been reported that the U.S. Army has tested chlorophyll as a detoxifying agent for radioactive contamination and found it very effective. This powerful green cleanser also helps rid the body of pesticide and drug residues.

Spirulina and Chlorella

Spirulina and chlorella are green microalgae, available from many health food stores in powder or tablets, which are rich in protein, chlorophyll, vitamins and biochemical elements. Spirulina takes its name from the spiral shape which shows up under the microscope. Chlorella is a single-celled microalga, round in shape. By weight, spirulina has four times as much chlorophyll as alfalfa, while chlorella has forty times as much. Both are high in quality protein, with all the essential amino acids. Although the percentages of the contents vary, depending on the chemical composition of the nutrient medium in which they are grown, the following lists of ingredients are impressive as anyone can see.

	Chlorella (%)	Spirulina (%)
Protein	63	71
Carbohydrates	14	13
Lipids	11	7
Minerals	6-10	7
Chlorophyll	2.1	0.8
Fiber	1.0	0.9
Ash	6.3	9.0

Amino Acid Content of Protein

	Chlorella (%)	Spirulina (%)
Arginine	3.36	5.98
Lysine*	3.40	4.00
Histidine	1.11	1.08
Phenylalanine*	2.89	3.95
Tyrosine	1.92	4.60
Leucine*	4.97	5.80
Isoleucine*	2.49	4.13
Methionine*	0.97	2.17
Valine*	3.46	6.00
Alanine	4.79	5.82
Glycine	3.31	3.46
Proline	2.58	2.97
Glutamic Acid	6.64	8.94
Serine	2.30	4.00

	Chlorella (%)	Spirulina (%)
Threonine*	2.91	4.17
Aspartic Acid	5.18	6.43
Tryptophane*	1.25	1.13
Cystine	0.63	0.67

Minerals (mg per 100 gm)

	Chlorella	Spirulina
Potassium	927	1540
Calcium	247	131.5
Magnesium	360	191.5
Iron	195	58.0
Phosphorus	1410	894.2

Vitamins and Others

	Chlorella	Spirulina
Vitamin A	86,200 IU/100 gm	—
Vitamin B-1	2.37 mg %	5.5 mg %
Vitamin B-2	6.15 mg %	4.0 mg %
Vitamin B-6	0.98 mg %	0.3 mg %
Vitamin B-12	—	0.2 mg %
Folic Acid	0.63 mg %	0.5 mg %
Vitamin C	21.4 mg %	—
Vitamin E	3.9 mg %	19.0 mg %
Total Carotene	51.7 mg %	190.0 mg %
Total Xanthophyll	268.0 mg %	100.0 mg %
Total Chlorophyll	2,110.0 mg %	760.0 mg %

Both spirulina and chlorella are whole, pure and natural foods, and both have been extensively tested in hospitals, with beneficial results in cases of stomach disorders, colitis, liver problems, slow healing wounds and anemia.

Other micronutrients are known among the algae, and some under investigation at this time may prove to be more potent than either spirulina or chlorella.

Evening Primrose

Evening primrose is one of the most fascinating and useful of the herbal remedies. The whole plant is edible. An oil is taken from the seeds (for internal use), and the plant can also be made into an ointment for rashes and other skin problems.

Evening primrose is mucilaginous and astringent, which helps make it effective in relieving coughs and inflammation in the throat. It is good for colds and has been used to treat depression with considerable success. Part of its effectiveness is thought to be due to its tonic action on the liver, spleen and digestion.

The oil of the evening primrose is primarily polyunsaturated fatty acids — 9% gamma linolenic acid and

72% linoleic acid. These fatty acids are vital to the formation of the prostaglandin PGE-1, which acts to lower blood cholesterol, lower blood pressure, prevent thrombosis and reduce inflammations in the body. In Europe this oil is reportedly used to treat multiple sclerosis, with a 30% success rate. Scientists are also studying its effects on arthritis, heart disease, schizophrenia and liver disease.

Recently, evening primrose has been given to hyperactive children and to children with learning disabilties. It worked well in relaxing the hyperactive children, while some improvement was noticed in the group with learning problems. I believe we have much more to learn about this unusual plant.

Lady Slipper

The list of functions for this particular herb is impressive indeed: nervine, relaxant, tonic, antispasmodic, diaphoretic and diuretic. We notice it is also called American valerian, perhaps because its primary use is often to sooth the nerves — as valerian does. As a nervine it is gentle and slow acting but very effective. Lady slipper is considered a good pain reliever and tonic for insomnia.

Its action on the nervous system has made it one of the priority choices for taking care of nervous disorders, even cases of hysteria. The diaphoretic action brings out the perspiration and, as a diuretic, it increases urine output. In its natural "live" state, lady slipper carries an oil which can be very irritating to the skin, causing an unpleasant rash if it is handled.

La Dean Griffin, an herbalist I hold in the highest regard, has pointed out that lady slipper has a normalizing effect on the choroid plexus, which maintains pressure in the cerebro-spinal fluid system. She has found that imbalances of the choroid plexus can lead to a variety of disturbances including neck pains, headaches, dry brain, whiplash conditions and digestive problems. Lady slipper is said to offer considerable relief and improvement for these conditions.

Colloidal Sulfur

Colloidal sulfur in its natural form has been appreciated for its healing properties since the time of the early Egyptian dynasties nearly 3,00 years ago. In more recent times, William A Caudill, a chemist and pharmacist, has investigated its contents and healing properties in some detail. Colloidal sulfur has been studied by medical researchers and universities as well.

Although sulfur has been used for hundreds of years in its chemical state, both by application to the skin and as an internal medication, very little of it is absorbed by the body. In contrast, colloidal sulfur is assimilated very well, effectively meeting the body's needs and eliminating any deficiencies.

Caudill has pointed out that the chemical constituents of natural colloidal sulfur do not account for its beneficial effect. Catalytic and electromagnetic properties developed by high temperatures, intense pressures and gaseous infusions of subterranean processes have resulted in healing powers not found in manufactured sulfur compounds or even in surface sulfur springs. The sulfur springs which carry the potentized suspension of chemical elements come from deep within the earth, not surface springs and pools.

A colloidal solution is a liquid in which microparticles of one or more substances form a homogenous state, not settling to the bottom of a container as ordinary mixtures would and not dissolving in the solution as soluble chemicals would. Colloidal sulfur can be taken in through the pores of the skin by adding it to bath water or can be taken internally and assimilated through the bowel wall.

Studies by Dr. Derric C. Parmenter, a medical researcher at Harvard University, showed that colloidal sulfur detoxifies the body, eliminating chemical and bacterial poisons. It is easily dissolved in the blood and carried to epithelial tissues such as the skin, lungs and serous and mucous membranes which need it for normal functioning. Colloidal sulfur is reported to normalize blood pressure, no matter if it is high or low to begin with, and to normalize cell metabolism.

Using colloidal sulfur on arthritis patients, the percentage of cures was 40% as compared to 10% with most standard forms of treatment. Researchers believed that colloidal sulfur was able to replenish lost sulfur in joints and cartilage, as well as normalizing overall body metabolism. Previously, some medical researchers stated that rheumatoid arthritis is basically a sulfur deficiency disease.

In diabetics, taking colloidal sulfur has lowered blood sugar, acting like insulin. In cases of hypothyroidism, it has increased the metabolic rate from 10 to 20%, acting like thyroxine. It appears to be useful in all diseases in which toxicity plays a part.

No undesirable side effects have been found among those who have used the colloidal sulfur orally or in baths.

In the human body, sulfur plays an important role in epithelial tissue, as stated before, and it is also an important constituent of the amino acid cystine. Cystine, in turn, is part of glutathione, which is critical to all cell respiration. Sulfur is found in every vital organ of the body and in many of the glandular secretions, including insulin. When small doses of colloidal sulfur are taken with insulin, the action of the insulin is tripled. Because of its affinity with the skin, sulfur often brings quick healing in cases of acne and eczema (caused by metabolic disorders). One researcher has shown that cell division is directly proportional to the amount of sulfur in the basil cell layer. These cells were deficient in sulfur in cases of chronic skin disease.

Dr. Jenor Wright of the British Public Health Service showed that vitamin deficiency diseases such as pellagra, beriberi and scurvy are more quickly healed when colloidal sulfur is used with vitamin therapy. Dr. Wright believed that vitamins are more efficiently assimilated by tissue when the proper amount of sulfur is present.

Perhaps one of the most interesting things about sulfur as a chemical element is that it takes on several electrical charges, which makes its electromagnetic properties unusually variable in solution with other positively and negatively charged ions.

Analysis

Specific Gravity at 15.6ºC 1.120
Reaction pH..............................8.5
Total Solids, by Evaporation
    at 80ºC grams per 100 cc 20.122
Total Sulphur as S, grams per 100cc 11.220
Monosulphide Sulphur, grams per 100 cc 0.728
Polysulphide Sulphur, grams per 100 cc 5.700
Thiosulphate Sulphur, grams per 100 cc 3.930

Sulphate Sulphur, grams per 100 cc 0.862
Carbonates, grams per 100 cc 0.192
Silicates as Silica, grams per 100 cc 0.561
Sodium, grams per 100 cc 5.150
Fluorides, mg/100 cc 0.796
Sulphated Ash, grams per 100 cc 20.967
Total Chlorides, grams per 100 cc .... .436
Magnesium, grams per 100 cc .... .023
Calcium, grams per 100 cc..................0.03
Iron and Aluminum Oxides, grams per 100 cc .0.0014

SPECTROGRAPHIC EXAMINATION

	Evaporated Solids (%)	Original Liquid (%)
Sodium	30.0	5.28
Calcium	0.093	0.016
Potassium	1.4	0.25
Magnesium	0.13	0.023
Boron	0.029	0.0051
Silicon	0.051	0.0090
Iron	0.0037	0.00065
Aluminum	0.0015	0.00026
Lithium	0.0053	0.00093
Copper	0.0012	0.00021
Strontium	0.0039	0.00069
Chromium	0.00066	0.00012
Barium determined by flame photometer	0.0023	

Strange Tastes of Other Peoples

All sorts of queer foods are enjoyed in different parts of the world, for instance:

Vindaloo, a Burmese savory dish of fish which has been buried in the earth for three weeks.

The Eskimos eat rotten fish and meat with no ill effect.

Connoisseurs in Britain will not eat meat unless it has been "hung" for several days.

Herman J. Almquist of the University of California found that chick bleeding could be cured by using putrid fish meal—high in vitamin K, the coagulative vitamin.

An old Burmese dying in hospital had been given up. His case was hopeless. Wanting sour pickles and rotten fish, these were brought to satisfy a dying wish. The old man ate himself full, sat up and recovered!

In European pharmacopeioas, there is a prescription of an "elixir of long life," the formula being a compound of aloes and other purgatives.

Chapter 43

What we can expect from foods

We have discussed many of the qualities and constituents of foods at some length, but we find there is still much more to learn. It was Dr. Brown Landone who talked so much about auxins, the plant hormones responsible for plant cell growth, and when we stop and think about it, we realize that there are foods necessary for the production of human hormones as well.

What are hormones? Scientists have found that hormones are complex chemicals secreted in extremely small amounts from certain glands in the body — glands such as the pituitary, thyroid, adrenals and so forth. They are extremely powerful in their effect on the body, so that an excess or deficiency can be dangerous or debilitating.

Several years ago at the San Diego Zoo, some species of animals were not reproducing, while others were giving birth to such unhealthy offspring that they lived only a brief time. Now, this was a very difficult situation for the zoo, because animals from other nations and continents have become extremely expensive. What did they do? They gave the animals fresh sprouts to eat. Apparently, the auxins in the sprouts rejuvinated all the animals with reproductive problems. They became more active and energetic. They seemed to come back to life again. There was no problem with reproduction or with healthy offspring after that.

Dr. Landone claimed that sprouts, especially mung bean sprouts, were richer in auxins than older plants. He believed that auxins played a role in keeping people looking and feeling young. Dr. Landone was the one who showed me that the greatest growth in sprouts take place in the dark.

We take for granted that if we eat the right things and live the right way, we will have plenty of energy, a radiant personality, beautiful skin, endurance, stamina, vitality virility or femininity, alertness, responsiveness, and youthfulness well into an advanced age. We expect these things when we are eating right, don't we? In many cases, hormones determine whether we have these qualities, and auxin-rich sprouts contribute to the health of the glands.

The chemical elements from sprouts and other foods we eat are taken by the glandular cells and, in the laboratory inside the cell, they are transformed into hormones — substances 80 million times more powerful than the foods they were derived from. In the processes of digestion and assimilation, then transformation into an entirely new substance in the cell, I believe there is a kind of alchemy taking place which raises the vibratory level of the chemical elements undergoing these various processes. The hormones are a kind of "inner food" in the body, feeding or changing the activity of glands, organs and systems, and they are more highly evolved than the "external food" of which they are made.

We Use Energy To Create Energy

When we stop and think about it, it takes energy to make energy. It takes energy to digest food, to assimilate nutrients, to circulate the nutrients in the bloodstream, to draw nutrients into the cells and to transform them into energy, protein, hormones, enzymes or any of the various other chemical substances of the body. This means we must take in considerably more energy than we use, or we could end up with an energy deficit.

If we use the best foods to begin with, less energy is needed to transform them into cell end products (such as energy) and we have more energy available for use. The better the quality of our foods, the better the quality of our bloodstream and tissues. We need the best possible foods to make hormones.

For example, adrenal exhaustion is characterized by fatigue and depression, conditions which often usher in diseases of one sort or another. The adrenal glands can be restored, but not by coffee and donuts. Not by cake and ice cream. We should have foods that are whole, natural and pure. Junk food won't do it, and anything less than the best foods will slow down the rejuvenation of the adrenals. That's the whole point.

To transform a fatigued, depressed body into an active, vitality-filled body may take more than foods, but without the right foods it can't be done at all.

When the hormones are flowing again, the body and mind are re-energized. With release of the right hormones, a coward can be transformed into a brave man. A shy girl can be transformed into a bold, confident young lady. A slowpoke may become a human dynamo.

The glands are important controls over many body processes. Pituitary malfunction can result in dwarfism or giantism. Lack of insulin from the islands of Langerhans in the pancreas can cause a type of diabetes. If the thyroid is underactive, the metabolism of every organ in the body is slowed down. All these functions can be restored if the glands have not been neglected too long.

We can tell when a person's glands are working well by the youthful appearance of the skin and the restoration of energy.

The Hormone Builders

Foods can work miracles for people if only properly used. One of the most vital steps in sustaining health and high level well being is to eat the right foods for keeping the glands in the best possible condition. The right hormone balance is not only essential in keeping the physical temple in good condition but also the mind and spirit. We find that the spirit can do very little with a depressed mind and fatigued body.

The building blocks for hormones and enzymes (the catalysts for chemical reactions in the body) are amino acids, which we get from the protein foods. Most of our energy on the planet is derived directly or indirectly from sunlight. Chlorophyll is a sun food, and most of our proteins are obtained from animal aources that use the chlorophyll-rich vegetation or from grains grown and ripened by solar power.

Lecithin and cholesterol are fatty foods used in building nerves and brain tissue and in building some of the glandular secretions. A high percentage of male semen is lecithin, while the adrenal hormones are largely made of cholesterol. Both lecithin and cholesterol are needed by every cell in the body, but they are essential to proper glandular function.

Lecithin is rich in phosphorus, the "light bearer" element so vital to proper brain function. It is the brain phosphorus that serves as the bridge between matter and mind, allowing the soul to bring through and develop its potentials. We need the highest evolved lecithin for this purpose, found in such foods as egg yolk and codfish roe. Lecithin is in most foods of animal origin, but it is destroyed when food is cooked at high heat. Vegetable lecithin, as found in soybeans, is not as highly evolved as the animal lecithin. We find that cholesterol is plentiful in the bodies of most persons, but we need to make sure we are getting enough lecithin to help keep the youthful qualities.

Algae such as spirulina and chlorella, rich in protein, minerals, vitamins and chlorophyll, are excellent gland builders. By taking a little of the algae each day we can help the body use its other nutrients more effectively and speed up the repair and rejuvenation.

Again, the point is to get away from foods which do little or nothing for the body and to concentrate on those which do the most good at the least expenditure of energy. We want to build up faster than we are tearing down. We have to stay away from dead foods. We need foods that build living tissue.

Food Chart

The following foods are good glandular builders.

> Almonds (no other nuts)
> Sesame seeds
> Eggs
> Lean red meat
> Raw milk
> Cheese (hard and crumbly the best)
> Spirulina
> Chlorella
> Sprouts

Enzymes, Minerals and Vitamins

Enzymes, as we have said, are the catalysts that drive many of the chemical reactions in the body. Under the influence of enzymes, digestive processes that might normally take 3 to 4 hours, are speeded up to 10-15 minutes. Although enzymes trigger chemical reactions, they do not take part in them and are "recycled" out of the series of steps at some point.

We find that enzymes are preserved in many of the raw, fresh foods we eat but not the canned, packaged or processed foods. Pasteurization kills enzymes in milk. These enzymes are of value in the foods we eat, but should not be confused with the fact that our bodies manufacture enzymes from amino acids as obtained in our protein foods.

Vitamins are like enzymes in that they catalyze certain chemical reactions and they are like hormones in that very small quantities act powerfully upon the system. Vitamins regulate certain physiological processes. For example, vitamin E prevents fats from oxydizing or growing rancid in the body. Vitamins A, C, D and folic acid aid in the assimilation of calcium and iron, an enzyme-like action. Natural vitamins, as I have said before, are superior in quality to synthetic vitamins. One of the most useful roles of vitamins is to help in the assimilation of minerals.

Minerals are chemical elements needed by the human body to perform particular metabolic or structural tasks. They are best taken in foods but must sometimes be taken in supplement form when serious deficiencies are found. Chelated minerals are easiest for the body to assimilate. So many of the inorganic mineral supplements are poorly utilized by the body that I seriously question their usefulness. I have had patients with severe calcium depletion who had been taking the chalk calcium for months without results. Some of them had open ulcers on their ankles. They were taken care of by using a lot of green leafy vegetables and green vegetable juices.

We find that many Americans are chronically deficient in calcium, iron and silicon. The complete story of the chemical elements and their effects upon body and personality is told in my book *The Chemistry Of Man* in great detail.

I do not want to end this discussion without mentioning that I believe natural sunlight also acts as a catalyst in the human body. Not only does it convert one form of cholesterol into vitamin D in the skin, but it irradiates the blood as it travels in the peripheral skin capillaries, keeping serum electrolytes charged with a high vibratory rate. Without sunlight, we could not make a body with the chemical elements alone.

We are sun-energized. The sun is a sodium star, and sodium is the youth element. So, we can say that the sun sustains youthfulness. Sun ripened fruits bring solar energy to the body, and so does chlorophyll. Chlorophyll has been called "liquid sunshine". It is a wonderful cleanser and deodorizer, and helps sweeten the colon to create a favorable environment for beneficial bacteria. All green leafy vegetables are high in chlorophyll.

To Sum Up

Plenty of energy calls for foods rich in calcium, iron, sodium, sulphur, magnesium and a trace of copper. We need iodine foods to keep the thyroid going, potassium to counter muscle fatigue. Leave sugar alone and get the natural sugars from fruits. Take a protein food once a day, a lecithin food and fruit and vegetables with vitamins B-1, C and D.

Increased radiance comes from well-toned muscles and nerves, which takes foods that have potassium, sodium, copper, silicon, calcium and iron. Magnesium guards against excess muscle tension and soothes the nerves. Manganese increases the heart activity, iodine and sodium prevent nerve problems, and phosphorus feeds the brain neurons. Take foods with cholesterol and lecithin.

Beautiful, youthful skin comes when we increase the growth rate of skin cells. The skin is an eliminative organ and to keep it clear we must see that the other channels are healthy and open, especially the bowel. Brush the skin twice daily with a natural bristle brush. Take a tablespoon of bran after breakfast for the bowel. Use foods with plenty of auxins for the silicon, also calcium, magnesium, sodium, potassium, sulphur, iodine and foods with vitamins A, B-1, B-2, C, D and G.

To increase body responsiveness, the nerves and endocrine glands must be activated. We need the protein foods to assure good brain and nerve function and to build up hormone values, lecithin foods to keep artery walls clean and to feed the brain and glands, cholesterol to build the steroid hormones. Foods high in potassium, calcium and phosphorus to keep the heart toned, iodine for the thyroid; manganese, phosphorus and calcium for the brain; foods with vitamins A, B-1, C, D and E.

Endurance requires a steady, sustained energy supply, which is assisted by stimulating the bone marrow to produce new red blood cells. So, we should take foods rich in iodine, phosphorus, potassium, sodium, iron, calcium, magnesium, manganese and vitamins A, B-complex, C, D, E and G. We need protein foods and some fatty foods.

Sexual vitality calls for special attention to the glands and bloodstream, but also the brain. If the sexual response center in the brain isn't activated, it won't matter what you do for the glands. So a clean bloodstream is necessary, and slant board exercises may help bring blood to the brain. We need iodine for the thyroid; zinc for the pelvic organs; protein, lecithin and cholesterol for the secretions; vitamin E for the reproductive system. Sprouts are excellent for revitalizing the sexual system. We also need foods high in calcium, iron, potassium, sodium, copper, manganese, and vitamins A, B-complex, D, E and G. After prolonged deficiencies, it may be best to go to the glandular protomorphogens.

Youthfulness, so they say, depends on the joints, which require a good deal of sodium to remain limber and to keep calcium from depositing out of solution. They also say we are as young as our glands. In either case, we can't go wrong by having plenty of sprouts in the diet to provide the auxins for cell stimulation. We need chlorophyll foods to keep the body clean, the bowel sweet and to help in the assimilation of iron. The heart and muscles need potassium to keep young and the brain needs lecithin and other phosphorus-rich foods. We'll need foods high in vitamins A, C, E and G. And, we'll need to be on a good exercise program to stimulate the circulation and keep the brain active.

Auxins contribute importantly to each of the preceding seven results that people look for from healthy living. When we stop and think about it, seeds are among the most powerful things on earth. In each seed is the genetic blueprint for a mature plant and enough nutrients to start the action of growing until the first root finds its way into the earth and the first pair of tiny leaves shoot out. When a seed becomes vitalized by soaking in water, enzymes are awakened which quicken the internal cells to prepare the vitamins and nutrients needed by the growing plant. A sprout represents the first quickening of youthful growth energies from the seed, and is highly nutritious. It has the life force still in it.

Tests with animals have demonstrated the restoring power of auxins from sprouts. The life force of the auxins is transferred to the animals and people who use them. We find that many Chinese retain their youthfulness well into advanced age, and I believe this is no random circumstance. The Chinese have eaten sprouts for hundreds, perhaps thousands of years, and that is why they stay young and vigorous.

Sprouts are easy to grow at home and many supermarkets now carry them too. You can find out how to home-grow them at your local health food store. If you have a garden, don't throw away the tiny young vegetables as you thin your rows. Wash and eat them. You can always grow three or four romaine lettuce plants inside or outside and pick the young outer leaves before they begin to mature. The lettuce will continue growing and producing new young leaves for a considerable time, so you will have a plentiful supply.

Auxins are one of the secrets to youthfulness. Make sprouts a regular part of your food regimen.

The Onliest and Deepest Secrets of the Medical Art

A sealed book of 100 pages, bearing the above title, was found among the effects of the celebrated Dutch physician, Dr. Herman Boerhave, after his death in 1738. The book was sold at auction for $10,000 in gold. After the seal was broken the buyer discovered that 99 pages were blank. Only the title page bore this inscription in the doctor's own hand: "Keep your head cool, your feet warm and you'll make the best doctor poor."

Unusual Food Facts

If lost in the jungle, a Malay native will use anything for food he sees a monkey eating, knowing the food will not harm him.

Every breed of domestic fowl is derived from the wild jungle fowl of India.

The banana is a vegetable when green, a fruit when yellow.

The expression, "as cool as a cucumber," is well founded because a cucumber is usually one degree cooler than air.

Honey is the oldest sweet known to man.

Lemons, so large that one fruit will yield a pint of juice, are grown in Africa.

An onion, found in the hands of a mummy of ancient Egypt, was planted in the Jardin Desplantes, Paris, and GREW!

All varieties of the apple are derived from the crab apple.

The Islanders of the Faeroes dry fish until hard, then beat it with a hammer into a powder—and eat the dust.

In 1960, England prohibited the sale of chocolate drinks without a license.

A popular method of teaching the alphabet to English children years ago was to bake gingerbread letters, the child eating each letter as he learned its name.

The ice cream of the Eskimos is made of seal oil mixed with snow, cranberries and moss blackberries.

In 1850, spinach sold for 50 cents a forkful in San Francisco.

A jar of rattlesnake meat won first prize for the most unusual exhibit in the Chicago World's Fair canning contest.

The country folks in Holland, when drinking tea or coffee, signify they have had enough by simply placing the cup upside down in the saucer.

Thirty people were required to serve Louis XV his dinner. Four people were required to give him a glass of water.

Pears with the stem on the large end grow in Australia.

Chapter 44

Is our water fit to drink?

In recent years we have become more water-conscious in this country due to drought, pollution, the acid rain in the Northeast, the issue of fluoridation of the public water supply and the deterioration of water quality almost everywhere in the United States. As long as we had plenty of clean fresh-tasting water, no one talked about it. Our needs — industrial, agricultural and personal — were being met, and the water that satisfied those needs remained out of sight, out of mind, out of public discussion. It seems only when something becomes a problem that we start talking about it.

Water has become a problem.

I have traveled around the world, frequently visiting countries where I was told, "Don't drink the water." Americans who have spent time abroad, as I have, learn to appreciate clean, pure water. We see what happens in countries that don't have it. We find cholera epidemics in areas where rivers are polluted with human waste. We find skin diseases, eye diseases, leprosy and other devastating conditions in countries where lack of hygiene, poor nutrition and filthy water are present.

Now that Americans are beginning to lose the purity of their water, perhaps they will begin to appreciate it.

Our Many Uses Of Water

First of all, the human body is between 70% and 80% water. The brain is 80%, the heart 75%, the lungs 86%, the liver 86%, the kidneys 83%, the muscle 75% and the blood is 83%. A 150-pound man is composed of between 105 and 120 pounds of water, and it is obvious that water is one of the most important constituents of the body. We could not survive long if the brain was not protected and cushioned in liquid, if the organs and tissues of the body were not fed, surrounded and lubricated by liquid, most of which is water.

A large percentage of everything we eat is water. Neither vegetation nor animals can exist without it. When I was traveling in Baja, Mexico along a road that ran next to the ocean, I counted 13 crosses marking the graves of persons who had died of thirst right next to water. Ocean water is undrinkable. We must have fresh water. But, close to the graves barrel cacti were growing which contained enough water for survival. Seagulls,

which require fresh water to survive, are found as far out at sea as 3,000 miles. How can they do it? Membranes inside their beaks filter the salt from the salt water they drink, a principle similar to one of the best available purification methods.

Our industries use immense amounts of water, and farms in arid parts of the country flourish by means of irrigation from local wells or from dams somewhere in the area.

Virtually everything we do requires water. Water, in many cultures, is a symbol for life, and we can understand why.

Is Our Drinking Water Safe?

In many parts of the world where the population density is high, such as China and India, rivers and streams are commonly contaminated with coliform bacteria such as E. coli, evidence that fecal material has been in contact with the water. Such water is unfit to drink without purification, or disease may result. The human body can defend itself against a surprising variety and amount of foreign substances, but when water or food is literally saturated with germlife or toxic material, our defenses may succumb to it. We cannot drink just any water; it must be sufficiently pure and clean for our bodies to assimilate and use without harm to any organs or tissues. Yet, as I mentioned before, we are so accustomed in this country to having plenty of pure, clean water that we have grown careless. We don't know, in many cases, what is in the water that pours from the tap in the kitchen or bathroom.

Is our drinking water safe? The U.S. Environmental Protection Agency doesn't believe it is. In the booklet titled "A Drop to Drink," the EPA has this to say: "There are thousands of toxic chemical compounds in use today. New chemicals are developed each year and many of these can enter and contaminate both surface and underground water. In large amounts some of these chemicals found in drinking water could cause cancer, genetic mutations, or birth deformities."

Among the contaminants found in drinking water are:

> Asbestos
> Bacteria
> Chlorine
> Colloidal matter
> Detergents
> Dissolved solids such as
> > sodium, calcium, magnesium, cadmium, sulphates, nitrates, and chlorides.
>
> Fluoride
> Hydrocarbons
> Industrial waste
> Pesticides
> Pyrogens
> Radioactive substances
> Turbidity
> Viruses

The following are some headlines found in major urban newspapers. *The Salt Lake Tribune:* **BILLIONS ARE WASTED IN PROJECTS TO CLEAN UP U.S. WATER**; *Los Angeles Times:* **MILLIONS DRINK CONTAMINATED WATER**; *The San Diego Union:* **WATER HERE FAILS '81 SAFETY RULES IN TESTS — Has 2-4 Times Level of Suspected Cancer Agents**. *Time* magazine ran a cover article titled, "The Poisoning of America," about our water while *Newsweek's* cover asked, "Are We Running Out Of Water?".

Most of us simply rely on our state and local governments to keep the water clean enough for us to use. But, the evidence shows that they have done little to curb the trend of lower water quality because so many complex socio-economic factors are involved. For example, to halt industrial pollution altogether would force many industries to shut down completely, with the resulting loss of hundreds of thousands, perhaps millions of jobs. To clean up pollution effects in one massive effort is such a tremendous job that they say it would bankrupt our nation, so it is being done step by step. Meanwhile, we all are exposed to varying levels of pollution in our water, air, foods, etc.

When this nation was founded, the Hudson River in New York was one of the most beautiful rivers in North America. Now, rats live on its banks, eating the garbage and filth that washes ashore. The San Lorenzo River in Northern California once teemed with trout and salmon; now few fish can survive in it, due to destruction of gravel beds needed by salmon for spawning and the high coliform bacteria count. Lake Tahoe in the High Sierra, once a cold, clear lake whose waters were pure enough to drink, is growing murky, with green algae slime along its North Shore due, it is suspected, from inorganic fertilizer runoff from the golf courses around

it. Near Sedona, Arizona, one of the cleanest areas in this country, a swimming hole in the beautiful stream that runs through the area is periodically closed due to high coliform bacteria count. In all major agricultural areas of the nation, massive amounts of inorganic chemical fertilizers have leached down into the ground water, altering its former chemical composition.

We find that local water treatment plants all over the country add chemicals to the water supply to kill bacteria, counteract turbidity, reduce high iron content, change the odor and so on. In some communities, fluoride has been added to the water to counteract dental cavities.

Fluoridation of Public Water Supplies

Some decades ago, it was discovered that a small amount of sodium fluoride in drinking water reduced dental cavities. The fluoride, according to authorities, hardens tooth enamel and makes it more impervious to decay. Some civic-minded individual then came up with the idea of reducing dental caries throughout local populations by adding sodium fluoride to the public drinking water. It was a commendable idea—but in theory only.

Further research showed that even minute levels of fluorine in drinking water could block or interfere with enzyme functions in the human body. Dr. Jonathan Forman has described fluorine as "a protoplasmic poison." Nobel prize-winning scientist Hugo Theorell has said, "As far as is known, the toxic effect of fluorine is due solely to its inhibitory effect on many enzyme systems.... The example of lipase inhibition by fluoride in such a small amount as one part to five million may be taken as an illustration." Fluoride inhibits glutamine and argenime synthesis as well as phosphate-transport enzymes. The systems affected by the blocking of these and other human enzymes are the genito-urinary system, circulation, the gastro-intestinal system, bones, teeth, skin and hair.

Because each individual is different, there is no safe way of introducing fluorine into the public water supply. What is barely sufficient to help one person can be toxic to another. Some scientists have suggested that fluorine can accumulate in the body, reaching destructive levels in time. It is possible to take fluorine supplements in tablet form or other ways without forcing other people to have a chemical in their water that they don't want, so the issue or debate that has arisen is largely spurious. Those who want to take fluoride supplements can do so.

We find that inorganic sodium fluoride does not have the right vibratory rate to harmonize with the human body. But the fluorine in raw goat's milk does. Biochemical fluorine is a natural germicide, wonderful for building resistance to disease and for keeping the body's natural immune system strong. Quinces also have considerable fluoride in them, but they must be taken raw. Fluorine is a gas and is easily driven out of foods by cooking, so we must get it from raw foods.

Fluoride, carelessly used and in the wrong amount, is considered responsible for discolored teeth, reducing the blood clotting capacity and increasing the number of birth defects. It is best if we leave this chemical alone, excepting for its use when we find it naturally in foods.

What Is the Solution?

If good sense and wisdom prevail, oiur government and people will soon learn that we must harmonize with Nature and return to natural principles. But, that could take a hundred years. Meanwhile, there are some things we can do.

Some nutritionists advocate using bottled mineral water, others say to use distilled water for drinking and cooking. My experience has shown that distilled water tends to leach minerals from the body, and this is supported by an engineering study into the contaminants found in water coming from the pipes of a desalinization plant on the West Coast. The desalinized water was found to be pure as it came from the purifying plant, but it dissolved chemicals from the walls of the pipes it flowed through after that. Water with a few minerals dissolved in it doesn't react chemically with the pipes it flows through. I have, on occasion, recommended the use of distilled water to arthritis patients and others with calcium deposits in the joints.

Various types of home water purifying or softening units are available. The standard water softener replaces the minerals it removes with sodium, which is bad for those with heart ailments, circulatory problems and others who must be on a low-sodium diet. Charcoal water filters improve the taste of tap water, but allow the growth of bacterial colonies in the carbon bed; they also do not remove dissolved heavy metals, minerals or germlife. Distillation equipment is available but expensive; substances such as chloroform and other contaminants with a lower boiling point than water can be taken into the finished distilled water. Boiling the water kills germs and boils off chemicals with low boiling points, but all other pollutants remain. The Environmental Protection Agency has found coliform bacteria in some samples of commercially bottled water, so we can't take its purity for granted.

One of the better approaches to water purification is reverse osmosis, which pushes water through a cellulose membrane that filters out virtually all chemicals and germlife. The cost is relatively low. However, the water pressure at the installation point must be at least 40 lb. per square inch.

As I have mentioned, very pure water may dissolve some minerals from the body, However, we can mix water obtained from distillation or reverse osmosis with a little fruit or vegetable juice and drink it that way.

It is also possible to get all the liquid we need from juices, and not drink water at all, excepting for herbal teas and other various decoctions and combinations.

We must do something, however, to assure that the water we drink is not harmful to health. One of the first rules I teach my patients is, "We must stop breaking down before we can build up." If your local water is high in contaminants, you should consider a purification unit, bottled water or staying with juices.

Our Last Frontier — The Ocean

Man's development in the past has constantly pressed him to new frontiers. The last frontier on earth is the ocean. Before we push any further our technological advancements and the inventions of man, let us consider keeping our oceans clean. It is here that we can obtain enough food to take care of us through any population explosion. It offers us the highest protein available to build strong bodies and an alert mind. It is the greatest source we have for the soluble minerals that man has been leeching out of his cooked foods. It is the reservoir for the soluble salts from our mountain sides, valleys and rivers. It is probably the greatest source we have for the trace minerals the body needs these days.

To have these elements and have them as clean and pure as God gave them to us is most necessary. Man has plundered and desecrated the earth, polluted the air and is now on the verge of poisoning the oceans. When we recognize that we have to be wary of man's inventions (those inventions can be the end of man), certainly it is time to take a moment out of our trespasses and transgressions to take care of our lakes, rivers and oceans. Man is capable; man is divinely endowed to have the "know-how" of caring for himself, but he has neglected this factor. To see us dumping the pesticides, herbicides, sprays and other poisonous chemicals on the soil, plus sludge is unbelievable. These, along with sewage from many ocean front cities, find their way into the oceans. Certainly, the scientists have given us the word to stop. The warning is out. It is time that man heeds it.

Our shrimp beds at the mouth of the Mississippi have now been destroyed; seal populations have fallen in Alaska. In other places, radiated fish are found belly-up—all of these due to man's inventions—and all throughout the world today. We have even dumped deadly nerve gases, radioactive wastes and liquids into the ocean which are bound to bring disasters at some future time. Not only will we as a country pay for it, but other countries will suffer along with us. The ocean currents, tides and animal life will carry the poisons of each country to others.

Our goal now should be to get rid of excessively destructive knowledge and technology — to unlearn and start again. This moment we must turn in another direction, reclaim our planet and live with God's richest garden. Even now, we will suffer from the sins of our fathers and those we have committed ourselves. For the good of the next generation, it is time to stop. Surely we can find economical and practical alternatives to polluting the ocean and many life forms in it.

Did You Know That

Alfalfa seed tea is excellent in relieving arthritis?

Avocado liquefied with milk is a good food to wean baby?

Carob flour gives a chocolate flavor to milk when mixed with it and this makes a good nutritional after-school snack for children?

You can use all the fruit juices for sweetening your teas?

The best weight-building foods are bananas, sunflower seed meal (3 or 4 ounces per day), soymilk and dried fruits?

It takes 14 muscles to smile but it takes 52 muscles to look "down in the mouth" and depressed?

A New Wrinkle for Getting Rid of Wrinkles

Are you tired of those "tired lines" in your face? Try this new wrinkle for getting rid of old wrinkles. The "Honey Pat" is the "new wrinkle" for getting rid of old wrinkles and helping you erase blackheads and whiteheads from your skin. Here is how it works: Pour a little honey in a saucer, dip your fingers in the honey and then apply it to your face, drawing the facial muscles out with the sticky honey. Don't pound your skin, let the honey do the work. This exercises the muscles and pores and helps develop the tone of the underlying muscles of the skin. Do this ten times daily for a couple of months.

Something to Think About

How old is old? Christian Jacobsen Dranberg, a Dane, was born in 1626 and died in 1772 at 146! At the age of 70, he was taken prisoner by Algerian pirates. He served as a slave for 15 years, then escaped and participated in a war against Sweden. At the age of 111, the Dane married a woman of 60 and outlived her. At 130, he proposed to several women, but was rejected. He lived another 16 years, during which his conduct was "far from blameless," but he simmered down at the age of 141 and died at 146.

"If one man can live a life as full as this," said Dr. Theodore Klumpp of New York City, "there is no reason why science cannot make it possible for many of us to marry at 111, propose and be accepted at 130 and live to 146. Middle-aged people should not prepare to be old, then they could take the aging process as it comes instead of hurrying toward it.

IV
A well being

Health Through the Kitchen

I believe that many people would like to live better but they don't know how! In the field of food science, they are ignorant. They can't balance the nutrition of the body by getting the proper chemical ratio and so build better health and eliminate disease. In order to do this, we have to start out with training in what foods to use in our kitchen and how to prepare them. We must learn a good healing way to live, how to make tonics, cocktails and entrees that are good for us instead of harmful. We must understand the importance of growing foods on healthy soil.

This is an advanced work but truly one that every housewife, every mother, every cook, every person who handles food for the public or has anything to do with food and the feeding of the human race should study. Only wise feeding of our bodies will enable them to continue the youthfulness of the young far into old age. We must realize that beauty is more than skin deep and that having beautifully functioning organs is necessary for good health. Nature is beautiful, and the body being the highest of all creations falls into this beauty category. To prolong life, to keep ourselves in good health at every age, to prepare our bodies for whatever may come their way in the form of accidents, epidemics or atom bombs, we must live according to the best we know. It is well we realize that balanced menus, health recipes, natural medicines, tonics, juices and fresh raw salads play a big part in giving abundant health and high efficiency to our bodies.

The preparation of food from breadmaking to ice cream must be taken care of properly. While the average doctor today is dealing with disease, this course of instruction deals with the building of good health. While experiments are being conducted on rats, plants, parasites and bacteria, this course deals with the living man. It deals with a living chemistry that builds good health, not disease. I know of no other course of study that puts so much material together for the person who wants to know how to have the best health level possible. It is time our scientific studies taught us to know our foods, their effects on the body, and what foods will keep us in good health. Only this knowledge put into practice will build the better generation to come.

The Chemical Nature of Disease

There have been scientific experiments using food to try and balance the nutrition of the human body. We have found that people in a state of disease are longing for certain chemical elements. Disease from a chemical standpoint means an altered body chemistry, a disorganized chemical balance. The body's demand for chemical nutrition is not being supported. I am convinced that no doctor will ever cure us until we have learned to eat properly. Neither can he cure himself. He must supply the food elements that are necessary for the various tissues of the body.

In following up medical techniques, seeing the results of operations and treating people who are filled with pills, we know that today we are treating them for the treatments they have had in the past. People's ailments haven't been treated properly until they have been taught how to eat properly. To heed the voice of nature and to hear the call of starving tissues in the body, one must be accustomed to the results of the lack of certain chemical elements in the body. To us, every disease is the symptom of a wrong diet. There may be other causes, but we never see a disease without seeing a lack of certain chemical elements.

Even though a bone has to be set when it is broken, and we know that the mechanical setting is necessary, the work that nature must carry on in the knitting process is chemical. There is a need for chemical elements if the knitting is to come. To wait until we have developed a clearly-defined disease and expect a well-meaning doctor to correct it with certain techniques, treatments, drugs, etc., is not getting at the fundamentals. We are truly a chemical being—one that repairs, regenerates and rejuvenates itself constantly. Nature can only do her work well when she has the materials to work with. We have seen diseases leave when we use the science of food chemistry applied to human needs.

We have found that whenever there is a lack of certain food elements the body changes, tissues change, bones change, the nervous system changes. Having experienced this time and again, we realize that disease is a call for certain chemical elements. All tissues must be fed. To heed that call, we have to find out what the natural foods are, the proper proportion of foods, what variety we need in the body, the proteins and the natural starches.

All the chemical elements have their story to tell. The individual symptoms, ailments, weaknesses and the sensations we suffer from whenever we live in hunger for these chemical elements is their language. It has to be understood before a true healing can take place in the body. Knowing the language and nature of these elements, in what form they are fit for human consumption, how to avoid their destruction in food preparation and when to apply them to meet human needs is the job of each of us. After all my days of practice in this chemical study, I am convinced that the average person wants to do the right thing but doesn't know what to do.

People Differ

Most rules for healthy living can be considered just common sense ideas. However, there must be room for a little latitude, because we know that convalescing people cannot take the same foods that robust, healthy people can. Those people who have a vigorous constitution, a resistive temperament, a strong stomach that is made like iron—you have heard of these people who can digest nails—have a truly healthy appetite. These people can eat almost anything. They can take heavy alcohol-treated foods, fat-saturated foods and other disease-producing foods. They can take stimulating foods and fancy food mixtures and they can live in restaurants for years before anything happens. Eating the devitalized manufactured products and those foods filled with chemical preservatives, artificial colorings and flavors, it seems that nothing happens to them. But there are others we have to consider—those who have the delicate, nervous stomachs. These people cannot take the unsavory dishes and heavily-spiced, indigestible foods. We must consider individual differences, even knowing the health purposes that proper foods are trying to accomplish.

My old professor used to say: "There are some people who will go for years without any disturbance in their bodies, but the lack of proper food will insidiously work upon the body like the everlasting drop of water, and this lack will finally show in a serious physical problem." He used to say that one couldn't live on foodstuffs that would injure a spook and kill a gorilla and get away with it forever.

Let us find a human way to live—the way that is meant to fit the human chemistry. Let us find the way that is approved by the all wise ones. Let us not feel that we are taking candy away from the baby forever. Let us grow up. Let us be interested in good health and produce

a new body, so that we may enjoy all the wonders of nature. Thus, we will make our occupation a success, make our marriage a success and our future will be assured.

What Your Body Needs Comes Through the Kitchen

In planning the operation of your kitchen, the first thing to recognize is that a kitchen has two doors—one through which food enters, the other through which it goes out into your dining room. Is it not criminal to bring in good food through the one door, subject it to murder and robbery in the kitchen and pass on what is left to yourself and those dearest to you? The kitchen is the go-between between Nature and the "family of man." Make sure, as a homemaker, that you do not send your husband to the operating table because of what you have done in your kitchen, that you do not bring up your children to become doctor's bills. In your kitchen is largely determined whether or not you and your family will enjoy good health. The choice is yours to make. Sickness is a matter of failure on our part to learn how to live. God is no respecter of persons. Haven't you seen more than enough of people who are sick? Isn't it time we become "sick" of being sick? Let us find out that nutrition has something to do with our well-being, and live for the higher and better things in this world.

In administering this part of your domain, whether your family be large or small or simply consists of you alone, the most important thing to see is that you have the best foods. If it is necessary to practice economy, do so on things other than nourishment. You and your family deserve the very best.

In purchasing foods, remember that natural methods of production give you fruits and vegetables highest in mineral content and other nutritional factors. Select variety. Buy in season. As foods become available throughout the growing season, you will get all of the chemical and vitamin elements, the vegetable sources of proteins, different whole grains and seeds, all in their natural form, and your body will derive the necessary materials for growth and the building of new tissue.

We need every element so that throughout life we keep our body ever renewed, youthful and vibrant with energy. To have foods as fresh as nature intended, grow your own. But if you cannot do this, select the greatest possible variety, according to freshness from dependable centers of distribution, and whenever trips are made through the country, arrange to purchase directly from the growers—preferably organic—who sell retail. Do your marketing at frequent intervals, each time choosing different varieties when available.

Chapter 45

Good earth—healthy people

It has been recorded that at one time "man was as tall as the cedars and as strong as the oaks." It was a time when man lived close to the earth, and a time when that earth was vital and young. It is said that "two men came out of the valley of Kadesh-Barnea carrying one bunch of grapes on a pole between them!" A wonderful bunch of grapes that were rich in the life-giving, health-giving qualities imparted to them by a soil that was fertile and "alive." The kind of grapes that could build "men tall as cedars and strong as oaks."

There are only a few places on the earth today where man lives a simple, natural life and maintains a healthy, hardy body. The Hunzas of Pakistan are one of the few peoples left of the "tall as cedars and strong as oaks" races of men.

Today, particularly in the so-called "civilized" areas of the world, people are living off soil that is demineralized, devitalized and so badly depleted that man is now a creature beset by physical ills and bedeviled by mental maladjustments. Man has consistently taken from the earth and not given in return. He has broken the spiritual law which demands he give in order to receive. Man, who should walk the earth like a king and be custodian of all he surveys, has degraded himself to the point where he is merely the despoiler of Nature. Nature, following the inexorable laws of life, takes her toll of man. Doctors find the vast majority of people are sadly lacking in minerals, mineral elements and vitamins. In short, they are suffering from malnutrition.

Speaking of malnutrition, Dr. D. W. Cavanaugh of Cornell University stated, "There is only one major disease, and that is malnutrition. All ailments and afflictions to which we may fall heir are directly traceable to this major disease."

It is time we realized that malnutrition goes deeper than just a bad combination of foods put together in our kitchens. It goes further than how you may cook the different elements out of your food by boiling, frying and oversteaming. It goes further than eating food which has been standing around from four or five days to two weeks with a resultant loss of its chemical elements. It even goes further than what foods taste good and look good. In the natural course of events, tissues are broken down in the body and must be renewed. When you work you become tired and hungry; the body then reaches out for the element-building-blocks to appease your hunger and replace worn out tissues. If these element-building-blocks are not supplied through food, the body begins to slowly die from lack of replenishment. We recognize this as malnourishment or disease.

In a dying body, you will have such ill-health symptoms as lack of appetite, abnormal cravings, pains, short breath, nervousness and a body that bruises easily.

It has been realized and recognized by many farmers, professors and doctors that the basic problem of getting an adequate mineral supply to our bodies through the natural fruit and vegetable kingdom can only be solved by a standard mineralized soil covering the range of minerals required by the body. This balanced soil would produce balanced bodies or bodies free from malnutrition and disease. We know that 70 or more minerals are needed to maintain our bodies properly.

The genetic pattern itself has evolved certain chemical elements in the human body and in animals. The supply of these elements must be kept in the body through the soil. We obtain the minerals which we need from plant life which subsists primarily upon the minerals obtained from the soil plus the chemical action of the sun and nitrogen and carbon dioxide from the air. It takes certain minerals to grow more wool on an animal, and healthy hair on the human head; specific minerals are needed for the different organs of the body.

When we know that our circulation must have certain mineral elements to function, that the contractability of the arteries is maintained by certain elements, that the softness of the tissues and the strength and pliability of the muscle structure requires certain elements to keep in prime condition, then we know that we must look to the soil for help. When we consider that obesity, high-blood pressure, goiter and many other diseases can be avoided and overcome wholly by taking care of the desired mineral balance in the body, then it becomes a necessity that we start with the soil as the basis upon which we must build the foundation for good health.

Your Life Is Rooted in the Soil

It seems that man has been trying to change his ways of living all through the centuries. Many changes have been made in his mode of transportation. His change in dress is almost seasonal and he has made many changes in living conveniences and even his mode of thinking has changed with the years. One thing is

ESSENTIAL ELEMENTS KNOWN TO BE NEEDED
FOR ADEQUATE NUTRITION

Air Elements	Twelve Major Mineral Elements		Trace Mineral Elements		
Carbon	Chlorine	Phosphorus	Cobalt	Cadmium	Barium
Oxygen	Fluorine	Potassium	Aluminum	Mercury	Strontium
Hydrogen	Sodium	Magnesium	Zinc	Germanium	Titanium
Nitrogen	Silicon	Manganese	Tin	Lead	Copper
	Calcium	Sulphur	Arsenic	Bromine	Zirconium
	Iron	Iodine	Vanadium	Boron	Cerium
			Selenium	Nickel	Thorium
			Beryllium	Lithium	Antimony
			Silver	Rubidium	Bismuth
			Gold	Cesium	Chromium

certain—the kind of air man needs to keep him alive today is the same kind of air he needed 10,000 years ago. We need sunshine today just as we needed it from time immemorial. The requirement of the body for certain amounts of minerals and vitamins from plant life, which comes from the soil, will always the be same.

In order to get these required mineral and vitamin elements from our foods, the foods must not only be prepared properly, but grown properly. The soil must be rich with vital minerals. Sunshine, air and water are also important in our consideration of supplying our bodies with the needed nutritional elements. We must take more thought in the matter than just to say we will eat certain yellow, green and red foods, and to say that we will eat plenty of protein and starch foods. It would not be safe to choose our foods by our depraved likes and dislikes and expect our bodies to respond properly. Such shallow reasoning would be beyond me in this day of soil depletion and mineral deficiencies.

In the body, we find iron in the blood iodine in the thyroid gland; calcium in the bones; phosphorus in the brain. To manipulate ignorantly or to wilfully change the chemical balance of food by processing it in any way so as to make a chemical imbalance in the body would lead us into the disastrous results of disease and chemical exhaustion.

There is one thing certain. We must look to the earth—the soil that is not depleted but which is rich with vital minerals. We must look to Mother Earth for the natural foods which were here before man was brought into this world. After all, we did not originally live without food. The food which comes from Mother Earth was prescribed for us by the Great Physician, just as our bodies were prescribed for the foods. The food was made for us and we were made for the food. We are inseparately connected with a life force which keeps us alive. Truly, we are the dust of the earth. That dust is made up of so many mineral elements and in different proportions that go to make a healthy or a diseased

plant. Let us emphasize the importance of having the proper soil and include a few suggestions on what can be done about it.

Man in his growth takes hold of the natural things that took so many years to grow and so many years to produce, and destroys it in a matter of minutes. Mechanized farming is ruining a lot of the topsoil today, because it is forcing the crops to take everything possible and very little is being returned to the soil. In the 20 years following 1914, according to soil men, there was more topsoil ruined than in the whole previous historical period. This is something to think about.

There is much to be learned from some of our primitive farmers; for instance, the Hunzas in Pakistan. Everything grown from their soil must be returned to it in its waste form. They even see to it that the human body goes back to the soil again. We find that they live to the ripe old age of 100 to 125 years.

In this country, we grow food and ship it to all parts of the world, but we do not replenish the soil properly. Consequently, our topsoil is becoming barren. This has become a problem which we must take care of.

There was a day when natural composting took place. The leaves and different growths from the soil were brought to the topsoil and planted there. Leaves and plants died out and became part of the topsoil again. Soil is like a bank. You can draw from it, but you cannot continually draw from it without leaving an exhausted condition.

In Switzerland, they use the urine and manure of their animals to spread over the land, because they contain many mineral elements. They put everything they take out back into the land. The humus which is developed with the straw and the feed from the barn is put back into the soil again. Their crops are beautiful, and we can truly say they are good organic farmers.

Topsoil is necessary to give us a proper plant life. Topsoil is robbed of certain mineral elements when plant life is grown from it. When this process continues

331

over a period of years, the soil becomes barren of the mineral elements needed by our bodies. A shortage of calcium or other minerals may develop, as the soil is leached of its elements by the different roots of the plant in its growth. When the plants are removed and the mineral elements are not put back into the soil again, we will have a mineral-poor soil. It may be short of calcium and be lacking in iron. Some plants take up more calcium than iron from the soil and this is one reason for the rotation of crops. Some plant life should always be restored to the soil again. It is this plant life or humus, which acts as a base for bacteria to develop. This is a necessary part of keeping any soil program.

When we realize that there are men today who have the knowledge to take the garbage of the city and use it for a constructive purpose, as for fertilizer, then we should investigate this matter for the good of our lives and for the good of our pocketbooks as well.

Los Angeles could do a great service to the community by establishing a compost company that could manufacture compost material to send out to growers in any part of the world because of our fine harbor facilities.

It is a sin against nature and a crime against humanity to spend such huge sums of money, as we are now doing, to burn up our usable waste material in the incinerator. This burning also pollutes the air and is slowly killing people as they daily breathe it in. It is so foolish and shortsighted to go on any longer burning this valuable material which should be going into the earth to replace the minerals taken out by the seasonal crops. We know that our earth is very deficient in the vital mineral elements and that the people are slowly starving to death from "hidden hunger." So the sooner we do something about it, the better.

Dr. James S. McLester, Professor of Medicine, University of Alabama, says, "The assumption is current that a diet, which in other respects is satisfactory, will furnish a sufficient amount of mineral elements. This is by no means true. Studies of the average American dietary have shown that the content of elements in food often falls far below the calculated optimum, and sometimes below the minimum. A striking example of this is the failure of many dietaries to furnish sufficient calcium." Calcium shortage could also come from vegetables grown in mineral-depleted soil.

This same principle applies to trace minerals as well as to major mineral elements, such as iodine, manganese, potassium. Some trace minerals are cobalt, copper, silver, nickel, etc. In the past, natural manure was supplied by the animals which roamed the forest and the plains, but today, we have gone into commercial farming and we are whipping the soil by adding the "three-element" commercial fertilizer. We are causing dust bowls and erosion by not replanting and rebuilding the soil into what it was originally. We

deplete the soil of water-soluble mineral elements by allowing water drainage to carry off these elements. Where there is no growth to tie down the soil, it is hard to absorb the rain and water coming over it.

Man is a usurper of all natural things. He has everything at his command and he changes everything on this earth from one substance to another. We recognize that nothing can be destroyed, but we also realize that as we change these different substances on the face of this earth, we may encounter problems which we have to live with and by. For instance, we recognize that the dust bowls we have today are the result of our not planting bushes, trees, etc., to hold the water in the soil.

It was said there was a time when half of the USA was covered with forests. When we consider that today only half of that timber exists, you can see how we are upsetting the balance of nature. This upsets the water balance and we do not get the proper rainfall where it is needed and many farms have been left barren because of it.

We find there are thousands of acres of topsoil thrown into the oceans and rivers yearly. I have read statistics stating that 80 years from now we will not have enough topsoil in the US to keep us from starving to death. While we were once rich in this topsoil, we are fast becoming poor.

Somehow or other, man has not studied nature enough to know how he can keep things the way they were in the beginning. So when we deviate from these natural laws, we are not going to get into trouble, we are in trouble. For in the deviation from natural methods, we are losing topsoil wastefully.

Parts of the country are very deficient in water-soluble iodine that is needed by the body. We call these "iodine belts." We find that people produce goiters through the lack of iodine. There are other water-soluble minerals that can be carried away when the soil has not been cared for properly.

Statistics show that 50 billion tons of topsoil is washed away yearly. It is stated that 700,000,000 tons go down the Mississippi yearly. It is no wonder that gardening our foods in the depths of the ocean is being considered.

I believe the dulse of the Atlantic Coast is very rich in the chemicals our bodies need and we should give this great consideration. Especially so when we see that in one day, May 11, 1934, a black cloud of topsoil moved into the Atlantic Ocean. This black cloud contained 300,000,000 tons of topsoil, bearning many of the trace minerals and iodine, iron, phosphorus and calcium—the minerals we need for building good bodies. In one day, 3,000 one-hundred-acre farms had their topsoil removed, thus preventing the growth of vitamin and mineral-rich plants.

Amazing Crops Produced by Virgin Soil

When the virgin soil of California, its richness untapped, was at last turned over, it yielded astonishing returns. When the second State Fair opened in Sacramento in 1855, Governor Harry S. Foote pointed out some amazing agricultural developments. In his address, he said: "But what, I pray you, would our friends and fellow citizens of the Atlantic States think or say to me were I to mention here, partly, of course, for their entertainment, a hundredth part of the wonderful things I have heard and which seem to me well attested, touching the results of farming in California?

"Suppose, for instance, I should say that in the year 1853, one of our California farmers raised from 99 bushels to the acre; that 600 bushels of potatoes had frequently been produced from a single acre of land; that upon another acre had been raised 40 tons of turnips; upon another an equal amount of beets; upon another 20 tons of tomatoes; and upon yet another that 100 dozen of cucumbers per day had been grown throughout the season, amounting in the whole to 9,000 dozen—should I not incur serious risk of being charged with gross exaggeration?

"Where beyond the limits of California, would a man be listened to with credence? Who should state—what no one present certainly would question—that delicious peaches had been known here to mature on trees only 2 years old from the pit? That repeated instances had occurred of a double crop, both of pears and apples, being raised in the same season?

"Whoever heard, save in California, of pumpkins weighing 120 pounds? Of beets 7-1/2 feet in length? Of a stalk of Indian corn 24 feet high?

"Where, except in California, can it be asserted or proven that strawberries ripen every month of the year, and that it is possible to bring to perfection 2,000 pounds of this delicious fruit from an acre of ground devoted to their cultivation?"—Sacramento Bee

Experiment after experiment has shown that we must take care of the soil before man can secure the proper health in his body. If we continue to ignore the soil problem, our greatest chance to be a strong and healthy nation will be overlooked. Most of us today cannot think correctly. Our alertness is gone. Our "decisive abilities" have been lowered and our vitality and strength is slowly being depleted by the malnutrition conditions ever on the increase. This can partly be laid to an unbalanced mineral soil; from failure to remineralize the soil by natural methods.

On top of this, the commercial foods are robbing our bodies of the health elements more than we realize. Then when this food gets to the kitchen, it is given a final blow to make our foods foodless. A University of Wisconsin bulletin says, "The introduction of synthetic and purified foods into the modern diet has tended to eliminate mineral salts. Science now finds these minerals are of greatest importance to the human organism, even though the amounts may be small, representing only a trace." So there is much to look forward to in correction, but let us first start with the soil.

Many of the diet books written in the past are not the best sources of information in trying to work out our soil problems today. We find that celery grown in New York is entirely different than that grown in Utah. The soil in Utah has more sodium because of the heavy salt content. Celery is a good sodium-storing plant and should grow very well in the Utah valley. It is amazing to see the difference in crops grown in the different soils throughout the country.

Long Island spinach has been tested for its iron content and was found to contain only 18 parts per million, while spinach grown in Indiana was found to contain 2,895 parts per million. This is quite a difference.

Stories have come out of the war about prisoners having been placed on virgin soil where they grew their own food. It was found that their physical conditions improved tremendously after eating food grown on this soil.

Down in the Louisiana lowlands, we find some of the finest growth in the country. This is due to the overflowing rivers that carry the topsoil down from the Northern states. The swamps have been receptacles for much of the topsoil which grows our best crops. I believe that much of our sugar cane grown in the south is rich in minerals, but it is robbed of these minerals in the processing and refining of the cane.

Experiments by Dr. E. E. Pfeiffer, in his laboratory at the Threefold Farms in Spring Valley, New York, were conducted with mice that had a susceptability to cancer. The survival rate was 64% among those that ate organically grown foods, but only 35% among those fed chemically fertilized food. When they painted a carcinogenic-producing agent (cancer-causing) such as is found aspirin, etc., on the skins of all mice in both groups, 71% of those fed on chemically fertilized foods became cancerous, while only 45% of those fed on organically grown foods came down with the disease.

Dr. James Asa Shield, Assistant Professor of Neuropsychiatry of the Medical College of Virginia, said in an address before the Southern Medical Association convention, as reported by the Associated Press: "Food produced from soil fertilized with chemicals has caused an increase in degenerative diseases throughout the United States."

Spray materials have been found to be injurious, not only to the insects but to all those animals and birds that kill insects. These birds and animals are not harmful to our orchards and plant life, yet whole colonies of bees have been destroyed when disinfectants and sprays have been used in this way.

Some birds can eat as much as 30 pounds of caterpillars and insects a day, which is to the farmer's benefit. But this cannot be done if we are going to continue to use insecticides and sprays.

Many of the fertilizers we use today are not made available to the plant. For instance, of the rock phosphates that are added to the soil, probably only 1/10th of this phosphate actually gets to the roots of the plants, where it is so needed. There are many people who have complained that, in spite of their soil having all the minerals, it still would not grow anything. Such soil is in need of humus and the proper bacterial activity. Organic matter is the most important of all in soil fertilization.

While I was in London a few years ago, there was considerable talk of how aluminum sulphate was causing a good deal of cancer when used as a fertilizer. We are wondering whether or not an excess of this chemical in its raw state will become an irritant when brought to the plant life itself. Certainly it is far from the natural way of remineralizing the soil.

I find from some of my own experiments that those plants that were fed properly and grown in the colloidal soil from Death Valley, grew tremendously and were of entirely different color from those grown in our depleted soil. There is such a thing as calcium, calcium and calcium. There is such a thing as flesh and flesh, diseased flesh and healthy flesh. There is such a thing as depleted soil and healthy soil—soil that will grow good vegeteables and good fruits for human consumption.

Many of the foods grown by farmers today can only be considered "colored foods," for they are lacking in the chemical balance of the mineral elements. We are eating foods that only "look good." They do not contain the vital elements to give us vigor, energy and health which we as humans are entitled to have. There are 50,000,000 farmers in this country who should be given a standard as to taking care of the many foods they are growing. We should have a standard for distribution; a standard for preserving these foods and a standard to live by in the kitchen, whereby the average housewife would know how to keep foods and prepare them in a manner which preserves all the vitamins and minerals.

Now to go still further with the idea of balancing the soil by using various ways of fertilizing. It has been brought out that we should take care of the soil through composting or adding to it a material that is broken down through bacterial activity. It has seemed as if nature planned things more or less that way.

Humus is a necessary part of rebuilding the soil. To rebuild it with chemical nutrients is not always enough. The proper bacterial invasion is necessary, for in this way, we find the life from which plants can grow. The soil must be a living organism in order to grow food.

Today, much of our plant life is lacking in some or all of the vital minerals that a good soil should have. For this reason, we have very little good soil which is rich in minerals. Our plant life cannot take up minerals which are not there and so they really are not healthy. If we were to use plant life for fertilizer, plants which were lacking in these minerals, it would be unsuccessful. But if grasses which have very long roots and which go deep down into the different stratas of earth to get their minerals were used as fertilizers, I believe we could build a good topsoil. Alfalfa and sweet clover are such grasses.

More on Earthworms and Composting

We have all observed the great amount of work an earthworm does, a burrowing terrestrial worm, useful for enriching the soil. The topsoil of the earth, which is built up by a very slow process of nature, upon which all plant life depends for its sustenance, must have humus. This is the natural organic matter of the soil, containing the decomposing plant residue, leaf mold and other materials. This soil is symbolic of the earth, our mother, and it is vitally alive with bacteria and living organisms. Maintained in a high degree of fertility and fed with the necessary elements for proper mineral content and given an adequate supply of water, it brings forth, with the cooperation of man, "our daily bread," the limitless variety of foods of greatly varied flavor, texture and smell which gratifies our appetites and nourishes and sustains our wonderful physical organisms—body and mind—and inspires our souls to thankfulness for the bounty of Nature.

This little creature, the humble earthworm, has an important part to play in this drama of the eternal process of growth and decay, the creation of new plant life and disintegration of plant residue, all of which material should be returned to the land to enter into the process of decomposition to feed the living soil. Together with the work of the earthworm, this aerates the soil, making it porous. The soil must be loose, granular, so that water can penetrate to the roots of plants and so that root systems can send their branches and fibers in every direction underground. The earthworm provides one of the fastest means of improving the condition of the topsoil. It has been termed by the ancient Greek philosopher, "The intestines of the earth." These little worms literally plow their way through the under surface developing a perfect medium for plant life to grow.

Historically and geographically, we have learned of the great importance to civilization of the Nile, that famed river of Egypt, whose annual overflow has through long ages deposited in the fertile Nile Valley the rich minerals and debris carried down by streams from the upper jungles of Africa. Earthworms utilize this organic material from bird and animal and dead plant life through their digestive processes to such an extent that they produce castings, an excellent form of manure, which aids in the improvement of the topsoil, as high as 120 tons per acre. In that rich soil, the natives need only scratch the surface and plant their seeds, and the harvest is "out of this world."

Natural soil fertility in America, whose generally rich, virgin land has been exploited by those who did not appreciate the value of the soil as our greatest natural resource, and a requisite for the sustenance of all life, is almost a thing of the past. Most growers have found ways of feeding the soil for the fast growing of crops, thinking primarily of producing and not enough of conserving, thinking in terms of the harvest and not of the processes of natural plant growth which precede it. Cultivated plants become increasingly inferior by the use of chemical poisons and artificial stimulants, necessitating a correspondingly increased use of these injurious elements. We are supplied with that which is represented as food for human consumption which the processes of Nature—if not interfered with by man through his "scientific" knowledge—would destroy. Nature will nourish and sustain only that which is vitally alive.

There are different kinds of earthworms. The ordinary gray worm is found in almost everyone's garden; however, cross breeding has produced new species which are being used in composting or breaking down kitchen refuse and material that has once had life and is being returned to the soil again. The average worm used in the worm gardens today is the red worm. It will travel as much as 100 feet in the dark in one night. The worms used in the domestic bed where castings are developed and used in the garden and other cultivated soil lay eggs once every 9 to 21 days. Each egg produces from 5 to 20 little worms. They must be fed or they will leave.

There are many different foods for this purpose and it is best to make sure there are different layers of various kinds of food for these worms to live on to keep them from migrating. Some of the best food material for them is just plain straw that has been ground through a hammer mill or shredder, sometimes adding a little molasses to better feed the worms. Use rabbit manure, as it does not attract flies; then, with the addition of a layer of dirt, you can leave the worms to their happy pursuit of burrowing and consuming their food. Within 90 days, you will have a topsoil that will grow food you will never forget! The average worm reproduces its weight in castings every 24 hours. If fed properly, he will live for some 15 years! It takes some 90 days for the baby worm to become mature and start laying eggs.

It has been found that worms will go as far as 15 feet deep into the soil. They are always coming to the surface, looking for the green pasture just as a cow reaches her head over the fence. The castings of the domestic worms are developed in a layer under the surface of the soil, not brought to the top of the ground as in the case of native worms. These little muscular beings can move objects weighing 60 times their own weight. A million worms will produce a ton of rich castings daily. You can use horse manure, leaves, grass clippings also in this compost.

Worms have been used to bore into red clay and adobe soil and have shown that in a matter of just a short time they converted it into black soil. Worms convert the minerals of different kinds of material in the soil into organic material, making this available to the feeder roots of plant life.

Castings are developed in the alimentary canal of the worm. It has been shown by Eric E. Sanders that when a worm takes in a mass of this material which is converted into castings, it is finely ground and worked through the internal secretions of the worm and ejected. Such material contains 5 times as much nitrogen, is 7 times richer in phosphates and 11 times richer in available potash than the material which the worm consumed. What better fertilizer can you buy for your garden, orchard or grove?

Worms aerate the soil so that the proper oxidization can take place from the atmosphere, keep the soil from getting hard so that moisture can be retained below the surface. An earthworm works 24 hours a day; no machinery on earth can accomplish what this little organism can do! He is the underground plow. Earthworm eggs, or capsules as they are called, are shipped to all parts of the world. These eggs will not dry out, can be stored for a long time and even kept under refrigeration for months. When they are placed in the soil or in their new home, they hatch out in 21 days. Many types of fertilizer are used—coffee grounds, oak leaves, etc. Earthworms help to neutralize the alkalinity of the soil as it is passed through their glands of secretion.

A simple method for composting is to dig a trench 2 feet wide, 2 feet deep, the length depending upon the number of cultures used. Mix 1/3 manure, 1/3 leaves, ground hay, straw, etc., 1/3 soil. The leftover soil can be added to the compost from time to time together with grass clippings, dead weeds, garbage or anything which has lived and died. It isn't necessary to turn the compost. The earthworms will take care of this. Just continue adding to the top of the pile and keep wet.

The worms are dumped on the top and covered with an addition of some of the same mixture used throughout the compost. When composting worms are transferred to trees, flowers or shrubbery or anywhere they are used, simply dip into the pile with a pitchfork and load into wheelbarrow, pickup truck or any conveyance. When you see that this has been developed into good topsoil, it is time to make the removal to the ground itself.

The abundant digestive secretions of the worms mix with the various materials that you are composting, are poured in as a solvent and neutralizing action. This semi-liquid mass is slowly moved through the long intestinal tract, mixing with valuable animal hormones and substances that man probably will have difficulty ever finding their true purpose or what they are made of. It is thrown both in the earth and on top of the earth as castings or earthworm manure; it is a humus; it is a finely-conditioned topsoil richly endowed with all the elements for plant nutrition in water-soluble form. You don't wait for months—dead vegetation, animal refuse, organic debris are converted in a matter of a few weeks, ready for their part in building the proper vegetable life we need.

Mr. Arthur J. Mason testified before the Committee on Flood Control of the House of Representatives, 70th Congress, stating, "The weight of the angle worms in this country is at least tenfold the weight of the entire human population."

Compost must be soaked 24 hours before using. Earthworms require plenty of water if they are to multiply rapidly. Compost must be kept moist but not soggy wet. Sprinkling should be carried out once or twice a week. Never allow the cultures to dry out.

When harvesting the eggs you can allow the material to become a little bit drier for easier handling. Temperatures of 60 to 70 degrees will be found favorable for best capsule production. Earthworms are originally water animals. They require plenty of water.

To sum up the whole story, provide earthworm culture materials consisting of a mixture of soil and organic (from the plant and animal kingdoms) elements, wet it down, keep it moist, add worms or egg capsules. Let nature take her course. All variations used in earthworm culture, whether they be a small box, tin container or a specially-designed culture bed or a 100-ton heap are subject to the same principle—wet food for worms—then put them in and they will start to work.

Hybrids—Better or Not?

For many years, scientists in agriculture have been cleverly crossing and culling every species of plant to produce new strains. They insist successful types give greater yields and are of superior quality. But are they better nutritionally?

In 1946, Spanish-American farmers in the Rio Grande Valley of New Mexico were encouraged to plant hybrid corn in preference to the poorer native variety. The higher yields and quality led more farmers to change over in the second year, but by the fourth year, only three of the sixty were still growing the hybrids in spite of these advantages. It was not just a matter of stubborn adherence to old customs. M. F. Ashley Montague, Ph.D., in *The American Journal of Clinical Nutrition* tells of the experiment. "The corn had not been popular from the first harvest. All the wives had complained. Its texture was wrong; it didn't hang well together for tortillas; the tortillas came out the wrong color. Few had cared for the flavor."

Could this be one of the reasons so many chemicals are used in bread nowadays? Old-time bakers will tell you that the modern flour is more difficult to work with than that of 50-odd years ago.

Unfortunately, standards today are based almost exclusively on yield and appearance. Even weight, size for size, is hardly considered. If you have ever compared an organically grown "natural" carrot with a similar-sized forced one, you will know what I mean. We are robbed of our inherent taste discretions because so many sugars and spices are used in cooking that the natural taste of the vegetable or grain is never allowed to come out. So we don't realize that we are getting less value tastewise. How could we possibly suspect, therefore, that nutritional value is inferior also? Hybrids lack vitamins and minerals.

Hybrids lack that dynamic spark of life so characteristic of nature. They have to be continually bred to keep restoring this living quality. We know that artificial fertilizers deplete the organic matter in the soil and reduce the quality of native species, but to the potency of hybrid seed this deals a death blow. Even the Spanish farmers who returned to their native corn are not getting yields as high nor taste and texture as perfect as were their great-grandsires with their old methods of putting back in the soil the organic matter to maintain fertililty.

Hybrids contain less protein and a poorer quality protein. Tests indicate that they have not the same number or proportions of amino acids. Even chickens have been found to grow faster and have more protein in their flesh on open pollinated corn than on hybrid. Man has again interfered with nature. When the internal balance of a plant is upset, how can good health possibly follow the use of such material for food? Certainly insect infestation is greater in hybrids showing that nature is not in favor of this intruder. Reproduction in animals is very dependent on their food, an important factor being the reproductive power of the plants. With their notoriously poor ability to reproduce, how will hybrids finally stand up in this respect?

Putting It All Together

If we could put all these methods together, it seems there is a way and means by which we can develop a standard for soils and have mineral-rich foods whereby all mankind would benefit.

When the soil has been depleted and the soil structure is unbalanced, we grow plant life which is diseased and underdeveloped. By making a more fertile and well-balanced soil, we are able to change diseased conditions. Do you know that most of us today are suffering from certain dangerous diet deficiencies which cannot be remedied until the depleted soils are brought into proper mineral balance? The alarming fact is that foods, fruits, vegetables and grains now being used on millions of acres of land no longer containing enough of certain needed minerals are starving us, no matter how much of them we eat!

The men in agriculture today are very much interested in this soil problem and they do not laugh at the ideas which have been brought up from the past.

The man who is trying to mineralize the soil properly needs a soil analysis. They use a spectrographic analysis today to determine all the trace elements that are present in the soil. The farmer finds that by adding a certain amount of whatever he finds lacking in his soil, he can produce a good, healthy plant stock again.

In our civilization today, we seem to need more calcium than anything else. Yet there are many soils today which are in very poor condition calcium-wise. In fact, I understand that there is less calcium in the California soil than in most other soils in the United States.

Research was made in the East, through some medical groups, which showed that out of some 4,000 cases tested for the calcium balance in the body, only 2 had the proper amount needed. It would be a wonderful thing if we could have a guaranteed analysis, showing the mineral and vitamin content of our foods as they come to us. Before we can do this, we will have to have a guaranteed analysis of the soil upon which our foods are grown and this would give us what we should know. This would determine a standard soil that farmers could go by.

We look to the farmer for a lot of good help in the future, for he will have to care for the badly nourished people. Most of the world today is sick, and I believe that our nourishment or malnourishment, is the beginning of a lot of our bodily ailments. We must look to a mineral-balanced soil to give us rich plant life and to keep our bodies minerally balanced and in good health.

Let's Make Farmers Our Doctors

Over 500-million dollars are spent on vitamins each year. If people only realized it, the farmer could give us more good health than all the drugstores combined, just by seeing to it that the soil is properly taken care of. A survey of the U.S. Department of Agriculture shows that over 75% of the population over 60 years of age (and many younger) are suffering from a calcium deficiency, a protein deficiency, an iron deficiency and some vitamin deficiencies.

We have definitely found that many of the minor elements are just as important to have in our bodies as some of the major elements, and we must have them in good combinations or we cannot be well.

In our own little way, we are trying to grow foods in our organic garden and we find it is wonderful to see how plant life can be grown which is rich in chlorophyll. How, when you break a leaf, you find that green juice overflowing. It certainly is different from the plant, just a few feet away. The plant grown in the soil which was not properly treated is certainly lacking in this rich, green juice, because it does not have the proper minerals in the soil to make the chlorophyll.

Magnesium is an important part of chlorophyll. That is how the plant gets its color. Boron increases chlorophyll. Boron is another one of those minor chemical or trace mineral elements, as they call them. Boron gives elasticity to the cherries, prunes and tomatoes. There is less cracking after rain when there is enough boron in the soil. Zinc aids root development and quickens germination, pollination of the plant and increases the keeping quality of some foods. Copper helps chlorophyll development and controls fruit splitting. These minor elements are very necessary to our bodies, just the same as they are in plant life. It has been truly said that there is only 1/1000 of an ounce of iodine between keeping us sane or allowing insanity to develop.

A recent magazine tells us about the red vitamin B-12. It is found in combination with cobalt, which is one of the trace minerals. When cobalt is lacking in the soil, the plant life, when fed to animals, interfered with the proper sex development and we find they cannot breed properly. Vitamin B-12 is used as a "pick up" for a person with a low blood count and it does it in a very quick way. Some 40% of vitamin B-12 is found to contain pure cobalt.

Years ago, when a man wanted to add the proper minerals to the soil, he was considered a "crackpot." Even today, he is not looked upon too favorably for his ideas in that respect. I remember a book written years ago entitled *Bread and Roses from Stones*; the author had much opposition. But he grew much better plants than his neighbor. This he did by using certain rocks and mineral elements, which he added to the soil. Adding this rock combination to his soils performed many miracles which other people could not understand. Some people even went to jail for selling these minerals as a fertilizer. Yet today it has become quite common to buy minerals to rebalance the soil.

Here at our Ranch, we worked many experiments to prove to ourselves that by the care of certain soils, we were able to produce different types of plant life that we could not have otherwise. Today, we have come to the conclusion, definitely, that those soils which are prepared properly do grow an entirely different food. We can tell the difference in effect almost immediately.

We have been using organically grown food in our sanitarium and we find that people like it much better. It has more flavor and we see health improved with its constant use.

There are so many things to consider when we are taking care of the soil. For example, we must consider the irrigation. There are ways of subterranean irrigation. We must consider this when we have to deal with soluble salts that we might carry away or deposit in the soil. It would be wonderful if we could throw the proper mineral elements back into the soil again through our irrigation system.

Plants have appetites. Plants have health and disease just as humans. They are controlled through feeding. Many times, animals have had better health by grazing on food grown out in the desert than when grazing consistently on ground which has been used time in and out, year after year, with constant and continuous cropping. Sometimes the animals will seek growth that comes from soil which has not been used constantly.

I would advise anyone interested in taking care of the soil to get Dr. Ehrenfried Pfeiffer's book on *Bio-Dynamic Farming and Gardening* and also to subscribe to "Organic Gardening and Farming."

Much credit must be given to the Savage Farms in Kentucky for the wonderful work they have done. I am indebted to Mr. Lyle for his generous help while at my sanitarium.

Let's Think "Prevention"

When we realilze that 97% of the money spent in the healing art is spent after a person gets into trouble, I think it is well that we realize that more time and money should be spent on the prevention of disease. Especially when we consider that less than 3% of the money spent in the healing art is for the prevention of disease. To begin to prevent disease, we must start with the soil. The doctor of the future will be the "man of the soil," the man who knows the mineral balance which will produce life more abundant.

It is to the children of the future, our next generation, that we owe the inheritance of a good soil. Certainly it is to our own advantage to see that the next generation is given the best to carry on. But we are going to give our children a very depleted nervous system if we have produced a bad constitution within ourselves, because we would be giving them a poor "inherent quality" by having a depleted soil condition.

Much knowledge and information is now coming to the front for our best good and for that of future generations. We should work unselfishly in carrying out our part in the great program for man's higher good. If we continue to live ignorantly on the coffee and donut diet, all the minerals and soil work cannot save us. It is well that we consider this mineral program all the way from the soil to our table!

Loss of fertility is vastly more extensive in its incidence than erosion.... Probably more soil has been lost since 1941 than in the whole previous history of the world.

It is well we know our bodies act like a plant, ready to absorb and take in the chemical elements necessary for the rebuilding of every cell and organ in our bodies. Many experiments have been worked with animals and they have found that natural food as God created it has always given the best health to the animal. A giant gorilla in one of the large zoos in our country died a short time ago because of cookies and sweets fed to it by visitors. We carefully feed our animals to make sure they are free of disease. Why shouldn't we do the same thing with the human body? If we have the right foods going into the body, we can rebuild broken down tissues and maintain that which has been worn out. When we eat sugar-high cookies, pickles and ice cream combinations, the ghost flours that are fed so prevalently in our restaurants today, it is no wonder our skins are broken out, our eyes lose their power and we lag in physical endurance.

Chapter 46

What foods are made of

Nutritional scientists are finding more and more constituents of foods beside the basic proteins, carbohydrates, fats, vitamins and minerals. There are enzymes, prostaglandins, neurotransmitters, neuroinhibitors and other factors which have specific functions in the body.

In this chapter, however, we will only be discussing the basic components of foods: proteins, carbohydrates and fats. Others are covered in other chapters.

We find that all growth and tissue repair is accomplished by means of foods, which provide us with the substance to build tissue and the energy to carry on life. It is important for all of us to understand a few of the basics about how foods work in the body.

Protein

All proteins are made up of a small unit, the amino acid. There are more than 20 different amino acids, and the body can synthesize at least 12. This fact was discovered by William Rose, a biochemist at the University of Illinois. Ten amino acids are known as "essential" because they cannot be manufactured and must be supplied in foods. These ten are: arginine, phenylalanine, valine, lysine, tryptophan , threonine, histidine, leucine, methionine and isoleucine.

Because vegetable proteins often lack one or more of the essential amino acids, they are classed as "second-class protein." Animal proteins, on the other hand, have all the essential amino acids (except gelatin, which lacks three), and are called "first-class protein." This classification is rather misleading. With a good variety of vegetable proteins, the vegetarian can obtain all the essential amino acids because any lacking in one food will be made up by others (the total of over 20 amino acids allows for combinations in 2,432,902,008,640 different ways!)

Tradition has accumulated a strong prejudice of the inferiority of vegetable proteins. Modern research shows this to be an unsound generalization. Chemically and nutritionally, soybeans, Brazil nuts and peanuts rank with animal protein. It is likely in the near future that others will also be added to this class. Nuts are the only protein of certain tribes in parts of the world, and that millions survive on legumes, poorer vegetable protein, shows that there are gaps in our knowledge. The only essential amino acids found in these in any quantity are isoleucine, threonine and valine. Monkeys and apes (our nearest relatives) live on shoots, berries, tubers, leafy vegetables and nuts; and some of them can shift half a ton. Gorillas are even stronger.

Flesh proteins are acid forming. Practice does not uphold the fact that eating much protein necessarily develops energy and vibrant health. Sometimes the opposite is true.

In 1948, Professor A. Fleisch, President of the Swiss Federal Commission for Nutrition, stated, "2,160 calories are enough unless a person is a very heavy manual worker (2,400 United Nations minimum daily requirement).

"These conclusions are based on large-scale experiments made with scientific thoroughness on 4,000,000 people in Switzerland. The experiments showed that the amount of calories, proteins and fats formerly considered essential iln civilized countries is utterly unnecessary.

"Our conclusion is that a standard figure of 1 gram of protein per kilogram of body weight (0.035 oz per 2 lb 3-1/4 oz) is correct, compared to the more than 100 grams a day advocated before the war, which was not only unnecessary, but harmful."

The body cannot get rid of excess protein, but must excrete it by way of the kidneys. Early this century, Professor Russell H. Chittenden of Yale University, carried out thousands of tests on nutrition and proved that the average man eats twice as much protein as he needs. No recent experiments have disproved this. Professor Hindhede endorses them. Working with professional men, whose occupations were mental rather than physical, he showed that a drastic cut in protein intake improved health, energy and resistance to fatigue. A group of soldiers gained in strength phenomenally.

There is a lot of talk these days about us needing more protein in our diet. It is something to think about, especially when people are eating so haphazardly and gambling with their digestion at the corner restaurants, baseball games and fast food drive-ins. We are making a living by straightening out people's dietary habits, teaching them how to live correctly and setting up new nutritional patterns that they may follow.

One of the most important things to realize is that our body must have a new beginning to get out of the predicament most of us are in. We must learn a new way of maintaining good health. Everyone seems to be dieting these days. Get off that diet. Learn a good, healthy way to live. Diets are useful for slenderizing and for the elimination of various toxemias, but let us also reckon with one fact: we must learn how to live correctly after we get off the diet. A basic way of living should include six vegetables, two fruits, at least; one starch and at least one protein every day. The average person who really wants to build his body and nervous system should consider adding extra protein value.

Many of the amino acid preparations we have today do not contain all the different amino acids our body needs. There have been experiments which show that glutamic acid is especially good for backward children. Children fed on this amino acid have far surpassed others in tests, showing that it is probably one of the factors missing in the diet or is needed in larger amounts when such a condition exists. Amino acids have various functions in the body besides being a main component of flesh tissue. Some are specific in action. For instance, one amino acid may assist the gallbladder, another the liver and still other different organs and expressions of the body. In order, therefore, not to run the risk of missing any essential factor, it is well to get a variety of proteins. Do not depend upon any one protein for all the amino acids. Soybeans probably have most of them, but not all, and to rely on soybeans entirely would lead you to find weakness in your health over a period of time.

It has been said that a person weighing 175 pounds would need 85 grams of protein a day, or the equivalent of 1/2 pound or 2 cups. It is foolish to say that these figures can be followed exactly, as there are no two people alike, either in physical makeup or temperament. Highly-strung persons would, no doubt, use more than the calm serene types. Tension, worry and fretting wear one out. The person who has found a tranquil way of living will not have to depend on food to pay back shortages in his body or build up a burned out chemistry in organs or tissues. So you cannot treat everybody exactly the same.

Now, if you feel you need directions to follow, here is a table to help you. Personally, I belileve that our protein intake is too high and we would do better to learn a way of living that would allow us to get along with much less protein in our bodies. But in this day and age of stress, tranquilizers and antacids, people need immediate help while learning a better way to live.

The most natural way to correct any of your bodily problems is to consider using the following foods because their protein is rich in amino acids. It is well to use two, three or four of them daily, in the amounts suggested, in a glass of tea, pineapple or any other juice. This makes an excellent protein tonic. Vary the drinks from day to day. Sweeten them with a tablespoonful of maple sugar, apple concentrate or grape concentrate.

Lecithin—1 tablespoon
Gelatin—1 tablespoon
Wheat germ flakes—1 tablespoon
Wheat germ oil—1 tablespoon

Brewer's yeast—1 tablespoon
Vegetable broth powder—1 teaspoon
Egg yolk—1
Soymilk powder—1 tablespoon
Dried milk powder—1 tablespoon
Skim milk powder—1 tablespoon
Raw milk—3/4 glass
Yogurt—2 tablespoons

Carbohydrates: How Much Do We Need in the Body?

Carbohydrate foods are those providing our sugars and starches.

Sugar found in fruit is more easily taken up by the body than sugar made by man. Nature's sugar is organized with other elements and is, therefore, more adapted to the body than the sugars that are bought at the grocery. Our body breaks down carbohydrates, starches and sugars, to a dextrose, which is a grape sugar; a levulose, or a fruit sugar; and a galactose, or a milk sugar. The fuel of the body is derived from carbohydrates and fats. Carbohydrates should be chewed very thoroughly.

Much of the caloric intake in our body is dependent upon the carbohydrates we eat. It has been said that some 85% is supplied by carbohydrates and fats. The amount of protein we need in our daily intake has been worked out from a scientific standpoint, but there has been nothing specific about the carbohydrates that we should have in our diet. We know that when we take an excessive amount of carbohydrates, we can develop body fat. We know that we can develop putrefaction in the bowel; we know, too, that a person can become lazy, indolent and inactive by taking too many starches. On the other hand, there are people who want to do without starches in their diet and this can be very dangerous. There are also many people who eat starches so they will not be hungry for the next meal. As starches form the greatest part of the American meal, this should be curbed, because they crowd out the nice greens and vegetables that are necessary to keep our body in good chemical balance.

Some carbohydrates are easier to digest than others and are readily absorbed and used by the system. There are many ways of preparing carbohydrates, which make it easier for them to be digested and utilized by the body. For instance, we can bake some starches, cook some or heat some. It is possible to do without carbohydrates, but it is better not to, unless one is prepared to go through a considerable transition period. There are some people who say we can live on proteins entirely, but we do not approve of this. We deal with many people and find that it is better to have balance.

We believe that everyone should have at least one carbohydrate every day. We have found in parious parts of the world that there are people who live on an almost complete protein diet. For instance, the Eskimos and people living in parts of Africa have been found to live on practically all meat and fat. The carbohydrates give us the calories for the body, and we find that many people increase their carbohydrates in order to get that extra fuel, energy and heat. However, if we overwork the digestive system that handles these carbohydrates, it can lead to many disease processes. Probably the most important one is diabetes. A good deal of the carbohydrate intake should be regulated by the demand for energy. A person working hard physically needs more carbohydrates than a person who works mentally. A growing child should have more carbohydrates than a well-developed, mature person. Doctors, scientists and nutritionists have not worked out a scientific formula as to how much carbohydrates we need. However, boys who are in the army, working hard physically, have run up their daily requirement to some 3,200 to 3,600 calories per day. This is made up mostly of starches.

There are some countries, such as Mexico, Guatemala and China, where the people use a good deal of rice and can subsist on it very well. But they take the whole grain, the whole rice, the whole corn, and one of the greatest of all gland and nerve builders is found in the germ of the corn, the germ of the oats, rice and wheat. The activity of the muscles in the body depends on vitamin E, and the greatest amount of this is found in the germ of grains. Reproductive ability is dependent upon the amount of whole grain we have in our diet. I believe a good deal of this depletion has come about in this country due to the fact that we have used devitalized, demineralized, polished starches. It is not only the amount of calories we have, it is a matter of whether we are getting a natural substance.

We can get 100% calories out of granulated white sugar, but that doesn't mean that it contains the vitamin and mineral values that our bodies should have. The main thing to understand in this diet work is that our body will mold to whatever food we give it. If we give it unnatural food, our body can end up in a disharmonious state. A nonchemical balance can be the result. We can end up with a nutritional shortage.

I think it is well that we have natural foods and let our bodies mold to these, because all the vitamins and minerals are found in natural foods. We can get along for some years on our own body, living on the fats, the carbohydrates and the protein storage, but eventually, we develop a chemical shortage that shows up in what we term disease or in symptoms of pain, aches and disturbances in various organs of the body. If we are going to use the nutritional science for keeping well, it is necessary to realize that a certain amount of good carbohydrates should be included in our everyday routine. We can have diets set up for us where we cut out

starches for the present moment to make up for the overuse in the past, or to make up for the abuse of certain types of carbohydrates which develop allergies because of a lack of whole foods. The reason wheat is probably considered one of the greatest offenders today in allergy cases is because of the fact that the whole wheat is not used to begin with, but only part of it. The way to counteract this is to turn to another type of grain entirely, leaving the wheat out of the diet for a short time. When we have changed the chemical balance, the chemical ratio of the acid-alkaline balance in the body, then we can come back to these natural foods and they will not cause allergies.

The most important thing to consider with starches is that we have to chew them well. The digestion of starches begins in the mouth. When we chew thoroughly, a generous supply of saliva is secreted to take care of the starch. Saliva supplies ptyalin, which is an enzyme that converts the raw starches into sugar, making it easy to digest and absorb in the body. We cannot bolt our food. Don't let the trap door allow food to go down, especially a carbohydrate, until it has been well masticated and broken down by the teeth. If you chew your food properly, you can get a taste from your food that you wouldn't otherwise enjoy. By chewing foods, the digestive centers of the brain which help to secrete the digestive juices, are stimulated, which, in turn, helps the digestion of foods as they are passed on to the stomach and the small intestines. Many people do not appreciate their foods because they do not chew them. They do not spend enough time with food to give it the right thought. There is a lot of bulk, a lot of cellulose in starches and sugars. We find that glucose or the grape sugar, is the easiest to digest of all sugars that go into the body.

Whenever taking starches into the body, it might be well to realize that starches will dry up in an oven very quickly. Whenever eating starches, we must have the water-carrying foods along with them. These are found in dried fruits and vegetables especially. Never eat sandwiches without also having vegetables. Starches can cause constipation in many people if they do not have enough vegetables along with them. One thing we should realize when taking a lot of starches is that we can get an excessive amount of carbons in the body, and we know that carbons slow down the body. Carbons are hard on metabolism. An excessive amount of oxygen is needed to handle the carbon foods, such as is found in sugar, starches, fats, etc.

Carbon is the cradle of creation—in the principal element of growth. This is necessary, of course, when children are growing. Whenever carbon and oxygen are at work, one upon the other, there is heat generated and carbonic acid gas. It supports the vital system, but when there is an excessive amount of carbon in the system, it leads to obesity. Carbon is the basic element of cell birth and cell life. However, most people eat an excess of carbohydrates and fats. An excess of carbohydrates in the body can result in boils, obesity, fatty degeneration, anemia and a hundred and one ailments that have all been translated into Greek and never been cured.

When we have an excess of carbon in the body, we dislike work and seek a soft bed. We become awkward in everything we do. We become clumsy, drop things easily, and our fingers always seem to be in the way. We grieve over insignificant things. We stumble because of our clumsiness. We can suffer from fermentative obesity, from asthma, toxic goiters, sleepiness, drowsiness, catarrhal and mucus problems can develop; pus formation, carbonosis, pyorrhea and carbon dioxide poisoning can result. Noises in the ear, vertigo, spasms and a thousand other disagreeable symptoms and sensations can result.

Our highest sugar and starch-containing foods are:

All bread stuffs	Rye
All baker's products	Pumpernickel
All white flour foods	Rice
Biscuits	Rice flour
Cookies	Rice pudding
Crackers	Wild rice
Cakes	Pancakes
Pastries	Hominy
Crullers	Oatmeal
Buns	Doughnuts
Lady Fingers	Ginger snaps
Graham crackers	Dried apples
Cracked wheat	Dried dates
Whole wheat	Dried pears
Yellow corn	Dried figs
Rolled oats	Prunes
Raisins	Sweet apples
Popcorn	Candy
Grape juice	Sweet drinks
Honey	Soda fountain drinks
Maple syrup	Spaghetti
Molasses	Macaroni
Sugars	Noodles
Sorghum	Most beans
Jellies	Barley preparations
Lentils	

Foods low in sugar and starch:

Muscle meat	Lettuce
Internal meat	Limes
Bone broths	Loquats
Wild game	Nasturtiums
Roquefort cheese	Dwarf nettle
Dutch cheese	Spinach
Goat whey	String beans
Swiss cheese	Tomatoes

Celery	Cucumber
Eggs	Fish
Egg white	Fish broths
Egg yolk	Codfish
Hickory nuts	All lake and ocean fish

Foods Lowest in Fats and Carbohydrates

It will be necessary to exclude from our diet foods that are high in fat or have any fat carbohydrates in them. We might consider the foods lowest in fats and carbohydrates such as:

Asparagus	Limes
String beans	Loquat
Cabbage	Nasturtium
Cauliflower	Nettle salad
Celery	Buttermilk
Endive	Bone broths
Kale	Green cucumber juice
Common lettuce	Beaten egg white
Winter lettuce	Egg shell broth
Young radishes	Dried olives
Spinach	All herb teas
Watercress	Fish
Chayotes	Gelatin

Foods High in Minerals and Alkaline Ash

Often when we take carbohydrates we have them in a refined state which leaves out a lot of the minerals or the ash material that is necessary in alkalinizing and keeping our body in good nutritional balance. Some of the foods high in minerals and alkaline ash are:

Egg shell broth	Rice bran extract
Chicken bone broth	Rye bran extract
Whey cheese broth	Rye bran muffins
Whey cheese dishes	Wheat bran tea
Whey cheese tonics	Swiss cheese
Goat whey	Roquefort cheese
Goat brown cheese	Extracts from dandelion
Extracts from watercress	Caraway seeds
Extracts from endive	Sunflower seeds
Dried tomatoes	Sauerkraut
Cherry juice	Blackberry juice
Juniper berries	Fish

Our bodies cannot adequately digest or eliminate devitalized foods. The body does the best it can—it molds to that food, but in time we find that the body becomes distorted, just as the food is that we have been eating. We should eat starches sparingly, and they should be natural starches, otherwise they can be called dead foods. They can be called adulterated. In this day and age, we should know what to eat, but we should also know what to leave alone. Certain foods can build us or kill us by degrees. Some foods, drinks and dope should be religiously avoided, because they are made of bleached and processed flour and because they contain adulterants that are actually useless or else harmful to health. They contain toxic preservatives; they are laboratory products and not real foods; they have been sulphured, fumigated or treated with poison and because they have been made of inferior food materials; they have been dyed, doctored up or doped. They have been treated chemically until they appear fresh and inviting to the innocent public.

Therapeutic Use of Carbohydrates

Starches, sweets, sugars, etc., can be used therapeutically. High blood pressures respond very well to the rice diet. This is a diet where a person has two meals a day of rice and vegetables. Of course, they should use brown rice.

We find that heart trouble responds very well when we use the supreme heart remedy, which is made of whole wheat. One of the finest remedies I have found for the heart, during my years of practice, is a whole wheat cereal. When freshly ground, whole wheat has the wheat germ and the oils intact. Wheat germ is a special heart builder containing vitamin E, the heart vitamin. Within 16 hours after the wheat is ground, many of the oils are dissipated. Use a fresh-ground hard northern wheat from Deaf Smith County in the following way.

One-half cup ground wheat to one-and-one-half cups hot water; put in a thermos bottle; cork the bottle, stand all night to soak. By this method, the cereal is not overcooked and the vitamins are not destroyed by the use of high heat, and since no air comes in contact with the wheat, there is no dissipation of some of the very essential vitamins. Use this as a cereal for breakfast every morning for three months or longer if you wish.

Honey and water is considered a wonderful energy-giver for the person who has a lack of energy due to any heart disturbance. Honey and water is also very effective in cases where the person cannot sleep well, as carbohydrates will tend to quiet a person if he is of a nervous temperament. In China and India, where they eat so much rice, there is very little heart trouble or mental illness. However, I don't think it is all due to the fact that they eat a lot of rice; I think some of it is due to their mental attitude.

Jerusalem artichokes should take the place of starch for people who are heavy potato eaters. It is an easy starch to digest.

Taking a colloidal sulphur helps the pancreas to digest the starches better. Huckleberry tea also helps the pancreas.

Fats

Fats, absolutely essential in the diet, are a wholesome and useful constituent of foods. More than any other food, the fats produce the sense of satiety or satisfaction after eating. They are the most concentrated form of energy of all foodstuffs, having a caloric value more than double that of either carbohydrates or proteins. If eaten in excess, fats usually produce a rapid gain in flesh, encourage intestinal putrefaction with rancid stools, and are apt to give rise to a troublesome and even dangerous condition known as acidosis. It is strictly physiologic that fats be eaten with cereals or breadstuffs, for the starch which is found abundantly in cereals is necessary for the proper utilization of fats by the body cells.

In the body, the blood carries 4% fat, the muscles carry 3% and bone marrow has 93%. Fats yield a certain amount of energy to the body and in addition, they protect delicate organs, prevent excess radiation of heat and keep us from having chilled blood by helping to cover the nerves from too much exposure to the elements. The fat which covers the nerves is made from lecithin and cholesterol. The mental worker has a greater need of nerve fats than the manual worker.

A subtle element, the growth-promoting vitamin A, essential for health as well as development, is often, though not always, associated with fats. When fat is lacking or deficient in quantity, this element is likely also to be lacking; and because of this association, which has only recently come to be understood, injuries resulting from the withholding of fats have very naturally been attributed to lack of the fat itself rather than to the absence or deficiency of the growth-promoting vitamin with which the older physiologists were not acquainted. This element is abundant in butter but is deficient in lard, in some vegetable oils and many other fats. It is also plentiful in greens.

Fats are derived from both animal and vegetable sources. They consist chiefly of carbon and hydrogen, with a small amount of oxygen. Every animal produces a fat peculiar to itself. Such fat is formed by the conversion of starch and other carbohydrates into fat by the action of the body cells.

When a surplus of food is eaten, the fat is deposited in the tissues in the same form as that in which it is swallowed. This is true of beef or mutton tallow and of other fats eaten by man. They cannot be transformed into the same sort of fat which the body makes from starch and sugar, but remain as is to be deposited in the tissues. It is an interesting fact that vegetable fats are more nearly like the natural fat which the body produces from starch and sugar than are the fats found in the ox, the sheep and the dog.

Some of the best fats to be used in the diet are from the nut and seed butters; such as sunflower seed, sesame seed or tahini, coconut oil, ripe olives, olive oil, safflower oil, raw cream, almond oil and sweet butter. Fish and fresh raw goat cream are also good. However, an excess of any fats going into the body will hinder the digestion and overwork the gallbladder and the liver, since all fats have to be taken care of by digestive juices which the body produces in the gallbladder and liver.

Whenever any fatty foods, such as egg yolk, are eaten, it is well to use a high iron food with them; e.g., cherry juice, blackberry juice, spinach greens or other tops of vegetables. These are necessary to accompany the fats to ensure their proper digestion. Dandelion tea helps to stimulate the gallbladder and will help throw off excess fats for a person who has accumulated them over a period of time because he has not or is not eating properly.

When grandmother used poached eggs on greens such as spinach, she probably had the best combination of all. Fried fats, as in fried eggs, are very indigestible and are very difficult for the gallbladder and liver to process. If cooking fats at all, they should be heated at a very low temperature, and any such heated fat will cause a disturbance in the body. It is my conviction that heated oil actually cannot be handled properly by the body and that such oil is responsible for much of the cholesterol deposits in many people today.

I believe that fats are used too heavily in the American diet, and I think that we could get all we need from natural foods such as avocado, yogurt, nut butters, sesame seed, milk, cream and eggs. Too much fat can hinder protein digestion and retard the secretion of our digestive juices so that the fats accumulate in the tissues where they cause considerable damage by settling around the vital organs, especially the heart.

Sometimes it is necessary to correct the harm already done. There are definite physical and chemical laws that control the building up of fat structure, so the correction must be to cut down on the fat intake so that the excess the body already has will be absorbed and finally eliminated.

Hindhede of Copenhagen had as one of his subjects an athlete who lived for 22 months on a diet from which fats of all sorts were rigidly excluded. The food consisted of bread prepared from the whole wheat, potatoes and greens. It was remarked that the consumption of large quantities of greens were found necessary to keep the patient in good condition.

When on a visit to Hindhede's laboratory in Copenhagen, Dr. John Harvey Kellogg had the pleasure of meeting the subject of this experiment, Mr. Madsen, and found him to be an exceedingly robust and athletic man, apparently enjoying perfect health, and in no way endangered by his long abstention from fats and the numerous other dietary experiments of which he had been the subject during the preceding twenty years.

The Liver and the Gallbladder

The liver and gallbladder are much talked of by the average patient today, as in nearly every disease we find an improperly functioning liver and gallbladder. Our liver is influenced by our ideas and emotions just as our mouth and stomach. Let us imagine a savory omelet, served piping hot. Not only must we swallow while reading this sentence, because the salilvary glands have filled the mouth with saliva, not only does gastric juice collect in the stomach, but a portion of fresh bile also flows from the liver into the gallbladder. Indeed the liver is subject to the influence of emotions to a greater degree than any of the other digestive glands.

The influence of emotions on the liver is quite remarkable. A feeling of joy produces moderate increases in the bile flow, sorrow increases it considerably, while anger results in a complete stoppage of the flow. If a person is overcome by a strong feeling of loathing and nausea, the bile duct contracts and inhibits the flow. Since the digestion of fat is impossible without bile, a fat-free diet is prescribed for persons with gallbladder disease.

The liver is the detoxifier of the body, and waste material is brought to the liver and transformed into

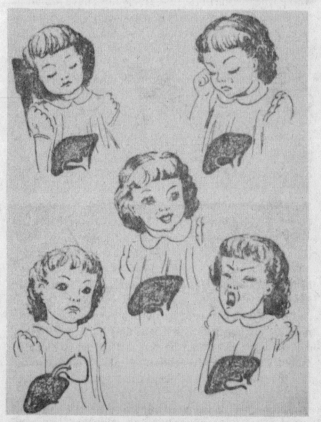

These drawings indicate the effects of emotion upon the gallbladder.

harmless compounds. The liver filters all the blood going through it. Daily our lives are saved through the blood cleansing activities of the liver.

Excessive alcoholic drinking over a period of years may produce a liver as hard as a board. It is a known fact that alcohol does great damage to the cells of the liver. The primary cause of cirrhosis is excessive consumption of alcohol.

The substance that the liver cells make from cholesterol and various salts is called bile. Bile is a golden yellow when fresh and turns a dark green when exposed to the air. Bile is very bitter and the expression, "bitter as gall" is well stated. This bile does not flow directly from the liver into the intestines but goes first into the gallbladder. As fatty food passes the opening of the bile duct, it activates release of a hormone which triggers bile flow into the intestines.

It is well known that gallstones form in the gallbladder and the older we are, the more subject to having gallstones we become. Many people have gallstones that never bother them but others suffer great pain when a stone is in such a position as to interfere with the normal flow of bile.

Gallstones are very lovely, beautifully iridescent ochre yellow or a shining malachite green, but they can be a serious problem in the gallbladder of a human.

The Value of Gréens

If I were going to bring out one particular food to cleanse and rebuild the body, it would be greens. If you are green inside, you are clean inside. Greens control the calcium in the body. They are high in iron and potassium. The more bitter they are, the more potassium they contain. Greens are one of the finest things known for neutralizing the acids in the body. The chlorophyll in greens is high in vitamin K, the antihemorrhagic vitamin. Also there is usually a lot of vitamins C and A in any of the green vegetables.

We can absorb greens into the digestive system faster than any other food. The least digestion is necessary for getting chlorophyll into the blood than of all the other chemical elements. There is nothing more wonderful to use than greens to sweeten the body, to clean the mouth, sweeten the breath, take away odors. It can be used for tonics by taking a teaspoonful of the liquid chlorophyll in a glass of water a day. Add it to a glass of cherry juice and you've got a wonderful blood builder and another wonderful tonic. If you add an egg yolk you have the ideal tonic combination for the brain and nervous system, as well as the bloodstream. Liquid greens can be used in many other different ways. You can get green liquids in nearly all raw vegetables. Never use a bottom vegetable without including the green tops. Green tops control the calcium in the body.

I heard of some poor fellow who spent over two thousand dollars to cure his halitosis and then found

that nobody wanted him around anyway. Now to sum up a few miscellaneous ideas. The individual who does a lot of physical work should have plenty of iron, calcium and silicon, and if they perspire a lot, they should add sodium. I can look at any person and tell if they are lacking in at least four chemicals. Namely, iron, calcium, silicon and sodium. I will watch him walk, his facial expressions, his hair and have him wink at me.

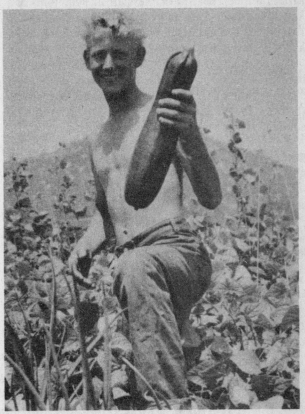

This zucchini squash is one of our bland foods, especially good in transition diets. It is very high in sodium, which makes it a good dissolving food for any hard settlements in the body.

Then I'll tell him he is lacking in all four. I can be sure I'm right because everyone is lacking in these four elements to some degree. The difference is that some of us, too many by far, are gravely deficient in iron, calcium, silicon and sodium. We must do something about it or lose our health, if only for insurance. It is every man's job to give attention and serious consideration to the business of maintaining good health. Isn't it better to pay the cost of keeping you well (prevention) rather than paying the bill for curing yourself until you die?

Sodium, chlorine and calcium are the three best alkalinizers. The history of what they can do in the body, and how they are used up is important. If we don't have enough sodium, toxic symptoms come in the body—any part of the body where an inherent weakness may be found. Drawing sensations in the tendons and nerves (cramps) may develop; bad breath and a feeling of discomfort after eating are other experiences, and the person who is constantly burping lacks sodium, as well as good manners.

When the voice becomes weak and the throat hoarse and sore, we are lacking sodium. When we cannot ride in an automobile or on a train without being sick, we need sodium. The skin becomes sticky, the feet and fingers fall asleep, dyspepsia sets in, as does intestinal decomposition and the growth of bacteria. Mouth blisters, heartburn, these are all symptoms of a lack of sodium; so are unnecessary wrinkles in the skin. Insufficient sodium destroys our look of youthfulness, and our love turns sour when this youthful element leaves our body. Our tempers become easily ruffled and happiness goes out of us for lack of sodium. We get sodium from goat milk whey, crisp celery, goat cheese (brown) and cabbage. Beaten egg white is high in sodium, as are okra, squash and strawberries.

Some Items You'll Want From Your Health Food Store

HERB TEAS: Oatstraw, alfamint, huckleberry, strawberry, mint, shavegrass, peach leaf, fenugreek.

CEREALS AND GRAINS: Whole grain wheat, wheat germ, rice polishings, brown rice, wild rice, lentils, soybeans, soymilk, seven grain cereal, barley, cornmeal, oats, millet, peas, beans.

SEEDS: Safflower, sesame, Guatemala squash, sunflower, pumpkin.

OILS: Safflower, sesame, peanut, olive, sunflower, soy, tahini.

POWDERS: Dulse, banana, coconut, carob, Health-A-Whey.

BREADS: Whole grain, millet, rye.

FRUIT JUICES: Black cherry, Concord grape, prune, apple, fig, pineapple, pomegranate.

NUTS: Almond, pine nuts, pecans, walnuts, cashews, peanuts, Brazil, coconut, malted nuts.

NUT BUTTERS: Almond, peanut, cashew.

SALTS: Vegetable, celery, mineral, garlic.

HERBS: Paprika, rosemary, basil, thyme, sage, flaxseed.

NATURAL SUGARS: Honey of many kinds, molasses, corn, date, raw and maple.

DRIED FRUITS: Apricots, dates, olives, prunes, raisins, apples, figs, pears, peaches.

Cherry concentrate or apple concentrate for flavoring, topping on yogurt. Make delicious drinks for the family with the concentrates.

Also include cheese of all kinds, gelatins, salad dressings, meat substitutes, lecithin spread, lecithin granules and dry cereals.

Our bodies have a tendency to mold to the excess elements we may be taking in our foods, or to chemical deficiencies due to improper food habits. Both conditions are imbalanced, and either will result in problems. We must always remember that chemical balance is necessary for good health, happiness and well-being. There is a relationship between mental activities and the physical body, such that chemical deficiency or excess affects the mind as well as the physical side.

How Will You Have Your Snake?

"A few years ago, any ordinary civilized person would have been disgusted at the mere idea of eating snake meat, yet today, canned Florida rattlesnake is a popular and fashionable dish and is served in the most highest-priced restaurants and hotels in New York and elsewhere. There are many other snakes just as palatable as the rattler, among these being the common black snake, chicken snake, bull snake, gopher snake, pine snake, while the boas and anacondas of Tropical America are deemed far superior to rattlesnakes when properly cooked. Alligators' tails are also excellent food....Epicures pay exorbitant prices for terrapin and the big savage snapping turtles of our ponds and lakes are deemed just as good as the diamondbacks."

Chapter 47

How we handle what we eat

Digestion is a marvelous process. All manner of chemical reactions take place within the gastrointestinal tract. Biochemists and physiologists have been studying these for years. But still we have much to learn. Digestion begins the moment the food is introduced into the mouth. Chewing is the first act in this remarkable drama. By this means, the food is broken down into smaller fragments, thus allowing the digestive juices to carry on their work more completely. Chewing is important for another reason. It helps to relieve nervous tension. It encourages the flow of gastric juices, thus increasing the nutritive value of the food. The food, which has been thoroughly mixed with gastric juices, flows to the deepest part of the stomach near the pyloric sphincter. The alimentary canal consists of four large divisions: mouth and esophagus, stomach, small intestine and large intestine.

The Importance of Saliva

The mouth is alkaline owing to the saliva; the gastric juice makes the stomach acid. Because of its secretions the small intestine is again alkaline. And, finally, the contents of the large intestine are acid because of the activities of the bacilli in it.

Within the mouth, an important chemical called ptyalin is added to the food. This enzyme is produced by the salivary glands. Ptyalin begins to digest the starches within the food, breaking them down into more simple forms of carbohydrate known as sugars, such as maltose and glucose. Most people fail to make use of these valuable enzymes within the mouth. They swallow their food without properly chewing it, and then they wonder why they suffer from indigestion.

The activity of the saliva in various people shows tremendous differences. In the average person, only a little of starch liquefied in the mouth is digested. However, digestion is completed in the stomach.

The chewing gum habit reduces the effectiveness of salivation.

When the saliva is not doing its job properly, stomach digestion is interfered with. The food arrives in the stomach in an imperfectly broken down form; also the undigested starch absorbs the pepsin of the gastric juice, thus leaving its acid free to give rise to gastric spasm, pain and other discomforts. It is, therefore, imperative that we chew our food well to at least give the saliva a chance.

While fruit acids, such as malic and tartaric, exert very little effect on the saliva, citric acid stimulates its flow greatly, aiding protein digestion very much. Acetic and oxalic acids (rhubarb and spinach) interfere with digestion. One to two teaspoons of vinegar or one part oxalic acid in 10,000 are sufficient to entirely stop the action of saliva. Tannic acid has a similar reaction. This is another reason why tea and coffee are not healthful.

The saliva possesses valuable antiseptic properties. Although typhoid fever and tetanus bacilli, colon bacillus or pus-producing organisms are not destroyed, many other pathogenic bacteria cannot survive in human salilva. That of goats and other rumminants, especially parotid saliva, has been found to have distinct bactericidal properties. Clairmont of Vienna, who conducted many experiments, concluded that the saliva maintains mouth conditions unfavorable for the growth of microorganisms which might otherwise remain there, causing decay or ulceration. It is well known that wounds in the mouth heal rapidly. Pickerill and Gies urge the use of salivatory stimulants as an excellent way to preserve the teeth.

The taste of food does much to aid digestion. The pleasure of food in the mouth stimulates the stomach, pancreas, liver and other organs of digestion to secrete their juices. This is accomplished by the nerves of taste-sending messages to the reflex centers of the brain. The longer the food stays in the mouth, the more gastric juice will there be in the stomach to receive it. Where the taste has not been perverted, it also acts as an automatic control on the body's needs, governing our desire for this type of food or that, according to our nutritional requirements of the moment. Thorough chewing is another prerequisite to the effectiveness of our built-in regulator, especially with regard to quantities. The uvula, or soft palate, at the back of the mouth is sensitive to solid food, rejecting any such particles and routing them back to the teeth for further breaking down. It also polices the entrance to the esophagus against any foreign and injurious articles eaten.

There is nothing simple about this digestive procedure. Most of our foods are very complicated in their chemical structure. Numerous steps are therefore necessary to reduce these complicated substances to more simple forms, so that they can be assimilated by the body. All of these many different chemical reactions are carried out within the gastrointestinal tract by means of enzymes.

Enzymes, the Work Horses of Digestion

Enzymes are organic substances produced by living cells, which have some particular chemical function to perform within the body. There are hundreds of different enzymes within the human body. Most of them operate within the cells. Only a microscopic amount may be needed by any one cell to meet its particular purpose.

In the digestive system, enzymes work in a different way. Here these powerful chemicals are outside of the cells.

The digestive enzymes are produced by certain glands. They are poured out into the digestive tract, where they go to work on the various food substances during the process of digestion.

The digestive enzymes do not actually enter into these complicated chemical reactions. They only make them possible. Thus, one molecule of an enzyme may change many thousands of molecules of the substance that is being acted upon. Each enzyme acts as a kind of catalyst. It operates on only one particular substance.

The mechanism of digestion is very intricate. It is largely dependent upon the nervous system. The sight and smell of food instantly cause the digestive juices to flow. Different parts of the nervous system are involved in these responses—the eyes, olfactory organs and the taste buds. Just let the mind think about lemons for a few moments. What happens? Almost instantly a thin, watery secretion begins to flow from the salivary glands. Other foods produce different reactions.

Since time immemorial, man has been eating and digesting food, yet it was only when, at the end of the 19th century, Pavlov made his remarkable discoveries that much of a definite nature about the latter process became known. His book, *The Work of the Digestive Glands,* gave medical dietitians a real foundation to work on. Previously, Beaumont, in 1834, and later Carlson, observing through gastric fistulas the workings of the stomach, were able to give a little knowledge about the secretion of gastric juice. Beaumont noticed that the stomach, at most, contained one to two ounces of gastric juice. Carlson upheld this observation, believing further that the secretion was continuous—usually one to two ounces an hour, but sometimes up to five. Recent experiments show that actually a maximum of nearly one pint can be produced in an hour, but it is usually secreted continuously at a rate varying from one third to one-and-a-half ounces every 10 minutes. The kind of food and the quantity greatly influences the stomach's activity. Several pints are needed to digest each meal (just under one-and-a-half pints for one such as a dinner). In a 24-hour period, about 3 pints are secreted. But people are individualistic, and even digestive juices show individual differences in rate and volume of secretion.

Gastric juice is the product of six different sets of glands. Three secrete the ferments pepsin, rennin and lipase (for fat digestion). Another secretes mucus, another acid, and there is also secreted a serous fluid termed diluting juice which regulates the acidity and digestive activity of the gastric juice. The juice secreted continuously is less acid than that produced during the digestion of a meal. At times of fever, stomach inflammation or gastritis, secretion ceases. Nature does not intend us to eat when we are not well.

How the Stomach Works

The stomach is a large, hollow organ with muscular fibers that are elastic or possess a certain tension. The stomach is capable of holding a considerable quantity of food. In healthy people, however, the stomach unfolds in all directions in response to the entering food until the normal capacity of the organ is reached. It expands gradually like a balloon without changing its original form. Its walls are much thicker than any other part of the digestive tract. It has been designed in such a way that it can knead and churn the food, thus aiding in digestion. The glands in the wall of the stomach pour out large quantities of liquid. These digestive juices contain hydrochloric acid, which is necessary for the complete digestion of some foods. Hydrochloric acid has five functions: It activates pepsin; accelerates the action of pepsin; stimulates the muscle fibers of the stomach wall; and aids the movements of the stomach. It also activates the digestive apparatus in the sections of the intestinal tract.

Powerful enzymes are also present within the digestive juices. Pepsin begins to break down the proteins in the food. It reacts best when there is sufficient hydrochloric acid present. Another important substance, known as the intrinsic factor, is also produced within the stomach. This acts on vitamin B-12. Pernicious anemia may occur when there is not enough intrinsic factor present.

The amount of gastric juice secreted depends upon a person's appetite. Tasteless, monotonous food produces little gastric juice. Attractive meals encourage the outpouring of larger quantities of digestive juices. This means that the nutritive properties of the food depend not only on the quality of the food itself, but also on how it is prepared and the atmosphere in which it is eaten. One's mental attitude is of great importance in good digestion. Be happy during meals.

What makes a person feel hungry? Usually there is a drop in the level of glucose within the bloodstream. At the same tiome, strong rhythmic contractions begin to occur within the walls of the stomach. These contractions begin at one end and pass slowly over the stomach. They last about 30 seconds at a time. These are what some people refer to as "hunger pangs." They can be clearly seen under the fluoroscope. They tend to become more intense when food is withheld beyond the accustomed time. These contractions are governed to some extent by the nervous system. Some people are much more aware of them than others. But they are also induced by chemical changes within the bloodstream.

Water and other nonirritating liquids do not remain in the stomach more than a few minutes. They pass immediately on into the duodenum and are soon absorbed. Solid foods are different. They tend to remain in the stomach for longer periods, up to four or five hours.

The stomach does not digest fats except milk fat, so the others are first digested in the lower sections of the intestine. Fatty foods take longer to digest and large quantities of fat slow down the gastric digestin because the fat covers the other foods and renders it difficult for the gastric juice to come into contact with the food. The greater the fat content of a food, the longer it remains in the stomach and the harder it is to digest. Milk fat contents remain there over an hour.

The most vigorous activity takes place near the pylorus. This is the outlet of the stomach. The peristaltic waves continually pass over this area, hastening the process of digestion. From time to time, the pyloric valve opens and allows small amounts of the now liquid material to pass out into the duodenum, which is the first part of the small intestine. Within the duodenum, many remarkable chemical reactions take place because of the various digestive juices that are added to the food. These juices are produced numerous glands within the gastrointestinal system.

The Importance of the Pancreas

The pancreas is the main digestive gland. It lies just behind the stomach and is almost encircled by the duodenum. Its secretions are poured into the duodenum through a small duct or tube. The pancreatic juices contain powerful enzymes, capable of digesting all three foodstuffs—proteins, fats and carbohydrates. The pancreas is activated by the brain. It is small, weighing only 1/20 as much as the liver.

The pancreatic enzyme that breaks down the carbohydrates, such as starches and sugars, is known as amylase or diastase. Another remarkable fat-splitting enzyme is called lipase. It works best in the presence of bile from the liver. The powerful enzyme that splits protein foods is known as trypsin. It requires the presence of another enzyme from the intestinal tract known as enterokinase to be fully active.

The pancreas does not function well unless the food has already been mixed with hydrochloric acid within the stomach. This liquid material is called chyme. As soon as this chyme enters the duodenum, the pancreas begins to pour out its secretions.

The discovery of this interesting mechanism gave us the first clue to another most remarkable group of chemical substances known as hormones. In 1902, Bayliss and Starling found that the pancreas poured out its secretions when food reached the small intestine. Further study revealed that this was not a mechanical arrangement—it was a substance that was apparently produced in the wall of the duodenum and then carried to the pancreas via the bloodstream.

They called this remarkable material secretin because it was produced in one organ and caused another to secrete. This was the first hormone to be discovered. Today, we know of many more. In fact, almost every activity of the body is, in some way, affected by the presence of hormones.

Another important digestive organ is the liver. It is the largest gland of the body and next to the approximately equally heavy brain the largest organ of the body. It weighs about three pounds on the average and fills the entire space under the right half of the diaphragm.

It has many important functions to perform. The liver is more particularly concerned with the food materials after they have been absorbed into the bloodstream. In the liver, most of them are changed and stored, ready for use when needed in other parts of the body.

What the Liver Does

The liver produces a clear, golden-colored liquid called bile. This bile is stored in the gallbladder, where it becomes more concentrated. This process changes its color from yellow to dark green. Bile has an important function to perform. It is necessary for the dissolving of fats so that the lipase from the pancreas can digest them prior to their being absorbed. Bile also increases the peristaltic movements of the intestinal tract, and thus keeps the colon regular.

The gallbladder is influenced by another hormone which, like secretin, is released into the bloodstream by the small intestine. This causes the gallbladder to contract and empty its contents into the duodenum to aid in the digestion of certain foods.

Digestion in the Small Bowel

The walls of the small bowel contain myriads of small glands, all producing enzymes that aid in digestion. Among these are maltase, sucrase, lactase, nuclease, phosphatase and enterokinase, all of which supplement the action of the pancreatic enzymes.

The inner lining of the small bowel looks and feels like velvet. Under the microscope, it is seen to consist of myriads of tiny villi. These are small branching processes through which many blood vessels pass. By this means, the small bowel presents an enormously large surface area, so that food materials are readily absorbed and carried to the liver.

The intestinal walls are composed of various muscle coats. Some are circular, others run lengthwise. These smooth muscle cells are largely under the control of special nerves that cause these cells to relax and contract at the appropriate times.

During digestion, the small intestine is in constant motion. Peristaltic waves continually move the food along, so it comes in contact with the various digestive enzymes.

The small bowel measures over 20 feet in length. It is one of the most important organs of the body. Without its continual absorption of food, the body would soon waste away and die.

The small bowel finally pours its contents into the large bowel through a special doorway, known as the iliocecal valve. Its function is to prevent the small bowel from emptying too rapidly.

The principal function of the colon is to absorb water. This organ arises low on the right side of the abdomen, extends up toward the liver, then across the abdomen and down the left side to the rectum. The colon is about five feet in length.

In addition to the waste products of digestion, the colon also contains myriads of bacteria, most of which are quite harmless. They seem to perform some function in providing certain vitamins of the B complex. Strong laxatives sweep these bacteria out and thus deprive the body of many products that might be important.

The colon is closely connected with the sympathetic nervous system. This is why frequent nervous tension often results in chronic constipation. Faulty bowel habits usually start in childhood, with the habitual use of strong laxatives. During the older years, many people do not drink enough water to keep the body in good health. Elderly people should be encouraged to drink plenty of water.

The human digestive tract is a marvel of organization. Every part of the body is dependent upon it for nutriment and the sustaining of life. All the way through, from the stomach to the colon, each part is constantly under the influence of the central nervous system. Such emotional disturbances as anger, fear and frustration, all greatly affect a person's digestion. For a more comfortable life it is important that we keep this wonderful network of organs in perfect operation at all times. This is the best way to live longer and enjoy real health and vitality.

Bacteria of the Digestive Tract

There are literally millions of bacteria in the digestive tract of every healthy person. When a few pathogenic (disease-forming) bacteria enter, they go unnoticed as they are quickly taken care of by these "home guard." A good, natural diet, however, rich in mineral elements is necessary for their welfare. With the absence of even one of the essential elements, a weakening of the chain results and the whole bacterial system breaks down to the point where a few invading pathogenic bacteria have an easy victory and disease appears.

Experiments have been carried out with streptococci bacteria and a soil culture, rich in soil bacteria. Later, under a microscope, it was clearly seen that battles were raging. These plainly illustrated the function of the natural bacteria in their defensive role of protecting our health against the invasion of disease-producing bacteria.

Further experimentation has shown that, by taking a green juice of a mineral-high plant such as alfalfa at frequent intervals, streptococci throat infection overcome, and arthritic and rheumatic pains have been known to subside. It seems reasonable to conclude that the plant extract, being very high in minerals, corrects the imbalance or deficiency in the human body, making it an undesirable soil for the habitation of the streptococci. The blood would be the first to be affected, then the nerves would register pains (arthritis and rheumatism) at the points where the missing elements are most essential. Local infection can therefore be traced to a deficiency. As we have said so often before, every disease is caused by a chemical imbalance.

Increasing Your Vital Energies

Many people cannot digest their foods or eliminate toxic materials properly. Their vital energy is so low they haven't the inner power to keep functioning properly. When any activity in the body is below normal (such as circulation, elimination or digestion), all of life's activities to build and repair our body become slow and, in many cases, our health goes downhill faster than we can repair and rebuild for good health.

One of the nicest ways to rebuild vital energy and pick up our digestive abilities is to keep the body warm. Sun heat without the overuse of the infrared rays and ultraviolet can be gained very nicely in the reflection from rocks.

To build your vital energy, lie on rocks at the end of the day, preferably after your evening meal when the rocks are still warm and there will be enough heat to bring your body temperature just slighly above normal. This will help those with depleted energies to pick up their vital forces and help them digest their foods more easily.

We have made experiments to show that the reflection from copper builds the blood count. We have seen plants growing in dark rooms, yet with the reflection of copper lighting, these plants grow to a beautiful green state. They do not do this with any other type of reflection.

We must raise the body heat of a sick person whose vital energies are always depleted to a low ebb. Their circulation is poor; their feet are cold because their extremities do not get enough blood. Heat from the rocks will help to keep just enough heat in the body over the period of an hour to help digest the evening meal properly. People with poor circulation, low metabolism, cold hands and feet improve tremendously by riding on a horse bareback. The heat from the horse greatly helps them, especially those with arthritic and poor circulatory conditions.

Also to build the vital energies in the body, it is well to use warm goat milk instead of cold. (The animal energy from the milk leaves in about three hours' time.) The strength of a devitalized person can be improved by using milk warm from the goat.

A cold body cannot digest foods properly. A slowly circulating bloodstream cannot digest foods properly.

Another way to pick up the vital energies in the body is to walk in warm sand, then in cold water. Keep the extremities warm. If the feet are always cold, wear ankle socks. Do not get chilled, especially after bathing. Swimming may be good, but standing in a cool breeze can devitalize the person quickly by using what little body heat he may have in reserve.

Many times we have to get a high blood count to increase our vital energies. We have to have the right companions, a good marriage, a cheerful disposition. Picking foods and eating them right from the garden, going to a higher altitude, living in a drier and warmer climate are other means of building the vital energies.

Eating Habits of Other People

The Yosemite Indian. To the Indians of the Yosemite Valley, acorns were the "staff of life." Gathered in the Fall, they were stored in interwoven deer brush granaries to be used throughout the year as gruel, mush or patties. Before using, they were first ground, then leached with several washings of water to remove the bitter tannin. Then the fine grindings were cooked into a thin soup, the middle meal into mush and the coarser material was shaped into patties and cooked on flat hot stones. The mush was cooked in large baskets: 2 quarts fresh leached meal to 6 or 7 quarts boiling water. The cooking method was to immerse hot stones into the basket. Upon completion, these stones were plunged into cold water so the congealed mush could be peeled off and eaten.

Quite a trade with the Tono Tribe was carried on with the insect delicacy, Ka-cha-vee. This peculiar pupae breeds in the salt Lake Mono in countless numbers. When waves washed mounds of the grub onto shore, the Indian women would scoop them up, dry them and rub off the skins. More drying preserved them for winter use. They tasted like mild shrimp.

Another article of trade was the caterpillar of the Pandora moth. As the caterpillars left the trees to go into pupal cases in the ground, they were trapped by the squaws in shallow trenches. They were dried for storage and used in stews. Grasshoppers and yellow jacket larvae were roasted in earth ovens for food.

Meats such as deer, squirrel, rabbit, fish and bird were cooked on hot coals by broiling or roasted in front of the fire in hot ashes or in an earthen oven. If the meat was whole, hot coals were stuffed into it to hasten cooking. Torn limb from limb, it was then shared out to the family. Meat was cured for the winter by cutting it in long, thin strips and hanging it to dry on bushes in the air and sunlight. Sometimes a rack 18 inches above a small fire was employed.

Miner's lettuce constituted a raw green. For flavor, red ants were encouraged onto them to add a piquancy from their formic acid. Our vinegar is a modern innovation of this. When beginning to uncurl, shoots of the Brake Fern were scraped of hairs and eaten raw or cooked. Tender young clover was eaten raw, and sometimes California's bay nut was munched with it as an aid to digestion. Several species of lupines were also used for greens, manzanita cider being a tasty addition.

Californian settlers referred to the Yosemite Indians as "Digger" Indians, so adept were they at digging for bulbs and edible roots. Squaw Root and various brodiacas were popular. They were cooked in pit ovens between layers of hot stones and leaves. A fire was built on the earth covering the pit and the bulbs left to cook overnight.

During April and May, mushrooms were plentiful and these were shredded and dried. They were cooked by boiling or ground in a mortar for soup.

Mineral salt was used by the Yosemite for seasoning. The Manzanita berry, with a pleasant acid tang, was made into cider and used as a seasoning with other foods or for drinking. The Manzanita berries were also eaten raw, as were wild raspberries and strawberries, thimble berries, currants, gooseberries, wild cherries and squaw berries. Pine nuts also added variety to the menu.

Mealtimes were social occasions where the family would gather around the one basket of acorn mush or other food and all dip the two front fingers into the dish. Sometimes just one finger would be stirred round and round in the mush. When served as an appetizer, Manzanita cider was sucked off a feather "spoon." A small woven basket dipper was also used as a cup for cider and water.

Unhampered by the attractions of the supermarket or drugstore, the Yosemite Indians enjoyed a varied and nutritious diet. They did not even cultivate any foods. Yet, Nature furnished them a bountiful supply. bountiful supply.

Acidity, the Enemy of Health

It is also to our advantage to know that there are some acid foods to religiously avoid. Any foods that have been fumigated, exhausted of their vital elements through bleaching and processing, had adulterants added to them or toxic preservatives used, are laboratory foods. They are no longer natural foods, God's foods. They are man's inventions and produce acids in the body which are difficult for us to overcome. These foods are producing sickness. So avoid those sulphured foods; avoid any doctored, artificially flavored and colored foods.

Often people are tempted to follow the market bargains rather than their body's needs. They rush in and over balance the diet with fruits or proteins and other acid-producing foods when these glut the market in a peak season and have to be sold at reduced prices. This is something we have to think about; something to be careful of.

We complain about rheumatism and arthritis jokingly sometimes declaring that "our hinges are getting rusty." Well, it is these acid foods that produce the acid joints. Acids lead to ulcers and bad skin conditions. An acid uterus leads to barrenness, leukorrhea, all female ailments, menstrual pains, menstrual colic, etc. Some sufferers from these conditions end up having surgery; others end up in the divorce court. People with acid kidneys and livers frequently become intemperate, perform wild deeds, perhaps develop into alcoholics. These tendencies may lead to toxemias difficult to handle or even murder and other crimes.

Acid-producing food can produce pressures in our body from gases. These gases can cause pressure against the spine causing lumbago, pressure against the heart causing heart disturbances and many others. The stomach hangs like a big bag, unable to digest foods that form gas. We develop a stupor that interferes with concentration; dullness begins to overcome us. Spasms may come on that send us to asylums. Science watches over us but can do nothing.

Importance of Bowel Health

If we are going to deal with bowel management, bowel health, food is very important. Yet, very few people will take the right foods unless they are mentally adapted to them. You have to want to do the right thing.

Many people don't desire to do so. We find that they will sit down to foods that just please their taste. They live in passion. We have people who have passions for many things: sex, drinking, smoking, food. These are passions that can only be changed by starting out from the right spiritual standpoint. So I say it is necessary that we get our minds straightened out, to start from the higher things to work out the lower.

Let Us Look at All Aspects

I don't like to talk about the bowel. My mother and father didn't like to either, so I just grew up. I grew up with faulty habits. I grew up not knowing what should be done; how to take care of myself. I didn't know I was supposed to have a bowel movement after every meal. But then again, we took the dog out after every meal. The bird had a bowel movement after he ate. The baby had to have the diaper changed after every meal; but do you know, somehow we get busy. Sometimes we find there are other jobs to do that are more important. We don't recognize that elimination is most important. So we get to the place where we find it is to our advantage to go back and take up a little study of this function.

I knew one lady who had not had a natural bowel movement in 27 years. After one week here, she came running up excitedly to tell me she had had her first natural bowel movement.

The Bowel Affects the Whole Body

In one of my books, I have a chart showing the comparative mortality rates due to the diseases of the digestive tract. We find there are many deaths attributed to bowel problems. These statistics were published by the Register General of England, who said that no group has contributed more to the death rate from intestinal diseases than doctors. Now, I didn't say that. But we find that 50% of physicians and surgeons die from intestinal disturbances while only 19% of people who are agriculturists do. This is something to think about. Inn keepers take second place; attorneys, solicitors and barristers third. Seamen are fourth. Then clergymen, priests and ministers; then the butchers, carriers, farmers and gardeners. Then came railway guards and porters, and agricultural laborers are last. Fewer agricultural workers die from intestinal disorders than any other people.

Bowel management is a subject everyone should be well acquainted with. I believe, very sincerely, there is nothing in your body that can move, act or rebuild, but that the bloodstream has something to do with it. Now in traveling throughout the body, the bloodstream touches every organ—organs such as the kidneys, stomach and the bowel. When it touches the bowel, is it possible it can pick up the waste material? There are a lot of doctors who say that the bowel eliminates toxic waste and that it is impossible to absorb it back into the body. But I believe this is absolutely wrong. I stand on it very sincerely.

By taking care of the bowel, I have seen results that have been phenomenal. I know if you take care of the bowel, the blood will be better. And as the blood travels to every organ in the body, I say that every organ is only as clean as the bowel function allows it to be. A clean, efficient bowel will lead to a clean bloodstream and clean organs. A sluggish bowel loads the bloodstream with toxins that affect every organ.

The Good Book tells us that the life of the body is in the blood thereof. Let us have clean blood. It will nourish the organs and make changes in every part of the body. We know that all the blood in the body travels through the thyroid gland every hour and a half. Is there any reason to believe that as this blood travels through the various organs, we couldn't look for regeneration if it was cleaner, better? This is what we have to look forward to.

I do know this, if you have arthritis, you will never get over it until your bowel is right. I don't care what disease you mention, there is a chemical relation in the body to that disease. And the chemical relation should be taken care of first through the bowel. I might go back a few years and tell of my experiences with Dr. Glen J. Sipes of San Francisco. He was one of my professors, and I remember one day he was called to see a lady. This lady's baby was about 6 months old and was all bloated. Other doctors insisted on having an operation immediately. But Dr. Sipes asked this lady for a feather. She took a feather from the feather duster. Dr. Sipes told her to hold her baby up by the heels. Using the feather, he tickled the baby's rectum. It didn't take more than half a minute, 30 seconds, before something happened. Such relaxation took place that there was a bowel movement, gas. It was unbelievable! An operation was avoided.

I wonder sometimes how important the relation is between relaxation and the bowel. I know some people are all tied up. I know the Mayo Clinic tells us that 9 out of 10 people with ulcers of the stomach get them from fretting, worrying, stewing, love troubles and financial difficulties. Well, where are we going to operate on these people? Are we going to operate on their heads? We know that in all cases of colitis there is definitely an emotional, mental factor. So we have to make sure that we get the head in order.

As Dr. Tilden of Denver used to say, "We are all toxic laden." Toxemia is the thing we have to take care of in the body. But toxemia to most people is an enigma. They don't understand what it is. They don't realize that when we have catarrhal congestions in the body they always come from a bowel that is not working right. When we have an acidity in the body, we can expect to find some form of bowel trouble. Doctors today don't pay enough attention to the bowel. Let's find out what can be done for the bowel and do it.

Bowel Pockets: Great Sources of Infection

First, I would like you to realize that we have about 6 feet of bowel at the end of our intestinal tract called the colon. Many times there develop what we call "pockets" or diverticula. These pockets are like the inner tube of a tire with a blowout. At these little balloon spots where it blows out, fecal material from the bowel lodges. But do you know, the best food in the world settling in these pockets, not being removed in a certain length of time, becomes a source of infection and throws toxic material back into the body? This is a source of infection that I know exists in the body. I have made an extensive study of this. I have traveled to Battle Creek Sanitarium and spent time with John Harvey Kellogg, who was a colon specialist. I have spent time with Sir Arbuthnot Lane, who was the king's physician in England. He was a bowel specialist. We find that Mechnikoff, who used fermented milk (acidophilus milk) was also a specialist with the bowel. These men have given us things to work with. I am convinced that if we could see the anatomy of the bowel, knew how it was built and what to expect of it, we could develop a good bowel program—not one to talk about at the table—not one to consider with every move we make in life—but just so we would know that things are all right or know where to look for trouble when we have sickness. I think it is to our advantage to take these few moments and look over this problem.

In 1954, I was given an award by the doctors' profession for demonstrating before a group of doctors in Portland, Oregon, that when these pockets had developed in the bowel, there was a definite reflex action to some organ in the body. For instance, we know that if you have a bowel pocket halfway down the descending colon, it can produce many catarrhal problems of the bronchial tubes. If that pocket is a little bit lower, it can cause a congestion in the breast area.

One of the cases we used in Portland as an illustration was a boy, who for three years, was treated for leg trouble. He had been adjusted by chiropractic, manipulated, given water treatments. They had given him all types of treatment, even to shots at times to take care of the pain. He was taking tranquilizers to get to sleep at night. When I looked in his eyes, I noticed signs of a pocket and a very emaciated condition of the bowel, especially in the sigmoid colon. Trouble in the sigmoid colon will cause trouble with the leg. I said, "It is time you had an X-ray of that colon because I am convinced the trouble is there." He said, "I have regular bowel movements and there is nothing wrong with my colon." I said, "I will not take the case unless you have an X-ray." We found cancer of the sigmoid colon. The boy died three months later of cancer.

The fact is we may be treating symptoms in our body when actually the colon is at fault.

While I was spending time with Sir Arbuthnot Lane in London, he told me about his great work which was accomplished by taking out sections of the bowel. Whenever there was an emaciated section, he would take it out. For instance, he found in one lady, who had a huge goiter, that after taking out a section of the bowel, the goiter was gone in six months. He hadn't changed the diet; he couldn't imagine what had happened. Another boy, who had been in a wheelchair 14 years with arthritis had a section of his bowel removed, and within 6 months, he was out of the wheelchair and walking. It was a shock to Lane when he found that after taking certain sections of the bowel out, some ailing part of the body responded and became well. We find that the last days of Sir Arbuthnot Lane were not spent in operating any more but in working entirely with diet. In spite of the fact that he did not operate, he changed these bowel conditions. Then the bodily condition changed.

Now if we could only realize that many of our headaches come from the bowel, that many times when we are treated for arthritis in the shoulder, we should have taken care of the bowel.

A newspaper article provided by the Los Angeles County Medical Association, said that diverticulosis is incurable—bowel pockets are incurable, there is nothing you can do for them. I am not going to say that we can cure this thing either, but if we get in and do our utmost to help these conditions, to get a 90% cleansing of the bowel, and the blood becomes 90% cleaner because of this, don't you thjink that every organ would be better off because of that cleaner blood? Well, we are able to demonstrate it day in and day out. Taking care of these pockets is not easy; it is not just a matter of saying, "Here is one thing to do." I know you can't get well with just diet when you have bowel pockets. If you don't exercise properly, you will never make it. But I know, too, that if you don't follow certain principles with foods, you will never get well either! There are some people with such a sweet tooth they will never get well. There are some people who must take care of their bodies by changing their physical habits.

The Beginning of Our Problems

How do we get into this trouble in the first place? Many times, I think it starts with the weaning of the baby. We start in with such atrocious foods for young children. I know that this is developing little gas bellies. I know we are beginning these gas pockets here. If you would have spent some time with me when I was in Italy after World War II, for instance, and could have seen the effects of white flour and white sugar sent over by our country to feed the Italians, you would understand. A revolution developed in the Italian intestinal tract from such foods with gas and diarrhea. They weren't used to refined carbohydrates. I believe a lot of our troubles come from the foods we eat.

To avoid trouble, I think it is well that we start from the very beginning of life and develop a good program. In our first three days of life we draw from mother's milk a product called colostrum. While in the mother's womb, the baby's bowels do not move, as there is no need. We are building tissues. We are building an embryo, a body. Nature is just interested in dividing, building up. What little toxic waste that is developed can be absorbed—taken up by the mother. But once that baby comes into this life, takes its first breath, starts its nursing program, the first thing that happens is an awakening of a friendly bacteria in the bowel. These friendly bacteria are awakened by the product colostrum found in mother's milk during the first three days of nursing. This is a most important part of baby's feeding. It is a most important part because it is here that we start out feeding lthe friendly bacteria responsible for developing normal bowel movements.

If the mother is not well, it is difficult for the child to get a proper start. When she hasn't been too good, is not strong, then baby fares none too well either. Pretty soon, the baby is weaned. We go from bad to worse. We get on formulas—artificial formulas—substitutes for the natural thing, the right food. The first thing you know we are developing intestinal disorders that eventually cause many diseases such as eczema, rashes, colds, bronchial trouble, etc., leading right to hay fever and asthma. I don't care what disease you mention, I think its beginning goes way back to the time we are born.

Even the dentists tell us today that if a child can be nursed until he is 10 months of age, he will probably have normal natural teeth at the age of 40. But this is the unusual thing today. I know many dentists are making a living by treating the teeth of children who haven't even reached the age of 3. They say that in this country, the average 5-year old has 5 cavities already. Mother's milk is the greatest calcium source we have. Teeth come from calcium. When we get an improper start in life, we cannot have good teeth.

When I speak of disease, you can mention any of the symptoms with all their variations—eye trouble, ear trouble, joint disturbances, fever, rheumatic disturbances—yet we can take care of many of these troubles if we look to the bowel.

It is easy for children to have three bowel movements a day. It isn't easy as we grow a little older. I think children are more normal than grownups. I had a woman patient, for instance, who worked in an attorney's office. There were seven attorneys there. If she didn't go to the bathroom before she left for work in the morning, she would not leave her office because of embarassment on her part. What crazy thinking! Yet, I mentioned in the beginning, children are not taught to respond to nature's call. We seem to forget that all of nature obeys this rule. Animals live a natural life when they are in the forest. They are living a natural life when they are outside.

We Must Learn to Heed Nature's Call

A few people still live a fairly natural life. I know a medical doctor in New York who spent a lot of time in Russia and various parts of Siberia. He was telling me about these long-lived people. He actually believes their longevity is due to the fact that they had no inhibitions whatsoever in having eliminations., If they had to have an elimination while they were waiting for an appointment, they would go outside and eliminate. It wasn't a matter of waiting. And why do I bring this up? Do you know that today I am treating pockets, rectal enlargements, that hold one, two, three or four meals before we have a call, before enough pressure is exerted to have a natural knocking at the door telling us that we must have a bowel movement? We wait until the very last minute. This is the reason why so much gas is developed in the bowels today.

Never go four or five days without a bowel movement, for in doing so, every cell in your body becomes as toxic as the condition of the bowels. In that way, disease will soon become the greater part of you and vital health becomes the lesser. Never miss one day as far as a bowel movement is concerned. It is wise to resort to an enema, if necessary. In case of constipation, it is well to drink more water, fruit juices and vegetable juices. Most cases of constipation are due to the inactivity of the bowels. This inactivity is usually the result of an impaired body produced by using our reserve energy beyond its power to recuperate. For example, this condition can be produced from a lack of sleep, not enough exercise, too much reading or overeating.

Many people have two or three bowel movements a day and think they are not constipated, even some people with protruding abdomens. This does not necessarily mean that they are constipated; but in all probability, they are. A person of this type is usually 10 or 15 meals behind. The larger the waistline, the shorter the lifeline. To overcome ill health in our bodies, we must acquire a good working and clean intestinal tract. It is impossible to throw off any disease unless the cell structure is perfect. Every cell is dependent upon the nourishment picked up in the intestinal tract.

In dealing with this now, the first thing we are going to have to do is to realize that we must work with these bowel movements mentally; that when the call comes we must be there. Get on the go. Move. Have that bowel movement. Now I am going to tell you ways of feeding the bowels, softening up the fecal matter. But what is the use if you don't answer nature's call? It is very necessary to see this.

Upon occasions, we are confronted with an opposite condition, diarrhea or a running off of the bowels. In every case, except in amoeba infection, it is well to let it take its course. When an extra amount of raw vegetable juices is added to the diet, many times diarrhea sets in. Allow it to take its course and it will last only a few days. In the retracing process of correcting chronic conditions in our body, a diarrhea is sometimes encountered which is perfectly normal. Some of our raw vegetables are grown in heavily manured soils. In many cases, they result in foods covered with parasites. Be sure that vegetables are well cleaned before using them.

Foods in the Bowel

One of the main things that causes bowel trouble today is eating too much bread. I am sure we should think twice about eating bread. Now, we do serve bread here at the Ranch, but I think there is such a thing as "good" bread. We serve the best we can get. But I still feel you can overdo it. If you are going to have bread, have good bread, but if you are sick, I would leave it alone entirely. Do I have to go into any long dissertation to tell you that there is bread that has life and bread that is lifeless? When I was going through Washington a short time ago, I heard a little child praying over a loaf of bread, saying "Give us this day our daily bread." It was a loaf of white bread that had 1.2% of life in it. In other words, 98.8% of the wheat germ had been take out—the life. The Staff of Life had gone.

You cannot look to that kind of bread as the Staff of Life. I know that a lot of people today are trying to get good out of white bread. Bread is foodless, especially if it is made from white flour. Devitalized bread ferments and putrefies in the bowel. On the other hand, the original grains will not ferment and cause as much indigestion as when they are made into bread. If you want rid of headaches, even migraine headaches, try giving up bread. I have experienced much improvement in people just taking away bread from them. I tell you this very sincerely. Get on a program providing the most natural starches possible. Natural millet does not ferment in the bowel like millet bread. Whole wheat will not putrefy in the bowel as whole wheat bread does.

Most natural foods do not ferment, do not blow up the bowel. You can prove this for yourself. If you put cooked cabbage out in the sunshine, in a couple of days, it will be rotten. But raw cabbage on the other hand, won't putrefy and break down nearly as fast. That is one of the reasons why I tell you that 60% of your foods should be raw. This will eliminate much of the putrefaction we had in the bowel before. Having only cooked foods will give you more trouble.

One thing we cut out in the diet is head lettuce. I do not believe in head lettuce, as it is very gas forming. It slows down digestion. It has a product in it similar in structure to a narcotic, and we find that it produces gas. Use romaine lettuce instead. Use endive, watercress and other greens. There is a hundred times as much iron in leaf lettuce as in head lettuce. During the war, the government wouldn't even allow the farmer to use the space in a freight car to ship head lettuce because there is so little nourishment in it. I can get romaine lettuce in a restaurant by pleading with the waitress. I tell her I am sick, that I am under a doctor's care and that he won't let me have head lettuce—I have to have romaine. I tell her I have the money to pay for it. I always get it, and I don't ever have to pay extra. I don't know but that is one time sympathy helps a little. The way I walk out of the reataurant, I guess she thinks I am well enough that I didn't need it, but I asked for it and got it. It is well to know what you should do for yourself.

One of the greatest putrefactive materials you can put in the bowel is meat. I don't like to be against meat. There are some values of meat that are wonderful. There are some marvelous things that can be done with it. On the other hand, I could talk for two hours on meat so that you would never eat it again! I can really fix it up. I can really flavor it for you. But I will tell you right now that if you have a lot of bowel trouble, cut meat down. At the Ranch, we serve meat two or three times a week, but I take it away from most people because they have had it two and three times a day. Truly, meat spoils in the intestinal tract quicker than any other food. It was John Harvey Kellogg who took a beefsteak, put it out overnight, and found next morning that it was filled with maggots. However, when he put beefsteak in buttermilk, he could keep it for a long time, and there was very little spoilage.

Meat will not spoil in an intestinal tract that has a lot of lactic acid, that has a friendly bacteria. That is good. That is perfect. If you are going to eat meat, you had better have a good bowel. Then to aid its digestion, I think a couple of papaya tablets would be the best thing you could take. Papaya will help digest meat better than anything else you could put in the body and keep it from putrefying longer than anything. So, whenever you have a good steak, take a couple of papaya tablets along with it.

Buttermilk is mostly cultured today. But it is the lactic acid in the buttermilk that has the value whether it is cultured or not. Personally, I don't think that nourishment we get out of milk after it comes through pasteurization is worth anything. But lactic acid is a most wonderful thing, especially for people who haven't good bowel tone.

Whenever we use the muscle structure of our body, we produce lactic acid naturally. But America is considered the softest nation in the world today. I don't think we exercise enough to produce lactic acid in our bodies. lactic acid is most wonderful for getting rid of nerve disorders. The nerves need lactic acids. They live on lactic acid. And if you have any nerve disorder, I think you should try to develop more lactic acids through physical exercise. This is how we balance our life. However, in the meantime, to get extra acid and have enough for the friendly bacteria, you can take acidophilus or buttermilk. There is a buttermilk powder that can be used in some liquefied drinks and may be of help to the bowel. Many times, buttermilk is very quieting to the nervous system, and it is also soothing to an erupting bowel. That is why we use it. Otherwise, I don't think it is the best, unless we can get a real home-cultured buttermilk. But who can? Our foods today have been so mutilated, and they have gone through such processes, that it is hard to recognize the food anymore. It is no longer food.

I don't think meat and buttermilk is a good combination. I think that dairy products don't work well with meat. But why shouldn't we have buttermilk along with meat if it preserves meat, the most putrefactive food? Well, you see, this buttermilk adds to the lactic acid in the intestinal tract, and it's this that we are more interested in than buttermilk as a food at this moment. Now, we find that the putrefaction that goes along with buttermilk and meat mixed together is not good, especially in the intestinal tract. Milk or any dairy product with meat is not a good combination. This was an experiment which used meat preserved in buttermilk. It shows that when we keep meat in lactic acid, it doesn't spoil. This is proof of why we have to have a good intestinal tract to keep the meat we eat from putrefying.

In discussing various things that take care of the body, let us consider milk. I think we have to have raw milk. Pasteurized milk can upset an intestinal tract quicker than anything else. We find that pasteurized milk cannot be digested properly. The protein element cannot be absorbed properly because it has been broken up. Pasteurized milk is no longer a natural food. It will spoil quickly, much quicker than raw milk. It may be germ free, but then we should get milk that has been inspected: certified raw milk. We should have inspectors, making sure we get good milk. Pasteurized milk, processed milk, is no longer a food. Children cannot be well on pasteurized milk. I would rather tell you to give up milk than have pasteurized milk.

There are milk substitutes you can use—nut and seed milk drinks. Find out how you can use nut butter. Mix it with some soymilk. It will not be catarrh producing. What can this nut milk do for you? John Harvey Kellogg was a great one for soymilk. He made his colon culture out of it. He thought that soymilk powder was one of the best foods for the friendly bacteria in the bowel. We use a product that I think is wonderful. It has been found that the acidophilus bacteria, that friendly bacteria in the bowel, will grow best in whey. So we use whey, and we use a lot of it. Whenever you make cheese, have the whey on your table. Recognize that this is one of the highest sodium foods that we can put in the body. Sodium is a bowel element. It keeps the stomach sweet and clean, and it is one of those great foods for the friendly bacteria we speak of. Get powdered whey, if you can't get fresh.

Now, I am leading up to one thing—that there is an intestinal flora comprised of friendly bacteria. These bacteria have to live. If the bowel flora gets out of proper balance, you will find that another bacteria type begins to develop, just as a putrefactive bacteria develops in meat, causing breaking down, a getting back to earth again.

I once made an experiment. I had the fecal material of 500 of my patients sent to the laboratory to be tested for the balance of bacillus E. coli to the acidophilus bacteria. According to Dr. John Harvey Kellogg, we should have about 85% acidophilus and 15% bacillus E. coli. I found in the 500 cases I tested the proportions were just the opposite! Each person had 85% bacillus E. coli to 15% acidophilus. Doesn't this just show that people who are sick need to take care of the bowel in order to return to good health again? When the bowel flora is out of balance, actually we are dying. That is why you have attracted that kind of bacteria in the bowel. It is a dying bowel. To keep the bowel alive, it has to be kept free of the bacillus E. coli, the gas-producing bacteria. This can be done by keeping the bowel sweet and clean. And you keep it that way by eating good food, by living on a proper diet.

Balanced Daily Eating Regimen

I hope that you know by now what a good diet it. I hope you have been following the laws for some time. Just to remind you, there are probably six laws we must follow. First of all, foods must be natural. Natural food putrefies in the body least and feeds the friendly acidophilus bacteria best. I want to qualify that by saying that we should have at least half of our foods raw every day. In my books, I say 60% raw food every day. Food that you can eat raw, don't eat cooked. We go further and find that we must have the right proportions of foods: 6 vegetables and 2 fruits daily. It is possible to live on all fruit but the reason I give you the proportion of 6 vegetables and 2 fruits is because people do not get real good fruit. You go to the market and get fruit that looks good but was picked green. You cannot eat fruits high in green acids and have a good intestinal tract. This is one of the reasons I cut out citrus fruits with most people. Green citric acid stirs up the acids in our body too much. The vegetable kingdom carries off the acids; fruit stirs them up. I am not against fruit; I am not against citrus fruit, but I am against fruit that is green.

With distribution, freezing, etc., the chances of getting good vegetables are better than getting the other foods good. Then have one starch a day and one protein daily. This balances up the proportions of the foods daily. The next thing is variety. My aunt is the best example of no variety; she always ate carrots and peas. That's all she ever had in her house. That is not enough. We will become only what carrots and peas can do for us, because we mold to our foods. It is necessary that we have a variety of vegetables and fruits.

The next thing is not to eat too much. People do overeat. Find out how little you can eat, not how much. The secret of life is in how little you can eat.

The last thing is combinations. I separate the starches and proteins. Have starches at noon and the protein at the evening meal. But combinations are at the bottom of the list. You could have the worst foods in the world in good combination, and it wouldn't mean a thing. Let's have natural foods. Raw foods combined wrongly wouldn't hurt you as much as man-handled foods correctly combined.

Dealing with Constipation

In working out problems with the bowel, I would like to give you some suggestions. There are various treatments to use. Get on the healthy way to live program and then start working for natural bowel movements. My book *Tissue Cleansing through Bowel Management* goes into these things in much greater detail, and I recommend it strongly to all who have chronic bowel problems.

There are many forms of laxatives. Personally, I don't like laxatives. A mild form is Garfield tea. I have used it for many years. Another mild, yet good one which causes the least trouble, is Celery King tea. But, not approving of laxatives, I think it is better now that we learn what the laxative foods are and begin to rely on what we eat to regulate our bowel, although there are many good herb laxatives.

The constipating foods are the fried foods, cheese, pasteurized milk, all denatured, refined, spiced, salted and unnaturally concentrated foods. Heavy cellulose foods can be constipating; rich foods also. Constipation results from eating foods improperly combined, such as starches without vegetables. Never eat starches without vegetables. Never eat a sandwich without a salad or salad sticks. Never eat any bread unless you have vegetables with it. It will putrefy, spoil, cause constipation and develop gas pockets quicker than anything I know.

Don't send a lunch to work with your husband expecting him to be well unless there is celery with it, also carrot sticks or bell pepper sticks, lettuce leaves and cucumber. Don't send a lunch to school with your children unless it has vegetables along with it. Doctor up the vegetables, if you like. There are ways of stuffing celery with nut butters or cheese spreads; stick carrots through olives; use grated carrot as a sandwich filling. If nothing else, package up some of the dried fruits, such as raisins or dates. There is date paste that can be used as a sandwich spread. Don't forget the lettuce, green leafy lettuce with your sandwiches. When my boy was in school, he always took his lunch with lettuce, and they called him a rabbit. At home I told him that he wouldn't have constipation if he used lettuce in his sandwiches. So when they called him a rabbit, he said, "Well, at least I'm not a constipated rabbit!" The boy had the answer.

For good bowel activity, try our internal water treatment. Take 3 or 4 glasses of warm water before breakfast, the first glass one hour beforehand, the second, half an hour beforehand, and the last immediately before eating. This not only aids sluggish bowels, but cleanses the genito-urinary tract as well.

One of the cheapest and best laxative foods I think you will find is flaxseed meal: A tablespoon of flaxseed meal with each meal. Don't use it dry—it will stick in your throat. Take some liquid along with it. It will add the proper bulk, lubrication and it is a wonderful supplement and adjunct. You can add it to your meals if you like. Flaxseed tea is also wonderful. It is not necessary to have it raw for lubrication; however, if flaxseed tea has been soaked and not boiled, it is higher in vitamin F. Vitamin F is a wonderful vitamin for healing the intestinal tract, especially when we have inflammation, colitis, ulcers, etc. Vitamin F is necessary to heal any inflammation in the body. Vitamin F is found highest in unboiled flaxseed tea. But you will find that if you boil it, this vitamin is destroyed. So, for these extreme enteritis conditions, colitis, etc., it might be well to use it after just steeping the seed overnight. Bring the flaxseed to a boil, then let it soak overnight after turning the flame off. Strain it next morning and use it that way to clean up these conditions.

Cherry juice is another wonderful laxative. So is grape juice. It is also excellent for the liver and gallbladder. Both are high in iron and anything high in iron is very good.

You have heard of chlorophyll, haven't you? It is one of these elements which sweetens up the bowel. I'm sure you have heard of chlorophyll being used for deodorizing. Well, there isn't anything that you can put in the bowel that will clean it up quicker than chlorophyll. Chlorophyll is the green coloring matter in plants. As you go through life, just remember that when you're green inside, you're clean inside. Greens will give you that correct condition in your body. Greens will do more for you than anything. I have seen more people get well with greens than any other single thing.

Alfalfa tablets are very useful in cases of sluggish bowels. Using 4 tablets each meal helps to give a little extra bulk which many bowels need; bulk holds water.

Now there are many laxative foods. Prunes have a laxative quality. The first thing some people think about when they get up in the morning is prunes. But I tell you, you can't use prunes all the time. We must have variety. Why not find out other laxative foods? Figs are wonderfully laxative. In fact, we find that all fruits have a laxative quality. Apricots, peaches, have laxative properties. Get plenty of beets into the diet to help the elimination also.

There are many laxative drinks you can take. Prune juice and celery juice together is good. So is prune juice with whey. Lemon and whey together makes a good laxative. Whey with grape juice is also laxative. Another wonderful combination is green juice from the tops of vegetables or chlorophyll mixed with fig juice. If you want something a little stronger, you can use molasses—blackstrap molasses, one tablespoon in one cup of hot water will be laxative. Taking molasses in cold water is usually not laxative. Blackstrap molasses is wonderfully high in iron and that is good for the liver and the bile formation.

Many have liver and bile disorders along with constipation. Anything that moves the bile along, helps relieve constipation. Chlorophyll is good for bile. All these laxative foods—yellow foods—are good for the bile movement.

A very good laxative is aloe vera. Cut up a 4-inch to 5-inch-long piece of the cactus and put the bits into a quart of water. Let stand 3 to 4 hours before using. Keep it refrigerated and each evening, pour off 1/2 cup of the liquid to drink. When all the liquid has been used, more water can be added, but you may have to chop up a little more aloes to give it strength.

In Switzerland, they have a simple way of regulating the bowel with the use of yogurt. I think yogurt is a wonderful food, though many times we take it away from those who have extreme catarrhal conditions. In Switzerland, they use a sauce dish of yogurt with a tablespoon of apple concentrate on it and it is really wonderful for constipation. It makes a delicious dessert. Use it every day for 30 days and see what wonders it will do. In Switzerland, dairy stores are called yogurt stores. In other words, that's the main item in the store, and it should be.

Mechnikoff has given us such wonderful enlightenment on the people who have lived long lives. He claims it is due to the fermented milk. It's the clabbered milk that has helped these people have wonderful intestinal tracts and therefore they live long lives. That is why Bulgaria has many people over a hundred years old. They use much of this clabbered milk, Bulgarian buttermilk, cultured milk. It is a very difficult thing to get this kind of culture in our milk in this country because different bacteria grow in different altitudes. The Trappist Monks in Canada tried to get the Bulgarian bacteria and culture milk, but they have had a very difficult time collecting it and keeping it alive.

I might say that if you want to do something wonderful for the bowel, think of an **acidophilus culture.** When people come to me with extreme intestinal disorders, that's the first thing I think of. If you are on a program which is not reactive enough, I think you should go to your health food store and get this culture. There are various kinds. In my opinion, they are all good. It might be well to try this acidophilus for a period of 2 months. If you have extreme problems, you might double the quantity for the first 2 weeks and then come back to your ordinary procedure. Follow through for 2 months; skip a couple of months—2 or 3—and then take it again. If you have a lot of bowel trouble, use it for 3 programs during the year. In fact, I think we should all consider acidophilus culture in our lives, because cooked foods destroy this friendly bacteria. Sprays on the vegetables destroy this friendly bacteria, and artificial fertilization of foods destroys this friendly bacteria. We find that we cannot keep a good bowel unless we have natural food, good food. Canned foods destroy this friendly bacteria; preserved foods destroy it; vinegar, salt, pepper and spices that don't belong in our intestinal tract destroy this friendly bacteria. Devitalized foods that start putrefaction draw to them the bacillus E. coli and crowd out the natural bacteria.

A lot of people ask me about acidophilus milk. Well, it is good. There is nothing wrong with it at all. The only thing is that if you want to use this material to overcome a bowel disorder, you will have to use 365 glasses of acidophilus milk to equal one bottle of the acidophilus culture. The acidophilus culture has millions of friendly bacteria to every teaspoon and there just aren't that same number of bacteria in the acidophilus milk.

Many times, in order to overcome constipation, we have to take away extreme roughage from some people who have a sensitive stomach and sensitive bowels. Sometimes roughage can cause the bowel to swell up. Celery strings we have to remove; we should also eliminate turnip greens. We turn to a bland diet.

Bland foods are soft foods. They are foods that do not cause a lot of gas, like our sulphur foods. We do not call cabbage a bland food; we do not consider it rough. One of the most bland foods you can take is zucchini or a nice summer squash. This is one of the finest foods you can put in the body, and it will not produce gas. Gruel—rice gruel, barley gruel—is another fine thing for the intestinal tract, and many times when we have these severe irritations, we have to take gruels.

Learn how to prepare bland foods without destroying them, without murdering them. Many bland foods have been treated to such an extent that they no longer have any food value. So much is dependent upon the one in the kitchen. It is unbelievable. The one in the kitchen controls the health of the whole family. Overcooked foods have little value. That is why the Chinese probably cook foods the best. They little more than dip their food in boiling water. Don't really cook them; don't boil the life out of them. You will find you won't destroy the coloring, so you won't have to add baking soda to make them green. And, by the way, baking soda is the greatest thing that destroys natural bacteria in the bowel. Get away from baking soda—especially stomach ulcer people.

Now, of course, we can use enemas—many types. A lot of people cannot stand water enemas, and I think using flaxseed tea is one of the finest things to get rid of inflammation in the lower bowel. There are some who have bleeding in that area. If so, we use flaxseed tea with a little liquid chlorophyll, the greatest healer we have for the tissues. Many other enemas can be used. Some people use lemon juice, but I don't particularly favor this. In his work, Father Kneipp used chamomile tea. I think that is also wonderful for an enema. We can use white oak bark tea whenever we have colitis, inflammation of the bowel. We can go still farther and use one of the things that neutralizes the lower bowel best and that is plain old buttermilk; use half buttermilk and half water.

Dr. Max Gerson was here at the Ranch once and he used coffee enemas to get the toxic waste out of the bowel and to stimulate the bile. I don't believe enemas serve any good purpose other than removing the toxic waste and getting a sweet, clean bowel; getting that bowel moving is so important. Many times we can use garlic enemas for stimulation, garlic powder or garlic oil in the water. Where children have pin worms and other lower bowel disturbances, we can use garlic enemas. Other times, you can insert a garlic oil capsule in the rectum every night. You will find that it can help get rid of pin worms in children. You can also give it to them orally. Nothing can live around garlic, you know that. It is very strong. Your neighbors will even leave you! So use it with care.

The Value of Colonics

Taking colonics is the quickest way to get rid of toxic waste in the bowel. I have seen many pain symptoms removed in just one treatment. I am of the opinion, however, that other means, such as reacidulating the bowel and changing the intestinal flora, are very important to the permanent change necessary to eliminate rheumatism and arthritis.

There are many forms of colonics and to use them without eating properly and exercising adequately, will deplete bowel activity, wash out the intestinal flora, and in the end, reduce us to a permanent dependence on colonics. However, used correctly, they are one of the greatest adjuncts I know of in working along with this program to clean up the body of accumulated waste and rheumatic acids.

Get Bowel Tone through Exercise

How do you get tone in the bowel? The only way is to exercise it. The best exercise for the bowel is the slanting board. So, if you do not have high blood pressure, use that board. It will give your bowel tone and power as no other exercise. If you use it every day, as we have instructed for three months, I will guarantee, without a shadow of a doubt, that you will have better movements. I know. I use it all the time with my patients, and I know the response that comes from it.

There are other exercises you can use. My Indian exercise is a wonderful one, the bending over exercise, the twisting from side to side. Get your hands above your head; move the torso around in a circle, everything from the hip up in a stiff position so that all the movement is in the bowel. It is very necessary to do that.

Now, getting the bowel in its normal position is necessary. Those people who have prolapsus have pressure on the sigmoid colon, the lower part of the bowel. They cannot move the waste along fast enough; gas backs up; pressure develops and we are in trouble. When we have this condition of prolapsus, we have what is called a "fish-hook" stomach. The stomach drops and goes down into the abdomen. Then we find that we carry acids in the stomach too long. Belching develops and we have that sour taste coming back into our mouth. This is due to prolapsus. We also have pressure symptoms developing on the prostate gland; uterine trouble develops whenever there is a prolapsus. Let us get this colon back into place and develop good tone.

People who cannot take the slanting board exercises and would still like to help the bowel, can do the rubber ball exercise. Get a rubber ball about the size of a tennis ball or a little smaller and roll it around the abdomen in a circle about 25 times. This will move the gas along and develop tone in the bowel. In 2 or 3 months, you are going to be surprised at the good tone and power you have acquired in the intestinal tract.

Although food alone cannot build tone in those muscles, you must feed them all the material to give tone. Unless you exercise also, you will not have it. So I have to emphasize here, how important both are to the bowel. It is necessary to be active; you cannot sit in one position all the time. Much of the bowel trouble causing heart trouble is because of the sedentary occupations. You can't sit in one position all the time and have good bowel tone.

I must bring out here that you cannot be well if you are tired. You cannot have good bowel movements if you are tired, and, by the way, most sick people are tired. Tired tissue does not work well. It lies down on the job. It cannot do the work. But all this goes along with good food.

Other Aids to Bowel Management

There are other things to be used for bowel disorders. Some use sitz baths. They are wonderful in bowel disorders and they also give much relilef to other organic structures of the body. You can alternate a sitz bath—hot and then cold: one minute hot, half a minute cold, for eight changes. If you want to just sit in the cold water, do it two or three minutes and then get out and walk around. Be sure you are warm while walking around because you will find that all the blood has been forced into the internal organs.

I use one of the wonderful Father Kneipp packs I learned about while I was in Worishofen, Germany. That is the water pack on the abdomen to dissipate gas or bring on relaxation of the bowel. It is also a great bowel stimulant. Dip a hand towel in cold water, wring it out and fold it to the size of the abdomen. Wrap a dry towel around it, pinning it tightly so that no air can get to the wet towel above or below it. You keep it on for one hour every day. If you have extreme gas, this is one aid that will help get rid of it. It will relax the bowel. This cold towel will first constrict and contract the tissues of the abdomen, but you will find that in two minutes, relaxation will start and the heat that comes from the body will warm the towel.

The Why of Whey

Whey is Nature's own delicious intestinal aid.

In the 12th century, the great physician, Maimonides, wrote on the subject of diet: "The ordinary ailment will yield to nature only if you take care of the patient's diet. The best any physician can do is to fortify the patient's strength and in this way help along the work of nature. Most physicians only hinder nature instead of helping it. *If a man is susceptible to disease, the thing to do is to build up his general resistance so that he may be rid of his susceptibility.*"

To this we would add that an important part of diet is to use foods liberally which contain the mineral sodium, the "youth maintainer."

While sodium is found in okra, celery, beets, cucumbers, string beans, asparagus, turnips, strawberries, oatmeal, cheese, raw egg yolk, coconut and black figs, we find whey to be the food with the highest content.

Whey is what remains after the cream and casein (protein) have been removed from milk when making cheese. One tablespoon of dried whey is made from almost two quarts of regular liquid whey. When it is added to the diet, we get the concentrated mineral food as a supplement.

Sodium is found and needed mostly in the digestive system (principally the stomach, which is the most important organ for holding sodium reserves) and in glands and ligaments. It is a blood builder and a great neutralizer. It aids digestion, counteracts acidosis, halts intestinal fermentation and purifies the blood. It holds calcium in solution to maintain the suppleness of youth in the joints. Whey is one of the finest youth foods available to us.

When we lack sodium, the first organ to show disorder is the stomach and this disorder gradually spreads throughout the body. This is a signal that we should increase our intake of foods high in sodium and whey is the answer to this problem. It is well to build and maintain a healthy body and avoid the suffering that goes with a body out of repair.

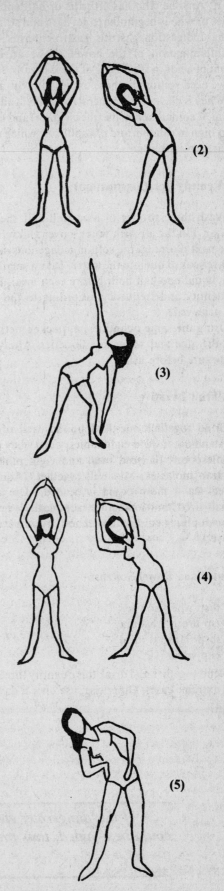

(1) **The Indian Walk (just a glorified walk).** Start with an exaggerated walk, toes turned in and arms swinging, hips going one way and shoulders the opposite. When there is a rhythm established, cross arms at shoulder level and keep swinging, still opposite to hips. Now turn head in opposite direction to shoulders.

(2) Feet apart—clasp hands while arms are stretched straight above head. Circle arms in big circles with hips still—body, from hips up, firmly stiff—bending only from hips. This is the liver twister.

(3) Feet apart—stretch one arm straight above head and keep straight while stretching other arm down and bending knee on same side. Keep other knee unbent and try to touch toes.

(4) Arms stretched above head and kept together—bend straight over at hips from side to side with upper part of body kept fairly stiff.

(5) Pat stretched abdomen quite vigorously with open hands while leaning to side and slightly back—first one side then the other—pat only the side that is stretched.

We are living in an age of arthritis, but we need not have it. Anyone who has arthritis or hardening of the arteries or who is beginning to get hard and stiff, anyone who has indigestion, gastritis, gastro-enteritis, colitis or any inflammation of the bowel shows an excessive amount of acids in the tissues of these organs. It is a sign that we need sodium in those tissues for neutralization.

Whey is classed as a mineral food and in addition to sodium, it contains chlorine (the cleanser) and lactase. It is also high in calcium and phosphorus, which are good for our nerve structures.

Aloe Remedy (for Constipation)

Wash three prongs of aloe well and slice into a quart jar. Fill the jar with water, cover and refrigerate. By the next morning, the soft, mucilagenous substance will have soaked out into the water. Take a small glassful of this liquid one-half hour before each meal. Regulate the quantity and frequency according to the laxative effect achieved.

Using the same quantities, a quicker method is to blend the aloe and water in a liquefier. Always shake this mixture before using.

Dried Fruit Laxative

Grind together one-third pound each of raisins, prunes and dates. Add eight tablespoons whey powder, six tablespoons flaxseed meal and eight tablespoons blackstrap molasses. Mix well together. (Add a little flaxseed tea if more liquid is needed.) Use about a "golfball-sized" portion before each meal. (When taken with acidophilus culture, bowel activity will eventually improve.)

Regulator and Bowel Softener

1 tbsp whey powder
1 tsp broth seasoning
1 tbsp flaxseed meal
1 cup water

Blend together and drink this quantity three times a day in extreme cases. Otherwise, use once a day before breakfast.

Changing the Intestinal Flora

4 oz apple juice
4 oz goat milk
1 tbsp whey powder

Beat together and drink this amount four times a day to sweeten the bowel.

Potato Milk Soup

1 smallish-sized potato
1 cup milk

Peel the potato, cut up and boil in milk until tender. Rub through a sieve or blend in liquefier to make "soup" consistency. (If more milk is required, it must be boiled.) This soup may be used for diarrhea.

Barley Gruel

Soak pearl barley overnight in cold water to cover. Bring to boil and simmer (in double boiler) until barley is tender. Rub through a sieve or liquefy. Add a little vegetable seasoning, a knob of butter or a little sweet cream for flavor. Soaked, peeled dates could be used.

Do not use all of these remedies at one time.

In Conclusion

There is much more that could be said in regard to bowel management, but I do feel that we have covered the basic factors.

There are many conditions that we may have to take care of personally. We find that in cases of colitis we often have to use special things or what we call "specific remedies." We use slippery elm bark, a "slickage." And many times, we have to use barley gruel. Other times we use the flaxseed tea as I have mentioned. Comfrey tea is wonderful for the bowel; very soothing. It also carries a slickage with it. We use comfrey regularly here. We grow it. We believe in it. We use the comfrey juice along with a little pineapple juice. This is a wonderful combination, wonderful food for the bowel. If constipation could be cured in the average American home, there would be almost no diseases for the doctors to take care of.

"If the 'dangerous' elements in food could be identified, they then could be avoided, thus preventing many cancers."
—Dr. Paul A. Marks

Chapter 48

Make food your medicine

Make Your Food Your Medicine

Let us look to natural remedies for the relief of many small ills. Here is a list of some foods that can be used and their values and remedial qualities. Paliative drugs have the power of giving temporary relief from pain and they may even reduce the suffering caused from nutritional starvation, but it is food alone that contains the necessary elements which can restore a normal condition.

ARTICHOKES have iron, otherwise they do not have too much nutritional value; however, they give a nice variety. The Jerusalem artichoke is one food that diabetic people can take because it has a natural insulin. To use Jerusalem artichokes as a remedy for diabetes wouldn't be the proper thing to do, but all those who have a pancreatic weakness can handle them much easier than they can potatoes, either white or sweet. I know of no other starch that is better for the body. Don't use them as a remedy for diabetes, but include them in your diet to contribute to reducing the work of the pancreas.

ASPARAGUS is a wonderful bulk food, high in chlorophyll. The best way to eat it is to break it off right from an asparagus bed in the garden and eat it raw.

BROCCOLI is a winter vegetable and is high in sulphur. If you don't want it to produce intestinal gas, steam it in parchment paper or eat it raw.

BEET GREENS contain oxalic acid, but not so much as spinach and Swiss chard. Have them raw in salad and also steamed. The stems contain more iron than the leaves. Suggestion: To prevent burning of food cooked in stainless steel pans, place some raw beet leaves in the bottom of the pan.

BRUSSELS SPROUTS, CABBAGE AND CAULIFLOWER are good winter vegetables containing sulphur. There is 40% more iron in the green base of the cauliflower than in the bleached head, so make sure to use the greens surrounding the head.

CELERY was a food given the early Olympic games winners as a prize. It was considered the greatest thing they could receive. It was the one thing that rejuvenated them more than anything after a long run or some arduous competitive game. It is the most cooling thing you can have in the body. Today, it is one of the foods you must be most careful of because it is sprayed. Brush it well. A wonderful food remedy that can be used in the summertime to keep you cool is celery and

pineapple juices together. It replaces the salts lost in perspiration on an extremely hot day. This may be mixed with prune juice, especially for the type who needs the nerve salts to help the nervous system.

CUCUMBERS are very valuable. Don't forget to eat the peeling, unless it disturbs you. You can get the equivalent value in other foods, especially greens. No drinks are better in the summer than cucumber and celery, cucumber and whey or cucumber and pineapple. In summer, they tell us to keep as "cool as a cucumber." Cucumbers are high in sodium, the cooling element.

DANDELIONS should be used for the gallbladder and liver. The finest beverage you can get is made of roasted dandelion root. Learn to use this in place of coffee.

FISH has long been called a brain food, which doctors have called "tommyrot," but from a chemical standpoint, we know that our brain and nervous system are built up of vitellin, brain phosphorus, lecithin, brain and nerve fat. These elements are found in highest concentration in ocean fish, particularly black bass. While it is not a complete food for the brain and nervous system, it has organized brain and nerve elements that cannot be found in the fruit or vegetable kingdoms.

KOHLRABI is especially high in vitamin A.

LEEKS are classified with onions and are good because of their powerful effect in driving out the germ life in the body. All onions have the wonderful effect of ridding the body of catarrh. As an external remedy, try onion packs for chest conditions, chest colds. Because of their iodine content, onion packs are beneficial for thyroid disturbances, so use on the throat.

While we are talking about onions, we have to include garlic. One of its best uses is for simple hemorrhoid conditions. Insert a clove of garlic into the rectum each night.

LEMON JUICE is nature's most powerful antiseptic—use internally and externally. Apply to corns, on scalp, on sores, use it for an eyewash, gargle, brush the teeth with it, drink it to purify the breath.

LETTUCE. There is almost no nourishment in iceberg head lettuce. It is very gas forming and contains an opium by-product which slows down digestion. Leaf lettuce has 100 times as much iron as head lettuce. Endive is a wonderful food, very high in potassium.

MUSHROOMS have very little nutritional value. I believe they have an effect on the body and there is some good in them, but they have no real value as they, like radishes, grow so fast. A rapidly-growing vegetable doesn't have the same value as a slow-growing variety.

NUTS are all good. The almond is the king, being highest in alkalinity. Black walnuts are the highest in manganese, which is the nerve element. Pine nuts are one of the highest in fat content (49%). They make a nice salad dressing, best mixed with fruits—especially with apricots.

ONIONS. Use both bulb and tops to avoid gas formation which may occur from eating the bulb alone. See Leeks.

PAPAYA is very good for stomach troubles. Make tea of the seeds as they contain natural papain which is needed by the stomach as a digestant. Tablets are good for pyorrhea. Papaya tablets disintegrate proteins when they are soaked overnight in the juice. This is why papaya tablets are so wonderful when left in the mouth after a meal to dissolve slowly. They break down toxic protein deposits on the teeth, such as occur in pyorrhea, and should be used after each meal. Following this, use a gargle of liquid chlorophyll, a wonderful mouthwash.

PEAPODS make a wonderful vegetable juice and may be mixed with celery and carrot to make a very tasty drink. Put in soup for flavoring (they may be discarded) or with any vegetable while cooking. There is a lot of value in them.

PUMPKIN SEEDS are an excellent food and a good source of vegetable protein. Fresh pumpkin seeds may be liquefied into a juice, strained and combined with other foods which would impart flavor. Use suitable sweetening agent.

RADISHES are good for gallbladder or catarrhal conditions. Whether they contain much mineral value or not, they add bulk. Black radish and horseradish have a beneficial effect on sinus disturbances and gallbladder troubles. Powdered horseradish is used as a remedy for gallbladder catarrh. Raphenon is an extract which has been developed from horseradish for this purpose.

RED FOODS are usually the red blood builders. From a remedial standpoint, it is always a food that looks like a gland that will build a gland or a red food that will build red blood. In fact, green chlorophyll as found in the tops of vegetables, alfalfa and other green leaves, contains the greatest amount of iron and is one of our best red blood builders.

SQUASHES are the mildest vegetable you can have in your diet. When baking squash, leave seeds in for flavoring. Never remove seeds unless you save them for planting.

TARO ROOT is a good remedy in case of intestinal distress or colitis, as it is an easily digested starch, native to the Hawaiian Islands.

TURNIPS are high in vitamin A. They come under the classification of a sulphur food. Being so high in this vitamin, they will fight any catarrhal trouble in the body. If you want to get rid of any such trouble, think of turnip juice.

WATERCRESS is the finest garnish for salads and can be used as a green base.

Body Conditions and Suggested Remedies

ACIDITY developed by muscular labor and activities. Celery will help to neutralize the acids in the body.

ARTHRITIS make "coffee break" a "nutritional break"—1 teaspoon broth powder, 1 tablespoon whey in a cup of hot water. Simmer for a few minutes.

BEE STING press an old-fashioned watch key firmly over the spot to force out the sting, then rub well with raw onion juice or moisten earth and apply as a poultice; secure with a bandage.

BLADDER pomegranate juice with whey. Barley water. Take 3 ounces pearled barley (not the kind sold by chemists), wash in cold water, then in hot. Boil in 2 quarts water until reduced to 1 quart. Strain. Dose: Small cupful three times daily.

BLOOD to build red blood cells, use greens. Any green vegetable is high in iron, the blood builder. Other blood-building foods are black cherries and strawberries. Black cherry juice concentrate may be used in molded gelatin salads. For coagulation of blood, use liquid chlorophyll (for vitamin K), 1 teaspoonful in a glass of water before breakfast. To promote circulation: spinach juice and celery juice. To direct the flow of blood to the head area, use a sulphur food (of the cabbage or onion family) with a protein, thus making this element more active in the upper extremities of the body.

Outdoor exercise is one of the finest things for building a good bloodstream. Sunshine is necessary. Spend some part of every day in the open air, inhaling lifegiving oxygen around growing things. You cannot be well unless you live among growing things.

BOWEL. For a laxative, the following formula has been used by a doctor from the famous Mayo Clinic. (It is also an aid in overcoming arthritis.)

Dried Natural Fruits
(One week's supply)

21 prunes	7 halves pears
14 teaspoonsful raisins	7 halves peaches
14 halves apricots	7 figs

Put in large pan, pour boiling water over fruit to cover entirely. Cover with loose-fitting lid; let stand for four days at room temperature, adding water to keep fruit covered; then store in lower compartment of refrigerator. Each day take: 3 prunes, 2 tsp raisins, 2 halves apricots, 1 pear half, 1 peach half and 1 fig. If desired, grind these dry with senna leaves.

Other laxative foods are whey, black cherry juice concentrate, flaxseed meal and flaxseed tea. The use of the slant board is helpful.

BRAIN AND NERVOUS SYSTEM. Stew together an ounce each of the following herbs: Vervain, valerian, skullcap and mistletoe in 2 quarts water for 20 minutes. When cool, strain and drink half a small cupful three times a day. Eat plenty of onions, raw, if you can digest them, preferably green onions with tops. Egg yolk (may be used in liquefied drinks). Wheat bran tonic (contains 16 chemical elements) called the "staff of life" is one of the finest nutrients.

CATARRHAL CONDITIONS. Turnip juice diet. Mix with pineapple juice. Proper altitude is to be considered, also a dry climate. In many cases, asthma and bronchial conditions may be corrected. To loosen catarrh in bronchial tubes and for the impending flu symptoms: Bake a lemon for 20 minutes. Use the juice of half of it to one cup of hot oatstraw or boneset tea. Then go to bed and perspire.

COLDS. There are many remedies for colds. This is a complex subject which has been dealt with independently, which includes bronchial asthma, sinusitis, bronchitis and influenza. Let us remind you that you should learn a way to live correctly to prevent colds. We do not want to compete with the nostrums and remedies of the drugstores. A word of caution should be sounded regarding the use of antihistamine preparations; their prolonged use may lead to asthma.

The condition of the skin, that vital organ of elimination of toxic waste from the body, is an important factor in the prevention of colds. The care of the skin is therefore essential for healthful living. An experiment which you may make to show how the skin is affected by atmospheric changes is to dip your fingers in water or blow on one side of your fingers and you will feel something akin to a cool current of air. This acts as a shock to the skin, causing the pores to close. Such a condition can bring on a chill. It is this change in the humidity of the surrounding atmosphere which causes a change in the condition of the reflexes that many times may be the beginning of symptoms of the common cold.

COUGHS, COUGH SYRUP. Over a chopped-up onion, pour one tablespoon of honey. Let stand four hours. Use one teaspoon of the juice every half to one hour.

EARS. To remove wax accumulation, use glycerineis the only oil that mixed with water. Warmed glycerine which is the only oil that mixes with water. Warmed glycerine in an eye dropper, dropped into ears and left overnight, will mix with and dissolve wax. in the into ears.

ENEMAS. Plain water enemas are the best to empty the lower bowel. If there is a little inflammation or irritation, use flaxseed tea, 1/2 pint to an enema. If it is very thick and heavy, dilute flaxseed tea with water. The knee-chest position is the best in the average person for taking the enema.

EYES. For watery eyes, when affected by smog, use sterilized raw linseed oil made from flaxseed (contains vitamin F, which is destroyed in cooking). Use one drop in each eye. This is good for conditions of inflammation.

One of the finest things to use as an eyewash is camomile tea, which must be carefully strained. Also drink this herb tea.

FEVER. Vital Broth (recipe in other section of this book).

FUNGUS. White iodine will help to kill fungus under fingernails. One of the finest natural remedies is aloe, a plant-like cactus, which grows more in Florida than here. A book has been written on the remedial uses of this plant by the University of Florida at Jacksonville. For skin troubles, burns or stomach-soothing, ointments are made of it. Apply a piece around infected fingers, bandage and leave on overnight.

GASTROINTESTINAL TRACT. To change the intestinal flora, one of the greatest remedies is acidophilus culture or you can use yogurt. Taro, one of the wonder foods of Hawaii, is especially good for colitis, inflammation of the bowel. It is a very easily digested starch, soothing to the bowel. Use especially where bland foods are indicated or where diarrhea or any bleeding of the bowels has occurred.

FLAXSEED TEA. Flaxseed tea is wonderful in stomach and bowel inflammations. It can be mixed with raw vegetable juices or flavored with a little lemon.

Flaxseed tea is made by using 1 tablespoon of whole flaxseed to 1 pint of water, boiling 6 to 7 minutes and straining off the seeds. Do not use the seeds. Just use the liquid. This flaxseed tea can be used for an enema whenever there is excessive gas, colitis or inflammation of the bowel.

HAIR. For hair and scalp troubles (loose, falling hair) use egg yolk with 1/4 teaspoon sea salt. Apply to scalp. This is your shampoo. For gray hair use parsley juice, a half glass daily, mixed with celery, pineapple or apple juice. Blackstrap molasses, 1 or 2 tablespoonsful daily is also useful. For baldness, people almost bald have grown healthy heads of hair by rubbing garlic oil well into the scalp night and morning. Or, if unprocurable, pour equal parts of rosemary, bay rum and olive oil into a bottle, shake well and rub into the scalp well night and morning.

HEADACHE (Migraine). For headache caused by tension in the neck and stiffness in the neck, use a halter stretch for 5 minutes every day.

HICCOUGHS. Hold a spoon on the tongue for four or five minutes, with pressure.

JOINTS. For arthritic conditions use one pint of alfalfa seed tea daily. A turnip juice diet is also beneficial. Avoid use of white sugar which is one of the things contributing to arthritic conditions.

For rheumatic conditions, wear a red flannel jacket at night to protect the shoulders from contact with cold air (in cases of shoulder pains). Wrap knees in red flannel for pain in knees. To relieve pain in joints, before retiring, wrap area with a heavy towel wrung out of cold water, then wrap with a dry towel to hold in the moisture.

LACTATION (Nursing Mothers). Diet high in greens.

LIVER AND GALLBLADDER. In cases of constipation, to encourage bowel movement and to help gallbladder to drain, beets are one of the finest foods.

Gallbladder Remedy

1 cup finely-shredded raw beet
2 tablespoons virgin cold pressed olive oil
Juice of half a lemon

Take 1 teaspoonful of this mixture every 1-1/2 hours during the day for 3 days. Continue this program 3 days a week for 1 month.

To aid liver in taking care of proteins, try black cherry juice concentrate.

MOUTH ODORS. Bad breath, coated tongue—use liquid chlorophyll, one teaspoon diluted with one or two parts water. Raw apples are the best thing for bad breath. Use them in between meals.

NOSE AND SINUS. To clear the sinuses of congestion, breathe deeply while walking. Take sage, rub between hands, breathe into nostrils to open passages. Carry a few bay leaves, inhale aroma while walking. Put some fresh horseradish on tongue, take some deep breaths, it will drain sinuses. For nose bleeding, use liquid chlorophyll, 1 teaspoon in a glass of water 3 or 4 times a day; gelatin 2 or 3 times daily. Make veal joint broth, use over a period of time for frequent occurrence of nose bleeding.

SKIN AND COMPLEXION. For a clear complexion, drink cocktails made of apple juice concentrate with cucumber juice. This is a very good summertime drink as cucumbers are high in sodium, which helps to keep the body cool.

SNORING. Apply oil in nostrils before retiring; 1 or 2 drops of any natural oil.

SPECIAL DIETARY REMEDIES. An elimination diet of grapes is a wonderful remedy. Turnip diet, carrot juice and acid-alkaline balance diet are also used.

TOOTH DECAY. To attempt to control this by means of fluoridation of water is a poor remedy for the condition, especially when we are not told how to get organic fluorine into our bodies through foods. People are getting breakdown of teeth from the pampered foods, the luxury foods. Sweetened, devitalized foods are also responsible for tooth decay. If we do not learn to stop breaking down our bodies before resorting to remedies, the remedy is going to be worse than the disease. It is possible that 10 years from now, we will look back and be sorry for fluoridated products, for this can accumulate in the tissues of the body and eventually cause problems that will be far worse than tooth decay.

STOMACH. For nervous stomach, use 2 tablespoons of powdered papaya in 1 quart water; sip slowly throughout the day. In the morning, have water.

WARTS. Use green papaya, make mark with fingernail. Take thick material from papaya and apply to warts.

WEIGHT GAINING. Use soybean milk and dried fruits between meals. These dried fruits should, of course, be soaked or brought to a boil and allowed to soak all night long, eating them the next day. A cup of flaxseed tea, taken at least 10 minutes before each meal helps one to gain weight also.

WEIGHT REDUCING. Exercise in a sweat shirt; perspire. Appease the habit of having to have something heavy to eat at noon by taking dry cottage cheese and one prune or yogurt and fresh fruit only. Select a low calorie diet; the varieties from the vegetable kingdom are lowest in calories.

Helps for Gaining Weight

When the body weight is abnormal, we must first find the cause. Our emotional state is very important. The nervous system may burn any food faster than it can be built into sturdy tissue. Slow down. A contented mind gives the body a good time. Usually when we come into the healthy way to live and get ourselves clean, we find our own weight without doing any more. If, however, there is nothing organically wrong, we can follow these suggestions to advantage.

Never consume calories without vitamins. Ice cream, doughnuts and pastries may be fattening, but there is nothing healthy about this kind of weight. Get on the regular diet regime with a bias towards the weight-building foods. Have a good whole-grain cereal for breakfast. Put a little flaxseed meal, sunflower seed meal, dulse and rice polishings on it, and cream or butter. Have a glass of goat milk or buttermilk. Choose more from the sweet and dried fruits as citrus fruits are slimming. Take a spoonful of nut butter with them. Have between-meal snacks of nut milk or sesame drinks, using carob, dried fruits, banana and honey for flavoring. Take a dish of yogurt with fruit. A small whole-grain sandwich with stuffed celery sticks occasionally will help. Rich cocktails of fruit or vegetable juices with an egg yolk and other supplements added will help or a drink of milk with fruit and cheese. On your luncheon salad, use a cream or oil dressing, sometimes adding an egg yolk. Favor more of the root vegetables, but don't neglect the greens. Choose a cream or legume soup or a soup thickened with barley or whole rice. Nibble on raw nuts, sunflower and pumpkin seeds at odd moments. Don't skimp on proteins. Drink cocktails with a flaxseed tea base. Before bed a hot carob-milk drink is permissible.

One little thing I have found which helps in gaining weight is to use one cup of flaxseed tea 20 minutes before each meal. Rather than use fresh fruit juice in drinks, use reconstituted dried fruits with soybean milk, nut butter, etc. When using raw vegetable juices, add one tablespoon sunflower seed meal or one tablespoon sesame seed meal so the drink will add weight to the body.

Weight gaining is not all food. Get plenty of exercise. Sleep and rest is especially important if you are the thin, worrying type. Live as much as possible out in the open air and sunshine.

Additional Health Building Suggestions

Some years ago, we became aweare of the fact that people in this country were ruining their stomachs and the nutritional balance of their bodies by taking only part of the wheat. Wheat has been called the staff of life, and it truly is, because when it is grown from the proper soil and served properly, it has most of the chemical elements that are needed for complete nutrition. However, man in his industrial methods and anxiousness to put out a product for a good price, has forgotten the health aspects. He has served his fellowmen with a product that is disease producing because so many of the elements have been taken away through the refining and devitalizing processes.

In 90% of the people in this country suffering from nutritional disorders, they could overcome some of these deficiencies by using a bran water. Bran was brought to my attention years ago by Dr. McFerrin in Florida. Since then, I have seen marvelous results accomplished by using bran as packs on various leg ailments such as eczema, pimples, boils, etc., and I am convinced there is a wonderful mineral value to bran if used properly.

I have seen great results when bran is used as a blood building tonic. It is one of our highest foods in silicon. Bran has the structural elements to give us the tone and power in the body that most of us are lacking. The 16 chemical elements can be found in very good proportion in bran if used properly. To get the greatest good from bran tonic, it can be made and taken as follows.

FOR THE BLOODSTREAM. Add one cup of sifted bran to three cups of cool water and bring just to the boiling point. Do not boil for even a moment. Remove from the stove and allow to cool. Strain off the liquid into a quart jar and refrigerate overnight. The starch will settle at the bottom of the jar. Pour off very carefully without disturbing the starch and stop pouring the moment the starch begins to rise. Drink three or four cups of this liquid daily, a half hour before meals. Do this for two or three months to get the best results. Add a little celery salt, garlic salt or vegetable broth powder. You may take this either warm or cool. By adding cherry concentrate to this broth, it makes a wonderful drink for the children and one they will not refuse. This is one of the finest drinks when liquid chlorophyll has also been added. It is a great tonic for the bloodstream. Be convinced by trying it over a period of one month.

Salt

Knowing what we know about the biochemistry of foods, which deals with the chemicals that are fit for human consumption, we have had our lesson in regard to salt. Foods that come directly from the garden are rich in chemicals, and we never go wrong when we use them for the health of our bodies. I have long been in doubt that the salt used in this country as a preservative of various foods and sprinkled so generously on the foods we eat, has any good effect in our bodies. It is a known fact that salt will cause hardening of the arteries. Doctors make a living treating people who have produced this condition in their bodies through the constant use of salt.

The salts that come directly through the fruits and vegetables are beneficial, but we do not approve of salt that comes from the sea or the earth. We are of the opinion, however, that there are some chemicals in sea salt that are of a colloidal nature and can be used in our human economy. There are many ways we can get these salts back into the body; for instance, by the use of juices, supplements and various tablets like chlorella or spirulina—but I don't think we need the ordinary table salt that is used so promiscuously.

I am of the opinion that the heavy salt many people use can hold water in the body, can produce lumps, nodes, cysts, high blood pressure, arteriosclerosis, arthritis and many heart diseases. It is the accumulation of this salt over a period of time that causes most of the trouble. When we consider that one type of salt can produce toxic acids in the body, overweight, degeneration of the arteries, loss of elasticity in the body and many skin diseases, it is well we consider what we put into our mouths.

Dr. George W. Crane has gone all out in telling people to use sea water. I partially agree with him. Good effects can be accomplished in certain cases where there is a loss or lack of specific salts in the body, but I believe also we can replace these salts by more natural means.

Salt in Your Food Can Bury You

Would you use sodium, a caustic alkali, to season your food? Or chlorine, a poisonous gas? "Ridiculous question," you say. "Nobody would be foolhardy enough to do that." Of course not, but the shocking truth is that most people do because they do not know these powerful chemicals constitute the inorganic crystalline compound known as salt.

For centuries, the expression "salt of the earth," has been used as a catchall phrase to designate something good and essential. Nothing could be more erroneous. For that apparently harmless product you shake into

367

your food every day can bury you. Consider these startling facts:

1. Salt is not a food. There is no more justification for its culinary use than there is for potassium chloride, calcium chloride, barium chloride or any other chemical on the druggist's shelf.

2. Salt cannot be digested, assimilated or utilized by the body. It has no nutritional value. Instead, it is positively harmful and disease-producing, especially in the case of kidney ailments.

3. Salt may act as a heart poison. It also increases the irritability of the nervous system, tends to aggravate epileptic conditions and lowers the bars against apoplexy.

4. Salt acts to rob calcium from the body and attacks the mucous lining throughout the entire gastrointestinal tract.

If salt is so dangerous to the health, why is it used so widely? Mainly because it is a habit that has become ingrained over thousands of years. Many people, and in fact, entire races of people such as the Eskimos, never eat salt and never miss it. Once a person is free of the habit, salt is as objectionable and repulsive to the taste as tobacco is to a nonsmoker. How did the habit originate? The biochemist, Bunge, explains that in the prehistoric times there was a proper balance of sodium and potassium salts in the earth, but continued rainfall over the centuries washed away the more soluble sodium salts. In time all soils and land-grown foods became deficient in sodium, but high in potassium. The result was that animals and human beings developed a craving for something to replace this deficiency. They found a poor, ineffective and highly dangerous substitute in inorganic sodium chloride or common salt.

Since salt is a chemical that is harmful to the digestive organs, we can understand why the stomach develops a sudden and abnormal thirst after salt is consumed. The stomach is simply reacting to a foreign substance and is taking quick action to wash it out of the body through the kidneys. Of all the body organs, the kidneys are the most subject to injury from salt. Salt eating, in fact, is known to pave the way for kidney disease. Just as salt is harmful to the kidneys, so it is injurious to the heart. The action of the heart muscle is governed by the relative concentration and balance of sodium and calcium salts in the blood. An excess of sodium will therefore tend to disturb this action, increasing the heartbeat and the blood pressure. In the same way, salt upsets the nervous system.

The decalcifying effect of salt has been noted by Dr. Uhlmann. He points out that it tends to rob the body of calcium by drowning calcium salts in thirst-quenching liquids and creating a predisposition to acidosis. For this reason, Dr. Uhlmann forbids the use of salt by persons with colds and sinus conditions. Salt starts its attack by biting into the mucous membranes of the mouth and then spreading its irritation all along the gastrointestinal tract.

Persons suffering from sexual hyperesthesia, manifesting itself in various types of perversion, are sometimes particularly addicted to salt, pepper and other condiments. The ban on the use of salt by epileptics is designed to curb their well-known sexual tendencies. The most dramatic case of salt injury occurred in a Binghamton, New York Hospital where a number of babies died when the chemical was inadvertently used in their food.

The body needs sodium chloride, but only when it is provided in organic form such as in celery, sea vegetation, etc., can this substance be utilized by living cells.

With all the talk of salt today, you might remember history shows people who were starving to death, those people who lived on unnatural, concentrated and dried foods, are the ones who craved salt. Their diet was poor in the first place. Animals that live on dry foods have salt licks. Man, who sweats heavily, is in need of extra salt in his body, but it is to his advantage to know how to replace the proper salt.

To Replace or Rebuild a Salt Deficiency

There are a lot of vegetable broth powders on the market that will help to replace the salts that have been lost in the body through sweating. Spring Green tablets are a fine biochemical source of sodium and chloride, and can be used as salt tablets for people living in hot countries or those who perspire a great deal.

The Salt Story

"Reason should direct and appetite obey."
—*Cicero*

The gist of the story regarding salt from my standpoint is that it does not belong in the body. I am speaking of sodium chloride or common table salt. People have become accustomed to using this as a seasoning for foods, and the average consumption is six pounds a year. I can usually tell the age of a restaurant cook by the amount of salt I notice in his food, for salt so deadens the taste buds that more and more must be used in order to be tasted. No matter how much the cook uses, however, most patrons add still more salt after the food is brought to the table. Scientists have found that inhabitants of the interior of China never use salt. In some parts of China, it is used for suicidal purposes. Fifty grains of salt have been known to kill a dog; it invariably kills birds.

The reason I do not approve of salt is that it is an inorganic substance which is not a food, and which I regard as harmful to the body—as harmful as most drugs. If salt is given to a person not used to it, it causes irritation and debility in such organs as the stomach, the intestines, the heart, the blood vessels, etc. The throat will become dry. When given to an infant, vomiting may result. When an isotonic solution is taken for the purpose of purging the intestines, this is accomplished through the drawing of fluid from the blood into the bowel to wash out the salt. Salt acts as a purge because it is an irritant to the bowel. Persistent use would result lin tissue degeneration. Some experiments have shown that salt given to dogs, rabbits and other animals caused the muscles of their hind legs to become paralyzed. Even cancer has resulted from the addition of salt to the milk fed to cats, while cats lilving under the same environmental conditions but without salt in the milk did not develop cancer. Salt may cause the retention of water in the tissues and disturbance of the water balance.

Back in 1944, a doctor at the U.S. Marine Hospital on Ellis Island, Dr. Michael M. Miller, reported that relief from insomnia and tension was obtained in 11 out of the 12 patients in whose diet he reduced the amount of salt. It has been known for some time that a salt-free diet will reduce high blood pressure. I believe salt tends to harden tissues that absorb and hold it, and that it can produce hardening of the arteries, which in turn, produces high blood pressure. In my opinion, salt is responsible for a lot of dry skin and hardened tissue conditions in the body. It can be responsible for many rashes and other skin disorders, and can interfere with the circulation by causing arterial changes.

Various sodium salts which are used as drugs for temporary relief of such conditions as rheumatism, stomach disturbances, acidosis, belching, etc., include sodium salicylate, sodium bicarbonate, etc. As a result, we have not only the disease to handle in the future, but have salt deposits to remove. I believe that some day table salt will be considered a suppressant drug and definitely harmful to the body. One doctor remarked in an article that salt was used by our forefathers for embalming purposes. An equivalent today is its use in the preservation of foods.

Of course, there are arguments in favor of using salt and some questions which it would seem necessary to answer in its favor. For example, an extra intake of salt is recommended, especially for persons doing active work during hot weather, to replace that which is lost through perspiration. The salt requirement for this purpose could be supplied from vegetable sources by adding a concentrated vegetable powder to drinking water which is high in sodium salts. Salt should be taken into the body gradually, in organic form, from vegetables and fruits. Tribes of pygmies who are famous for their salt hunger also are cited as an example to justify the ingestion of salt. Egon V. Ullman, MD, in a book called *Diet in Sinus Infections and Colds*, says there are races whose languages contain no word for salt, the East Finns, the Kamtchadales, the Tunguses and Kirgises, the Tudas, the shepherds of South American Pampas and Fire Islands, the natives of New Holland and the Fiji Islanders. A Dr. Dickey, who studied natives in South Africa, found that by feeding them greens, he could overcome their craving for salt. Benjamin Rush studied Indians and said they had no such craving.

Some persons believe they have you stumped when they point out that certain wild animals, such as deer, will travel miles to sources of salt known as salt licks. They should be interested in the explanation given by Dr. A. C. Morrow in an article read at a meeting of the American Pheasant Society. He said: "Under normal conditions, birds and animals migrate temporarily, seasonally or permanently to those places containing the minerals they need. The deer lick was utilized by many wild animals and by our range stock before they were fenced off. Deer licks often are soils containing more than the usual amount of potassium or magnesium sulphate, and not common salt, as is usually supposed.

"At French Lick Springs, Indiana, I have observed birds, rabbits, squirrels and a raccoon drinking the overflow water from the famous Pluto Spring, and drinking with an apparent gusto. Whether these birds and animals were natives or migrants, I do not know. I do know that at the time, I was unfamiliar with mineral requirements for birds and animals and was greatly puzzled as to why they drank a water I heartily disliked, while other sweet water was available.

"Later, observing cattle and sheep eating so-called alkali dirt to the exclusion of good stock salt, a chemist's report explained the seemingly depraved appetite was desire and a need for the magnesium and potassium sulphate in this soil."

We are not trying to say that salt is not needed by the body, but we maintain that it should be in the organic form found in vegetables and fruits. We have stated the body's need for all the mineral salts such as sodium, calcium, potassium, silicon, etc., and we also include chlorine. Both vegetables and fruits contain sodium and chlorine, which are the constituents of our refined salt, but from these sources, they are in organic form. The mineral salts that have passed through the vegetable and fruit kingdoms and become organic have a different colloidal, electrochemical effect in the body. When they are eliminated from the body, they have left behind an electrical, vibratory effect which the body can use for cell repair and growth, and which it will not obtain from inorganic minerals such as those contained in table salt.

369

Honey and Pollen

Of the 60,000-odd bees in a beehive, the workers are the most important to us. The Queen merely lays eggs; the drones, the only males in the hive, mate with the Queen; but the thousands of workers tend the young bees, make wax, clean and air condition the hive and finally learn the intricate process of foraging for nectar and making honey.

The nectar from the flowers is collected in the bee's honey sac where it mixes with acid secretion. Back at the hive, it brews in the honey house until condensed to half its weight.

It takes millions of bees to satisfy our appetite for honey. A worker bee produces about 1/2 teaspoon of honey during its short 4 to 8 weeks of life. But much as we experiment, honey has never been produced artifically.

What Is Honey?

Percentage Composition of Honey

Water	17.0
Levulose	39.0
Dextrose	34.0
Sucrose	1.0
Dextrin	0.5
Protein	2.0
Wax	1.0
Plant acids: malic, citric, etc.	0.5
Mineral salts	1.0
Residues: gums, resins, pollen, etc.	4.0

Honey is one of the most natural of all sweetening agents. Not only does it add delicious flavor to foods, but it is an easily digested, nutritious food. Dextrin, a gummy substance, makes honey so digestible.

The protein is removed upon any clarifying of the honey.

Honey is rich in vitamins.

Dr. Schuetter, University of Wisconsin, stated that honey has nearly all the minerals comprising the human skeleton.

Honey from the flower is 75% water, 20% cane sugar and 5% oils, gums, etc., which give the flavor.

Honey improves as it is stored.

History

From times dating back to antiquity, honey has been mentioned in the writings of all races. It must have been one of the oldest edibles known to man. For centuries before sugar gained popularity, honey was used by rich and poor alike. It was found in an Egyptian tomb 3300 years old—as good, if not better than the day it was put there.

Processing

The beehive is hot. If a bee keeper can get the combs out quickly, the honey can be extracted easily without artificial heat. A filter removes solid debris so that this extracted honey is a clean, natural food, though perhaps not as completely natural as comb honey, which has a valuable laxative property for the bowel as well.

The next process is quite ruinous from a health standpoint. The honey is heated to stop it crystallizing. However, this changes the nature of honey. Bees cannot live on heated honey. Better to have sugary honey and stand it in a pan of hot water to liquefy again.

Be careful of honeys such as orange and alfalfa, because cases have been reported in which allergies have developed in people due to the sprays on the blossoms from which the bees collect the honey. Wild sage, eucalyptus and mountain lilac are safer honeys.

Uses

Honey is hydroscopic, so its use prevents baked goods from drying out. However, heated honey is "changed" honey, so we do not recommend its regular use in cooking. Use raw sugar; keep honey for uncooked dishes or sweeten at end of cooking.

Royal Jelly

The queen bee lays eggs in proportion to the amount of Royal Jelly she is fed. This wonderful food is converted immediately into living tissue. Sometimes the queen lays over 2000 eggs in a day. Yet she is able to more than duplicate her own weight with Royal Jelly in a 24-hour period. Royal Jelly appears to have the property of normalizing cells. It has been reported to have had amazing effects in some serious cases. Much else has been written in its praise. Many experiments with dogs and other animals have proven that it stimulates the glandular and nervous systems.

Royal Jelly contains 17 times as much pantothenic acid (a B complex) as is in dry pollen. It is thought that this is synthesized in making Royal Jelly.

Honey for Therapy

Down through the ages, therapeutic uses of honey have multiplied. It has been widely used as a cleanser and purifier. Long-standing ulcers have responded to honey. All over the East, it has been used along with soap to cure boils. It soothes pain, hastens healing—especially burns. Its preservative powers are well known in the East.

Today, hospitals in England have begun to use it on dressings. It is an antiseptic.

Many doctors say that honey is one of the finest foods for the heart. It stimulates with no after effects.

Honey is a good diuretic.

Its volatile essences prove valuable in relieving asthmatic attacks.

Honey is an energy food. For athletes and anyone needing quick, lasting energy, honey is much better than glucose. It offers no possibility of harm.

Tupelo honey is even said to be safe for diabetics.

Bee Bread

Bee bread is fermented pollen. Mixed with honey, pollen may be stored in the comb cells where it ferments due to lactic acid formation to become bee bread. Very much better than hand-collected and dried pollen, bee bread keeps indefinitely, remaining rich in all the elements of the fresh pollen. In addition, it contains vitamins E and K. Fed to bee larvae, it multiplies their weight 1500-fold in 6 days.

Bee's Way

This is a by-product of metabolism. A bee must consume 6 or 7 pounds of honey to make 1 pound of wax. The yellow color is due to fat-soluble pigments.

Pollen

Pollen itself is one of the most complete foods found in nature. Date pollen was used by some of the Arabs in Egypt as a supplementary food. Near Burma, the Chinese make pollen honey cakes which are dried and stored as survival foods during famines—and also used in the regular diet as cake or candy. Hunters often take honey cakes along with them as their only sustenance together with roots and fruits gathered enroute. Pollen is also used by these people as medicine and antiseptic.

The debris which collects at the bottom of the beehive is pollen and propolis, the resin-based substance bees use to seal their hives. This is commonly eaten in Russia.

Authorities in the USSR recently stated that of the 200 people authentically found to be between 110 and 150 years of age, nearly all were or had been bee keepers and ate a fair amount of honey.

Pollen is mentioned in the ancient writings of Persia, China and Egypt. The Koran, Talmud and Bible all refer to the wonderful properties of honey and pollen.

Nearly all the vitamins known have been found in pollen. Pollens richest in carotene may contain 20 times as much as is present in an equivalent weight of carrots. It has been suggested as a source of pro-vitamin A and also as a natural food coloring. Its mineral content varies, but the average compares to grains and seeds.

Pollen is very high in free amino acids. Again, it varies but is 5 to 7 times as much as an equal weight of eggs, cheese or lean beef. So a small quantity of pollen is capable of supplying enough of each essential amino acid, as well as a variety of the others.

Pollen is as rich in enzymes as yeast.

Sugars account for 30-40% of pollen's composition; fats for 5%.

One to three tablespoonsful a day is recommended as a food supplement.

The life cycle and the miraculous attributes and abilities of the bee are a constant source of wonder to those who understand nature best. The following is an exciting example of research on the subject.

"When a worker bee returns from a new source of nectar, she tells the other bees in an intricate descriptive dance. Turning first one way and then another, she reveals the direction of the honey source by the angle in which she dances in relation to the ultraviolet rays of the sun at that time. Between each turn, she wiggles, each wiggle indicating a specific distance. Her excited watchers then are able to leave the hive and fly directly to the nectar source, from the directions they have received."

—*"Honeybee-Master Chemist"*

Our Healing Food

We often mention foods used for specific purposes. For heart trouble, we need potassium. Sun-dried olives, for example, are high in potassium; they will combat fatigue. When climbing hills or mountains, or just taking a walk, we would certainly do better to chew some dried olives than consume a chocolate bar for stimulation. We might call the dried olive the "hiker's best friend." They also make a refreshing tea. The recipe is as follows:

Steep 10 dried olives in an average-sized teapot of boiling water for 10-15 minutes. Skim the oil off the top and the remainder is a potassium tea of real vitality.

This tea is a fine remedy for heart trouble. Another high potassium drink can be made from alfalfa. In fact, anything that is green and bitter is high in potassium.

Do you know that horseradish is one of the best vegetables a catarrhal sufferer can resort to? In powdered form, put in the mouth and wheeze into the nose. Its pungency stimulates the mucosa of the nasal membrane. This aids in throwing off acids that cause catarrhal congestion. It also makes a tasty dressing for many protein dishes, such as eggs or meat. Secure it in powdered form, add a little lemon and a bit of sour cream and you have something unusual for your recipe file. Also try mixing this combination with nut butter or cheese for a sandwich—well worth the trouble.

Sage leaves of the sagebrush and bay leaves stimulate the nasal passages just as horseradish— through a pungent odor. Crush these leaves together or separately, in the palms of your hands, then breathe deeply of the aroma. The volatile oils may, figuratively speaking, "take the top of your head off," or make you think so, but you will feel better instantly.

Tomato packs outside the body are healing to such skin diseases as eczema, pimples and boils. Potato packs on the body bring out toxic materials. Apple packs, especially after the apples have begun to degenerate and turn brown, are wonderful in cases of milk leg or phlebitis. Leg ulcers and varicose veins respond to packs of green curly cabbage and packs of oatstraw. (So save your oatstraw after using it for a silicon tea, if you are bothered with either of these conditions.)

Try onion packs on the throat for catarrhal troubles and on the chest for bronchial disturbances. Flaxseed and flaxseed tea are soothing in the highest degree for the intestinal tract; using the tea in enemas is recommended. For inflamed and bleeding bowel conditions or colitis, add a few drops of chlorophyll, the highest source of vitamin K (antihemorrhagic vitamin) to the flaxseed tea enema. It is not only healing but also soothing.

Our food can and should be our medicine. (Hippocrates, Father of Medicine, declared that in 400 BC.) The Plymouth Diet, consisting almost exclusively of rice with only a few vegetables from time to time has proved its worth by bringing down blood pressure. There is more than meets the eye behind these proven diets. The body works in cycles and in vibration. There is a positive and negative activity—the right side is positive and the left side is negative. Starches are negative; proteins are positive. Therefore, when the left or negative side is broken down, we need negative food to build it up. Rice is negative; so is wheat. Let us consider wheat for a few moments as a supreme heart remedy and learn a new way to prepare it. Add one-half cup of freshly-ground wheat to one-and-a-half cups of boiling water and pour into a prewarmed thermos bottle. Leave the mixture corked overnight. In the morning, we have a cereal mush with all the vitamins intact. We have a negative food for healing the heart, an organ on the left side of our body.

none of us is competent to run the kitchen. We should learn what a balanced meal consists of, how to prepare what has been carefully selected, how to combine and how to serve it. It is not easy. We have to put our minds to it sincerely. But the reward is worth every effort, and every moment of time dedicated to it—the health of ourselves, our families and everyone we contact who shows an interest and willingness to learn.

I read once of a civic uplift project in Oklahoma City that, high-minded as it may be, will, in my opinion, do more harm than good. Along with every marriage license issued, a free cookbook was included. I haven't seen a copy of the book—I don't want to. I'm afraid to when I think of the white flour and the white sugar recipes the average, run-of-the-mill cookbooks are filled with. I shudder to think of the cake fillings and frostings,

icings and other desserts that will come out of that cookbook to disrupt what should be happy wedded bliss. Sound like a wet blanket? Permit me to paraphrase and mix up the slogan of a widely-circulated women's magazine, "Never underestimate the power of a good digestion to insure tranquility in the home."

In all sincerity, I believe the city fathers could have done a better job by issuing a booklet emphasizing nutritional values of foods, not their external beauty on the table and catering to distorted taste buds.

Foods for Health

The skins of other fruits, besides the apple, as well as the skins of certain vegetables have valuable properties to affect different parts of our bodies. They should be in tonics and liquefied drinks. In every glass of carrot juice, there are 15,000 units of vitamin A. Turnip juice is a wonderful catarrhal eliminator. Every asthmatic and bronchially-affected person should know the value of turnips. My experience alone in using turnips to build health would prove it one of the finest foods available. I will not say it is the greatest, but I will say that with turnips alone, you can do more for bronchial ailments, more for lowering the blood pressure and for getting vitamin A into the body than with any other food I know.

Soon after World War II, I met two soldiers, just discharged, who had spent four years in a German concentration camp. This pair lived on turnips and nothing else for the entire four years they were in prison. You will find it hard to believe, but they were both in perfect health. I might add that I never found cancer in any person confined in concentration camps during the war. That is because, when they did get food, it was simple food, not very good to taste, true, but not detrimental either. The effects of a steady turnip diet among war prisoners is extraordinary. In many cases, they had better teeth when released than when captured. Of course, they were thin; turnips do not build fat on the body. Many of them had better complexions and better fingernails and hair. Their bodies were so influenced by the chemical elements in turnips that they had regular bowel movements. I have prescribed turnips for a number of people. I grow turnips on my Ranch—white turnips with the purple tops. Turnip greens were one of the nine greens we used in treating the little girl whose legs had been covered with ulcers for three years. The combination of greens healed them in three weeks.

One of our patients at the Ranch suffered from asthma, catarrhal trouble and a 240 blood pressure. We put him on a 30-day diet of nothing but turnips. We gave him turnip greens, turnip juice, raw and cooked turnips. Nothing but turnips for 1 month. When taken off the diet, he no longer had asthma or catarrhal trouble; his blood pressure was normal and he was down to his normal weight after losing 40 pounds. He was a picture of health. Compare this with the pills and potions he had been taking for years.

I could cite case after case where turnip juice has succeeded when other things have failed. When my wife's sister developed bronchiectasis, turnip juice helped most to correct her condition. As far back as 1915, turnip greens were found to be the best method then discovered for controlling pellagra, and it is still used for treatment of the disease in the South where it is most dangerous. Pellagra is the result of a lack of calcium in the body and turnip greens are high in calcium.

Besides turnips, there is another widely used food which I, myself, have used with considerable success. It is garlic or, in many cases, a garlic and onion combination. Like the turnip, these odorous vegetables are a wonderful thing for catarrhal problems. They can be used for packs on the chest and throat, and they can be chopped, mixed and fed to the patient. One of the best remedies I know of for a catarrhal throat is a cough syrup of chopped onions and honey. There is nothing better. Put a tablespoon or two of honey in a dish of chopped onions, let it stand for three or four hours; drain. Sip a teaspoonful every hour or, if necessary, every half hour. It may not sound like it, but it is a very soothing syrup and children will not object to it.

Another use of garlic and onions is in the treatment of tapeworms. In one of my books, we have a picture of a tapeworm close to 30 feet long that we eliminated from the intestinal tract with garlic and onions. Germ life cannot live with this combination. At one time, I studied with a San Francisco doctor who had many clever means of going back to nature for remedies. This doctor did not believe in many of the modern methods of healing. We called upon a patient suffering from tapeworm. He was put on an exclusive garlic and onion diet for three days. The fourth day he was given an enema of powdered garlic and water, then a severe herb laxative. To climax this strenuous treatment, he was seated in a tub of warm milk. The tapeworm was almost immediately eliminated in its entirety. The efficiency of this method will be easily recognized by any physician who knows that ordinarily the tapeworm is cut off through the elimination, perhaps only six inches at a time. When this happens, the tapeworm continues to grow and reproduce. If you do not want a tapeworm, put milk at one end and garlic at the other. It may sound crude, but it is effective.

Suppose now we return to more palatable sounding foods. The apple is charged with malic acid and glucose, which are both wonderful for the neurogenic principles of the body. They are wonderful for the nervous system because of the nerve salts they contain. Another excellent food is prunes. Because of their acid, prunes are sometimes not recommended, but I recommend them. Like the apple, they contain a high content of nerve salt. Apples and prunes are essentially valuable for growing children because of their benefit to the bowel. It is also helpful in cases of colic.

Figs, too, are excellent for the bowel if taken when fresh (one to three days old). They contain a high amount of magnesium, potassium, oxygen and papain. I have obtained excellent results in the treatment of arthritis and rheumatism with raw goat milk and fresh figs. Figs, ripe from the tree, are wonderful energy foods. They are high in a natural sweet and the seeds have a natural laxative coating which is important when a patient is in distress.

A walk through the garden at my Ranch would show you a number of herbs wonderful for the body. Fresh peppermint has a forceful gas alleviating effect. It can be made into tea, used as a flavoring in different foods. It soothes the stomach and helps other foods to be less gas forming. Fresh mint is the best, of course, but as it is not available at all seasons of the year, the dry peppermint will suffice. It is procurable in that form at the health food stores.

When studying the value of herbs, we might remember that all vegetables were originally herbs. Breeding through generations has resulted in making larger vegetables with more cellulose, more strings, bigger seeds, more skin and more pulp, but these vegetables contain less of the powerful materials found in herbs.

Take a peppermint or spearmint cluster, squeeze it and rub your hands together, then smell your hands. What it does for them it will do for your entire body. What it will·do for the nasal passages alone is unbelievable. You cannot make that experiment with celery, although it is a very fine food itself. Celery, like many of our larger vegetables, has lost some power in developing size. Herbs are the power-packed foods. Basil and marjoram have a wonderful effect on the kidneys and the heart.

Now, as to peaches and who doesn't like this lovely, luscious fruit? They are high in potassium and phosphorus content, also in oxygen and magnesium. They are also a good laxative; in fact, all of our Spring fruits are high in magnesium and sodium—the bowel foods. These two chemicals, along with chlorine are essential for the intestinal tract. For the muscular system, we need potassium, sodium and calcium. Food for the brain and nervous system includes iodine, sulphur, phosphorus and manganese. So again I say, we treat the system through different chemical elements and all these elements have their effect on the different organs of the body.

We'll now consider a few vegetables. Cucumbers are good for the blood. They get rid of pus tendencies developed by some individuals in the form of rashes, boils, pimples and carbuncles. Cucumbers are a wonderful Summer food because they are cooling. In lettuce, we find iron, potassium and sodium content high. However, there are different kinds of lettuce; some with more chemicals than others. During wartime, the government allowed no head lettuce to the shipped, claiming there was not the nourishment in it. As far as I am concerned, they could still ban its shipment. I do not use head lettuce. There is 100 times as much iron in leaf lettuce as in head lettuce. Head lettuce contains a property somewhat like opium, in effect, that slows down the digestion. Most people's digestion is slow enough without retarding it still more. Head lettuce is also gas forming and the nourishing value is poor. It is just bulk, and bulk is something most of you have been getting too much of for a long time anyway.

Mulberries favor reduction of high temperatures in the body. Those of you who are chronically inclined to fevers, should eat mulberries. They are also good in cases of stomach disorders, such as ulcers. The heavy dew in mulberries stains the intestinal tract so that the stomach acids cannot attack the linings as readily. The juice of mulberries reduces the heat of the body without causing excessive perspiration. Mulberries also contain a lot of natural sugar, which we should use instead of unnatural kinds.

Eucalyptus honey is one of the best honeys we have. It is the most powerful of all. The eucalyptol it contains is especially good for catarrhal problems, consumption, tuberculosis or swollen tonsils, if used with a combination of onions, as explained previously. This combination goes deep into cells to release harsh materials of a toxic nature that settle in the body. Failure to release this harsh material is the reason the skin breaks out so often in the healing process. It is why catarrh runs when we are cleansing the body. It is well to recognize that we are driving for a clean body in recommending all these foods. To get a clean body, we must eliminate the old. What a blessing it would be to us to learn to use only the good foods, rest, sunshine and all the other forms of natural healing.

We must learn that we cannot use drugs or any harsh treatment that will drive the wrong elements back into the body. Nature has the upper hand when it comes to healing. Let's see that she has a free hand.

Celery is our highest sodium food.

God has given us food for every purpose and for every ailment. It is up to us to learn these different foods and how we can remedy specific conditions by their use. We have to learn the different ways to prepare these foods, to cook them less and keep them close to their natural state. We should know the special dishes we can make for desserts with gelatin and the different juices that are so good for us.

For a dessert with a high copper content, use apricots. The apricot whip, made with egg whites and gelatin, is one of the many ways of serving apricots.

Homemade sherbets or ice cream prepared in the liquefier make fine desserts. For sherbet, we can use a different kind of fruit: strawberries, peaches, pears or bananas. Ice cream made from frozen grapes is good tasting and good for you. Grapes placed in the deep freezer, when they are in season, can be used the rest of the year.

Now to vegetables made into broth. For high sodium broth, use beets, celery, carrots and turnips. For broths high in both sodium and potassium, try apple peelings or better yet, the jelly from veal joints. This veal joint broth will do more for arthritis and rheumatism than all other foods combined. The sodium that has been made into the gelatin of the bones of the animal is virtually the same as that found in the human body.

For some time, science has known that the chronic alcoholic is lacking vitamin B, but few of them seem to know that this vitamin is found in rice polishings in its highest and most potent form. It is also found in wheat and rice grains. Anemic persons lack cobalt, which is found in the highest amount in the skin of the almond. These are but two of the foods so necessary for us to learn about. There are many others. Let us learn them all, not just a few. We cannot learn only Greek and Latin and feel we know all there is to know about languages, nor can we learn Sanskrit and French, Math and Music and forget everything else. We have to learn more than the specialization the universities are teaching today.

We should learn much more of the universal sciences, evidences of which surround us. What is found in the ocean contains iodine or is predominant in magnesium or manganese. We should know what is above the ocean and what is below it, as necessary for our balanced knowledge as knowing what is on top of the earth and in the bowels of the earth. We should know this from a food standpoint. We cannot study Agriculture in only one point.

In a community just a few miles outside of Los Angeles, there has been an animal experimentation farm operating for years. On this farm is a hospital for pigs, and there are never less than 500 "patients" of all sizes. There are giants and runts, scrawny pigs, pigs with intestinal disorders, skin disorders and every other disorder that a pig can acquire. This hospital has learned how to wipe out these disorders almost entirely through proper foods. They discovered a long time ago something that should have been known long before; namely, that pigs cannot live on garbage or leftovers. They have to get good food, whole food. Our hospitals for humans could learn a lot from this animal hospital. We could reduce the population of our hospitals and mental institutions by at least 50% by feeding the inmates properly.

Some years ago, I visited a mental institution in Utah. I saw the patients served fried foods, mashed potatoes and dessert, which is made up of 86% sugar and artifically-flavored and colored with a coal tar extraction. Is it any wonder that these people are not recovering? We do not offer them a cure. We do not offer them hope. In the last 25 years, there has been a more than 25% increase of population in mental institutions in the US. This is a crime. It has been calculated that 70 years from now, unless something is done about it, there will not be enough sane people to take care of the insane. This may be somewhat of an exaggeration, but it gives us something to think about. Poor health is on the increase outside of mental institutions, too. Diabetes, for instance, is increasing so steadily that within 25 years, every third person will be suffering from it. If we would only realize that we have our life and health in our own hands, and if we could know *where* to seek our health, it would be a wonderful thing.

The Why of Supplements

We have heard so much about hidden hunger, foodless foods, devitalized, demineralized, commercialized, artificially grown, chemically fertilized and sprayed foods that sometimes I wonder how the health-minded person can keep a balanced mind. There are so many personalized ideas in the health field that it is difficult for the average person to know what to do so far as food is concerned.

There is really only one answer. I have never gone wrong in my teaching concerning foods, for I know the natural way of living; the balanced life is the way for a man to live. It is not broken down in scientific terms or taught with laboratory analysis, but in the laboratory of life, in the stomach, in our everyday work, in our treatment of hundreds of thousands of people it has never failed to make improvement in those who try it. Furthermore, I have seen thousands who have eliminated the problem of mineral and vitamin deficiency and many times corrected conditions associated with constipation, catarrhal problems, rheumatic conditions and the like. I am not supposed to say cure, but in many instances, I believe that there are cases of deficiency corrected when following my advice.

We realize that science does not have all the answers. In fact, science can only express the brains that are running it. There are no brains to fire, chemicals, missiles, torpedoes and bombs. I believe wholeheartedly that there was an all intelligent, all powerful force that put together a whole wheat berry, whole rice, whole sugar, whole milk that no laboratory could ever duplicate or that science could ever construct, reconstruct, break down and put together again, add to or subtract from, that will ever have an inkling of a chance to compare with nature or the God-given foods that we were meant to live on in the beginning. I believe that God gave us foods to build, repair and maintain our bodies. I believe the Garden of Eden is still here, but man has made a mess of it.

This brings us to the point of what vitamins and minerals or supplements we need for our bodies. Let us first answer why we should need any additives in the form of vitamins, minerals or supplements. Man has mistreated God's natural foods through his commercial enterprise, his refining and pickling. What has he done to the soil on which his food is grown? How has he altered God's plan? We are only having half a loaf of bread. That is why we have only half health. We cook our food too much which is why we have only half the vitamins we need for our body. Of course, I do not mean that this is the only way we destroy vitamins.

Now from the above, I have come to the place where I feel that in our commercial way of life, our "business" foods, our supply is short of what we need to build a good body.

Most of the vitamins and minerals used are also a man-made product and to tell you the truth, I believe which has built up the left shoulder, I know you will life we are living and are not part of the whole life we need. They are just to get by. They are answering the whims of our scientists. They are palliative and can never be the answer to the whole shortage that develops from unnatural living. There are no substitutes for right living. There is no right way to do the wrong thing. Now you may say, here is a case against vitamins and minerals. I do know this, that if you are going to live the unnatural life, they will get you by until you can straighten out your life, think differently, until you know how to cook differently or cook less.

If you have been eating the polished white rice and it has been one of the foods you build your right shoulder with, if you have been eating the white flour which has built up the left shoulder, I know you will have complaints. Now that you have learned or are learning the way to live, the supplements to add to your diet to make up for the shortage in the past, especially for the white rice and white flour are vitamins B and E. There is a natural vitamin B from rice polishings, there is a natural vitamin E from wheat germ flakes. These are two natural vitamins to make up for the unnatural food you have lived on. Now you can get vitamins B and E from a hundred different sources, all the way from these most natural vitamin products.

Always try to get the most natural products. Remember in taking vitamins that they do not build the body. It takes minerals to build the body. Minerals are more important than vitamins. In my teachings, I try to get the vitamins and minerals from the most natural sources possible with the least manhandling possible. This is why I say, "Get your iron from black cherry juice, blackstrap molasses, greens and chlorophyll." I consider these as food supplements that can be taken in between meals or with a meal.

In case of emergencies, when vitamin and mineral deficiencies show up as definite symptoms in the body, we can turn to health store vitamins and minerals for the most natural supplements possible to help overcome this emergency moment.

I do not believe in vitamins made from coal tar; those that always carry the highest potency; those that are made from abnormal or inorganic substances. These prostituted vitamins will cause another disease in the body, and one of these days, we will have to be treating you for that type of vitamins and minerals.

I believe in vitamins and minerals, but I believe in natural vitamins and minerals from properly grown and prepared foods. Man is not equipped to take care of the concentrated, fortified supplements that are being supplied to him today.

To make up for deficiencies in the body, I believe we should remember these points:

1. Find out what a healthy daily eating regimen is and follow it.

2. Consult with a doctor who knows how to determine chemical deficiencies in the body or learn how yourself.

3. Find out the natural foods that are high in the vitamins and minerals in which you are deficient.

4. Make sure that all you add to the body, and everything that goes in the mouth is close to what God created and meant for you to have.

What Is Man—A Chemical Analysis

Man is clever; he knows lots of things. He can diagnose and dissect his fellowman and come up with all the answers—he thinks. "I know what man is," he says profoundly. "He is hair and bones and flesh. He is 96 compounded elements, including calcium, silicon and iodine. He has chlorine, magnesium and manganese. He has some oxygen and some hydrogen. He has a spot of cobalt and a trace of copper. He has all the natural elements of the earth—even a little natural aluminum and a little natural arsenic."

Having said this, clever man continues in his analysis of his fellowman. He takes him apart and starts putting him in little bottles. In one vial are 3-1/2 ounces of silicon and so on until he has 96 different parts of Mr. Fellowman in 96 bottles arranged on a laboratory shelf. "There, my friend, is man," he says. But he is very wrong.

Man is able to take man apart, but he is unable to put him back together, any more than all the king's men could put Humpty Dumpty back together again. Man is not 96 bottles on a shelf—he is a soul created by God. It is from our soul qualities we get life, and all that has been promised us for a more abundant life. Man cannot create or recreate the soul of man as God does; but he can live and enjoy God's creation by treating his physical being as it should be treated. To do this, he must look to physical foods, the effect they have on the body and which ones are most necessary. He must know which foods digest easily and which ones have a laxative effect. He must know the necessary food for an ailing body, and the one to conserve energy. Once these things are

learned, he will realize his "river of life," his bloodstream, is affected by every thought he thinks. Each one of us must realize our "river of life" contains our life, our energies, destiny, hopes, pictures of the past and of the future. It is the way we treat our "river of life"—what we feed into it that expresses each of us as an individual human being.

That wonderful bony structure of ours—do you know it must have calcium to keep it from collapsing like a tent in a storm, and to carry us from place to place? Our muscles must contract so our joints will bend. There must be elasticity in our arteries to keep the blood flowing to the machinery in our body, the nervous system, which carries messages from the brain to every cell in the body. One hundred thirty barrels of blood are pumped through the heart every day we live. We must breathe so much oxygen (but not too much), circulate so much blood (and again, not too much). *Believe It or Not*, Ripley had a field day with these statistics. Our body mechanism can construct two new brain cells a second, but not four; although such uncontrolled emotions as anger, fear, hatred, etc., can destroy them at that rate, leaving us depleted of needed vitality. That's something to think about the next time you start hating someone. Our body does not appreciate the "kindness" of people who talk us into eating and drinking what is not good for us. So, here again, I repeat that the most important thing in maintaining the proper functioning of all these organs, tissue masses, etc., this fantastic "believe it or not" phenomena is the knowledge and proper use of nutrition.

I stress nutrition because it is vital, but to enjoy its full value, we must embrace the complete triangle: the physique of an athlete is still not complete without love excellent digestion, a good heart and the beautiful plhysique of an athlete is still not complete without love in his heart for others. He must possess and express other attributes to give him soul quality.

Not long ago in Stockholm, Sweden, a group of noted scientists and physicians conducted a series of studies of the human body. They came up with some interesting conclusions, including seven remarkable ones. Among their findings was that we have a "heart brain" and a "stomach brain." They found that the pancreas is dependent on the brain, that a kidney disturbance could easily be a nerve depletion coming from the brain. From that, they concluded it was often necessary to repair the nervous system before starting on the kidney, stomach, heart or any other organ.

The Swedish professors made a thorough study of ganglionic tensions in the spinal cord. (For years, competent chiropractors, naturopaths and mechanotherapists have successfully tapped and eliminated these ganglionic obstructions along the spinal cord.) These men of Sweden reported the necessity of a free flow of the medullary or dynamic force from the brain to the different organs. This is a cellular source of energy communicated by the cerebellum, in the physical brain, which develops a continuous circle of each organ depending upon the other. For example: Respiration, which, in turn, is dependent upon oxygenation and respiration, *ad infinitum.*

Care of the Hair—Hair Culture

In taking care of the hair, we have to recognize that the hair is part of the bloodstream. It belongs to our body, just the same as our eyes. It must be fed by the digestive system. It is a part of the foods we eat. It is taken care of by the circulation of our body. We find that it lives. It has its being; it has its roots right in the blood, as well as in the scalp. In order to get a good plant to grow, we must nourish it, care for it and see that it has a balanced ration in the amount of sunshine and water it is given. This is also true of the hair—it has to be nourished and cared for.

There are many things that we neglect in our body and in our daily living habits which point to the fact that people are losing their hair, because they do not take care of it in the way they should. Hair must have more care than just the average combing or brushing it gets each day. Besides the food and the diet, it is well that we consider that the hair has a function as far as beauty is concerned. It is a receptor; it helps to keep us magnetically balanced. It is truly the one organ that keeps and holds the greatest amount of silicon in our body. Silicon is the "feeling" element of our body. Silicon is the magnetic element in the body.

I believe that women today are much more nervous than the women of the past when they wore long hair. I personally do not believe in cutting the hair of men or women; but in the society we live in today, the one who walks down the street with long hair is the odd one. I hope this fashion will come back again, and I am sure we will have a better balanced nervous system if it does.

It is best not to use a nylon brush on the hair. One hair in the head is worth two in the brush. The only thing I know that will stop falling hair is the floor. Some people think eating a good diet will make hair grow on a cue ball.

I know of many doctors who take care of hair, and they all have the same idea; the hair must be taken care of the same as the teeth. When the hair begins to deteriorate, the whole body is also deteriorating. Anything that interferes with the bloodstream getting to the head can be considered one of the first things that prevents the proper development of good hair. When we are tired, it is difficult to get the blood to the head. Tired tissue cannot force the blood against gravity or rather it cannot force the blood uphill very well.

If we went to Mexico, we would find very few national Mexican workers who are bald. We find they are people who do not work hard when they are tired. "Manana" is their favorite word. Whenever there is baldness or the hair starts to turn gray or the hair gets brittle, which starts with that early thinning, it is a definite sign that a person is not eating enough of the proper chemical elements or that he is burning them up too fast. A breakdown of the nervous system will cause thinning of the hair. Fevers often produce an extreme thinning of the hair. When the cerebellum of the brain is broken down, we find one of the main causes of thinning of the hair. When hair roots have been destroyed entirely, there is no way of growing new hair; just as when teeth are gone; or when a leg has been cut off, a new one cannot take its place. We must hold on to what we have. People who eat properly and have proper circulation can do much to rejuvenate this organ.

There is much research going on these days showing that the pituitary gland is largely responsible for both the growth of the hair and for baldness. They are finding out that the men who have masculine tendencies are the ones who are bald, while those who have more female hormones in their bodies and are more on the feminine side of life, small stature, small bones, etc., are the ones who have a full head of hair. Old Dr. Rocine used to say: "The cerebellum is responsible for the growth of the hair." This is a brain center, and I believe it is very closely related to the pituitary gland function.

Every hair has a hair-bed in the skin with a bulb at the end of the hair root, through which the hair draws its nutrition from the blood. The hair contains a food substance called keratin, which contains great quantities of sulphur. The scalp, which is made of muscular material, should be relaxed so blood will circulate well beneath it. We find that a tight scalp keeps the blood from circulating to the hair root. We also neglect the hair and scalp when we do not sleep enough. Sleeplessness is one of the causes for a lack of hair growth; also overstudy, worry, insufficient oils and nutrition in the blood. Baldness can come from a lack of lecithin, which is a brain and nerve fat. When we lack sulphur, silicon and iron in our food, the hair shoots will not develop and grow properly.

Typhoid fever and many of the childhood diseases can bring on loss of hair. Many people, in old age, find that the top of the head is not properly nourished because their tissues have become flabby and do not allow proper circulation of the blood.

The thyroid gland has a lot to do with this also, for when the thyroid becomes underactive, the circulation is slow and the tissue is flabby. An extra amount of iodine in the diet can help this condition; which will, in turn, help the hair. Strong acids and alkalies, when applied to the hair, can destroy it. Germ poisons, diseases, lack of nerve force or certain parasites, which generate poisonous gases and gnaw at the hair roots or infect the sabaceous glands, can use up the vitality of the hair roots. Dandruff can smother the hair shoots and the scalp in general. This is caused by a weakness in the sabaceous glands from a lack of skin fat in these glands.

To have a beautiful head of hair, one must give it care and attention. Learn what diets are good for the body and find out how to feed the various weaknesses in the body which prevent it from circulating good blood. Live on nutritionally balanced foods; stay away from devitalized foods and especially demineralized starches. The demineralized starches take away the outside layer (or silicon layer) of the grain, which is specific for hair growth. The finest foods to get into the body and into the bloodstream for helping the hair are found in the following: oakstraw tea, rice polishings, rice bran syrup, wheat bran tea, shave grass tea, radishes, horseradish, sprouts, sole, black fish, smoked blue fish, white fish, shad roe, bran bread, strawberries, avocados, cucumbers, steel-cut oatmeal, graham bread, seaweed, the shell of grain, nuts, fruits, dandelion, leeks, romaine, parsnips, whole barley meal, tender raw carrots, marjoram, pamerain, collards, caroway, whole rice and wheat or oatstraw broth cooked slowly for one hour.

Graying and Thinning Hair

There are many things we have used in the diet to help the hair, but we feel that the one thing that gets the greatest result is Nova Scotia dulse tablets. Also the use of three or four parsley tablets, three and four times a day or drinking about one half glass of parsley juice daily. This along with the massage on the slanting board, we feel will change the hair considerably in a period of six months.

Shampoo

One shampoo that is very stimulating to the hair and to the scalp is made of an egg yolk and a quarter teaspoon of sea salt. Rub this well into the scalp and let it set for 10 to 15 minutes; then wash it out with a castile soap. This can be done twice a week. Watch your elimination, make sure that the kidneys and bowels are functioning well. Be sure the skin is cared for by brushing it. It might be well to stimulate the circulation in the head areas at times, by using hot and cold packs while lying on the slanting board. Use the packs 1/2 minute hot, 1/4 minute cold. Make about 6 or 8 changes while on the board. Do this once a day.

To revitalize the hair, we must conserve our energy, control our imagination, stop working when we are tired and use a lot of silicon foods. Give your hair a 30 minute massage twice a week, for at least 6 to 8 weeks and a noticeable result will be observed. However, hair that is put under extremely hot hair dryers and subjected to the use of some of the dandruff cure-all remedies these days is having much of its hair growth destroyed. The itching

of dandruff can also be helped a good deal through the use of the above methods.

If there is a fungus growth in the hair, a good remedy would be to use sheep fat and a little garlic oil. Leave it on the hair for a period of 20 minutes, then shampoo. Washing the hair in soft water and castile soap is wonderful. The gentle friction as mentioned of the massage, will bring the proper heat and blood to the surface and help the hair shoots develop and grow the proper head of hair.

Tonics

We know that an egg yolk in grape juice is a great tonic to help the glands and to help the circulation. Whenever there is any hardening of the arteries, it is advisable to use whey and vegetable broth together. Onions, horseradish and the sulphur foods will help to drive the blood to the brain areas and to the scalp.

Dr. Rocine used a wash made of the roots of the ordinary grape vine once a week. He believed that drinks made of honey and tonics made of celery with Concord grape juice were good for the hair. Weak tea made of the roots of the grape vine should be taken occasionally. Remember that hair is like a vegetable growth. It resists dyes and colors of every kind. One can take the color out of hair but you cannot put it back. Gray is not a hair color; it is an aged hair and it indicates that the hair is dead to pigments. Hair can be dyed, but the dying will never be finished. Sage tea washes darken the hair, as do grape vine root and leaf tea, although the coloring is poor. Take care of your hair as you would any other organ in the body. Remember that a good, strong, healthy body will help to give you a good head of hair. If you are nervous, feed the nervous system; if the digestive system is not working properly, the hair will improve by taking care of the digestive system.

We had a nice experience at one time with a man who was called the strongest upside-down man in the world. His name was Joe Tonti. He lived in Oklahoma City. He told me years ago that he had a severe fever when he was a child and lost his hair. He also had blemishes on his face, an eczema that was very difficult to get rid of but he went into weight lifting and athletic activities. He did a good deal of his work upside down and found that in getting more blood to his head the blemishes on his face left and his hair returned. I have seen hair turn white from shock and I have seen hair turn from gray to black again in a couple of years, when using the methods described above. I do not think that any one thing is the real remedy for either dandruff, eczema or loss of hair, but I do believe that the combination of all these things will help the hair tremendously.

The Teeth

The human tooth is actually very similar to a fish scale. A shark's scale and a human tooth correspond completely in their basic structure.

A tooth is a projection of the skin which has entered into an intimate union with the skeleton, in particular with the jaw, so as to obtain support. The part situated within the socket of the jaw is known as the root, the portion projecting beyond the gums is the crown and the portion between these is called the neck.

Through the root canal, a passage remaining at the base of the root, the cavity of the tooth is invaded by blood and lymph vessels and by nerves.

The principal mass of the tooth is composed of a bony substance known as dentine. On its outer surface, the crown of the tooth is covered with enamel, as a finger is by a thimble. The enamel has no nerves or blood vessels and is the hardest, most compact tissue of the entire body.

Chemically, it consists of phosphate of lime, fluoride of calcium, carbonate of lime, phosphate of magnesium, as well as traces of other salts.

At birth, a human infant is without teeth. After 6 months, the first teeth appear in the center of the lower jaw, and in the course of about 2 years, a total of 20 teeth appear. These are known as milk teeth. Beneath these, rest a second series of teeth (32) that begin to come out at about 6 years of age when the child begins to lose his first set. By the age of 21, all of the 32 permanent teeth have usually come into the mouth, with occasional exceptions of the third molars or wisdom teeth.

The most frequent dental disease is dental decay or caries. When a defect appears in the enamel, the bacteria present in the mouth wander into this break in the enamel and set to work destroying the denture.

The basic cause of tooth decay is a diet deficient in calcium; or a diet containing an excess of concentrated carbohydrates which indirectly causes the calcium level in the blood to be lowered.

America's Dietary Deficiencies Show in its Citizens' Teeth

The problem of tooth decay is one of the major problems of the dental and medical professions today, to say nothing of the expense that must be added on to the family budget to take care of the family's deteriorating teeth. A recent survey by the Public Health Service shows that more than 21 million Americans have lost all their teeth.

There are innumerable research programs being conducted in laboratories all over the world with just one idea in mind: "The prevention of tooth decay." Most of these research programs have recognized that the most glaring fact discovered to date is that this decay is caused from faulty diets and nutritional deficiencies.

Dr. Michael J. Walsh, Director of Clinical Nutrition courses at the University of California Dental Extension in San Francisco says, "Americans are waterlogged and are suffering from dietary deficiencies—but don't know it. What the public mind looks upon as three square meals a day is likely to be a starvation diet and one that will decay the toughest tooth."

False Living—False Teeth

One of my own recent experiences brought this home to me plainly. An 11-year-old boy was sent in to me by another doctor and upon checking this boy, I found that he had a complete set of dentures! When we have to face the fact that a boy of 11 has to have dentures, it is time to start doing something about this horrible scourge! Every sincere and thinking medical man or healer today should be giving a great deal of his time and energy to this problem.

Eat Greens

We know that teeth are broken down and deteriorated when a person does not live right and follow a proper diet. In our diet, greens are most important as they control the calcium in the body. The Hunzas, who had such beautiful teeth and kept them until they died at over 100 years of age, followed a diet in which they ate a lot of greens and the tops of vegetables. We should eat more parsley, beet greens, watercress, spinach and the many different greens which we can get in our salads daily. These will help keep our teeth right.

Papaya and Chlorophyll

If we have tooth troubles and we find that tartar forms very easily, we get some papaya tablets. They are an aid to digestion but they will also eat away any abnormal tissue growth or abnormal bacteria breeding grounds. Put a papaya tablet on each side of the mouth after a meal and keep them there until each is dissolved; this will take care of many of the acid-producing germs.

We have also found chlorophyll effective in halting tooth decay. Chlorophyll is best known for its mysterious action in the process known as photosynthesis, which is the complicated chemical process in which a green plant converts the energy of the sun's rays into stored food energy. Science has never been able to break down this process and discover exactly how it works, but it has long been known that without chlorophyll, neither plants nor animals, including humans, could live. We know chlorophyll best as the substance that gives the plants their green color.

We can get chlorophyll by making juice drinks from the tops of vegetables. The liquefier comes in very handy for this purpose. Green kale, turnip tops, carrot tops, beet tops and other green vegetables run through the liquefier and made into a drink for the entire family should be a part of your program. It is much easier to do this than to suffer with an aching tooth or to pay the dentist's bill.

Take Time to Learn: Save Money

We cannot give the best to our job if we are suffering from an aching tooth. This, of course, goes for all dietary deficiencies as well. It has been stated by health authorities that billions of dollars could be saved by employers each year if the employees were better fed through improved nutritional programs, because better fed people work more efficiently. Americans can be better fed if they will only take the time to learn how.

The physiological symptoms of malnutrition are about the same as those of headache, burning sensations of the eyes, apprehension, pessimism, nausea or blood-shot eyes. Medical men have recognized that nutrition has as important a function in the rehabilitation of the drunkard as does psychiatric treatment.

We all know that millions of dollars are spent each year to improve personal appearance by having teeth straightened or a cap put on a discolored tooth, as mental attitude is so much better when we are satisfied with our personal appearance. Is it not smarter, then, to learn how to produce these beautiful teeth we so earnestly desire by finding out which chemical elements and vitamins are required in our diet to make them this way?

The Bloodstream

High altitude is a great help in building a healthy body; it quickens the thyroid glands so more oxygen can enter the bloodstream. We must remember, however, oxygen demands the chemical iron, because iron attracts oxygen. You could breathe from now on until infinity and never have oxygen in the body unless you have enough iron in the blood. The tissues will never be oxidized without iron.

Moving air is live air and still air is dead, stale. It is the same with water; we must find the running water.

The higher the altitude above sea level, the greater amount of oxygen we develop. Consequently, when we have heart trouble, we must live in a lower altitude. At ocean level, we can have a blood pressure of 4-1/2 to 5 million, while at the higher altitude, we can go as high as 8 million. For example, those living on the shores of Norway average a blood count of 5 million. In Peru, where elevation reaches 12,000, the average blood count runs from 7 to 8 million. While we need a high count for good health, our body cannot respond to too high an altitude. We will likely end up panting, nauseated and vomiting. We must be careful about this; we should not overlook or ignore it.

The blood does five important things we should be aware of. It distributes the food; stores the food; collects waste distributed throughout the body; and helps eliminate it. The blood regulates the heat in the body; kills the germ life and above all things, carries its secretions to the various organs that need it.

We respond immediately to the adrenal gland substance which is carried by the blood through the circulatory system to every cell. Blood travels at the rate of 30 feet per second. Every bit of blood in the body travels through the thyroid glands every hour and a half. Silicon in the blood, for example, speeds through the body to reach the toenails, the hair and other extremities where it is so vital. Bones that need calcium are bathed with blood-carrying calcium. The same blood that is depositing the calcium in the bones will also deposit whatever calcium is needed in the transverse colon to keep it from developing atosis or a prolapsus. Chronic colds, pneumonia, bronchial troubles and catarrhal disturbances lower the resistance of the body and take away the vital force of the blood. Above all, the important thing for us to learn is that bad food takes away the good from our body. We should not only seek better foods, but know the bad foods. Just for an example, the tannin in tea breaks down the bloodstream; it should be kept out of our diet. Use only herb teas.

children. Cold feet affect the entire body and we cannot sleep or for that matter, do anything comfortably. The whole circulation is dependent upon keeping the feet warm. Living in the sunshine, breathing plenty of good, fresh air, sleeping where the air is active and in other ways getting close to nature, are the life-building principles.

"The real arsenal of democracy is a fertile soil, the fresh produce of which is the birthright of the nations."

—Sir Albert Howard

Chapter 49

More money-saving tips and recipes

What is food? It is all in the point of view. Something to think about, isn't it? Do we have to have the kind of diet we have today? Where is this economy in food? What does the body need? With all these various ideas, I sometimes wonder how we are going to look at foods and say, "What is right while we are living down here in Escondido — or Denver — or New York?" What kind of foods do you get?

The first thing I'd like to tell you is that there are such things as famine foods. There are pestilence foods. There are starvation foods. I think it is poor economy, from a long-term standpoint, just to get by on foods. Why don't we know what foods are better than others? If I could put in front of you in one hand a food which could produce arthritis and rheumatism and foods which could produce good health in the other hand, which would you eat? If I put a poisoned pickle in this hand and a good ripe plum in the other, which would you eat? Of course, if you like pickles, I know what you would say. On the other hand, it is known that vinegar can destroy the red blood cells. We find that if you are going to put up foods like cucumbers in pickle form, you will never make them any better. Man can't make a natural apricot better than has been given us in the beginning. Man can't take anything away from food and make it better, except possibly a rotten spot in an apple.

As we look to these various foods, I believe that we have many diseases today which have come upon us because we are living in "these last days" the Bible talks about. We are living in famine and pestilence. There was a day when we had trouble with sanitary conditions — a day when we didn't drain the cities, didn't get rid of the toxic waste. It just flowed right down through the center of the street. Plumbing was poor. I have been in Java where all the waste from the toilets flows right down a center canal in the street. Dogs get in it, carry it around, drag it home. Is it any wonder that disease breaks out every once in a while? But we have gotten over that; this is a sanitary day. In fact, we have become so sanitary-minded that everything has to be white as drifted snow — flour, sugar. Haven't you seen that ad: it has to be white as aspirin? Do you know that while aspirin looks white and clean, it is made from the blackest material that exists? It comes from coal tar — the same thing that is used to pave our streets. Now, all that is white is not always pure and clean; least of all it is an indication of nourishment. So, I am bringing out that if we are to find the finest foods in the world, they are going to come first as very simple god-like foods, such as we have in the very beginning when we go out and pick them from the ground, from the trees, the very finest we can get.

When you know that when first picked beans are alkaline-forming and in four days' time they are acid-forming, you must realize that you cannot even get the very finest in the stores. A change is going on. When the changes go too far, of course the food breaks down and spoils. Man cannot afford to allow these changes to take place. He has found ways to prevent them by methods of preserving. Canning of foods started way back in Napoleon's time. There is an old saying that man cannot fight a war unless he is fed. So Napoleon worked out a way with his ministry to put up food in cans. Food was put up all over France so that it could be taken from one country to another. Napoleon's armies were so successful because they were able to carry their foods along with them.

I went out to see a young man only 27 years old who had developed a stroke. I know it is going to take 10 trailers to carry away the cans in his yard. I can't imagine a young man of 27 accumulating all these cans. Of course, as he was a bachelor he didn't have anyone to cook for him. But trash containers full of cans are not unusual. They say that today when a girl gets married all she needs is a husband and a can opener.

We don't do our own cooking any more. I have a little card passed out from a downtown restaurant. It says, "Please help us stamp out home cooking." They are not interested in your eating at home any more. But do you know, I make a living from people who eat in restaurants. I make a living from people who do not live on natural foods. Can you get natural foods in a restaurant? Very few people are putting up foods for your health. A large-circulation national magazine published an article about health foods some time ago. They talked about the 5 billion dollars that were being spent in this country annually on health foods, and what a lot of quackery and nonsense for people to spend 5 billion dollars on health foods. They tried to show how big 5 billion dollars is. But over 12 billion dollars is spent on alcohol in this country annually. What nonsense! Which is the most economical thing? What good are you doing? This is what you have to think about — survival. What are your ideals? What are you going to be tomorrow? Is this going to be a blessing to you in years to come? What builds your bones? What builds your heart structure?

Years ago I took part in an experiment back East where they took the potassium salts and ran them through a heart. They could actually keep that heart beating for 3 hours. Then they put sodium salts through the heart, and it could beat for 15 minutes only. Now, I am just wondering, do we need potassium? Do we need sodium? Do we need certain foods? Yes. We need these elements for the body's economy. Do you suppose we can take a substitute and get by on it? No, there is no substitute for the right and natural thing.

A drug tested some years ago stimulated people into sensing far more than normal. One of the experiments showed when you took this drug that if you stepped on a dime you could tell whether it was heads or tails, the feet became so sensitive. When you look at a flower, it can be so stimulating to you that you go into extreme ecstasy. They say there are ten thousand million brain cells. They say we use only about 10%. After discovering this number of cells, the psychologists and psychiatrists tell us we use only 1% of our brain cells. That is why we don't have the stimulation that we should have. There is a possibility that someday we may find out that it is *less* than 1%. I don't know how low it can get, but I think that for some they are going to find it to be pretty low. I will say this, we could extend our senses, extend our minds a little bit at least.

Lifeless Foods, Lifeless People

If we could find out how to buy properly, buy economically, and buy for our bodies' good, I think we would have something. Foods are doctored today. They are doctored, not by doctors but by men who are in business. They are in business for the dollar. When a man buys a bushel of potatoes, they may cost $6. He makes $48 on a bushel when he turns them into potato chips. This is a good business. They have to make food a good business, otherwise no one wants to handle it. But we should know ways of keeping, storing and shipping food so as to give it to people the cheapest way possible.

There was a time when 90% of our income went on the foods we bought. Today, about 70 years later, we find that we spend only 20% of our money on foods. The rest of it we spend on our clothes, on luxuries, etc. We don't have to spend so much on foods today because ways have been found of keeping the foods on the shelf. Foods don't spoil the way they used to. You can get a T.V. dinner now and keep it for six months. You find packaged foods are the order of the day.

But one of our greatest contemporary problems is what we find on the grocery shelves. These foods must have an eternal life. How long is eternity? I have some biscuits up in my home. They are white Uneeda biscuits. They are 11 years old, and they are as good today as the day I bought them. They will never spoil. They are in-destructible. But you will find too, that when you take the life out of foods and feed them to animals, they cannot be well. They develop diseases from lifeless foods. When foods have been treated, preserved, pickled, when they have been polished and devitalized, they can no longer produce good health.

So the first thing we have to learn now is what kind of foods we should have. Our life comes from the food we eat. Yes, we build our bodies around these foods. I say yet again, what you eat today will walk and talk tomorrow. It is going to be part of your memory, part of your bones, your teeth, your hair, part of your heart structure. All of the functions of our bodies depend upon our organs, and these organs depend upon the blood. The blood depends upon our food. So the first thing we have to do is get natural food.

Economy In Buying

We had some persimmon whip here one spring Sunday. Where do you suppose those persimmons came from? We froze them last January. We dipped them in hot water to peel before freezing them whole. They made a wonderful dessert, very high in a natural sugar.

Let me give you a suggestion if you are going to freeze some of these fruits — cherries, strawberries, etc. Recently we brought home 6 crates of beautiful strawberries, organically grown. You can't get everything you want when you want it, so when the opportunity comes, buy them and fix them up the way you want them. They must be ripe to begin with, of course. Clean them then freeze them individually on a tray. Put them in your deep freeze, let them freeze solid, then pour into plastic bags for storage. Do not put them all in a bag at once, as they will not freeze properly this way.

Here is a good way to freeze apricots or peaches. Make peach or apricot nectar by taking the ripe fruit and putting it in a liquefier with a little honey, a little ascorbic acid—a vitamin C tablet—or lemon juice. Then you slice the peaches or apricots into this nectar. Don't put them in too big a carton. They must "quick freeze" to be successful. This is the finest dessert you can have. No company can ever put out as good a food as you can put out for yourself. You can do the same with nectarines, or strawberries, or cherries or any other fruits.

You can freeze your surplus vegetables. You can do so with a lot of the leftovers that you have. If you have made too many sandwiches, don't throw them away, deep-freeze them. It isn't economical for you to fix up these things and then throw them away.

I have talked about freezing foods. You can also dry them. We have had dried cherries at the Ranch the last couple of weeks. You can dry cherries just as you can apricots, as you do peaches. One way is to put them in an oven having a low heat and open the oven. Use one of your cookie sheets to put the fruit on. (If you want to take the pits out of the cherries you can, but you don't have to.) Leave them there for a day at a time. When they have dried out pack them away in glass jars. Then you will get these foods at summertime prices. Winter prices are very high because somebody else has done these things for you—preserved them, dried them. Why don't you do it for yourself? I have made this statement many times—you are the best nurse for yourself. You must take care of your own foods. If you do it this way, you can do it nicely.

Seeds And Skins For Value

When you buy a papaya, you pay so much a pound. Do you throw the seeds away? Don't! Save them. Dry them and they make a wonderful tea which can be used to help digest proteins. Most people after the age of 40 or 50 can't digest their proteins well. Find out how to use seeds. Usually we buy seeds whenever we buy fruits and vegetables. But what do we do with these seeds? In most cases they are thrown away. In our classes we show people how to use the seeds of cantaloupes to prepare a milk. Learn how to use these seeds. Do you know that the seed is the first thing you should take if you want to survive? If you have to go underground, take seeds! Sunflower seeds, sesame seeds, wheat seeds. Life for your body can be found in seeds more than in any other item.

The reproductive life cycle is in the seed. The most valuable glandular extract you can put into your body is the seed. If we could realize it, we have the whole tree in the seed. If there is not everything in that seed, you cannot have the whole tree or the whole bush. The tree is only as complete as the seed.

If you want to have something wonderful to come into your life, just stop and think about watermelon seeds. Each year they send airplanes down from Canada to Florida to pick up watermelons. They grind the seeds for incurable cases of kidney trouble, an ailment called nephritis. There isn't a finer thing for kidney disturbances than the watermelon seed. People want to get rid of body odors; they also want to have something that will build up the bloodstream, something with a lot of iron. Well, chlorophyll and iron are found in everything that is green. Did you know that the outside of the watermelon is the highest source of vitamin K? And that the chlorophyll in the outside of the watermelon is easy to assimilate by the body? And yet you throw it away! The white is the highest source of sodium. Sodium is the element you need for your joints. And yet you throw that away! Maybe you came from a Danish family as I did. We used to pickle the melon rind, then it was alright, but raw it was hog-fodder, we thought. Now, if you want to do yourself a good turn, cut up the whole watermelon.

Why throw away what you've paid for? Put it in a liquefier or juicer. It makes a delicious cocktail. Sweeten it if need be; add a beet for coloring. It is one of the most wonderful things I can tell you of.

I speak of seeds. There are many kinds of seeds we can use. Pumpkin seeds are wonderful. Don't ever throw pumpkin seeds away. They are used with honey for driving worms out of the intestinal tract. There isn't anyone who couldn't use this occasionally. They have a wonderful effect on the intestinal tract. Do you know that pumpkin seeds are wonderful to use for prostate gland trouble? Doctors are finding out that they have a wonderful effect on the prostate gland.

It is very, very necessary that we consider using the skins of foods also. A lot of these peelings can't be used. Some people have an idea that you can use orange peeling, lime peeling, and other citrus peeling, but I don't see any good in them. However, many peelings are very valuable, especially the green ones. You say you don't eat papaya skins, but did you know you could make a tea of them? Apple skins make a most wonderful tea. We should learn how to use these things. Don't throw them away. You are paying for them. If you are poor you can't afford to throw things away. But I don't care how much money you have, if you throw things away, you are going to be poor; you are going to be poor in health. So, from an economical standpoint, you can't consider the money value of a purchase. You have to consider whether it is food or not.

Man-Handled Foods Are Costly

It is not an economical thing to take any food into the body from which some doctor is later going to make a living. Do you know it is possible to produce an excessive amount of catarrh in the body with pasteurized milk, processed cheeses, buttermilk, butter and other dairy products? If you are really wise, you will experiment with nut milk drinks. You will find that they are very economical healthwise. You will have much better health using them. In the nut milk drinks we have just as much calcium as in cow's milk and it is easy to assimilate. Before you use the nuts, always soak them overnight. Never use them dry. The next morning put them in your liquefier and blend. Nut milks are easy to make. Let me tell you also that you should always buy the nuts which grow a hard shell, and shell them yourself. The hard-shelled nuts have a lot of oil. The soft-shelled nuts dry out. Keep the oil intact as much as you possibly can.

I say we shouldn't eat bread because I don't think this an economically sound practice. It causes more gas, more intestinal disturbances than anything I know of. But I can't tell everybody these things. One of the things I know are bad for you is pickled pigs feet.

Raw Food

Perhaps this will help convince you how important it is to have plenty of raw foods in the diet. I am sure God meant us to use unchanged the foods Nature sets forth so deliciously. We cannot improve on a peach by stewing it; a carrot is not made better by boiling.

Heat produces marked changes in the chemical composition of food. The food value is lowered. Food is "killed" by cooking. It is the presence of enzymes in foods which gives them their "liveness." Enzymes are catalysts which enable cells to carry on their existence. All enzymes are destroyed by heat. Destruction begins at about 118° F and by the time 140° F is reached, all enzymes are lost. This must render cooked foods less able to sustain life, for although certain enzymes are manufactured by the body, a plentiful supply in foods would seem to lessen the burden of work our cells have to do.

We have spoken of the loss of vitamin C but most of the other vitamins and minerals are also affected by heat. It has been estimated that losses vary from 5 to 100%, average commercial methods destroying about 50%. If minerals and vitamins are not destroyed by the heating processes, they are so changed as to render them less assimilable. Losses occur because some are soluble in water. Oxidation destroys others. The shorter the cooking time, the less heat, the smaller the loss. Waterless cooking where the heat is distributed evenly brings the least loss.

Any heat causes coagulation of proteins making them less digestible. Some protein factors are destroyed by cooking, others are changed, the transformation making them less available. Some essential protein factors are not to be obtained from cooked protein sources.

Fats, too, are rendered less digestible by cooking. In frying, the fat so coats the other foodstuffs as to make their digestion impossible until the fat envelope is dissolved off. Fats digest at a later stage in the alimentary canal than other types of food. Over-heated fat has been found to be a carcinogenic agent. In fact, any food which is scorched to the stage where a soot is formed contains tars which are also carcinogenic (cancer producing).

Though well cooked vegetable food would seem to be more digestible it is found that it fails to stimulate peristalsis in the way that cellulose-rich raw foods do. Such material moves slowly in the bowel, fermentation is apt to set in and the resulting putrefaction is a prime cause of auto-intoxication. Raw food moves very quickly along the alimentary canal, allowing no stagnation.

Until recently, scientists considered the increase in white blood corpuscles after eating, a normal digestive reaction, but now it is known that this only follows a cooked meal, never a complete raw menu. In the bloodstream, the white corpuscles, our body's defense force, are augmented as soon as any cooked food enters the stomach. In medicine, this indicates that some disease process is going on in the body; for instance, it always occurs during infections. Even very small quantities of food call forth the same response. What is a cooked food in this sense? Experiments show that each food has its own temperature at which its state alters. Plain water can be heated at 87° C for ½ hour without changing the blood, but heat it to 88° for a moment and the white corpuscles increase! This has therefore been named the "critical temperature." It ranges from 87 deg C. for water to 97 deg C. for carrots, strawberries and figs.

Food	Critical Temperature (°F)
Drinking water	191
Milk	191
Cereals, tomatoes and Cabbage	192
Bananas	192
Butter	196
Apples	197
Oranges	197
Potatoes	200
Carrots, strawberries and Figs	206

There are other phenomena. For instance, if a cooked food is eaten with some of the same food in its raw form, no blood reaction occurs. The raw food can counteract the negative qualities of the cooked food it would seem, so long as the cooking temperature has not exceeded 212° F. Also, a raw food of the same or higher "critical temperature" can re-establish a different cooked food. If several cooked foods of the same critical temperature are taken along with a raw food, the law reacts similarly; but an augmentation of white corpuscles occurs if cooked foods of varying critical temperatures are taken along with raw food, irregardless of its critical temperature.

Raw foods can also over-ride the disturbing influences of man-made foodstuff such as sugar, chocolate, etc. But it takes two raw foods of different critical temperature to do it.

What is the quantity of raw food necessary to prevent the reaction of cooked foods? There is a definite minimum. For water, it is 50%. "Raw food" has been found to include all those foodstuffs in the state in which they exist in nature, for example water, mineral water, salt, vegetables, fruits, cereals, nuts, honey, raw eggs, raw meat and fish, raw milk and sour milk, butter...

Much has been written on the value of raw food. For instance, Professor Ziegelmayer, European nutritionist, says "It is certain that cooking alters our colloidal state of food; it decomposes highly molecular compounds... The uncooked state secures the maintenance of some food substances, prevents alterations of the proteins, preserves the original mineral salts in their optimum concentration."

Arnold de Vries says, "It is clear that all heat-processed foods undergo important changes in chemical composition. They lose a part of their mineral and vitamin content; their proteins are partly destroyed and rendered less digestible and nutritious; their fats become less digestible and assimilable and sometimes become toxic. The starches and sugars are altered, and some may become toxic. The complete chemical reaction to the cooking process covers considerable scope, as may be seen, and it is of definite importance in the science of nutrition, determining to some extent the value of practically all known foodstuffs."

There are plenty of experiments with foods going on today that we can learn from and apply to our own way of living. In the University of Denver for instance, a Home Economics group experimented with rats, giving them the foods they prepared in their cooking classes. They fed the rats bread, cake, pie and other cooked foods over a period of time. Another group of rats was fed natural foods. The rats fed on the natural foods were found to live more than twice as long as those fed on the cooked foods. There is something in natural food that is spoiled in cooking. This something is necessary for our bodies and for long life. One essential mineral that can be lost in the cooking of foods is iron. We need iron for the liver. It is necessary that we have natural food in order to obtain this iron.

Other tests have been done with animals. A pig may require up to 50% more food to produce a pound of gain in weight when food is cooked than when it is raw, one such experiment showed. Weill and Mouriquant of France fed pigeons whole raw grains and noticed their great activity and vigor. However, a similiar group on the same grains well-cooked became paralyzed within 90 days. They suffered acute symptoms of beri-beri which eventually killed them. One third raw grain was sufficient to give complete freedom from beri-beri symptoms.

McCarrison of India fame carried out revealing experiments with white rats. One thousand were fed a raw diet of cabbage, carrots, milk, meat, bread and sprouted legumes. They remained remarkably healthy, suffering no disease whatsoever. Two thousand rats were fed white bread, margarine, canned meat, canned jam, boiled tea, boiled potatoes, cabbage and a small amount of milk. They soon began developing every sort of ailment in the medical dictionary. Common were tuberculosis, arthritis, Brights's disease, gastric ulcers, duodenal ulcers, glandular enlargements, inflammation of the eyes, anemia, loss of hair, infected teeth, infected tonsils, middle-ear disease, corneal ulceration and skin diseases. Their dispositions were badly affected. Whereas the first group was affectionate and friendly, these rats were ill-tempered and vicious.

Dr. Francis Pottenger is a famous food scientist. One of his experiments involved cats. A group fed entirely upon raw meat and raw milk remained in excellent health in all cases. However, those fed cooked meat scraps were smaller in build, their skeletal and tooth development was progressively degenerate in each succeeding generation, reproduction was greatly lowered. Labor being difficult, kitten mortality was high and some mothers became unable to provide milk for the young. Sex interest and virility decllined, and cats were irritable and vicious. No cat lived longer than 3 months in the third generation.

Lunches, Salads, Snacks

When you are packing lunches to send out of your kitchen, see that they contain foods in the proper combination for best digestion and assimilation. For growing children a carbohydrate may be needed which will be provided in a sandwich, but make the sandwiches interesting, using the most nutritious varieties of bread, and try different vegetable fillings. Heavy proteins should not be included in the same meal with a starch. It is important to have succulent vegetables along with bread so it does not dry out in the bowel and become constipating. Have celery or carrots, whole if tender, otherwise cut into sticks; green pepper; a small zucchini squash; a small cucumber — these varieties have a higher percentage of water in their cell structure. Lettuce packed loosely in waxed paper to be eaten plain, along with a sandwich, is preferable to that between slices of bread where it loses some of its crisp quality. Bread is the least nutritious form in which to get your carbohydrates. Lunches without it can be interesting and satisfying. Try cabbage leaves for sandwiching hearty fillings. Use various stuffings for celery, and vegetables of different texture and colors. If a lunch kit is carried, the thermos bottle can contain hot rice or barley, or the surprise of an uncooked soup or one of the highly nourishing liquefied drinks cannot be improved upon.

Out of your kitchen must come a salad for luncheon and one for the evening meal. Have a chef's salad for either of these meals — a meal in itself. Determine this according to your particular situation. For those who don't like salads, prepare something which will be especially tempting after the salad has been eaten — for we should at least begin a meal with raw food to stimulate the flow of the digestive juices which the stomach must have to function properly. Make your salad at the last minute, as cut surfaces exposed to air allow oxidation, one of the "robbers" against which we should be ever vigilant. Vegetables juiced or liquefied, which may also be sieved to eliminate bulk, will take care of those sensitive organs unable to tolerate coarse vegetable material. At least 60% of your daily food intake should be raw. The addition of steamed raisins or cut-up dates to salads adds taste appeal for those who do not realize the deliciousness of vegetable flavors. Vegetable juices may be taken in different ways—liquefied cocktails are wonderful. For greater palatability, you may combine pineapple, papaya juice or guava juice with a vegetable juice.

Snacks that you prepare in your kitchen should be healthful—real "pickups." You can never go wrong in serving a liquefied drink if energy needs to be revived. Children particularly should have them — one of the soaked nut or seed varieties flavored with plenty of nutritious carob powder (St. John's Bread), and macaroon coconut, or with a soy milk base. Do you know there is a natural vanilla (no alcohol content) which delightfully flavors the soy base drink?

Seeds, Nuts, Sweeteners

Seeds and nuts are among the most "complete" foods we have. Seeds are going to be the foods of the future. Today we have found that many of the seeds have the hormone values of male and female glands. Seeds carry the life force for many years, as long as they are enclosed in the hull. Some found in tombs, known to have been there for thousands of years, when planted have grown. They are a very potent food, high in this glandular material, rich in proteins, and tiny storehouses filled with minerals and vitamins. Getting these seeds and nuts into the body in the form of a drink gives us the finest form of nutrition.

Sesame seed milk is one of our best. Almond milk, too, makes a very alkaline drink, high in protein and easy to assimilate and absorb. Sunflower seed milk makes a nutritious drink from the vegetarian's best source of protein, sunflower seeds. These milks can be used in place of regular milk and are not catarrh forming.

In the selection of sweetening agents there is not only natural raw honey of many flavors, but maple syrup and maple sugar, the latter made into interesting shapes as a confection for those who have a "sweet tooth". There are also Louisiana molasses and old-fashioned, unsulphured New Orleans molasses, both "good enough to eat from the spoon", and blackstrap molasses, one of the long-recognized basic health foods. Again, carob powder has a sweet taste and many uses. Have different varieties of dates, which may be stuffed in interesting ways as a confection.

Breakfast need not be the same type of menu the year round. All through the season when fresh fruits are available enjoy one variety after another — have a liberal serving, and, if desired, one good protein. In the cooler seasons, for heat and energy, have a whole grain, thermos "cooked" overnight, with one variety of dried fruit.

Include in your equipment a small electric nut grinder — keep it on the dining table when you serve whole nuts and seeds and grind each portion as it is served so that there is no loss through oxidation, as occurs when you buy ground grains and seed meals.

The foods on your pantry and cupboard shelves should be in as whole form as possible. Whatever processing is required according to individual need should be done in one's own kitchen. It is better for our nutrition to make such preparation ourselves, as is necessary — and let the children help with these activities and learn to enjoy working with these life-giving things. Don't rely on "quick" methods and processed foods. We are paying for man's inventions and his labor on foods. These open the way for trouble. We have to get the food before man gets hold of it. You can't find any substitute for what God has given in its natural form. We should be very careful when we have to pay for our health. Somebody is making a living — and more — from all the operations of food processing, and you are only buying troubles. It is a crime that man should make his livelihood and profit at the expense of our health. A notable example of this is the foods containing coal tar derivitives for artificial flavor and color.

Plan your meals ahead. Before you finish preparation of one meal, know what you will serve at the next. While preparing the evening meal, put to soak those foods which require this softening for the following day. Nuts must be soaked at least ten hours to get the good of the protein value out of them. The digestive juices will then start to work on them as soon as they reach the stomach. Vegetarians, for the most part, are starving for this element, as nuts are often ready for elimination by the time they can be assimilated.

Supplementary Foods

I have never found anyone who would not benefit from the daily addition of the following supplementary foods. Keep them by your table.

Nova Scotia Dulse — Take about ¼ teaspoon a day (or one tablet). Only minute quantities of iodine are required by the body, but dulse, being a high iodine food, supplies this need. Iodine keeps us from getting goiter. It prevents wrinkles. Lack causes mood swings, tiredness, dry and brittle hair and skin.

Rice Polishings — Use a teaspoonful a day. This is high in Vitamin B, a vitamin for nerves, appetite, and muscle coordination; and the mineral element silicon, the youth element. We become magnetic, vivacious, fast of thought, a "dancer" with this element. It is so necessary for beautiful hair, nails, and skin. Silicon is the "cutter" in the body, cleaning out all pus and debris. For cold feet and skin diseases take extra silicon.

Sunflower Seed Meal — Use 1 teaspoon three times a day. This is one of the finest vegetarian proteins you can have. If the body is protein-starved, perhaps due to overuse of mind in your studies or job, feed the brain and nervous system. All seeds are for glands too. Sunflower seed is high in silicon too. Consider the beautiful rainbow hues in the feathers of the parrot. The sunflower seed feeds the color in our different organs.

Wheat Germ — Use 1 tablespoonful daily. This is high in Vitamin E, the specific vitamin for the heart. It gives tone to the muscle structure, strengthening the veins (varicose veins) and helping circulation. Wheat germ also feeds the glands and nerves.

Flaxseed Meal — This meal is wonderful bulk if you are troubled with constipation, irregular bowels or if you feel the need of a little help. Be sure you drink water with this, or blend it with a liquid or it will stick in your throat. Take 1 teaspoonful at each meal.

Whey — This is one of the greatest of foods. Be sure you always have a bottle of the powder to make up. A very good habit to develop is to take a glass of whey at each meal. It is our highest sodium source. Sodium is known as the ''youth maintainer'', allowing our joints to remain supple. It also aids digestion and builds the blood. Whey is friendly to the acidophilus baccilli in the intestinal tract which are important to good intestinal management. It also has calcium, the tone-builder and strengthener, and chlorine, the cleanser. People on slimming diets need not be afraid of whey. Taken before meals, it partially appeases hunger.

Buying

Quantity purchase — by the lug — is an economical way to buy fruits if you can dry or freeze the portion which you cannot use while fresh. The difference in price for quantity purchase will enable you to have some things stored away, which, in comparison to purchase by the single pound, would cost you practically nothing. There will come a time when we can dehydrate our own fruits. If you are lucky enough to own your own freezer, follow my methods for healthful ways of home-freezing (see Chapter No. 35) and save all your excess food for out-of-season use. Those fruits which become too soft for freezing whole may be liquefied with a little honey and this puree frozen. It makes an excellent sauce for desserts.

Include soups very often in your menus, trying to have them raw. The liquefier will enable you to make interesting varieties. Try corn cut fresh from the cob, asparagus, celery, Borsch made of grated raw beets. Dried corn may be soaked and after liquefying pressed through a sieve. Always consider whether the food you intend to serve may be raw rather than cooked.

The fresher the fruits and vegetables, the more alkaline — the longer they are kept the greater the acid content becomes. It is, therefore, good if one of your kitchen doors leads out into your own garden. If your plot is small, at least try to grow your own greens, which

suffer the most on storage. Have small nooks and crannies planted with a variety of herbs for seasoning and to make into teas. These can even become an ornamental addition to your window boxes, or an indoor plant. If you have the room, grow enough to dry for winter use.

Remember that in the body fruits stir up acids, while vegetables carry off acids. Vegetables have varying stages of maturity, but fruits have a prime stage of ripeness at which they should be picked, and not before. Commercially marketed ones are invariably picked green, although they may look ripe. Vegetables may be used at any stage of maturity. If you can grow your own fruit, you can pick it when ready to eat — provided you find ways to keep the birds and bees from getting it first!

Sandwiches

Sandwiches are a traditional American lunch today. Sandwiches seem to have grown into an American institution because of our having to take something along with us to school and to work. In both restaurants and lunch counters, they have fallen in with the idea. It seems to be a "quickie" method of getting something to eat for a person at midday. In fact, it has become an assembly line of hamburgers and hot dogs — a bun with a wiener between; two pieces of bread with a slice of cheese, ham or bologna between.

There should be an art to sandwich making, that would make sandwiches appealing, tasty and above all, healthy. When we forget these things, then the sandwiches are not doing the good they should and they are not nourishing our bodies properly. If sandwiches have the addition of mustard, vinegar sauce, catsup, artificial colorings, preservatives, spices, canned, smoked, devitalized, devitaminized, inferior grades of fillings and materials — it is no wonder that we have undernourished children and rheumatic complaints from folks a little older.

Dr. George M. Uhl, City Health Officer, warned both the parents and teachers ''to be on the lookout for fatigued and inattentive children.'' These symptoms may be the result of poor nutrition at lunchtime. Too many children have developed a habit of consuming candy, cakes and soft drinks instead of a balanced lunch. A good lunch should include a sandwich, fresh vegetables, fruit, milk and dessert. (A chewy vegetable or fruit at the end of a meal helps to clean the youngsters teeth). He also warned parents to beware of using custards, custard filled desserts or milk puddings, unless they are refrigerated, because of the possibility of food poisoning bacteria growing easily in these foods when they are out of the refrigerator.

We have no objection to sandwiches, but we must consider the material from which they are made. We cannot afford anything but the very best. You deserve the very best — your health requires it. Every function in your body, every activity depends upon the food you eat and as the noonday lunch constitutes one-third of your daily intake, then one-third of your health depends on what you have in your lunch basket or what you eat at noon in the corner drug store.

You cannot afford "spook" bread. It must be made of the finest quality whole-grain material. The grains, such as rye, barley, millet, cornmeal prepared as muffins, rolls or bread for sandwiches, are starches and we have to consider them in relation to the other starches in your diet for the rest of the day. Most American meals have bread for breakfast in the form of toast, or pancakes, cereals, waffles, muffins, etc. Then the evening meal is made up of more starches — bread, potatoes, rice, noodles and many times, starch desserts. Therefore, it is to our advantage to cut down on the starches at lunch-time, if the other meals contain starches also. (Cut the bread as thin as possible, for the minimum amount of starch.) However, if the lunch-meal is your main starch meal and you are going to reduce the starches in the other meals, then you may have more starch for lunch. If you are able to choose what to have for your lunch, plan it in relation to your other meals, and try to follow some of these suggestions:

Make the fillings of satisfying and nourishing ingredients. Above all things, have *plenty of vegetables or vegetable fillings.* The reason is that bread of itself can be constipating. Breadstuffs will dry up in the heat of the abdomen and in the digestive process. Bread has already gone through an oven process and dries out quickly when put through the intestinal tract. However, vegetables are water-carrying and never dry out as the starches do in the digestive system. Their fibrous material, the cellulose which carries the water, taken along with bread or starches, will prevent their becoming constipating and will not allow a hard material to develop. This is the most important principle in regard to bread in the diet, so it may be considered a rule that whenever you send sandwiches to school with your children or with your husband to work, or for yourself, always have either carrot sticks with them, celery sticks, stuffed celery or lots of extra lettuce or any other succulent vegetable, for their water-bearing elements.

The tradition of using lettuce leaves in sandwiches is probably one of the greatest life-saving, healthful procedures used in the making of sandwiches. However, we do not believe in using head (iceberg) lettuce. It is better to use leaf lettuce, romaine, watercress, endive, bibb lettuce, chicory or prize (bronze leaf) lettuce. These assure us of getting more iron and other chemical elements for health-building than is found in iceberg head lettuce.

The second thing to be careful of in sandwiches is the combinations. The traditional peanut butter or cheese fillings, hamburgers and hotdogs, are an improper combination of starch and protein. (Try to avoid the starch and protein sandwich combination as much as possible.)

The best combination with the starch would be a filling of vegetables, such as you will find in the following recipes, or dried fruits, which are also permissible with starches. When using nut butters, we should use either dried fruits or vegetables which help supply the water-carrying cellulose with the starches. There are some suggestions for protein fillings, which may be used occasionally, but try to balance it by using plenty of dried fruits with it.

Instead of the familiar peanut butter, why not try almond and cashew butters? Peanuts are not nuts...they are a legume, and you will find them a little more difficult to digest than the nut butters. However, in using nut butters, always use the 'raw'; if you are going to use peanut butter (especially for the hearty and healthful person) always use 'raw' peanut butter.

Why can't we cream our own cheese? You can cream your own in your liquefier, using unprocessed cheese, such as Munster, Cheddar or Roquefort to make a cheese spread, instead of the usual oil spread of butter or margarine. Find ways of mixing yogurt and cheese to make it of a spreading consistency. Remember, variety is one of the laws in the selection of foods, so we should not constantly use one particular type of food. We believe that avocados make a wonderful spread. This may be flavored with the addition of vegetable broth powder seasoning, a sea vegetation such as dulse powder, celery salt or onion salt.

There are times when it is difficult to keep the combinations perfect, but it isn't what we do once in a while that counts. It is what we do most of the time. The main idea is to make a nutritional pattern for foods and make it as natural as possible, having as much raw foods as you can — at least 60%. With sandwiches, always remember to have cellulose material with the starch (bread) element.

For additional sandwich suggestions, refer to Dr. Jensen's book "Vital Foods For Total Health". This book should be in every kitchen to help organize the important activity of preparing better food for better health.

An interesting variation in the sandwich theme is to substitute for bread thin slices of unprocessed cheese, particularly if you wish to reduce the carbohydrate intake. A type of filling for this should be of consistency that will not leak (because the cheese will not absorb liquid as bread does) such as olive-nut filling or egg salad. This makes a complete protein sandwich which is a better combination than bread (starch) with a protein filling; another good filling would be a vegetable filling, such as grated or chopped vegetable, green beans, peas, asparagus; or cut up green, leafy vegetables and stews and combine with a dressing, which is a good way to get the less tender varieties in raw form for use as a sandwich filling. Again we say, try to have as much raw food as possible.

Another "slimming" sandwich, one of my favorites, is my apple and cheese special. Wash a whole apple and core it. Then cut it into thin slices and put two slices together with a piece of cheese between. Thick nut butters also make a delicious filling. (Apple slices may need dipping in lemon to prevent browning.) This would take care of the old adage *An apple a day keeps the doctor away*. In a three-year experiment by Michigan State University researchers, they reported "about 1,300 university students ate an apple a day—and they further reported one-third fewer respiratory infections and only one-sixth as many pressure and tension troubles as were had by nonparticipating students."

Sandwich Suggestions

Avocado Savory Spread

Mash an avocado with a little vegetable seasoning and quickly spread between two slices of whole-wheat bread.

Avocado and Tomato

On buttered herb bread, slice thin tomatoes and avocados. Place second slice of bread on quickly to prevent avocado browing.

Cucumber Sandwich

Coat freshly sliced, unpeeled cucumbers in salad dressing, place on whole-wheat bread or crackers, spread with almond butter.

Cucumber and Radish

Slice cucumbers very thin and place on bread. Cover with thinly sliced radishes.

Cottage Cheese Filling

To 1 Tbsp cottage cheese, add 1 tsp thick cream. Mix well. Add dash of grated nuts. Spread on whole wheat bread or crackers.

Green Pepper & Cream Cheese

Slice green pepper and mix with cream cheese. Spread on rye bread.

Celery Nut Filling

Slice celery and mix with chopped nuts.

Almond Butter & Tomato Juice

Cream almong butter by adding a few drops of tomato juice at a time. Spread on whole-wheat bread. Add a couple of leaves of lettuce.

Almond Butter Spread

Spread two slices of bread with a thin coating of almond butter. Cover with chopped dates and press together. A dash of lemon juice may be added.

Tomato, Lettuce And Filbert Butter

Place lettuce leaves on bread. Top with sliced tomatoes. Spread nut butter on the other side of bread.

Ripe Olives And Cashew Butter

Cream cashew butter with a few drops of tomato juice. Add ripe olives—spread on bread, adding a couple of leaves of lettuce.

Peanut Butter And Prunes

Add prune pulp to peanut butter to form a thick cream. Add some grated carrot if desired. Serve on rye.

Honey And Sunflower Seed Meal

Blend honey with sunflower seed meal to a spreading consistency and use as a sweet filling on soy bread.

Maple Syrup And Dates

Chop dates and mix with maple syrup to a cream. Serve on whole wheat bread or crackers.

Raisin Sandwiches With Cream Cheese

To ½ cup finely chopped raisins, add ½ C grated nuts and ½ cake cream cheese. Mix thoroughly and spread.

Open Face Sandwiches

On Whole Wheat Bread place a Lettuce Leaf. Then, finely shred some carrot. Garnish with sliced hard-boiled egg and some mayonnaise.

Spread Soy Bread with Herb Butter. Thinly slice Jack cheese over it. Place some alfalfa sprouts on this. Dot with French Dressing.

On a nut bread, spread cream cheese. Pile grated apple (mixed with lemon to prevent browning) on top. Garnish with sunflower seeds.

Season buttered bread with a little celery salt. Place slice of avocado and sprinkle with grated coconut and grated orange rind.

Take a slice of plain whole-wheat bread, butter and sprinkle with broth powder. Cut hard-boiled eggs on it. Top with chopped olives and garnish with paprika.

On a slice of rye bread, slice some cheddar cheese very thin. Down the middle, place a raw of radish slices. Garnish with chopped parsley.

Butter rye bread with nut butter. Place a layer of alfalfa sprouts over it.

If you cannot make your own bread, go to your health food store to obtain the next best bread, made from freshly ground whole grain products, shortened with natural fats and oils, and unadulterated by the numerous chemicals found in the usual breads today.

Fillings And Combinations For Sandwiches

Butter Spreads

There are many ways of preparing good, quick sandwich spreads with a butter base. Beat butter until soft. Add the other ingredients gradually. Chill the butter mixture until it is of a good consistency to spread. Beat until soft: 4 Tbsp butter. Add the butter slowly to one or more of the following:

½ tsp Lemon Juice
½ tsp Minced Garlic
2 Tbsp Chopped Olives
¼ C Soft or Grated Cheese
½ tsp Dry Mustard
2 Tbsp Chopped Chives
2 Tbsp Horseradish
½ tsp Grated Onion
2 Tbsp Chopped Parsley
2 Tbsp Chopped Watercress
¼ tsp Curry Powder
1 Tbsp Chopped Herbs, (fresh basil, tarragon, chervil, oregano, etc.)
Cream Cheese
Sour Cream
Yogurt
Cottage Cheese
Mayonaise

All of these combine well with the following:
Eggs, Dates, Figs, Raisins or Nuts, Herbs — dried or fresh, Ripe Olives, Chopped Vegetables: Celery, Carrot, Watercress, Parsley, Green Onions, Mushrooms, Pimento, Nasturtium Leaves and many others, not quite as popular.
Blends of Cheese, including Roquefort and Cheddar.
Nut Butters, such as Almond Butter, Filbert Butter, Peanut Butter, Sesame Seed Butter and Sunflower Seed.

"Typical" Co-Eds Live On Diet That Kills Rats

Ft. Collins (Colo.) — A "typical" co-ed's diet won't keep a rat alive.

A menu of chocolate cake, candy, pickles and soft drinks, declared by students and teachers in the nutrition laboratory of Colorado State College to be "just about typical" of what the college girl of today exists on, is slowly killing several white rats.

The food has been ground together, dried and fed to the rats for three weeks by 25 girls taking the nutrition course in the home economics division of the college. And for three weeks the rats have gained only a few ounces, have lost most of their hair, have turned yellow and in general show definitely that they are on the way toward death from lack of proper food.

School Lunches

If it is impossible for a child to go home for the midday meal, he may have a well-balanced lunch of a sandwich, salad, and a warm health drink carried in a pint thermos in the lunch box. A health dessert may be added occasionally for variation.

Here are a few suggestions:
Sandwiches
1. Avocado and romaine on whole wheat or pumpernickle bread.
2. Lettuce, grated carrot, and chopped raisin on date and nutbread.
3. Dates and nuts on whole wheat bread.
4. Romaine with celery and carrot, chopped fine.
5. Nut spreads with olives and chopped watercress on whole wheat datebread.
6. Mashed banana with cashew nutspread, honey or freshly grated coconut.

Simple salads may be put in a tightly covered glass jar and eaten from the jar with spoon or fork. Salads with sandwiches make an excellent combination.

Milk, nut or soy milk, and milk soups, or Vital Broth with any of the variations are an important addition and should always be included.

Once in a while a custard, agar gelatin dessert, homemade health candy or soaked dried fruits may be added as a pleasant surprise and should be included occasionally in the child's lunch.

The Working Man's Lunch

Sandwiches
1. Cucumbers, sliced very thin, marinated with French dressing with lettuce on brown bread.
2. Watercress, put into small pieces and marinated with dressing.
3. Watercress, chopped fine, creamed with butter, and spread on bread.
4. Cottage cheese, Spanish or green onion, mayonnaise if desired.

5. Cottage cheese or cream cheese with jelly or jam, health made.
6. Cream cheese with shredded pineapple.
7. Cream or cottage cheese and nuts.
8. Cream cheese, nuts, and raisins. Mayonnaise if desired.
9. Carrot, nut, and celery with mayonnaise.
10. Nuts and chopped olives.
11. Nut spreads and raisins.
12. Olives, nuts, salad dressing, and lettuce.
13. Avocado or avocado with olive.
14. Chopped raisins.
15. Chopped raisins with nuts and cream cheese.
16. Chopped raisins, dates, and figs, with or without nuts or mayonnaise.

Add dry or fresh fruits to the lunchbox to be eaten at ten or three o'clock to keep your man from starving while he waits to get at those fresh surprises in his lunchbox or on the dinner table when he gets home. The evening meal should be especially planned with enough protein to offset the starch consumed at the noon meal, and to give sufficient energy.

Thermos Bottle Suggestions

1. Vital broth, varied according to taste and desire.
2. Buttermilk or goat milk.
3. Oat straw tea or Hollywood Cup.
4. Thin cream soups and clear broths.
5. Veal joint broth variations.

The ideal lunch for everybody where sandwiches are included also includes a raw green vegetable salad and health drink.

Thermos Cookery

If you don't know what it is to cook in a thermos, you have missed something wonderful. No method could be more healthful, yet so simple. We are being warned of the destructive effects of high heat. Here is a way in which cooking takes place well below the boiling point. This is the long, slow, gentle cooking, with absence of air recommended so strongly by health authorities.

You will need a wide-mouthed thermos or it will be difficult to get the food out. Rinse the thermos with scalding water and quickly spoon in the food. Then fill to the top with boiling water, close tightly and leave to cook. Do not be afraid of expansion bursting the thermos. Plenty of water-space will take care of this and any extra juice after cooking can be used as a drink or in soups, casseroles, etc.

Do you like to stay in bed in the morning until the last possible moment? Do you have time to do your exercising and deep breathing? Wouldn't you also like a hot, nourishing cereal? Here is the answer to nutritionally inferior, pre-cooked, package-prepared cereals. Put the grain of your choice to cook in your thermos the night before and when you are ready to sit down to breakfast — serve!

What else can you cook? Lentils, peas and beans cook nicely after a preliminary simmer, as do soups and stews. If you can call it "cooking", your thermos is an ideal place to brew yogurt and other cultures requiring a steady and warm temperature.

GRAINS:
Use ½ cup to 1½ cups of boiling water. This is a good proportion for a pint thermos.

(I) WHOLE:
This is a simple procedure.
(a) To wash: Measure your cereal into the thermos
Add water and wash
Drain off water. If necessary, use strainer.

(b) To scald: Pour in boiling water and leave a few moments to heat both grain and thermos. Drain again.

(c) To cook: Immediately fill to the top with boiling water. Close tightly and leave 12 hours for most varieties.

1. **Wheat:** Results are excellent if the above method is followed. Use ½ cup wheat to 1½ cup water. 12 hours will cook it.

2. **Barley:** Using a scant ½ cup of barley and proceeding as above, the barley will be nicely cooked in 12 hours.

3. **Brown Rice:** Same proportions; same procedure.

Quick Cooking rice method for other meals
Short grain rice cooks completely in 2 hours following the above method.
Long grain rice takes longer — about 3 hours.

4. **Buckwheat:** Use a generous 1/2 cup buckwheat groats. Proceed as above, only 2 hours in the thermos is necessary to cook buckwheat completely.

5. **Millet:** This must be brought to the boiling point and simmered for 5 minutes before putting it in the thermos or the hard hulls will not be broken. After this, 2 hours in the thermos will complete the cooking.

(II) GRITS:
For greatest value, fresh-grind your own grain. Preheat thermos. Put in ½ cup grits and fill with boiling water.

Give it a quick, gentle stir so that no uncooked grits remain at the bottom. Close and leave 2-3 hours, depending upon the fineness of the grain.

I highly recommend a fresh, coarse-ground wheat left in a thermos overnight. The long, slow-cooking of the thermos does not overcook the grits.

Try a steel-cut oatmeal, rye-grits and 7-grain cereal this way.

(III) MEALS:

Again, grind the meal yourself just before using. Take 1/2 to 3/4 cup meal, mix to a cream in a warm bowl, using hot water, then pour into pre-heated pint thermos.

Top with boiling water, then close and leave 1-1/2 to 2 hours or overnight. Vegetable seasoning may be added prior to cooking. Add butter, honey or seasoning to taste on serving.

LEGUMES:

It is necessary to bring dried peas, beans and lentils to a boil and simmer gently 10-15 minutes before enclosing in a pre-heated thermos, in order to thoroughly cook. The bigger the seed, the longer the preliminary cooking. Also, soaking about 12 hours beforehand gives a more tender product. Very large beans are not suitable for thermos cookery.

Again, ½ cup dried seed to 1½ cups water is a good proportion.

The addition of a small minced onion or clove of garlic, plus vegetable seasoning before cooking will enable you to serve your legumes to be added. Experiment with various herbs in your thermos-cooked pulses.

Legumes for Vegetarian Loaves: Invariably, when a vegetarian loaf or roast is to be made from legumes, the recipe requires that these be ground or minced after preliminary cooking. As an alternative, soak them overnight, grind *before* cooking, bring to a boil with sufficient water, pop immediately into your pre-heated thermos. Close tightly and leave to cook 2-3 hours depending on fineness of grind.

SPROUTS:

Bring your seeds back to green life by sprouting them before cooking. This reduces their starchy nature, increases vitamins and improves digestibility. The flavor is altered somewhat, but it is a pleasant change. Lentils, beans, whole grains, etc. sprout sufficiently if kept moist for two or three days.

SOUPS AND STEWS:

Finely cubed vegetables in the form of soups and stews will cook satisfactorily in the thermos if simmered 5 minutes first to heat them through. Grated ingredients need only to be brought to a boil. Pre-heat thermos and leave to cook for 12 hours. Include onions, garlic, herbs — such as bay leaves, vegetable seasoning and vegetarian bouillon cubes for added flavor. Soybean cheese, 'muttose' and other meat substitutes can be used for protein value.

Traveling? Going on a picnic? Don't stay at home half the day in order to have a nice hot dish to serve. Give your soup or stew a good start on the stove while you pack the sandwiches, then your thermos will finish the cooking in a few hours.

Thermos cookery is an exciting new field. We have put you on the way. Experiment yourself. Buy a quart thermos — two pint ones — several different sizes to suit your various needs. If you have a tiny apartment with only one burner, here is your solution. Save time and fuel. If you are the normal sort of person who occasionally scorches the rice or has lumps in the porridge, you have found a new friend.

Kitchen Rules

We have given you much to think about in the planning and organizing of your kitchen routine. To recapitulate, let us now list a series of rules which we hope will pinpoint all the finer details, as well as the main considerations and turn you out a Health Queen of the Kitchen.

RULE NO. 1. The most important rule in the kitchen is to have fresh food.

RULE NO. 2. Try never to cook any food which can be eaten raw. As you study, you will find there is a life principle in food which is destroyed in all cooking and preservation. Stay away from the can opener. If you use canned or preserved foods, know how they are canned. If possible, learn to do it yourself in the best manner. Use unsulphured dried fruits. Those foods which come in glass containers are to be preferred to canned foods. Frozen foods are still better, especially if you have put them up yourself.

RULE NO. 3. When preparing raw food for your family, make sure it is washed thoroughly and rinsed well under running water before eating. Diseased leaves should be eliminated, soft and rotten berries discarded, and brown spots on apples and various fruits cut out. There are various preparations in health food stores that help to counteract sprays and contaminated materials which can remain on your fruits and vegetables. Avoid green, immature fruits or vegetables.

RULE NO. 4. Undercook your vegetables whether they are baked, steamed, broiled or roasted. Learn a low-heat, waterless way of cooking that allows no air to get to the vegetables. Experiment with thermos cookery. Learn to cook in a double broiler. Try to get your foods cooked under the boiling point of water. Don't cook over a direct flame, if you can help it. Do not use aluminum foil in cooking or baking. Learn why these methods overcome and eliminate the *three robbers* in the kitchen.

Avoid foods which have been overheated, pressure cooked, pasteurized or fried. The molecules in these foods have been disorganized—their chemistry is altered—the vitamins are stunned or destroyed. These foods are out to injure you, and even kill you. They cannot support life and have no place in the kitchen and above all, they should never be in a hospital.

Cut vegetables and fruits the way the fibers grow in them, because if you cut across the fibers, they bleed and you lose the valuable juice that has been stored in the cell life. When any juices come out of vegetables or fruits, these are immediately oxidized and begin to deteriorate.

RULE NO. 5. Use distilled water for drinking and cooking as much as possible. Use this in your fruit juices or when you can or preserve fruits and vegetables.

RULE NO. 6. Keep your kitchen immaculately clean. Your working tables and sink should be scrubbed and scoured. The hair should be put up, fingernails cleaned and hands kept scrupulously clean when handling food.

RULE NO. 7. Use glass containers. For refrigeration and to hold your foods in overnight, to preserve and can your foods, glass containers are best.

RULE NO. 8. Learn to read the labels on foods before they come into your kitchen. There should never be anything on the shelf that doesn't furnish you the maximum of health. Everything going into the mouth should nourish the various tissues so that you work, walk and talk well tomorrow. Demineralized, devitalized, scorched, embalmed and salted foods should not be in the kitchen.

Avoid as much as possible the foods that have been milled, pared, peeled and cooked. Avoid the ghost-like products of the baker. Keep away from the drugstore. Grow your own foods—get close to the orchard. Get clean, fresh, live foods from your farmer; stay closer to the organic farmer than to the supermarket.

RULE NO. 9. If God made the food, it can be considered good for you. Be careful of man-handled foods. Man's labor on foods usually destroys them. Live closer to nature than to the baker and the manufacturer of foods. They are not health specialists. They are not in business for your health. Get foods directly from your garden, if possible. Eat them as soon as they are picked. Eat the foods that are in season—the seasons offer us the various chemicals we need. It is after we have taken all the different foods that each season has to offer that we can begin to get well. We build up a reserve of chemical elements in our bodies by partaking of a variety of foods that grow at different times of the year.

RULE NO. 10. Use goat milk products, if possible. They are much better than products of cow milk. Live closer to the goat than the "milk king" and his plant. Learn to make your cheese, buttermilk and butter, too, if possible. Also use yogurt.

RULE NO. 11. Greens are most important in repairing, rebuilding and regenerating the tissues of the body.

Nuts are very important for their protein values. Soak them overnight in fruit juice or honey water. Learn how to prepare them in nut milk drinks. Strive to use them in good combinations.

Homemade rye muffins, yellow cornmeal, natural fruits, berries, nuts and goat milk products are foods which can help to lengthen your life, raise your health level and give you the strength and beauty you seek.

RULE NO. 12. Meals should be very simple—simple in combinations, simple as far as dressings are concerned, simple in preparation—but above all things, there should be variety. Aim at a change at every meal.

RULE NO. 13. Never fry foods. Never use heated oils in the kitchen.

RULE NO. 14. It is best to keep your foods in a room where the temperature does not vary much. A refrigerator is useful but too often jammed with foods much better eaten immediately. Every kitchen should have a food grinder, a liquefier, juicer and should be completely outfitted with stainless steel cookware. A nut grinder, salad shredder and other pieces of equipment can be added as funds arise, for convenience in the preparing of foods for your family. Many times, this kind of equipment makes the foods more palatable and favors their digestion.

RULE NO. 15. Do not force your food ideas on anyone in your family. Learn to enjoy your meals. Be patient with the children and the husband who do not see eye to eye with this new way of living.

If you are going to use up all your vitality, if you are going to worry, burn out, develop a temper and end up in the divorce courts—all this health work isn't going to be worth it. You may have to decide between coffee and doughnuts and your husband!

RULE NO. 16. You should eat only when you are hungry and never to satiety. Never eat to keep from getting hungry. If you can eat the same meal you have just finished all over again, then you have had enough. The secret of a long lilfe is to see how *little* you can eat—not how much you can get down.

RULE NO. 17. Frozen desserts and ice cold drinks with the meal or after it keep you from absorbing and assimilating the foods you have eaten.

RULE NO. 18. Take vegetable juices with a straw—chew your drinks. Masticate your food well and move the food you are chewing against the roof of the mouth with your tongue, develop the taste centers of the brain, smell your food, think well of your food; enjoy it. Fast eating leads to gas and intestinal disturbances.

RULE NO. 19. Avoid foods which are artifically colored, artificially flavored or preserved with many of these coal tar products used today. These foods are carcinogenic; that is, cancer producing. They have no place in the economy of the body or for building good health. Cut out fats, greases and excessive amounts of oils in your diet. Man was not made to take a lot of fats and oils. A fry cook, grease cook, fat cook is one to stay away from. He will cook you into the hospital and into an early grave.

RULE NO. 20. Have only one protein in a meal and have only one starch in a meal. Do not mix starches and proteins at the same meal. Do not have sulphur foods with your starches. Have them with proteins. Make sure that at the end of the day you have had one starch, one protein, six vegetables and two fruits. They can be had in any way that is healthful.

RULE NO.21. Avoid white sugar and doctor's bills. Add honey to foods after cooking or at the table. Use the natural sugars, the natural fruit juices. They may be dehydrated, concentrated or made under a vacuum or low heat so that the vitamin values haven't been completely destroyed. An excess of sugars or any sweets in the body will eventually lead to acidity, the grim reaper of old age.

RULE NO. 22. Keep your foods well covered, for as food begins to deteriorate and break into the dust of the earth again, nature's undertakers come in the form of bacteria and microscopic clouds of germs. These take over in helping to destroy and will contaminate your foods. So be sure to cover them properly. Germ life has a mission to accomplish. It is here to eat up tissue, foods and even bodies that are breaking down. Germs have been created by nature for a purpose and they have their place.

RULE NO. 23. We should average about 80% alkaline foods per day and 20% acid. Get completely away, if possible, from foods that are exhausted, bleached, adulterated, processed, preserved, useless, harmful, toxic and acid forming.

RULE NO. 24. Never have head lettuce in your kitchen. It is gas forming and contains an opium-like product. If you have stomach and bowel disorders, do not use any bread. Only use the natural grains as they do not produce gas.

RULE NO. 25. Market fruits are usually picked green so that many times after 4 or 5 days in the market, they look ripe on the outside but are still green on the inside. Often you may have noticed that the tomato looks ripe but when you cut it up, inside it has green seeds. Citrus fruits are the most difficult to get completely mature. These include oranges, grapefruit, lemons, limes and tomatoes. Do not have too many citrus fruits when you are trying to get well, or if you have an excessively overacid body. It is better to use vegetable broths and vegetable juices. If the juices produce too much gas, you can mix them with milk, soy milk or various teas, with other foods and liquids that are not gas producing; e.g., flaxseed tea, peppermint tea, etc.

RULE NO. 26. Drinking too much milk will crowd out the blood building foods, and you will eventually become anemic. Milk lacks iron. All cola drinks spell death to the bloodstream.

RULE NO. 27. Don't snack all day. Give your stomach a rest occasionally.

RULE NO. 28. Don't disturb your digestion with occupational problems, temper, overseriousness. Laugh and enjoy yourself at mealtime. Leave out discipline. Do not talk about money troubles at the table. Pray before your meals—get into the mood to handle your meal properly. Sometimes a 10-minute rest before meals will calm that nervous stomach. Prepare yourself for a feast: sit down to the Lord's supper and enjoy the gracious beauty and wholesomeness of God and nature.

RULE NO. 29. It doesn't hurt to miss a meal occasionally.

RULE NO. 30. We favor vegetarianism, especially so when you know your proteins, the combinations and adequate varieties that can be used. People can starve to death eating meat, for it only feeds part of the body, especially when the meat has been cooked. Eventually as we progress in life and go through the transitions that the world must still go through mentally, spiritually and physically, I believe we will all be vegetarians.

RULE NO. 31. For people without the strong, robust body to handle raw foods, we sometimes have to cook foods. We steam them to break down the bacteria and food cells, thus making the food more easily digestible and also liberating toxins. Broiling is another good way of taking care of a lot of foods; baking or roasting is also good—however, never use oils. Never fry. Avoid boiling foods. Boiled food is dead—water logged, altered and minus the vital life that is necessary for good health.

Decorating A Health Salad And Plate Suggestions

Even before the discovery of fire itself, prehistoric man was eating salads made from tender green shoots of young plants. The fact that today's cook, especially in our country, commands such a vast variety of ingredients, makes her potential achievement in the kitchen so much more inspiring and her failures, when made through carelessness or indifference, so much less excusable.

There is no substitute for the best. Good food cannot be made of inferior ingredients, masked with high flavor. It is true thrift to use the best material available and to waste nothing. Plan ahead. Planning ahead saves money as well as time and steps. Give as much care to simple dishes and humble foods as you do to elaborate dishes and fancy menus.

The best prepared dish will go unhonored if it is badly served, coupled with unlikely companions. It isn't magic that makes some hostesses so calm and cool. It is careful advance planning. Fine cooking is a very individual matter. Once the fundamental techniques and a reasonable range of recipes are mastered, each cook cannot help but create an endless series of exciting variations. Not only the food, but also the table setting in any home should reflect the special imagination, taste and whims of that particular house.

There is often no one technique for performing a certain task nor one recipe for a given delicacy. A general rule never to be broken is that the ingredients must be of excellent quality, but they need not be expensive. To add an exciting flair, the cook should also have a fine and warm feeling for colors that are compatible. A good recipe is half the secret of being a good cook, the other half of the secret is compounded of your own enthusiasm for cooking and good food.

The salad is often the first course. Sometimes it accompanies the entree or sometimes takes the place of the vegetable. A few extra trimmings, an accompanying extra or two and the salad becomes a meal in itself.

The most popular and most frequently served is the mixed green salad. "Greens" are available in great variety, adding color and texture to a mixed green salad. More people have come to know that there are other greens besides lettuce. The mixed green salad changes into a hundred salads with different flavorings for variety and pungency. Herbs, spices, vegetables, fruits, nuts and cheese are good salad accessories.

Everybody likes salads, likes the looks of them. Ah, there is the catch! How can they be beautifully arranged? How can they be done quickly and effectively? Any clever person can take a few vegetables or fruits and glorify them into a tempting salad. Fresh crisp greens are an absolute must in successfully making a fine salad. The Spanish proverb recommends "a spendthrift for the oil, a miser for the vinegar, a counselor for the salt and a madman to stir them up".

There are salad secrets of all kinds and varieties, including salads and dressings with international reputations. The minute you add tomatoes or radish slices to greens, or any other colorful crisp or cooked vegetables so good in a tossed salad, it is no longer a "green salad". But be sure it is a good and beautiful one. The mixed green salad arranges itself with the natural grace and color contrast of the pine woods in the country. With colorful vegetables added, you can have a "premeditated" beauty in picture salad bowls.

When being served, food must be well composed and attractive on the dish, for well prepared food deserves that introduction which will brighten the curious eye, excite the palate, then the imagination and the appetite.

Favorite Recipes

Spring Salad

Torn lettuce
Shredded carrot
Minced green onion
Tomatoes
Cucumber slices

Celery salt
Broth powder
Raw sugar
Oil
    Shake together and use to marinate salad.

Salad Combinations

1 cup chopped tomato
½ cup chopped ripe olives
Dressing

2 cups diced celery
½ cup chopped nuts
Dressing

A Dressing

Egg yolk
Vegetable salt
3 tbsp. thick cream — whip in
1 tbsp. lemon juice — add last

Green Bean Salad

String beans, cooked. Serve cold with garnish of:
    Cuban onion rings
    Green pepper strips
Dress with garlic-cream dressing

Fruit-Nut Salad

2 apples — diced
1 cup pecans — chopped
1 cup dates — cut up
Lemon dressing — enough to bind
    Mix together well and serve in lettuce cup. Garnish with whipped cream and strips of date to form a star. May use cherry in center.

Stuffed Cucumber Boats

(a)
⅓ cup chopped nuts
⅓ cup ripe olives
Green pepper — minced
Mayonnaise
    May also be used to stuff tomatoes

(b)

Halve cucumbers lengthwise and remove seeds.
Filling:
Chopped celery
Chopped onion
Chopped ripe olives
Chopped nuts

Moisten with mayonnaise.

(c)

Grated fresh coconut
Mayonnaise

Sprinkle with chopped nuts
Serve on lettuce leaf

Recipes

Lentil Loaf

1 C Cooked Millet
1 C Cooked Lentils
1 Tbsp Raw Peanut Butter
2 Eggs
1 Tbsp Minced Onion
2 tsp Vegetable Broth Powder
½ C Vegetable Broth
1 Carrot, Chopped

Liquefy chopped carrot with vegetable broth. Mix all ingredients together and put into a well-buttered baking dish. Bake in a moderate oven until firm.

Country Beans

2 lbs Green Beans
1 Small onion
(Cook together. Save liquid.)

To the bean liquor, add water to make up to 1½ cups of liquid.

4 Tbsp Arrowroot
1 tsp Vegetable Broth Powder

Mix to a cream with a little of the bean liquid. Heat remainder and add arrowroot and cook, stirring, until thick. Add beans and onion and allow to heat through.

Stir In:
2 Tbsp Butter
½ C Thick Soy Milk
½ tsp Paprika

Rosy Salad

1 lb. Fresh, Ripe Peaches
½ lb. Cranberry Sauce (Mock health variety)

Stuff peach halves with cranberry sauce, place a dollop of sour cream on each and add grated orange rind to garnish. Serve in crisp lettuce cups.

Dressing

½ C Finely Chopped Celery
½ tsp Vegetable Broth Powder
Pinch of Paprika
½ C Crumbled Bleu Cheese
½ C Sour Cream
¾ C Health Mayonnaise or Dressing

Combine and chill.

Good-Flavor Lima Bean Soup

1 C Dried Baby Limas — soak overnight
2 C Oatstraw   Tea, add and cook 1 hour

1 Medium Onion, Sliced
1 Medium Carrot, Sliced
1 tsp Vegetable Broth Powder
Add and cook until tender

May be rubbed through coarse sieve or liquefied slightly.

Add:
1 Tbsp Butter
1 Tbsp Chopped Parsley
1 tsp Baker's Yeast

Add with milk to make right consistency. Serve hot.

Millet Souffle

1 C Cooked Millet
2 C Milk
1 tsp Vegetable Broth Powder
½ C Grated Cheddar Cheese
1 Tbsp Minced Onion
4 Eggs, Separated

Bring millet, milk and vegetable broth powder to a boil. Stir in cheese until it melts. Separate eggs, beat yolks into hot mixture. Beat whites until stiff and fold in. Turn into well-buttered casserole. Bake in a dish of water in moderate oven until firm and golden brown. Serve at once.

That Festive Occasion

Your drinks can have more real "kick" than the highest highball imaginable, with no let-down later. Just because you don't believe in filling your body with cocktails and 'hot' hors d'oeuvres, there is no need for your parties to be dismal affairs of a lettuce leaf and a glass of milk. It is not what you do once in a while that matters, you know; it's what you do most of the time.

However, there are many tempting, and tasty ways of making canapes, appetizers and cocktails from wholesome ingredients. Here are some suggestions for going 100% healthwise, if you wish, when friends drop in on holidays or for your next festive occasion.

Plain fruit and vegetable juices are always acceptable, or combine different ones for delicious cocktails. Make punches from natural ingredients. Serve spiced herb teas, foamy nut milk shakes and 'heady' fruit nectars. Serve side dishes of raw unsalted nuts, squash, pumpkin and sunflower seeds and roasted soybeans.

For appetizers and hors d'oeuvres, veer towards the vegetable and fruit types. Just hollowed-out watermelons and pineapples for holding toothsome bites of cheese, olives, tiny onions, nutmeat cubes, pieces of pineapple, cubes of carrot, cucumber, turnip and green pepper; apple and cheese; pear and gouda cubes; dates and celery pieces, or attach these to a big grapefruit or half a cabbage with toothpicks.

Use whole-grain breads and rye crackers as bases for canapes. Spread with a variety of butters such as cheese (4 Tablespoons of grated cheese to 4 Tablespoons of Butter), chili (chili powder), chive, onion, lemon and horseradish. Make your own health spreads — they can be 'zippy' without catsup and pickles. Instead of all bread and cracker bases, prepare very thin slices of carrot, cucumber or zucchini, or apple rings with cheese spreads, nut butters and savory mixes. In place of pastry cases, brush thin whole-grain bread slices of varying shapes and sizes with melted butter and bake in patty tins (to give cup effect). Fill with wholesome fillings.

Pack your sandwiches heartily with vegetable fillings, or serve salad sticks along with them. Fill big green peppers or serrated orange 'shells' with your own homemade dips.) These are for the more ravenous appetites of the men, but you may also want small, lady-like sandwiches, cut in a variety of shapes with pastry cutters or sharp knives for dainty service. Go with open-face, ribbon, club and rolled sandwiches for attractive variety.

If you need cakes, cookies, muffins and waffles, don't buy the usual "mixes" and prepared packages. Use fresh ground, whole-grain products, raw sugar, unheated fats, etc. Eat plain, decorate with fruit and nuts or frost with cream cheese.

Have ice cream, if you wish, but make it at home from a healhful recipe. Don't decorate with chocolate sauce, but drizzle cherry concentrate attractively over it, use sliced fresh fruit or berries for accompaniment. Skip most of the fancy desserts. Use fresh fruits, or serve natural whips, sherbets or gelatin desserts.

Replace the usual "goodies" and candies with much more delicious stuffed prunes, 'marzipan' dates and sweet cheese 'eggs'. Roll dried fruit balls in coconut, tinted with cherry concentrate or chlorophyll.

The Unusual Sesame Seed

We can trace the use of the sesame seed back as far as the Roman empire. They used a sesame seed meal and honey for cakes. The Romans would dry the sesame seeds in the sun and make a cake of it to feed their athletes because it gave them great strength. Sesame seed is 49% protein.

We should learn the value of our different foods because there may be times in our life when we will need to use these foods for their particular values. Some countries use sesame seed a good deal more than others. Sesame seed oil is exceptionally good for the skin as it is very high in Vitamin F and can be used in cases of sunburn and in skin troubles. A dry skin is always improved when we use sesame oil both internally and externally.

The oil can be used as a dressing or the seeds can be ground with other cereals and used raw or in the cooked form. We find our greatest life-giving properties in the seed, in many instances, rather than in the full grown plant. An example of this is the egg. Most of the chemical elements that go to develop every part of the chicken is found in the egg yolk. The same thing applies to the seed as the seed is the glandular, or reproductive part of the original plant and carries most of the chemical or mineral elements to develop the whole plant. We can make up many shortages in our body by using seeds of plant life.

If you went to Turkey or Syria you would find that the sesame seed is one of their basic foods. It is very high in Vitamin C and the calcium content runs from 50% to 53%. Its valuable fat contains a lot of lecithin which is very good for the brain and nervous system and is also very high in Vitamin E. Sesame seed can be ground and used in the liquefier, served in salad dressings and it can be used for thickening soups and broths. Sesame seeds can be used with nuts and grains very successfully and served either raw or cooked. It is an alkaline food and is not putrefactive in the system and because of its high oil content helps in bowel conditions and in cases of constipation.

Sesame Seed For Lecithin And Vitamin E

Although it is the soy bean from which the commercial lecithin is prepared, other seeds contain appreciable amounts, especially the sesame seed. It is a seed high in calcium and of an alkaline reaction, making it an excellent lecithin food. If you are run down, sleepless and chronically tired and nervous, you lack this nerve fat. Sesame seed is obtainable as a meal, or may be made into liquid form as sesame milk or cream. This milk may be left to sour and used as such, as yoghurt.

Sesame Seed Oil is extracted without heat or refining, so contains its full vitamin value. It is more digestible and less acid forming than olive oil—in fact than any other vegetable oil on the market. It makes an excellent skin salve, as well.

Buying Sesame Seed

It is very important to buy fresh seed. If procuring the hulled seed, this is extremely necessary as on hulling, the flavor, vitamins and value begin to be lost on exposure to the air. Like any seed, rancidity begins and insect infestation is hastened.

Liquefied Salads

To the young and healthy, nothing is more pleasurable than chewing on the hearty, raw salad. This exercises teeth and gums and assures salivation, so necessary for good digestion. However, when teeth are missing, digestive systems below par, or conditions such as colitis, ulcers and spastic colon have developed, one must be careful not to irritate delicate linings by too much roughage and coarse foods such as salads often must be broken down. Never give up and go on a 'bread and milk' diet because a bland diet is called for. Raw foods are even more important to the sick than to the well. The irony is that you cannot get well without raw foods, yet most raw foods are too fibrous and rough. Blended in a liquefier, though, they can be reduced to a smooth, fine pulp which is usually harmless to the most sensitive digestive tract. In extreme cases only is it necessary to pass liquefied salads through a strainer to remove the last trace of fibre.

Never get the mistaken idea you are merely drinking. Liquefied salads are concentrated foods and must be sipped slowly and 'chewed' to salivate for good digestion. Taking through a straw is a wise policy. Do not drink ice cold either. Sometimes liquefied salads can be warmed over hot water, making them into raw soups of the richest and best.

Most salads are good liquefied. However, sometimes one which tastes delicious in its usual form, lacks palatability when the flavors run together in the blending. In this case, you will need to add a few dates (soaked), a little honey, pineapple juice, apple or grape concentrates, sunflower seeds, coconut powder, mayonnaise, carob, a tablespoon of nut butter, vegetable seasoning or others; even a dash of soy sauce.

Do not always be satisfied with plain water as a base. Try to incorporate other valuable liquids, such as any of the herb teas, whey, fruit and vegetable juices, sesame, soy and nut milks or salad dressing. Aim to match the base with your salad ingredients for correct combination. (Keep vegetable juices for vegetable salads, on the whole, and fruit juices for liquefied fruits; tea, milk or buttermilk are suitable any time. Fruits and proteins combine well, salads and proteins, vegetables and starches. Try to separate wet or acid fruits and the dried.) Consider flavor and color. Make liquefied salads thick or thin consistency, varying with your preference.

Many times, supplements such as rice polishings, dulse, wheat germ, amino acids, yeast, gelatin or egg yolks can be added to liquefied salads as a suitable way of taking these. The vegetable powders, e.g., alfalfa, okra and celery are very useful, especially when the fresh vegetables are not available.

Liquefied Green Salad

2 Romaine Leaves
Small bunch Alfalfa Sprouts (remove seed hulls)
Sprig of mint
2 rings of Green Pepper
½ Avocado
¼ Baby Zucchini Squash (chopped)
Few Alfalfa Leaves
½ Stalk Celery (chopped)
2 tsp Whey Powder
1 to 2 tsp Honey
1 C Nut Milk to liquefy

Fruit Salad

1 Small Apple
½ Banana
1 Small Peach
2 Dates (soaked)
2 Tbsp Sunflower Seeds
1 tsp Rice Polishings

Chop fruit. Use a suitable cream dressing in which to liquefy. (A scoop of health ice cream could be added as a special treat.)

Protein Liquid Salad

2 leaves Lettuce
1 leaf Beet
1 leaf Comfrey
1 Turnip Top
1 leaf each of several fresh herbs e.g. bay, rosemary, basil
2 sprigs Parsely
1 stalk Celery (chopped)
¼ Carrot (chopped)
2 tsp Gelatin
1 Tbsp Soy Milk Powder
1 Tbsp Apple Concentrate
1 Egg Yolk
2 Tbsp Cottage Cheese
2 tsp Nut Butter
1 C Mint Tea to liquefy (or more)

Carrot Salad

1 C Carrot (chopped)
¼ C nuts
¼ C Raisins (soaked)
¼ C Parsley
Enough Pineapple Juice to liquefy and blend.

Liquefied Corn Salad

1 C Corn off cob
1 tsp Vegetable Seasoning
1 or 2 fresh leaves of Sweet Basil
1½ Tbsp sweet or sour Cream
1 C Celery Juice to blend
Strain to remove hulls, if necessary.

Herbs In Cookery

APPETIZERS
Canapes, Crackers, Etc.
Anise, caraway, celery seed, chervil, fennel seed, mustard, oregano (pizza), parsley, poppy seed, sesame seed
Spreads
Chervil (butters and cheese), cumin (cheese), dill (avocado, cheese),oregano (cheese), parsley (cheese, avocado), poppy (cheese), sage (sharp cheese), savory (cheese), sesame (sesame butter), tarragon (cheese, sea food), thyme (sea food)

BAKERY GOODS
Bread
Anise (sweet bread, rolls and sandwiches), caraway (rye bread), cardamon, celery seed, (celery toast, seed rolls,) cinnamon, coriander (buns, bread), cumin, fennel (roll topping), poppy seed, saffron, sesame seed (bread, rolls, sandwiches)
Cakes and Cookies
Allspice, anise (coffee cake, etc.), caraway, cardamon, gr., (coffee cake and cookies), cinnamon, cloves, coriander, ginger, mace (coffee cake), nutmeg, poppy seed, sesame seed.
Pastry
Cardamon, gr.; coriander, gr.; mace (cherry pie); poppy seeds; sage
Pizza
Capsicum pepper, oregano

BEVERAGES
Cocktails
Basil (seafood and tomato juice), cardamon (fruit cup), dill weed (seafood), ginger (milk), marjoram (fruit juice, fruit punches), oregano (tomato juice), peppermint (fruit juice, tea, punches), rosemary (punch, fruit cup), sage (hot milk, tea), summer savory (tomato, vegetable juice), tarragon (seafood, tomato juice), thyme (sea food).
Juices
Basil (tomato), celery seed and salt (tomato), dill (tomato), oregano (tomato), summer savory (tomato, vegetable) tarragon (tomato)
Teas
Anise, peppermint, spearmint, rosemary, sage.

CANDIES
Anise, cloves (carob).

CHEESE
Anise (cottage cheese), basil, caraway, cayenne, chervil (cream cheese, rarebit), chili powder (cottage cheese), gr. coriander (cream and cheddar), cumin (spreads), dill, fennel (bel paese), fine herbs, marjoram, mustard, oregano (Welsh rarebit), parsley, peppermint (cream cheese), poppy seeds (spreads), saffron (cream cheese) sage (cottage cheese and spreads), thyme (cottage cheese, spreads, Welsh rarebit).

DESSERTS
Compotes
Basil, mint, rosemary, saffron, thyme.
Custards
Anise, bay, thyme, nutmeg, cinnamon, mace, fennel.
Frozen Deserts (Ice Cream)
Anise, mint, cinnamon, nutmeg, ginger.
Gelatin
Anise gr. cardamon, fennel, cinnamon.
Baked Apple
Allspice; caraway; ground cardamon; ground coriander; nutmeg; cinnamon; caraway and ground cardamon (baked pears); fennel seed (baked fruit)
Fruit Pies
Allspice, anise, cumin, cinnamon, nutmeg, gr. coriander, dill seed, fennel seed (apple pies).
Stewed Fruit
Anise, gr. coriander, summer savory (pears).
Sauces
Anise, bay, fennel, nutmeg, mace, sesame (subst. milk), ginger.
Puddings
Anise, cinnamon, gr. coriander (rice), fennel seed, nutmeg.

EGGS
General
Cayenne, chervil, chili powder (chili peppers), cumin, curry powder, dill, marjoram, nutmeg (eggnog), paprika, tarragon.
Creamed
Bay leaf (creole), caraway (devilled), cumin (devilled) dill, marjoram, gr. mustard, parsley (devilled), rosemary (shirred and devilled), sage, savory (devilled), tarragon, thyme (devilled and shirred), tumeric.
Custard
Cinnamon, nutmeg, mace.
Omelet
Basil (Spanish), chervil, dill, fennel seed, marjoram, oregano, parsley, sage (Spanish), savory, tarragon, thyme.
Scrambled
Basil, celery seed, dill, marjoram, oregano, rosemary, saffron, savory, tarragon.
Soft Boiled
Dill, oregano.

FISH
General
Basil, bay leaf, cayenne, celery seed and salt, chervil, dill (halibut, salmon, boiled fish, shell fish), fennel, fine herbs, green ginger (oriental), mace, marjoram (all broiled), mustard, oregano (melted butter sauce), paprika, rosemary (creamed shellfish), sage (chowder, baked, stuffing), savory (chowders, baked or broiled), saffron (halibut and sole), tarragon (in sauces), thyme, tumeric.
Chowder
Sage, thyme (clam and oyster stew).

MEAT
General
Bay leaf, caraway, cayenne, celery seed and salt, chili powder, curry powder, dill, green ginger (oriental), juniper berries (game), mustard, paprika, sage, savory (in gravy), sesame seed (oriental), tarragon (game, sweetbreads), thyme
Beef
Allspice, anise (stew), basil (stew), bay leaf, caraway, chervil, chives, chili powder, ginger (pot roast), marjoram (pot roast), mint, mustard, oregano (Swiss steak), parsley, rosemary, sage (stews), thyme, tumeric.
Lamb
Basil, chervil, chives, curry powder, dill (chops), fennel (stew), marjoram, mint,

oregano, parsley, rosemary, saffron, savory (roasts), thyme.
Liver
Basil, bay leaf, caraway (kidneys), fennel
Meat Loaf
Basil, celery seed, cumin (chili con carne), poultry seasoning with paprika, savory, thyme.
Poultry
Basil (duck), caraway (goose), chervil, chives, cumin (chicken), dill (creamed chicken), fennel (duck or goose), oregano, paprika, parsley, poultry seasoning (sage, thyme, marjoram, savory and sometimes rosemary), rosemary, saffron (chicken), sage, savory, tarragon (chicken and turkey).
Stews
Anise seed, basil, bay leaf, caraway, capsicum pepper (use whole), celery seed, cloves, cumin, dill (lamb), garlic powder, marjoram, oregano (especially kidney), rosemary, sage.
Veal
Mint, oregano, saffron, savory, tarragon.

SALADS
General
Basil, bay, caraway, celery seed and salt, chervil, chives, coriander, dill, fennel seed, garlic, marjoram, oregano, paprika, parsley, rosemary, saffron, savory, sesame seed, tarragon, thyme.
Avocado
Dill, sweet basil.
Beet
Caraway seed, sweet basil.
Chicken
Marjoram, thyme.
Coleslaw
Caraway seed, dill, sweet basil.
Cucumber
Dill.
Egg
Saffron, sweet basil.
Mixed Green
Basil, fennel seed, rosemary, savory.
Potato
Celery seed and salt (aspics), dill, oregano, savory, sesame seed, sweet basil.
Seafood
Fennel seed, marjoram, oregano, saffron, thyme.
Tomato
Basil and bay leaf (aspics), dill.
Fruit Salads
Anise, gr. cardamon (orange), cinnamon, mint, nutmeg, poppy seed (pears), rosemary (orange and grapefruit).

DRESSINGS
    Caraway, curry powder (French), dill, sage,
    sweet basil, tarragon.

SAUCES
    General
        Bay leaf, cayenne (hot), chili powder (cocktail),
        fine herbs, garlic powder, green ginger,
        mustard, nutmeg, saffron (butter), tarragon
        (Bernaise, tartar).
    Creamed
        Marjoram (for vegetables), sweet basil,
        tarragon.
    Tomato
        Allspice, basil (Italian), bay leaf, capsicum pep-
        per (hot), cayenne (hot), oregano (Italian),
        savory, tarragon, thyme (creole).

SOUPS
    General
        Basil, bay, caraway, celery seed and salt, cher-
        vil, dill, garlic and powder, green ginger, mace,
        mint, paprika, parsley, rosemary, saffron, sage,
        tarragon, thyme.
    Cream
        Anise, whole fennel.
    Stock
        Bay leaf, saffron.
    Almond
        Ground coriander.
    Bean
        Bay leaf, cumin, dill, oregano, peppermint,
        savory, tarragon.
    Beet, Borsch
        Dill, thyme.
    Cabbage
        Caraway seed, dill, sweet basil.
    Chicken
        Cumin, saffron, savory.
    Lentil
        Savory, sweet basil, cumin.
    Minestrone
        Basil, oregano.
    Mushroom
        Oregano, tarragon.
    Onion
        Marjoram, oregano, savory.
    Pea
        Basil, cardamon (gr.), coriander (gr.), cumin,
        dill, peppermint, rosemary, sage, savory, tar-
        ragon, thyme.
    Potato
        Rosemary, sage, garlic, sweet basil, caraway.
    Spinach
        Basil, marjoram, rosemary.

Tomato
    Basil, dill, marjoram, oregano, sage, tarragon.
Vegetable
    Basil, oregano, savory, sage, tarragon, thyme.

RICE
    Cumin, curry powder, green ginger, saffron
    (Spanish chicken and rice), tumeric.

NOODLES
    Basil, poppy seed.

STUFFINGS
    Celery seed, coriander, mace, marjoram
    (poultry), poultry seasoning, sage, savory,
    thyme.

VEGETABLES
    Artichokes
        Dill, garlic, lemon juice.
    Asparagus
        Celery salt, dill, lemon juice, nutmeg, paprika,
        parsley, tarragon, thyme.
    Avocado
        Chili powder, dill seed or weed (spreads,
        salads), lemon juice, marjoram, oregano (dip).
    Beans — green
        Basil, bay leaf, chili powder, dill weed, garlic,
        mustard-dry (browned butter), marjoram,
        nutmeg and onion, rosemary, sage, tarragon,
        summer savory, thyme.
    Limas
        Cayenne, chives, savory (browned butter), mar-
        joram, sage.
    Limas - dried
        Basil, cumin (Mexican beans), mustard (baked),
        parsley, sage, savory (baked beans), thyme.
    Beets
        Bay leaf, caraway seeds, chervil, cloves, cor-
        iander (spiced beets), dill weed, fennel seed
        (pickled), lemon juice, mustard, tarragon,
        thyme.
    Broccoli
        Garlic, lemon juice, oregano, thyme.
    Brussel Sprouts
        Celery seed, lemon juice, marjoram, oregano,
        paprika, savory.
    Cabbage
        Allspice, basil, caraway seeds and/or browned
        butter, cumin, curry powder, dill, nutmeg,
        onion, oregano, paprika, parsley, tarragon.
    Cabbage — red
        Allspice, caraway, cloves, dill.

Carrots
    Allspice, anise seed, bay leaf, cloves, dill weed, dill, garlic, ginger, marjoram, mint (browned butter), nutmeg, parsley, rosemary, sage, thyme.
Cauliflower
    Basil, caraway, marjoram, nutmeg, parsley, rosemary, savory.
Celery
    Chervil, chili powder, chives, dill weed, horseradish, onion, parsley, rosemary, tarragon (celery root).
Celery Root
    Caraway, chili powder, chives, onion, parsley, rosemary, tarragon.
Chard
    Celery, chili powder, garlic, lemon juice, onion, oregano, rosemary.
Chayote
    Chives, parsley, tarragon — alone or in combination.
Corn
    Chili powder, dry mustard, garlic, oregano, paprika.
Cucumber
    Burnet, chives, dill seed and weed, onion, parsley, rosemary.
Eggplant
    Allspice, basil, bay, dill, garlic, marjoram, oregano, rosemary, savory.
Endive
    Basil, chives, tarragon.
Kale
    Marjoram, nutmeg.
Leeks
    Bay, oregano, parsley.
Lentils
    Fennel seed, savory, cumin, sweet basil.
Lettuce
    Chervil, chives, parsley, tarragon, any delicate herb.
Mushrooms
    Chives, dill, garlic, nutmeg, oregano, parsley, rosemary, tarragon, thyme.
Okra
    Bay, garlic, green pepper, lemon, onion, parsley, thyme.

Onions
    Basil, bay leaf, cloves, dry mustard, ginger, marjoram, oregano, paprika, saffron, sage, thyme.
Parsnips
    Dill, lemon, marjoram.
Peas
    Basil, borage, chervil, cinnamon, cumin, marjoram, mint, rosemary (cook with a little lettuce leaves or button onions), tarragon, thyme.
Peppers — green
    Basil, garlic, onion, oregano, rosemary.
Potatoes
    Basil, bay, caraway seed, celery seeds, chervil, chives, dill, garlic, marjoram, onion, parsley, poppy seeds, rosemary, sesame seeds, tarragon, thyme.
Potatoes — sweet
    Allspice, cinnamon, cloves, dill, parsley.
Pumpkin
    Ginger, cloves, cinnamon and ginger (pumpkin pie)
Rutabagas
    Dill seed or weed, fennel, parsley, rosemary.
Salsify
    Chives, parsley, shallots, tarragon, thyme.
Spinach
    Basil, chervil, dill, lemon, mace, marjoram, nutmeg, peppermint, rosemary, tarragon.
Squash — winter
    Allspice, basil, bay leaf, chives, cinnamon, cloves, dill, parsley, saffron, savory.
Tomatoes
    Basil, bay leaves (stewed), celery seed and salt (juices), chervil, chili powder, dill (juice), garlic, green pepper, onion, oregano, sage, tarragon (in cooked or raw).
Turnips
    Basil, bay leaf, ground caraway, dill weed, fennel, onion, rosemary.
Zucchini
    Basil, bay leaf, caraway, curry, dill, fennel, garlic, lemon, marjoram, oregano, peppermint, thyme, saffron, savory.

Sulphur, like nitrogen, is obtained solely from proteins, according to J. I. Rodale, and both are acid forming. About half of one percent of all brain solids are sulphur.

Life-Building, Youth And Beauty Diet

Life foods are fresh, living, thriving foods, direct from nature's trees, bushes, gardens, plants and soil.

Foods containing the principle of life are:

Edible buds
Fruit blossoms
Alfalfa buds
Clover buds
Hop buds
Sprouts that bloom
Growing greens
Ripe fruit
Ripe berries
Nasturtium
Parsley
Celery hearts
Romaine lettuce
Leaf lettuce
Cabbage sprouts
Fresh tomatoes
Wilted spinach
Raw tender carrots
Collard
Shad roe
Blueberries
Blackberries
Wild cherries
Sprouts
Goat cream
Fresh goat milk
Raw fresh milk
Chard
Fresh currants
Raw egg yolks
Guavas
Mandarines
Raw nuts
Peppermint
Celery
Fresh asparagus shoots
Winter lettuce
Cos lettuce
Lambs lettuce
Green onions
Raw spinach
Raw okra
Cucumbers
Roe
Genuine honey
Elderberries
Black huckleberries
Barberries
Bilberries
Fresh buttermilk
Goat butter

Cottage cheese
Curly cabbage
Chayote
Fresh blackcaps
Raw egg white
Fresh leeks
Mangoes
Grapes
Grape concentrate
Nettle salad
Papaya
Fresh pineapple
Fresh plums
Tender radishes
Wild strawberries
Swiss chard
Oranges
Goat milk whey
Fresh dates
Fresh apples
Apple concentrate
Fresh pears
Tamarinds
Avocado
Chervil
Chinese cabbage
Marjoram
Yeast
Sun dried figs
Loquats
Endive
Green peppers
Garlic
German prunes
Fresh fruit juices
Raisins
Muskmelon
Salad greens
Fresh peaches
Fresh prunes
Fresh raspberries
Strawberries
Sugar beet leaves
Tangerines
Watercress
Roquefort cheese
Olives
Sun dried apples
Persimmons
Thyme
Celery bulbs

Chives
Edible greens
Mulberries
Fresh figs
Cowberries
Kumquats
Zante currants
Shallot
Turnip leaves
Caraway seed
Cole slaw
Gherkins
Sapotes

Fruit sauce
Casaba
Adriatic figs
Mint
Bananas
Nectarines
Life tonics
Codliver oil
Vegetable broth
Parsley
Yellow tomatoes
Papaw
Pecans

Extreme Low Calorie Reducing Diet

Monday:
Breakfast
Weak tea
Lunch
1 Bouillon cube in ½ cup diluted water
Dinner
1 Pigeon thigh — 3 oz. prune juice (gargle only)

Tuesday:
Breakfast
Scraped crumbs of burnt toast
Lunch
1 Doughnut hole (without sugar)
Dinner
2 Jellyfish skins; 1 glass dehydrated water

Wednesday:
Breakfast
Boiled out stains from tablecloth
Lunch
½ Dozen poppy seeds
Dinner
Bees' knees and mosquito knuckles salted in vinegar

Thursday:
Breakfast
1 Lobster antennae
Lunch
1 Guppy fin
Dinner
Jellied vertebrae ala mode

Friday:
Breakfast
Shredded egg shell skins
Lunch
1 Bellybutton from navel orange
Dinner
3 eyes from Irish potato

Saturday:
    Breakfast
        4 Chopped banana seeds
    Lunch
        Broiled butterfly liver
    Dinner
        Filet of soft shell crab claw

Sunday:
    Breakfast
        Pickled hummingbird tongue
    Lunch
        Prime rib of tadpole; aroma of empty custard
        plate
    Dinner
        Tossed paprika and cloverleaf salad

NOTE: All meals are to be eaten under a microscope to avoid extra portions. No substitutions.

Raw Food Recipes

Museli

1 tablesp rolled oats
3 tablesp water
    Soak 12 hours

2 apples, medium-fine grated
juice of ½ lemon
1 tablesp top milk
honey to sweeten
    Stir into oats quickly

1 tablesp grated nuts — sprinkle on top of each dish
    Serve immediately.

Avocado Soup

1 ripe avocado
1 cup warm, sweet milk
1 stalk celery
few sprigs parsley
    Blend in liquefier to make a pleasantly warm, nourishing soup.

Variations:
(a) Vegetable stock can replace milk
(b) A little cooked brown rice or barley can be used
(c) The soup can be gently heated in a double boiler.

White And Bright Salad Platter

2 carrots, finely grated
½ head white cabbage, shredded
parsley
leaf lettuce
    Arrange lettuce on salad platter. Alternate rows of carrot and cabbage across leaves. Use parsley sprigs to garnish.

Mint Dressing

2 tablesp oil
2 teasp lemon juice
1 teasp cream
1 teasp honey
1 teasp grated onion
1 teasp minced mint leaves
dash of crushed garlic
    Place in bottle with secure lid and shake well. Serve over slaw.

Chili Sauce

¼ cup tomato juice
2 cups sliced tomato
⅜ cup aged cider vinegar
    Blend smooth in liquefier.

¼ cup diced green pepper
½ cup sliced onion
¼ cup old-fashioned brown sugar
3 teasp vegetable seasoning
¼ teasp celery salt
¼ teasp dry mustard
¼ teasp chili powder
    Add and blend to chop vegetables — about 2 seconds only.

Classifying Your Foods

There are many charts for learning about various foods. This chart shows the amount of calories per pound of various foods. Using it, you will be able to choose those foods heavy and high in calories for wintertime use. Be careful about using foods heavy and high in calories in the summertime, and above all, be sure to use natural foods.

While many foods are listed in this classification that are not exactly good for the average person, it is well to use it as a means of comparison and for the knowledge you would like to have in your library.

When this chart lists hours of time required for digestion, this means digestion time in the stomach only. It does not tell whether or not foods are toxic or laxative.

There are many other requirements to consider in the diet other than calories. Consider combinations, making sure they are 80% alkaline, and 20% acid.

This list does not tell whether a food is high or low protein, only telling whether or not it has more protein than starch, or more starch than protein.

Peach Dessert

6 ripe peaches — mash or puree in liquefier
1 cup whipped cream — fold in
2 tablesp honey
½ cup chopped nuts
  Add and chill.

  Place in dessert dishes, topping each with a spoonful of ice-cream.

Almond-Fruit Milk

1 cup unsweetened pineapple juice
¼ cup soaked almonds
  Blend in liquefier to a smooth, satiny drink.

Sun Glow

½ cup sliced carrots
honey to sweeten
1 cup pineapple juice
1 cup milk
  Blend in liquefier to creaminess.

Fruit-Nut Candy

1 cup seedless raisins
1 cup figs, dried
¾ cup soaked almonds
½ cup walnuts
little lemon rind
  Put through food grinder, then roll into balls in fresh-grated coconut.

Chemicals such as choline, glutamine, tryptophan and tyrosine are being found to be very important in brain function. Brain cells turn tryptophan into serotonin, which determines the quality of our sleep, and tryptophan helps those with obsessive-compulsive neuroses. Glutamine increases brain efficiency, improves learning and speeds healing of stomach disorders. It has helped some—but not all—alcoholics dramatically. The body makes norepinephrine, another neurotransmitter, from tyrosine, which aids, depression. Choline is needed to form acetylcholine, a major neurotransmitter that can improve memory, especially in the elderly.

The population of the country is 180 million, but there are 64 million over 60 years of age, leaving 116 million to do the work. People under 21 total 59 million, which leaves 57 million to do the work. There are 31 million government employees, leaving 26 million to do the work. Six million are in the armed forces, leaving 20 million workers. Deduct 17 million State, County and City employees, leaving 3 million to do the work.

There are 2,500,000 people in hospitals, asylums, etc., leaving 500,000 workers, but 450,000 of these are bums or others who will not work, so that leaves 50,000 to do the work.

Now, it may interest you to know there are 49,998 people in jail, so that leaves just 2 people to do all the work, and that's you and me, brother, and I'm getting tired doing everything by myself, SO LET'S GET WITH IT!

	Acid	Alkaline	Proteins	Starches	Fats	Vegetables	Fruits	Hours of Time Required for Digestion	Caloric Value Per Pound	Vitamins found in these Foods
Agar-agar		X				X		1½	75	E
Almonds		X			X			2½	3000	A B
Apples		X					X	2¾	275	A B C
Apricots		X					X	2¾	300	B C
Artichokes		X				X		2	350	A B C
Asparagus	X					X		2¼	150	A B C
Avocados—										
Alligator pears		X			X		X	1¾	835	A B C
Bananas		X		X			X	3	350	A B C E
Barley—whole grain	X			X				3¾	1500	A B E
Barley—pearled	X			X				4	1250	B
Beans—dried		X	X			X		3	750	A B E
Beans—fresh string		X				X		3¼	100	A B C
Beans—green Lima		X				X		2½	600	A B C
Beans—dried Lima		X	X			X		2½	750	B E
Beans—kidney		X	X			X		3	750	B E
Beans—soy		X	X			X		3	750	B E
Beechnuts	X		X		X			3	2800	A B
Beef—lean	X		X					3½	1000	E
Beef—dried	X		X					3½	1000	E
Beef—raw juice	X		X					3	1000	E
Beets		X		X		X		2¾	150	A B C
Beet tops		X				X		2	150	A B C E
Blackberries	X						X	2½	250	B C
Blueberries	X						X	2	300	B C
Bran		X						2¾	1100	B E
Broccoli		X				X		3	160	A B C
Brussel sprouts		X		X		X		4	250	A B C
Butter	X				X			3¼	3700	A D E
Buttermilk		X			X			2¼	150	A B C D
Cabbage—white, raw		X				X		3	160	A B C E
Cabbage—red, raw		X				X		3¾	160	A B C E
Cantaloupe		X					X	3¼	300	A B C
Carrots		X		X		X		2¼	700	A B C D
Carrots—raw		X				X		3	240	A B C D
Cashew nuts	X				X			3¼	2500	A B
Cauliflower		X		X		X		2¼	150	A B C
Celery		X				X		3¼	90	A B C
Celery root		X		X		X		3½	250	A B C
Cereals—whole grain	X			X				3	1800	B D E
Cheese	X				X			3¼	2000	A B
Cherries—red		X					X	2	350	B C
Cherries—white		X					X	2	350	B C
Chestnuts	X				X			2¾	2500	A B
Chicken	X		X					3¼	500	E
Chocolate	X			X				2	2900	B
Cider	X						X	1¼	275	B C
Clams—round	X		X					4	200	A B D
Clams—long soft	X		X					3¾	200	A B D
Cocoa	X			X				2	2400	B
Cocoanut—dried natural		X			X		X	3¼	2800	A B
Cocoanut—fresh		X			X		X	2¾	2000	A B
Cocoanut milk		X			X		X	2	500	A B
Cod liver oil	X		X		X			3	2500	A D E
Cottage Cheese	X				X			3¼	2100	A B C D
Corn—sweet		X		X		X		3	490	A B C
Corn—dried		X		X		X		2¾	800	A B C
Cornmeal	X			X				3½	1800	A B C
Cottonseed meal	X			X				3¾	1000	A D E
Cow peas	X			X		X		3¼	600	A D E
Cranberries		X					X	3¼	225	B C
Cream	X				X			2½	900	A B D
Cucumbers		X				X		3¼	100	A B C
Currants—fresh	X						X	3	300	B C
Currants—dried		X					X	2½	1500	B C
Dandelion		X				X		2½	235	A B C E
Dates		X		X			X	2½	1600	A B C
Dill		X				X		3¼	250	A B C
Egg plant		X		X		X		3½	150	A B C
Egg whites	X							2¼	300	
Egg yolks	X				X			2¼	1700	A B D E
Endive		X				X		3	100	A B C
Farina	X			X				3½	900	B E

	Acid	Alkaline	Proteins	Starches	Fats	Vegetables	Fruits	Hours of Time Required for Digestion	Caloric Value Per Pound	Vitamins found in these Foods
Figs—dried		X					X	2½	1400	B C
Figs—fresh		X					X	2¼	350	B C
Flaxseed		X				X		3	875	B E
Flour—buckwheat	X			X				4	1000	B E
Flour—gluten	X				X			3¼	600	B E
Flour—graham	X			X				3	1800	B
Flour—rye	X			X				3¼	1100	A B
Flour—white	X			X				4	12000	
Flour—whole wheat	X			X				3	1700	B D E
Frog's legs	X		X					4	500	E
Garlic		X				X		2	200	A B C
Gooseberries	X						X	2½	300	B C
Gluten feed	X				X			3	600	B E
Grapes—white	X						X	1¾	350	A B C
Grapes—Concord	X						X	1¾	350	A B C
Grapefruit		X					X	2	200	A B C
Guava		X			X		X	3	450	B C
Halibut	X		X					2½	450	E
Ham	X		X		X			4	1900	A B
Hazelnuts	X				X			3	2400	A B
Herbs		X				X		2½	200	A B C
Hominy	X			X				3	800	B E
Honey	X			X				2¼	1600	B
Horseradish	X					X		4	100	A B C
Huckleberries	X						X	2¾	200	B C
Irish moss		X				X		1½	100	E
Kohlrabi	X			X		X		3	200	A B C
Kelp salt		X				X		3	100	E
Lamb	X		X		X			3	1000	A B
Leeks		X				X		2½	200	A B C E
Lemons		X					X	1½	200	B C
Lentils		X		X		X		3	1700	A B
Lettuce		X				X		2¼	100	A B C E
Limes		X					X	3	200	A B C
Linseed meal	X			X		X		4	1000	B E
Lupins—dried		X		X		X		2¾	1500	B E
Mackerel	X		X					3¼	450	E
Macaroni—white	X			X				3¾	1200	B
Macaroni—whole wheat	X			X				3	1700	B E
Mango		X			X		X	1¾	450	B C
Maple syrup	X			X				1¼	1400	B
Milk—cow's (skimmed)		X			X			2	300	A B C
Milk—(cow's whole raw)		X			X			2¼	1200	A B CDE
Milk—condensed	X			X				4	1500	A B C
Milk—human		X			X			1½	1800	A B CDE
Milk—goat's		X			X			2	1600	A B CDE
Millet	X			X				3¼	950	A
Molasses	X			X				2¼	1800	B
Mushrooms		X		X		X		2½	200	A B
Muskmelons		X					X	3¼	300	A B C
Mustard greens		X				X		3½	150	A B C E
Oats—whole grain	X			X				3¼	1900	A B E
Oatmeal	X			X				3½	1800	B E
Okra		X		X		X		2½	200	A B C
Olives—ripe		X			X		X	1¾	400	A E
Olives—dried		X			X		X	2	800	A E
Olive oil		X			X			3¼	4000	A D E
Onions		X				X		3¼	200	A B C
Oranges		X					X	2	200	A B CDE
Parsley		X				X		1½	270	B
Parsnips		X		X		X		3½	380	A B
Peaches—fresh	X						X	2½	200	A B C
Peaches—dried		X					X	2¾	1200	B C
Peanuts	X				X			3¼	3000	A B E
Pears	X						X	2¼	350	B
Peas—fresh green		X		X		X		3¼	500	A B C
Peas—dried		X		X		X		3½	1500	B E
Pecan nuts	X				X			2¾	3500	A B
Peppers—fresh green		X				X		3¼	450	A B C
Persimmons		X					X	3¾	350	B C
Pignolias	X				X			2¾	2700	A B

	Acid	Alkaline	Proteins	Starches	Fats	Vegetables	Fruits	Hours of Time Required for Digestion	Caloric Value Per Pound	Vitamins found in these Foods
Pineapple		X					X	2¼	200	A B C
Plums	X						X	2¾	250	B C
Pomegranates	X			X			X	3¼	450	B C
Pork	X		X		X			4	1200	A B
Potatoes—Irish		X		X		X		2	400	A B C
Potatoes—sweet		X		X		X		3¼	400	A B C
Prunes—fresh	X						X	2¾	350	A B
Prunes—dried	X						X	3	1550	A B
Pumpkin		X		X		X		3¼	160	A B C
Peppermint leaves		X				X		2½	100	A B C E
Quinces	X						X	3¾	400	B C
Radishes		X				X		3¼	100	B C
Raisins		X		X			X	2	1650	B C
Raspberries	X						X	1¾	150	B C
Rhubarb	X						X	3	1000	B C
Rice—natural brown	X			X				2	1600	A B E
Rice—white	X			X				2½	800	
Romaine		X				X		2¼	100	A B C E
Roquefort cheese	X				X			3¾	1600	B
Rutabagas	X			X		X		3¼	200	A B C
Rye—whole	X			X				3½	1100	B E
Sauerkraut	X					X		4½	200	A B C
Sage		X				X		2¾	150	A B C E
Sago	X			X				3	1800	B
Salmon	X		X					3¾	450	A B D
Salmon—smoked	X		X					4½	400	E
Scallops	X		X					3¼	450	E
Sea grass		X				X		1½	100	E
Smelt	X		X					3½	450	E
Smoked herring	X		X					4½	450	A B D
Sorrel		X				X		2¾	100	A B C E
Sole	X		X					2¾	450	E
Spaghetti—white	X			X				3½	1200	B
Spaghetti—whole wheat	X			X				3	1700	B E
Spinach		X				X		3	100	A B C D
Squab	X		X					3¼	1000	E
Squash—Italian		X				X		3	150	A B C
Squash—summer		X				X		2¾	150	A B C
Squash—yellow crook neck		X				X		3	150	A B C
Squash—Hubbard		X		X		X		2¼	200	A B C
Squash—banana		X		X		X		2¾	200	A
Squash—other winter varieties		X		X		X		3	200	A
Strawberries	X						X	2¼	150	A B C
Sugar—raw		X		X				1¼	1800	B
Sugar—white	X			X				1¼	1500	B
Swiss chard		X				X		3	150	A B C D
Syrup	X			X				1¼	1400	A B
Tapioca	X			X				2½	1800	B
Tomatoes—cooked	X					X		1¾	100	A B C
Tomatoes—raw		V				X		2	100	A B C
Turnips		X		X		X		4	200	A B C
Turnip tops		X				X		3¼	150	A B C E
Turkey	X		X					3¼	1000	E
Vegex		X				X		2½	1000	A B E
Vegetable oils		X			X			3½	2000	A D E
Vinegar—cider	X							2¼	100	
Walnuts	X				X			3	3000	B
Watercress		X				X		3¼	100	A B C
Watermelon		X					X	2¾	120	A B C
Whole wheat grain	X			X				3¾	1700	B D E
Wheat bran		X		X				2¾	1100	B
Wheat germ	X			X				3	500	A B E
Wheat gluten	X				X			3¼	600	B E
Whey—cow's milk		X			X			3	150	A B C
Whey—goat's milk		X			X			3	150	A B C
Wine	X						X	1¼	150	C
Wild berries	X						X	2	150	B C
Whiting fish	X		X					3¼	50	E
Wintergreen		X				X		2¾	100	A B C E

408

The paragraph on Nutrition below
has been excerpted from the 186
page report submitted in September
1948 to President Truman. The report was titled:

the nation's health

a report to **THE PRESIDENT**

by OSCAR R. EWING

Federal Security Administrator

NUTRITION

Despite our progress in acquiring knowledge about nutrition, people are still dying from the effects of nutritional deficiency. The widespread effect of inadequate diets is evident in poor resistance to disease.

It is necessary to increase our knowledge in certain directions: (1) To develop satisfactory methods of appraising nutritional status of representative population groups; (2) to discover all human nutritional requirements; (3) to identify more clearly the effect of different levels of nutrition upon the degenerative diseases; (4) to develop improved methods of measuring all nutrients; and (5) to understand the functioning of nutrients in the body.

GROWTH...
a measure of good nutrition

Two weeks old, each rat weighs 22 grams. Note soft, fine hair; plump, well-shaped bodies.

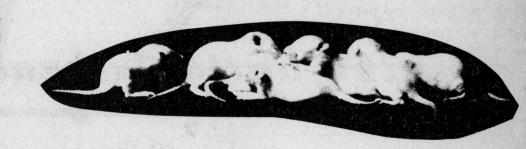

Four weeks old, rat weighs 47 grams. Fur and body shape are good. Appears bright and lively.

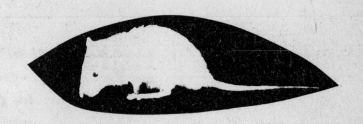

Twelve weeks old, mature rat weighs 193 grams. Weight, posture, shape, fur, eyes—all show signs of good nutrition.

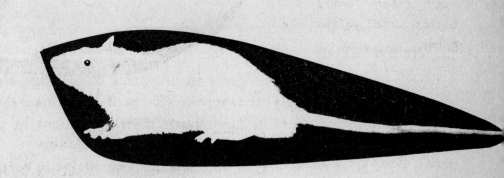

Rats are used for nutrition studies because they will eat the same foods we do and quickly show the effect of good and bad diets. A rat grows up 30 times as fast as a child and usually lives less than 3 years.

NUTRITION CHART No. 1

410

FOOD makes the difference in these twin rats

This rat ate only meat, potato, bread, and butter.   He
has poor fur and weighs only
89 grams.

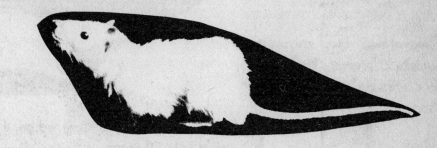

Bones show diet was poor—
lacking calcium and vitamins.

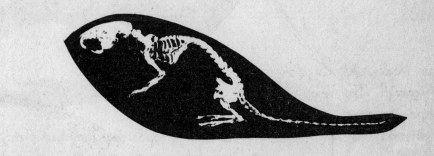

This rat ate plenty of milk
and vegetables, besides the
meat, potato, bread and
butter. He weighs 194
grams.

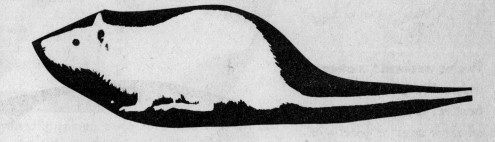

Skeleton shows diet was
good.   Bones are strong and
well-formed.

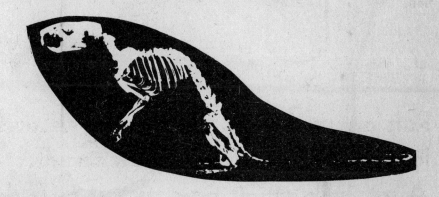

The following charts show the importance of some of the better known nutrients essential for human health

NUTRITION CHART No. 2

PROTEIN builds muscles, blood; is needed for growth

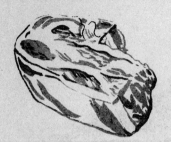

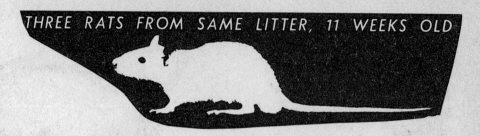

THREE RATS FROM SAME LITTER, 11 WEEKS OLD

This rat ate foods that furnished good quality protein, but not enough. It weighs only 70 grams.

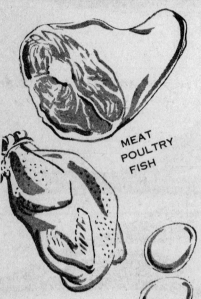

MEAT
POULTRY
FISH

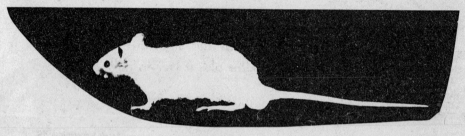

This rat ate foods that furnished plenty of protein, but not the right combination to give good quality. It weighs only 65 grams.

EGGS

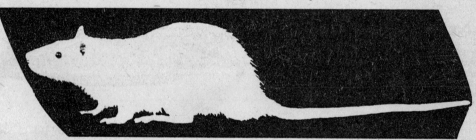

This rat had plenty of good quality protein from a variety of foods. It has good fur, well-shaped body, and weighs 193 grams.

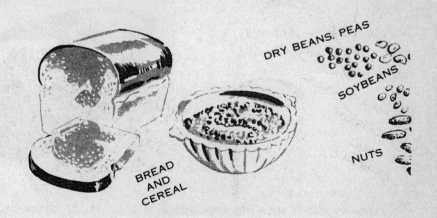

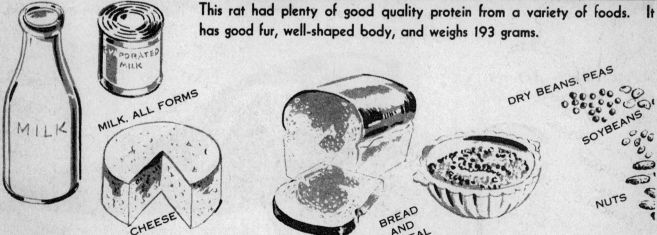

MILK

MILK, ALL FORMS

CHEESE

BREAD
AND
CEREAL

DRY BEANS. PEAS

SOYBEANS

NUTS

NUTRITION CHART No. 3

412

IRON, needed by the body to build red blood

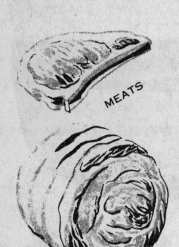

MEATS

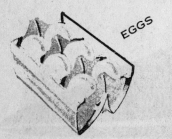

EGGS

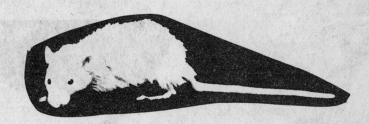

This rat did not have enough iron. It has pale ears and tail. Eight months old, it weighs only 109 grams.

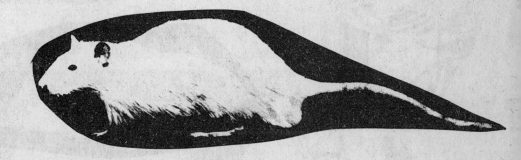

This rat had plenty of iron. Its fur is sleek and its blood has three times as much red coloring as the rat above. Though only 5½ months old, it weighs 325 grams.

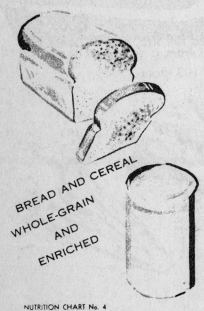

BREAD AND CEREAL
WHOLE-GRAIN
AND
ENRICHED

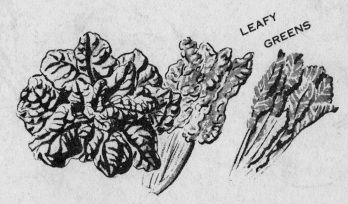

LEAFY GREENS

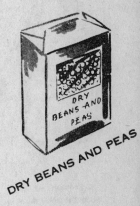

DRY BEANS AND PEAS

NUTRITION CHART No. 4

413

CALCIUM, builds bones, teeth, and is needed by all tissues of the body

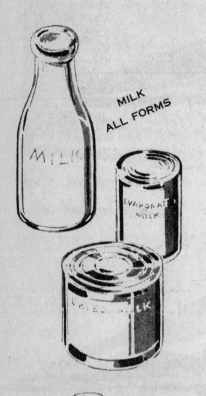

MILK
ALL FORMS

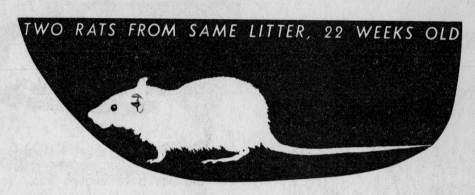

TWO RATS FROM SAME LITTER, 22 WEEKS OLD

This rat did not have enough calcium. Note the short, stubby body, due to poorly formed bones. It weighs 91 grams.

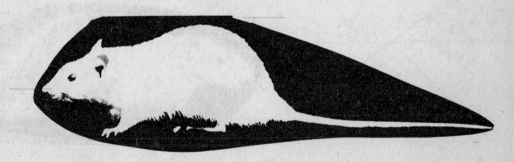

This rat had plenty of calcium. It has reached full size, and its bones are well-formed. It weighs 219 grams.

CHEESE

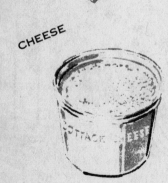

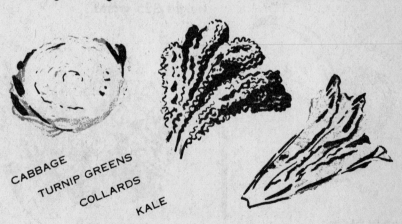

CABBAGE
TURNIP GREENS
COLLARDS
KALE

NUTRITION CHART No. 5

VITAMIN A . . .
needed for growth, healthy eyes, skin and other tissues

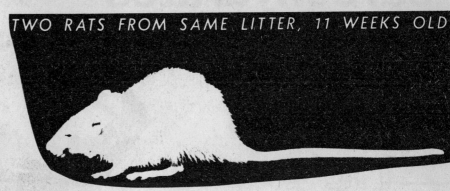

TWO RATS FROM SAME LITTER, 11 WEEKS OLD

This rat had no vitamin A. Note the infected eye, rough fur, and sick appearance. It weighs only 56 grams.

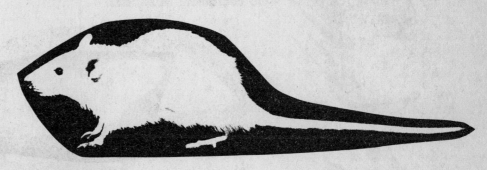

This rat had plenty of vitamin A. It has bright eyes, sleek fur, and appears alert and vigorous. It weighs 123 grams.

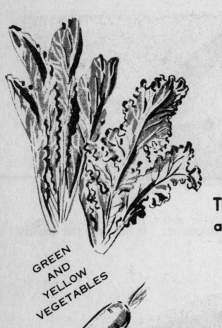

GREEN AND YELLOW VEGETABLES

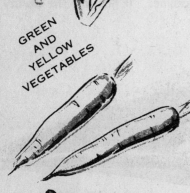

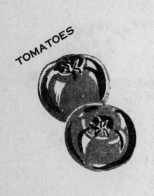

TOMATOES

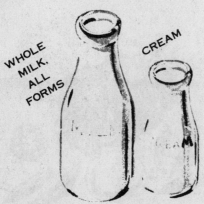

WHOLE MILK, ALL FORMS

CREAM

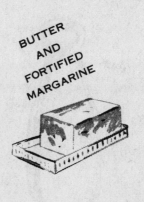

BUTTER AND FORTIFIED MARGARINE

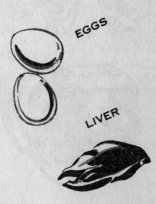

EGGS

LIVER

NUTRITION CHART No. 6

415

THIAMINE (vitamin B₁) . . .
needed by body cells to use carbohydrates

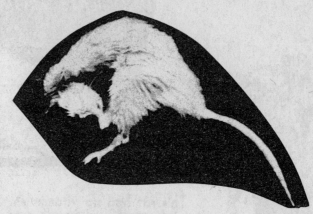

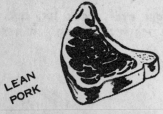

BREAD AND CEREAL
WHOLE-GRAIN
ENRICHED

This rat, 24 weeks old, had practically no thiamine. It has lost the ability to coordinate its muscles.

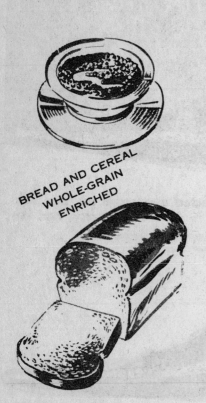

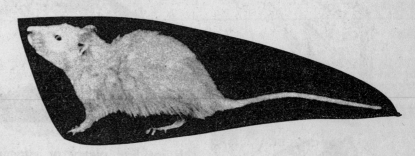

The same rat 24 hours later, after receiving a food rich in thiamine. It has already recovered.

LEAN
PORK

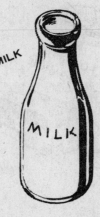

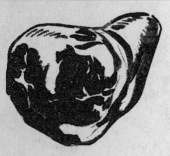

MILK

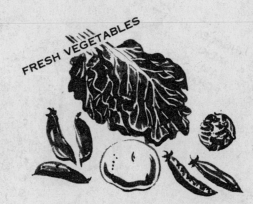

FRESH VEGETABLES

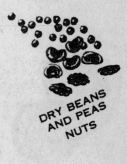

DRY BEANS
AND PEAS
NUTS

NUTRITION CHART No. 7

416

RIBOFLAVIN . . .
promotes health by helping body cells use oxygen

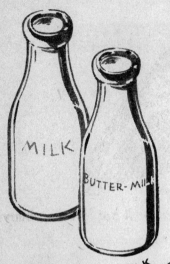

MILK
ALL FORMS

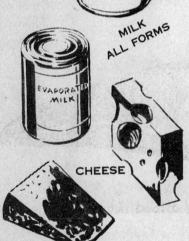

EVAPORATED MILK

CHEESE

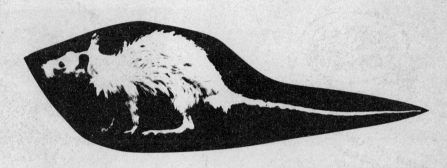

This rat, 28 weeks old, had no riboflavin. It soon became sick, and lost hair, especially about the head. It weighs only 63 grams.

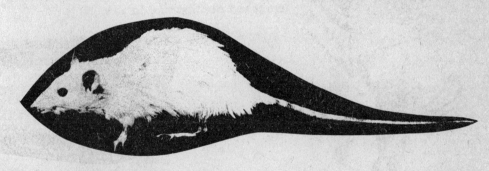

The same rat 6 weeks later, after receiving food rich in riboflavin. It has recovered its fine fur and now weighs 169 grams.

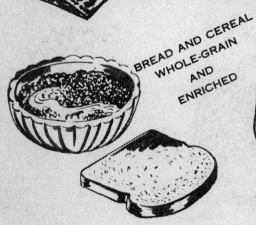

BREAD AND CEREAL
WHOLE-GRAIN
AND
ENRICHED

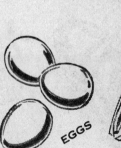

LIVER

LEAN MEAT

EGGS

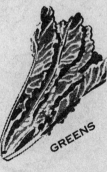

GREENS

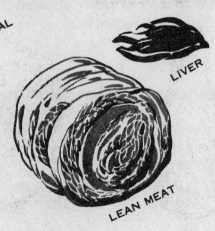

NUTRITION CHART No. 8

417

ASCORBIC ACID (vitamin C) helps to build healthy gums, teeth, and bones

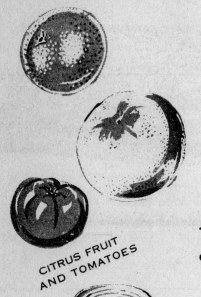

CITRUS FRUIT AND TOMATOES

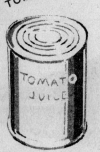

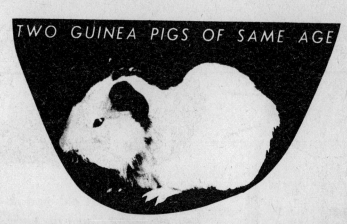

TWO GUINEA PIGS OF SAME AGE

This guinea pig had no ascorbic acid and developed scurvy. Note crouched position due to sore joints.

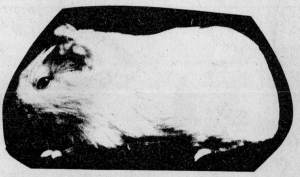

This guinea pig had plenty of ascorbic acid. It is healthy and alert; its fur is sleek and fine.

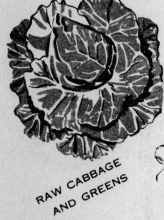

RAW CABBAGE AND GREENS

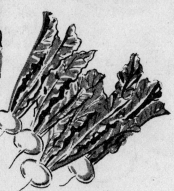

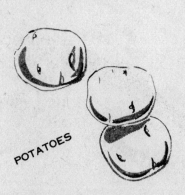

POTATOES

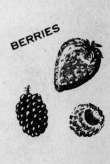

BERRIES

NUTRITION CHART No. 9

VITAMIN D . . .
for well-formed bones, teeth; and to prevent rickets

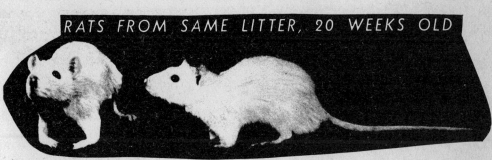

RATS FROM SAME LITTER, 20 WEEKS OLD

SUNSHINE

FISH OILS

This rat had no vitamin D. Its poorly shaped body and bowlegs are typical signs of rickets.

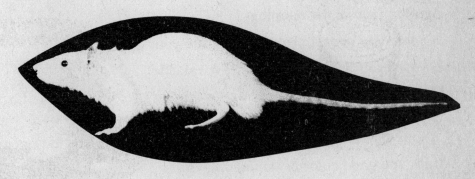

This rat had plenty of vitamin D. It has grown to normal size and its bones are strong and straight.

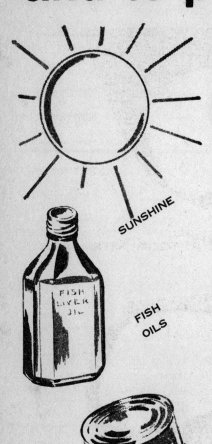

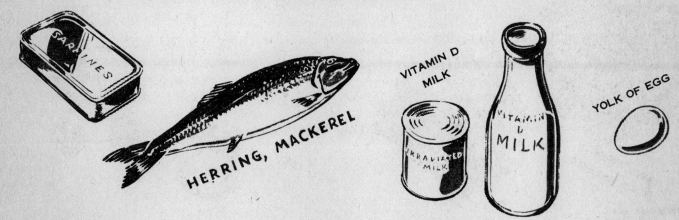

HERRING, MACKEREL

VITAMIN D MILK

YOLK OF EGG

NUTRITION CHART No. 10

HEALTH QUIZ

(Points are for each "Yes" answer.)

	POINTS	
Do you always feel perfectly well, free from pain, headache or dullness and wide awake, ready for work, study or play?	20	_____
Do you have a good appetite and relish for your food at every meal?	5	_____
Do you use laxative drugs or mineral waters?	5	_____
Is your tongue clean and your breath sweet?	10	_____
Do you have sound natural teeth? Do you have toothache?	5	_____
Do you get out of breath easily? Can you hold your breath half a minute?	5	_____
Do your kidneys act normally?	5	_____
Do you tire easily?	5	_____
Are you round shouldered, flat chested or in any other way deformed?	10	_____
Is your sleep sound without medicines?	5	_____
Are you tired in the morning?	5	_____
Is your sight perfect? Does reading tire your eyes?	4	_____
Is your hearing good? Do you have earache?	1	_____
Do you have frequent colds or sore throat? Do you breathe through your mouth or snore?	2	_____
Is your skin healthy, free from pimples, rough or do you have itching spots?	1	_____
Have you good color of skin and lips?	2	_____
Are your hands or feet cold or moist when they should be dry and warm?	2	_____
Have you had smallpox, scarlet fever, measles, diphtheria, typhoid or any other infection?	1	_____
Do the bowels move one, two or three times a day?	2	_____
Is your weight considered normal for your height?	5	_____

Your Total Points for Yes Answers: _____

Perfect Score: 100 Points

HEALTH DUTIES
(Points are for each "Yes" answer.)

POINTS

Do you take your meals at regular and proper hours?	4
Do you eat an abundance of fresh fruits and fresh vegetables daily?	4
Do you take at least two glasses of milk or buttermilk daily?	4
Do you take greens of some sort, such as lettuce, spinach, beet tops, cabbage every day?	4
Do you chew your food thoroughly and eat some sort of hard or dry food at each meal?	10
Do you eat whole grain cereals, such as wheat flakes, oatmeal and graham bread and bran, avoiding fine flour breads?	4
Do you drink three or four glasses of water daily between meals?	4
Do you visit the toilet and evacuate wastes at least three timies a day?	10
Do you sleep eight or ten hours a night in a room with open windows?	4
Do you exercise daily in the open air?	4
Do you live, work or play in well-ventilated rooms?	4
Do you hold your chest up and head erect in sitting, standing and walking?	10
Do you practice deep breathing, expanding the whole chest?	4
Do you take a warm, cleansing, soap and water bath at least once a week? A cold water or air bath every morning?	3
Do you dress properly, avoiding tight and high-heeled shoes and always keeping the extremities warm and dry?	4
Do you cleanse the mouth and teeth at least twice a day?	3
Have you had your teeth cared for by a dentist within a year?	4
Are you careful to avoid to avoid infection of every sort?	3
Are you careful to avoid spreading infection?	3
Are you sincerely endeavoring to care for and improve your bodily health by right living and the avoidance of injurious habits?	10

Your Total Points for Yes Answers: _____

Perfect Score: 100 Points

HABITS WHICH INJURE HEALTH

(Points are for each "Yes" answer.)

                                                                    POINTS

Do you drink coffee, tea, cocoa or cola drinks?   **10** _____

Do you use tobacco in any form?   **25** _____

Do you eat meat for breakfast, lunch, dinner?   **20** _____

Do you eat candy often?   **10** _____

Do you eat pickles, vinegar, pepper, mustard or hot sauces?   **10** _____

Do you eat too much often?   **5** _____

Are you irregular about your meals?   **5** _____

Do you eat hurriedly?   **5** _____

Do you drink too much water at meals? (More than one glassful?)   **5** _____

Your Total Points for Yes Answers: _____

Perfect Score: 100 Points

READER: All index references to pages after page 287 are two previous pages back. (Example: Ginseng 317, 318 should be 315, 316.)

Index

I

H

J

K

Kale 25, 41, 81, 85, 139
Kellogg, John Harvey, Dr. 36, 98, 171, 344, 356, 357
Kenan, William R., Jr. 290
Kidneys 12, 16, 32, 33, 36, 42, 47, 49, 165, 167, 171, 177, 182, 301, 303
Kitchen Rules 392-394
Kleen-Raw 172
Kleptomania 28
Kneipp Baths 37, 118
Kneipp, Sebastian, Father 37, 359
Koenig, Dr. 24
Kouchakoff, P., Dr. 108
Krebs, Ernest T., Dr. 156
Krishnamurti 50
Kronprinz Wilhelm 90, 92
Kut, Siege of 89

L

Lactic Acid 356
Lady Slipper 320
Landone, Brown, Dr. 322
Lane, Arbuthnot, Sir 153, 170, 353, 354
Laughter 122
Laxades (Cleansers) 308
Laxative 13, 18, 33, 36, 61, 69, 85, 112, 171, 300, 301 357, 362
Lead 157, 158
Lecithin 16, 17, 25, 34, 47, 52, 53, 75, 84, 147, 166, 273, 287, 288, 323, 397
Lederberg, Joshua, Dr. 186
Lefthanded 52
Legumes (see: Peas, Beans, Lentils, Garbanzos) 18, 156, 166, 236
Lemon Grass Tea 33
Lemons, Lemonade (see: Limes) 88, 301
Lentils 18, 156
Lettuce 45, 46, 85, 129, 355, 363
Li Chung Yun 8, 317
Limes (see Lemons) 88
"Limeys" 89
Lindberg, Robert 64
Lindlahr, Henry, Dr. 98
Linoleic Acid 288
Linseed Oil 34
Liver 17, 18, 26, 32-36, 41, 42, 47, 84-86, 90, 119, 167, 171, 182, 200, 303, 304, 311, 344, 345, 349, 366
Lofholm, Paul, Dr. 168
Longevity (see also: Geriatric) 19, 116, 147-152
Lunches 385

Lungs 36, 42, 119, 167
Lymphatic (also: Lymph Glands) 35, 115, 116, 177

M

McCann, Alfred 90, 91
McCarrison, Robert, M.D. 88, 93, 95, 104, 166, 385
McCay, Clive, Dr. 95, 100
McCollum, E.V. Dr. 101, 159
McLester, James S., Dr. 332
Magnesium 18, 25, 33, 73-75, 85, 86, 109, 112, 131, 147, 159, 255, 288, 295, 301
Malic Acid 32, 33, 79, 301
Malnutrition 148, 1151, 165, 295
Malva (Mallow) 311
Manganese 17, 20, 25, 76, 85, 364
Marks, Paul A., Dr. 362
Mason, Arthur J. 336
Masor, Dr. 103
Mayo, Charles, Dr. 111
Meat 18, 37, 89, 108, 127, 137, 152, 166, 209, 210, 212, 219, 227, 229, 306, 356, 400
Medulla 30
Memory 25, 148
Mendelsohn, Robert, Dr. 167
Menstrual Problems 303
Mental Illness 163-165, 374
Menus 278, 279, 281
Mercury 158, 161
Metchnikoff 108
Methyl Parathion 166
Milk Packs 34
Milk, Cow 290-299
Milk, Goat 295, 296, 351
Milk, Nut and Seed 304, 305, 356
Milk, Pasteurized 290-299, 304, 356
Milk Products (raw) 17, 18, 24, 27, 43, 46, 47, 81, 82, 147, 148, 225, 287, 290-299
Millet 18, 19, 35, 82, 115, 131, 156
Mineral Water 300
Minerals 58, 78, 80, 81, 85, 87, 89, 108, 117, 176, 185, 187, 206, 211, 225, 226
Miracles 22, 121
Molybdenum 110
Monosodium Glutamate (MSG) 157, 159, 162
Montague, M.F. Ashley, Dr. 336
Moon Cycles 256, 257
Morris, J.N. 166
Mother's Milk (also: Breast Feeding) 139-141, 366
Mouth Odor 366
Muesli 179, 270
Mulberries (and Juice) 301
Multiple Sclerosis 320
Mushrooms 363
Myopia 167

Y

Z

THE AWAKENED SOUL

At last I left the world behind
One path was all I could try
Sunlight—a breeze—the earth beneath
Was all that encased my God and I

The closest thing I could feel was space
My weight told me something was below
The sun made the shadows and forms about
But I was the one to sit and know

Spirits of trees know more strength than the wood
The petal of the daisy lifted for the above
The earth was dressed in her finest garb
I had all this and more, a Soul to Love

The world seemed big as she closed in on me
She couldn't push me out of my appointed place
I walked as a King and one with Him
an Awakened Soul, beloved by His Grace

The sun went down and the darkness came
My passage in life narrowed down to a trace
But I kept on going for I knew I was right
Because I followed the Light that glowed from His face.

—Bernard Jensen

(The above poem was written by Dr. Jensen in August 1948, while he was studying in Affoltern, Switzerland.)

For Your Good Health

Build a library of right living with Dr. Jensen's books, tapes and attractive wall charts explaining the natural way to happy, healthy living. If they are not available in your local bookstore, write for our free catalog and price list to: Dr. Bernard Jensen, Route 1, Box 52, Escondido, CA 92025.

Our Current Best Sellers!

Iridology: The Science and Practice in the Healing Arts, Volume II. Textbook, Practical Manual, Self-Study Course, Exhaustive Reference Work. Send for our free color brochure.

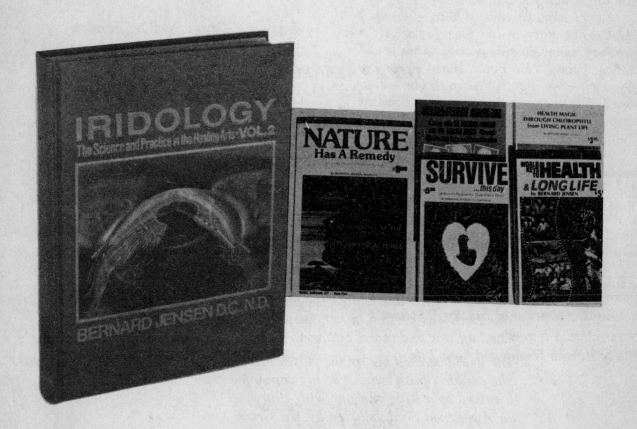

Iridology Simplified. Introduction to the Science of Iridology and its relation to Nutrition. Ideal for the beginner—color pictures, charts, case histories, 38 pages.

Tissue Cleansing Through Bowel Management, including the Ultimate Tissue Cleansing Program. Illustrated, 179 pages.

Newest Books and Products!

Breathe Again Naturally—How to Deal with Catarrh, Bronchitis, Asthma— by managing lung and bronchial conditions through a natural living and eating program. Illustrated, 128 pages.

Charts—Beautiful color charts on Iridology, Body Systems, Nervous System, Vitamins-Minerals-Herbs.

Coming Soon!

Video Teaching Tapes—Bring Dr. Jensen's lectures right into your home, clinic or classroom with this series of VCR tapes, now in final stages of production!

The "Man" Series—The Chemistry of Man will soon be joined by:

Food Healing for Man—Chock full of tips, instructions and practical wisdom on using food to get well and stay well.

The Healing Essence of Man, Volumes I and II—The story of the finer forces of the vibratory realm and their relation to health and healing. Foods, Vital Force, Herbs, Nutrition, Iridology, Love, Sex, Children, Light, Color, Sound, Music, Radionics, Homeopathy, Kirlian Photography and much, much more! Many beautiful color illustrations.

Arise and Shine: The Spiritual and Mental Healing of Man—Spiritual and Mental Keys, essential aspects of wholistic healing. Illustrated.

Complete Your Library !

Other Books by Dr. Jensen:

Science and Practice of Iridology, Volume I
Nature Has A Remedy
World Keys to Health and Long Life

Survive This Day
Blending Magic
Creating A Magic Kitchen
Doctor-Patient Handbook
Joy of Living and How to Attain It
Overcoming Arthritis/Rheumatism
Vital Foods for Total Health
You Can Feel Wonderful
You Can Master Disease
Health Magic Through Chlorophyll
A New Lifestyle for Health & Happiness
  (My System)

Cassette Tapes by Dr. Jensen (60-90 minutes—Inspirational)

Chemical Story
Building A Better Way to Eat
Replacement Therapy
Regularity Management
Divine Order
Seeds
Natural Healing
Key to Inner Calm
Breathing Exercises
Pathways to Health
Arise and Shine

Now retired from active practice, Dr. Jensen offers a few Iridology seminars, Internship programs, Rejuvenation seminars and the Ultimate Tissue Cleansing classes several times each year. Write for details.

Dr. Bernard Jensen
Route 1, Box 52
Escondido, CA 92025

Notes